Second Edition

Textbook of
Human Embryology

with Clinical Cases, 3D Illustrations and Flowcharts

As per the latest NMC Guidelines | Competency Based Medical Education (CBME) Curriculum under Graduate Medical Education Regulation

Now Clear your concepts thoroughly with CBSiCentral App

CBSiCentral App aims to cater to all the students from various educational segments and backgrounds with complementary digital content as supplement to print editions. The digital content is available in the form of videos, image banks, 3D videos and animated videos.

It contains the ancillary material uploaded for free viewing by the registered customers. Most of the Medical UG and technical books are augmented with online availability of valuable reference material, available through scratch code in the print editions.

What all you will get

 Animated videos
 MCQs
 Handwritten notes

and much more...

 Scan the QR Code to download the App

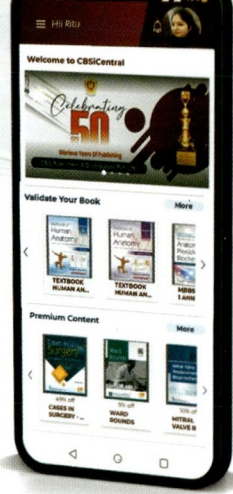

Second Edition

Textbook of Human Embryology

with Clinical Cases, 3D Illustrations and Flowcharts

As per the latest NMC Guidelines | Competency Based Medical Education (CBME) Curriculum under Graduate Medical Education Regulation

Yogesh Sontakke MBBS, MD

Additional Professor
Department of Anatomy
Jawaharlal Institute of Postgraduate Medical Education and Research (JIPMER)
(An Institution of National importance under the Ministry of Health and Family Welfare, Government of India)
Puducherry, India

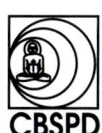

CBSPD

CBS Publishers & Distributors Pvt Ltd

New Delhi • Bengaluru • Chennai • Kochi • Kolkata • Lucknow • Mumbai
Hyderabad • Jharkhand • Nagpur • Patna • Pune • Uttarakhand

Disclaimer

Science and technology are constantly changing fields. New research and experience broaden the scope of information and knowledge. The author has tried his best in giving information available to him while preparing the material for this book. Although all efforts have been made to ensure optimum accuracy of the material, yet it is quite possible some errors might have been left uncorrected. The publisher, the printer and the author will not be held responsible for any inadvertent errors, or inaccuracies.

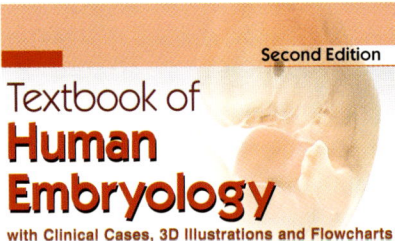

ISBN: 978-93-90709-10-6

Copyright © Yogesh Sontakke and Publisher

Illustrations: © Yogesh Sontakke

Second Edition: 2022
  Reprint: 2022, 2023
  Revised Reprint: 2024, 2025

First Edition: 2019
  Reprint: 2020

All rights reserved. No part of this book may be reproduced or transmitted in any form or by any means, electronic or mechanical, including photocopying, recording, or any information storage and retrieval system without permission, in written, from the author and the publisher.

Published by Satish Kumar Jain and produced by Varun Jain for

CBS Publishers & Distributors Pvt Ltd
4819/XI Prahlad Street, 24 Ansari Road, Daryaganj, New Delhi 110 002, India
Ph: 011-23289259, 23266838
Website: www.cbspd.com
e-mail: delhi@cbspd.com;

Corporate Office: 204 FIE, Industrial Area, Patparganj, Delhi 110 092, India
Ph: 011-4934 4934   Fax: 011-4934 4935   e-mail: publishing@cbspd.com; publicity@cbspd.com

Branches

- **Bengaluru:** Seema House 2975, 17th Cross, K.R. Road, Banasankari 2nd Stage, Bengaluru 560 070, Karnataka, India
  Ph: +91-80-26771678/79   Fax: +91-80-26771680   e-mail: bangalore@cbspd.com
- **Chennai:** 18/8B, Subbarayan Street, Shenoy Nagar, Chennai 600 030, Tamil Nadu, India
  Ph: +91-44-2032115, 26681266   e-mail: chennai@cbspd.com
- **Kochi:** 42/1325, 1326, Power House Road, Opp KSEB, Power House, Ernakulam, Kochi, 682 018, Kerala, India
  Ph: +91-484-4059061-65   Fax: +91-484-4059065   e-mail: kochi@cbspd.com
- **Kolkata:** 147, Hind Ceramics Compound, 1st Floor, Nilgunj Road, Belghoria, Kolkata 700 056, West Bengal, India
  Ph: +91-33-25633055/56   e-mail: kolkata@cbspd.com
- **Lucknow:** Basement, Khushnuma Complex, 7-Meerabai Marg (behind Jawahar Bhawan), Lucknow 226001, UP, India
  Ph: +91-522-4000032   e-mail: tiwari.lucknow@cbspd.com
- **Mumbai:** PWD Shed, Gala no. 25/26, Ramchandra Bhatt Marg, Next to JJ Hospital Gate no. 2,
  Opp. Union Bank of India, Noorbaug, Mumbai 400 009, Maharashtra, India
  Ph: +91-22-66661880/89   e-mail: mumbai@cbspd.com

Representatives

• **Hyderabad** 0-9885175004	• **Jharkhand** 0-9811541605	• **Nagpur** 0-8692091830
• **Patna** 0-9334159340	• **Pune** 0-9664372571	• **Uttarakhand** 0-9716462459

Printed at Magic International Pvt. Ltd., Greater Noida, UP, India

Preface to the Second Edition

This edition of *Textbook of Human Embryology* has been revised to fulfil the requirements of students and teachers as per the latest Competency Based Undergraduate Curriculum for Indian Medical Graduate.[1] The topics are divided in small chapters to generate the confidence in the learner in the pattern of the Miller's pyramid.[2] It helps to train the students to achieve the required levels of the given competencies: Knows (K), knows how (KH), and shows how (SH), with the help of included domains of learning, Knowledge (K) and skills (S). To fulfil the need for curriculum, requirements of the students and the field of medicine, this textbook characterizes the following features:

- **Concise text** with clinical correlation for quick recapitulation during examination.
- **280 Color atlas 3D illustrations** to provide easy imagining of developing structures.
- **105 Line diagrams** (practice figures) are easy to draw figures for theory examination.
- **110 Flowcharts** help to revise and memorize the text and to overcome the difficulty of summarizing the facts and developmental sequence in theory examinations and consolidation of knowledge.
- **61 Tables** to summarize essential facts.
- **Summary (examination guide)** to overcome the difficulty of summarizing the facts in theory examinations.
- **NEXT, MCQ, Viva, High yielding facts and Clinical facts** markings for preparation of various upcoming academic entrance examinations.
- **81 Boxes** to focus on important topics.
- **Interesting facts** to isolate them from the main text, so that these facts should not be missed by readers and ease the reading burden.
- **40 Scanning electron micrographs** to give real insight into developing structures.
- **76 Clinical cases** for *early clinical exposure* of various clinical anomalies encountered by eminent clinicians (vertical integration).
- **Special topics** such as assisted reproductive techniques (including *in vitro* fertilization) and ultrasonography in embryology, fetal viability, surrogate motherhood, contraception, sex ratio, teratogenesis, abortion, infertility, sterility and pregnancy tests are also included to give orientation toward clinical aspects.

I am hopeful that this book will help to fulfil all the requirements of students and teachers.

Students are suggested to read the book in the following sequence:

Color atlas 3D illustrations → Stages of development → Flowchart → Table → Summary (Examination Guide) → Practice Figure

Any suggestions from the readers are welcome.

Yogesh Sontakke
dryogeshas@rediffmail.com

---

[1] Medical Council of India, Competency Based Undergraduate Curriculum for the Indian Medical Graduate, 2018. Vol 1; pg 41–80.
[2] Miller GE. The assessment of clinical skills/competence/performance. Acad Med 1990;65(9 Suppl):S63–7.

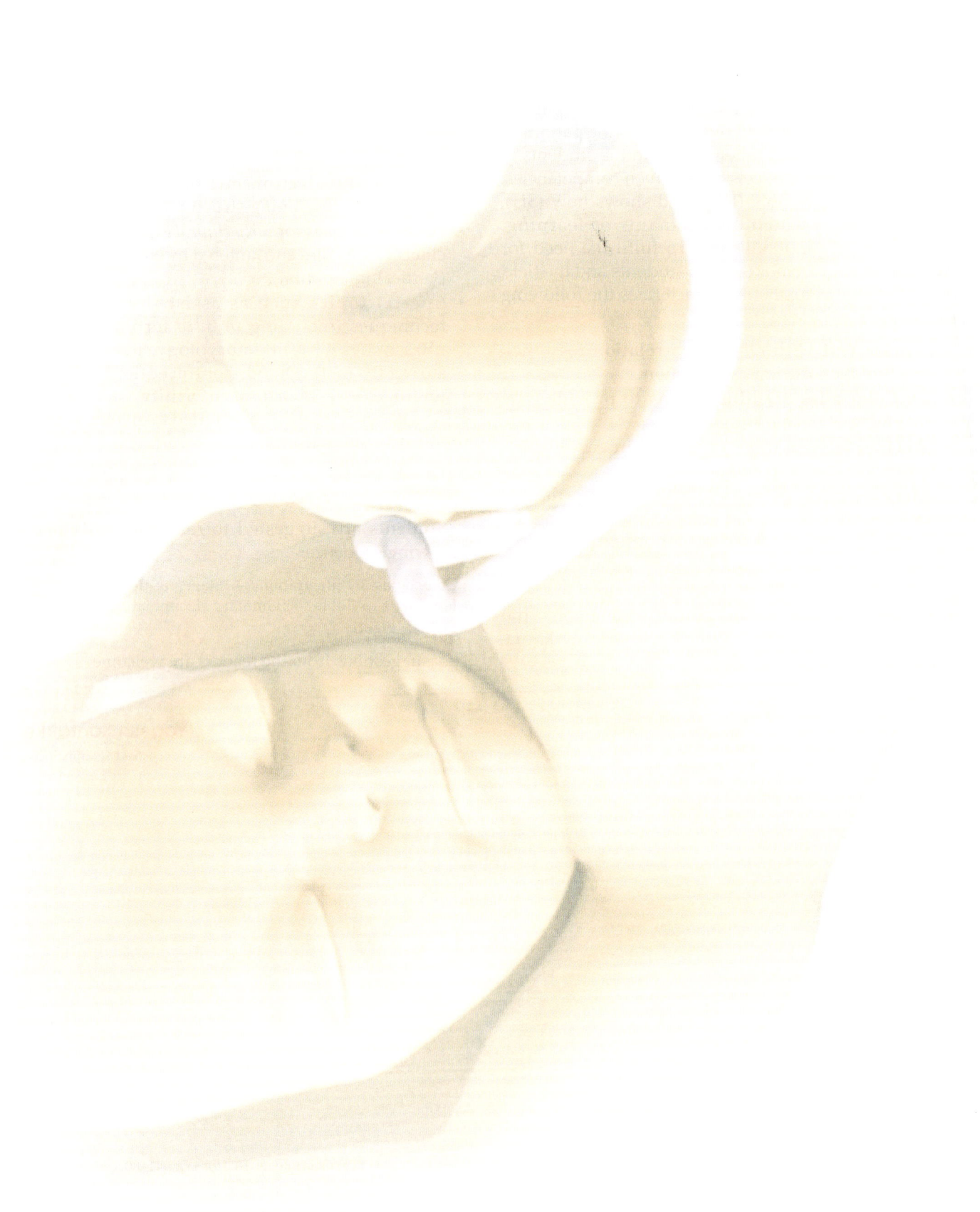

Preface to the First Edition

This *Textbook of Human Embryology* has been written keeping in mind the requirements of students and teachers. Due to the complexity of the subject, readers face difficulty in understanding and imagining the developing human structures. Hence, in the present book, the attempt has been made to provide all necessary information for easy understanding.

User-friendly features of this book with their purposes are as follows:

- **Concise text** is given in easy language; unnecessary details are avoided.
- **3D illustrations** to provide easy imagining of developing structures.
- **Flowcharts** to revise and memorise the developmental sequence.
- **Tables** to summarise essential facts.
- **Summary (examination guide)** to overcome the difficulty of summarising the facts in theory examinations.
- **Neet, MCQ, Viva Voce and Clinical facts** markings for preparation of various upcoming academic entrance examinations.
- **Boxes** to focus on important topics.
- **Interesting facts** to isolate them from the main text, so that these facts should not be missed by readers.
- **40 Scanning electron micrographs** to give real insight in developing structures.
- **70 Clinical cases** for early clinical exposure of various clinical anomalies encountered by eminent clinicians.
- **Special topics** such as assisted reproductive techniques (including *in vitro* fertilisation) and ultrasonography in embryology are also included to give orientation towards clinical aspects.

I am hopeful that this book will help to fulfil all the requirements of students and teachers.

Students are suggested to read in the following sequence:

Illustrations → Stages of development → Flowchart → Table → Summary (examination guide) → Practice Figure

Any suggestions from the readers for rectification and improvement are welcome at dryogeshas@rediffmail.com

Yogesh Sontakke

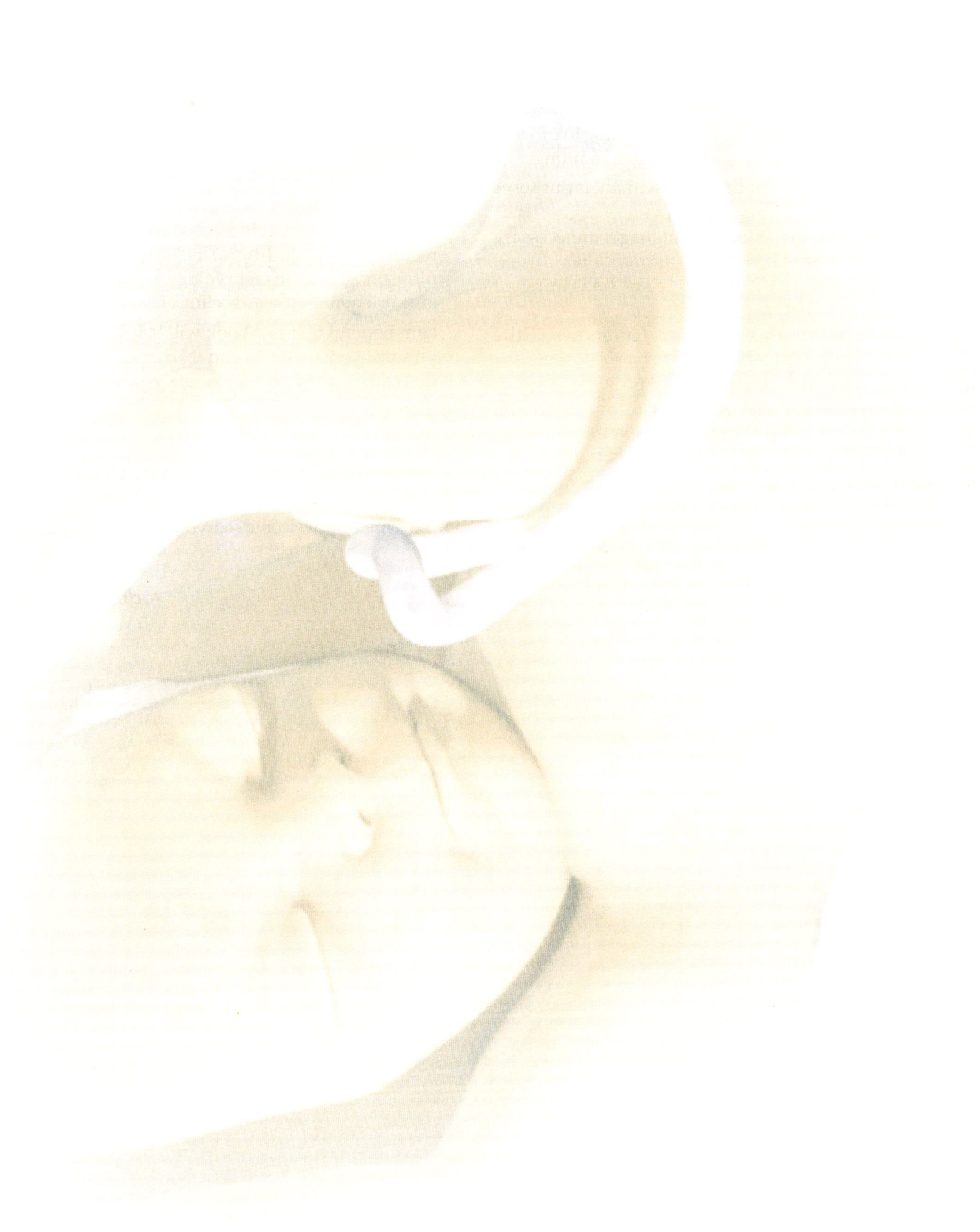

Acknowledgements

I am obliged to Prof Kathleen Sulik (Chapel Hill, North Carolina, USA), Dr Kumaravel S (Paediatric Surgery, JIPMER), Dr Bibekanand Jindal (Paediatric Surgery, JIPMER), Dr Uday Kumbhar (General Surgery, Puducherry), Dr Adhisivam B Neonatology, JIPMER), Dr Subashini Kaliaperumal (Ophthalmology, JIPMER), Dr Haritha Sagili (OBGY, JIPMER), Dr Mamatha Gowda (OBGY, JIPMER), Dr Keshav Malhotra (Rainbow IVF, Agra), Dr Saikat Chakraborty (Oral Pathology, Puducherry), Dr Rohit Rao (Ophthalmology, Raipur), Dr Prakhar Mohniya (Paediatrics, Jhansi) for their contribution of scanning electron micrographs, clinical images and suggestions.

I acknowledge the encouragement and continuous unconditional support from Dr Sarasu J, Dr Raveendranath V, Dr Suman Verma, Dr Sulochana Sakthivel, and Dr Rajasekhar SSSN. I am especially thankful to Dr V Gladwin, Vice-Dean (Academics), Dr Dharmaraj Tamgire, Dr Dinesh Kumar V, Dr G Dhivya Lakshmi, and Dr Mrinmayee Deb Barma for their critical suggestions.

I also acknowledge Drs Chandan Lal Gupta, Surraj S, Arun Prasad (senior residents) for their support. I also acknowledge Drs Sankaranarayanan G, Jahira Banu T, Lavanya R, CH Chaitanya Kumar, Raju Kumaran T, Srinivasan S, Sivasakthi M, Abbirami GR, Regina C, Sandy S, Urvi Sharma, Grace Suganya, Nandhini R, Nithya D, Kalaivani K, Jakkula Akhil (junior residents) for their help. I am thankful to Mr S Kirubanandan for his help in the typesetting of this manuscript.

I am thankful for the acceptability of views and support of Mr SK Jain (CMD) and Mr Varun Jain (Director), CBS Publishers & Distributors Pvt Ltd. I am obliged for continuous support from Mr YN Arjuna (Senior Vice-President—Publishing, Editorial and Publicity) and his entire team, especially Ms Ritu Chawla (GM—Production), Ms Ritu Tiwari (DTP operator), Mr Neeraj Prasad (graphic artist), Mr Neeraj Kumar Sharma (Editor). I appreciate the entire team of CBS Publishers & Distributors in the shaping of this book.

I am thankful to the support of entire CBS team for making the success of this book espically: Mr Deepak Rao (Bangalore), Mr Prasun Bhattacharya (Kolkata), Mr Sarkar (Mumbai), Mr Dinesh Dheek (Delhi), Mr James KC (Kochi), Mr S Ramesh (Chennai), Mr Sarbajit Gon (Bangalore), Mr Sumit Behl (New Delhi), Mr Ramesh (Hyderabad), Mr Jacob Joseph (Cochin), Mr S Muralidaran (Chennai), Mr B Jothi (Chennai), Mr BL Pradeep (Bangalore), Mr Ajay Kumar M (Bangalore), Mr Vikrant Shah (Uttarakhand), Mr Dinesh Giri (Rajasthan), Mr Javed (Mumbai), Mr Anand C (Bangalore), Mr Manish (Mumbai), Mr Dipam Chatterjee (Bihar and Jharkhand), Mr Krishnendu (Kolkata), Mr Pravin S Dhotre (Nagpur), Mr P Rajan (Chennai), Mr T Shinod (Calicut), Mr Narendra Singh (MP), Mr Somnath (Kolkata), Mr Sunil Pandey (Lucknow), Mr Vijay Pratap Singh (Lucknow), Mr Sujeet Morabad (Belgaum), Mr Balraj (Mangalore), Mr Tarak (Kolkata).

I thank my wife Dr Anindita for editing, proof-reading, and her continuous support. I appreciate my little girl Aripra for her unconditional love and support. My sincere regards to my family for moral support. I thank all my supporters who made this possible. I thank the Almighty for giving me strength and patience to continue my work.

Acknowledgements for Image Courtesy

I am grateful to the following academicians for their suggestions and contributions of clinical images (indicated in front of their names) in the present book.

- **Professor Kathleen Sulik,** PhD, Emeritus Professor, University of North Carolina School of Medicine, Department of Cell Biology and Physiology, Chapel Hill, North Carolina, USA.

  Scannning electron micrographs: 7.1 to 7.5, 8.1 to 8.5, 11.1 to 11.3, 12.1 to 12.4, 13.1, 14.1, 14.2, 15.1, 18.1 to 18.4, 19.1, 20.1, 21.1 to 21.3, 22.1 to 22.4, 23.1, 23.2, 24.1, 24.2, AV.1, AV.2.

- **Dr Kumaravel S,** MBBS, MS, MCh (Paediatric Surgery), Professor, Department of Paediatric Surgery, JIPMER, Puducherry, 605 006, India.

  Clinical images: 7.2, 9.5, 10.1 to 10.3, 11.1, 14.2 to 14.7, 17.1, 18.3, 20.1, 20.2, 21.1 to 21.5, 22.1 to 22.3, 26.1, 30.1, AV.1 to AV.3.

- **Dr Uday Kumbhar,** Professor, Department of Surgery, JIPMER, Puducherry, 605006, India. Clinical images 11.2, 21.6, 21.7, 27.1

- **Dr Adhisivam B,** Professor, Department of Neonatology, JIPMER, Puducherry, 605 006, India. Clinical images: 12.2, 14.1, 22.4A, 22.5 to 22.7.

- **Dr Subashini Kaliaperumal,** MBBS, MS (Ophthalmology), FRCS, DNB (Ophthalmology), Professor and Head, Department of Ophthalmology, JIPMER, Puducherry. 605 006, India.

  Clinical images: 23.5 to 23.9.

- **Dr Haritha Sagili,** MBBS, MD, MRCOG, MFSRH, European University Diploma in Operative

Gynaecological Endoscopy, FICS, CIMP, FIMSA, Professor, Department of Obstetrics and Gynaecology, JIPMER, Puducherry, 605 006. India.

Clinical images: 9.1 to 9.4, 18.1, 28.1, 30.2.

- **Dr Mamatha Gowda**, Additional Professor, Department of Obstetrics and Gynaecology, JIPMER, Puducherry, 605 006, India.

  Clinical images: 7.1, 18.1, 18.2, 22.8 to 22.11, 29.1 to 29.4, 30.3.

- **Dr Keshav Malhotra**, MBBS MCE, Director, Rainbow IVF, Rainbow Hospitals, Agra, Uttar Pradesh, 282007.

  Clinical images: 3.1, 4.1, 4.2, 4.3, 5.1.

- **Dr Rohit Rao**, MBBS, MS (Ophthalmology), IOL and Anterior Segment Fellowship (Aravind Eye Hospital), Anterior Segment Surgeon, Shri Ganesh Vinayak Eye Hospital, Raipur, Chhattisgarh, India.

  Clinical images: 23.1 to 23.4, 23.10.

- **Dr Prakhar Mohniya**, MBBS, MD (Paediatrics), Fellowship in Neonatology. Senior Resident, Maharani Laxmi Bai Medical College, Jhansi, UP, 284128. India.

  Clinical images: 12.1, 22.4B.

- **Dr Saikat Chakraborty**, Resident, MDS (Oral Pathology), Mahatma Gandhi Postgraduate Institute of Dental Sciences, Puducherry, 605 006, India.

  Clinical images: 13.1.

Yogesh Sontakke

Acknowledgements

I would like to thank the following teachers of anatomy for their constant blessings, encouragement, support, and kind words for this as well as my previous books.

- Dr Shakuntala Pai Former Associate Dean, Professor and Head, Kasturba Medical College, Manipal, Karnataka
- Dr Ashok Patil Principal, Professor and Head, SMBT Dental College and Hospital and Postgraduate Research Centre, Sangamner, Ahmednagar, MS
- Dr Ashutosh Mangalagiri Medical Superintendent, Chirayu Medical College, Bhopal, MP
- Dr Azhar Ahmed Siddiqui Dean, JIIU's Indian Institute of Medical Science and Research, Badnapur, Jalna, MS
- Dr B Naveen Kumar Vice-Principal and Professor, Mamata Academy of Medical Sciences, Bachupally, Hyderabad, Telangana
- Dr Deepti Shastri Deputy Dean (Academics), Professor and Head, Vinayaka Mission's Kirupananda Variyar Medical College and Hospitals, Salem, TN
- Dr Jaedeo Ughade Professor and Head and Academic Dean, Parbhani Medical College, Parbhani, MS
- Dr M Chatterjee Dean (Academics), Shree Balaji Medical College, Raipur, CG
- Dr M Sivakumar Former Dean, JIPMER, Karaikal; Professor, SRM Medical College, Trichi, TN
- Dr Muthukumaravel Narayanaswamy Professor and Associate Dean, Sri Venkateshwaraa Medical College Hospital and Research Centre, Ariyur, Puducherry
- Dr Nava Kalyani Vice Principal and Professor and Head, Government Medical College, Mahabubnagar, Telangana
- Dr Rajneet Guha Principal and Professor, Indira Gandhi Institute of Medical Sciences, Sheikhpura, Patna, Bihar
- Dr Shivaji B Sukre Dean, Government Medical College and Hospital, Parbhani, MS
- Dr Soumya Chakraborty Bhattachrya Director cum Dean, Nagaland Institute of Medical Sciences and Research, Kohima, Nagaland
- Dr T Rajan Vice-Principal, Professor and Head, Aarupadai Veedu Medical College and Hospital, Puducherry
- Dr TK Rajashree Vice-Principal (Academics), Professor, Malla Reddy Institute of Medical Sciences, Hyderabad
- Dr Aaditya Madhusudan Tarnekar Professor and Head, AIIMS, Nagpur, MS
- Dr Bertha AD Rathinam Professor and Head, AIIMS, Bhopal, MP
- Dr Biswabina Ray Professor and Head, AIIMS, Kalyani, WB
- Dr Brijendra Singh Professor and Head, AIIMS, Rishikesh, Uttarakhand
- Dr Joy Ghoshal Dean Professor and Head, AIIMS, Mangalagiri, AP
- Dr Kumar Satish Ravi Professor and Head, AIIMS, Gorakhpur, UP
- Dr Simmi Mehra Professor and Head, AIIMS, Rajkot, Gujrat
- Dr Manisha R Gaikwad Additional Professor and Head, AIIMS, Bhubaneswar, Odisha
- Dr Mrudula Chandrupatla Additional Professor and Head, AIIMS, Bibinagar, Hyderabad, Telangana
- Dr R Sarah Additional Professor and Head, AIIMS, Madurai, TN
- Dr Mrinal Barua Additional Professor, AIIMS, Rishikesh, Uttarakhand
- Dr Mukesh Singhla Additional Professor, AIIMS, Rishikesh, Uttarakhand
- Dr Nidhi Puri Additional Professor, AIIMS, Bilaspur, HP
- Dr Padamjeet Panchal Additional Professor, AIIMS, Patna, Bihar
- Dr Prashant Chaware Additional Professor, AIIMS, Bhopal, MP
- Dr Rashmi Malhotra Additional Professor, AIIMS, Rishikesh, Uttarakhand
- Dr Soumitra Trivedi Additional Professor, AIIMS, Raipur, CG
- Dr Gayatri Muthiyan Associate Professor, AIIMS, Nagpur, MS
- Dr Reeha Mahajan Associate Professor, AIIMS, Vijaypur, Jammu, J&K
- Dr Rohini Motwani Associate Professor, AIIMS, Bibinagar, Hyderabad, Telangana
- Dr Sumit Patil Associate Professor, AIIMS, Bhopal, MP
- Dr Alka V Bhingardeo Assistant Professor, AIIMS, Bibi Nagar, Hyderabad
- Dr Bhagyashree Assistant Professor, AIIMS, Bilaspur, HP
- Dr Ruchi Ratnesh Assistant Professor, AIIMS, Deoghar, Jharkhand
- Dr Sachin Soni Assistant Professor, AIIMS, Bilaspur, HP
- Dr Sunita Nayak Assistant Professor, AIIMS, Patna, Bihar
- Dr Sushant Swaroop Das Assistant Professor, AIIMS, Bilaspur, HP
- Dr Ujwala Bhanarkar Assistant Professor, AIIMS, Kalyani, WB
- Dr A Hima Bindu Professor and Head, GITAM Institute of Medical Sciences and Research, Visakhapatnam, AP
- Dr AK Singh Professor and Head, Soban Singh Jeena Govt Medical College, Almora, Uttarakhand
- Dr AK Srivastava Professor and Head, Saraswati Dental College, Lucknow, UP
- Dr Alka Singh Professor and Head, Rajashri Dashrath Autonomous State Medical College, Ayodhya, UP
- Dr Alka Udainia Professor, Government Medical College, Surat, Gujrat
- Dr Aloka Sharma Professor and Head, Jawaharlal Nehru Medical College, Bhagalpur, Bihar
- Dr Amar Jayanthi A Former Professor and Head, Government Medical College, Idukki, Kerala
- Dr Amit Mehta Professor and Head, Government Medical College, Chindwada, MP
- Dr Amrut Mahajan Professor and Head, Dr Ulhas Patil Medica College, Jalgaon, MS
- Dr Amudha Mohan Ram Professor and Head, Katuri Medical College, Chilkarutpeta, Guntur, AP
- Dr Angela A Viswasom Professor and Head, Travancore Medical College, Kollam, Kerala
- Dr Anil Rahule Professor and Head, Government Medical College, Ramagundam, Telangana
- Dr Anita Fating Professor and Head, Dr Rajendra Gode Medical College, Amaravati, MS
- Dr Anitha V Professor and Head, Government Medical College, Kanyakumari, TN
- Dr Anjali Aggarwal Professor and Head, PGIMER, Chandigarh
- Dr Anjali Sabnis Professor and Head, MGM Medical College, Navi Mumbai, MS
- Dr Anju Partap Professor and Head, Indira Gandhi Medical College, Shimla, HP
- Dr Anne George Professor and Head, Government Medical College, Kottayam, Kerala
- Dr Annie Doley Professor and Head, Tezpur Government Medical College, Assam
- Dr Anuj Ram Sharma Professor, Muzaffarnagar Medical College, Muzaffarnagar, UP
- Dr Anupama Doddappaiah Panagar Professor and Head, St Peter's Medical College, Hospital and Research Institute, Hosur, TN
- Dr Anurag Professor, VCSG Govt Medical College, Srinagar, Uttarakhand
- Dr Aparna K Vedapriya Professor and Head, Government Medical College, Siddipet
- Dr Aparna Professor and Head, NIMRA Medical College, Vijayawada, AP
- Dr Archana Goel Professor and Head, Adesh Medical College, Ambala, Haryana
- Dr Arindam Banerjee Professor and Head, IQ-City Medical College, Durgapur, WB
- Dr Arun Kasote Professor and Head, Government Medical College, Nagpur, MS
- Dr Arun Prasad Singh Professor and Head, Patna Medical College, Patna, Bihar
- Dr Arun Pundlikrao Kasote Professor and Head, Government Medical College, Jalgaon, MS
- Dr Arunabha Tapadar Professor and Head, Sarat Chandra Chattopadhyay Govt. Medical College & Hospital, Uluberia, WB
- Dr Ashwini Jadhav Professor, Grant Government Medical College, Mumbai, MS
- Dr Asis Kumar Ghosal Professor and Head, Deben Mahato Government Medical College and Hospital, Purulia, WB
- Dr Ausavi Siraz Mustapha, Former Professor and Head, Mahavir Institute of Medical Sciences, Vikarabad, Telangana
- Dr AV Kulkarni Professor and Head, SDM Medical College, Dharwad, Karnataka
- Dr Avanish Kumar Professor and Head, Indira Gandhi Institute of Medical Sciences, Patna, Bihar
- Dr Avinash Rudrajwar Professor and Head, Maitri College of Dentistry, Durg, CG
- Dr Bashir Ahmad Shah Professor, Government Medical College, Srinagar, J&K
- Dr Beena Nambiar Professor and Head, Government Medical College, Pariyaram, Kannur, Kerala
- Dr Bharat Patel Professor and Head GCS Medical College, Ahmedabad, Gujrat
- Dr Bhaskar Pal Professor and Head, Icare Institute of Medical Science and BC Roy Hospital, Haldia, WB
- Dr Bhaudas Khanderao Jadhav Professor and Head, Terna Medical College, Mumbai, MS
- Dr Bindu Singh Professor and Head, BRD Medical College, Gorakhpur, UP
- Dr Bipinchandra Khade Professor and Head, Chirayu Medical College, Bhopal, MP
- Dr BR Singh Professor and Head, Datta Meghe Medical College, Nagpur, MS
- Dr BS Lala Former Professor and Head, Sri Aurobindo Medical College and Postgraduate Institute, Indore, MP
- Dr C Kishan Reddy Professor and Head, Prathima Institute of Medical Sciences, Karimnagar, Telangana
- Dr C Lalitha Professor and Head, Kempaguda Medical College (KIMS), Bengaluru
- Dr Ch Jayamma Professor and Head, Government Medical College, Nandyal, AP
- Dr Chitti Narasamma Professor and Head, Kurnool Medical College, Kurnool, AP
- Dr Chittynarsamma Professor and Head, Kurnool Medical College, Kurnool, AP
- Dr D Sudhakar Babu Professor and Head, Government Medical College, Nizamabad, Telangana
- Dr D Asha Latha Professor and Head, Government Medical College, Machlipatnam, AP
- Dr DAVS Sesi Professor and Head, Ranga Raya Medical College, Kakinada, AP
- Dr Debjani Roy Professor and Head, Midnapore Medical College and Hospital, Medinapore, WB

- Dr Deepa Bently Professor and Head, Govt Medical College and ESIC Hospital, Coimbatore, TN
- Dr Deepa Deopa Professor and Head, Dr. Sushila Tiwari Govt Medical College, Haldwani, Uttarakhand
- Dr Deepali G Vidhale Professor and Head, Dr Punjabrao Deshmukh Memorial Medical College, Amaravati, MS
- Dr Deepali Onkar Professor and Head, NKP Salve Medical College, Nagpur, MS
- Dr DH Gopalan Professor and Head, Tagore Medical College and Hospital, Chennai, TN
- Dr Dimpal Patel Professor and Head, AMC Met Medical College, Ahmedabad, Gujrat
- Dr Dipali Trivedi Professor, BJ Medical College and Hospital, Ahmedabad, Gujrat
- Dr DV Singh Professor and Head, Rajshree Medical Research Institute, Bareilly, UP
- Dr Fatima M De Souza Professor and Head, Goa Medical College, Goa
- Dr GA Jos Hemalatha Professor and Head, Government Medical College, Virudhunagar, TN
- Dr Ganesh Khemnar Professor, Vishwa Bharati Institute of Medical Science, Kurnool, AP
- Dr Garima Pardhi Assistant Professor, ABV Government Medical College, Vidisha, MP
- Dr Gautam A Shroff Professor and Head, MGM Institute of Health Sciences, Aurangabad, MS
- Dr Ghulam Mohammad Bhat Professor and Head, Government Medical College, Srinagar, J&K
- Dr Gnanavel A Professor, Meenakshi Medical College, Kanchipuram, TN
- Dr Gunapriya Raghunath Professor and Head, Department of Anatomy, Saveetha Medical College and Hospital, Chennai, TN
- Dr Gunwant Chaudhari Professor and Head, Zydus Medcal College and Hospital, Dahod, Gujrat
- Dr Gyan Prakash Mishra Professor and Head, Autonomous State Medical College, Basti, UP
- Dr Haritha Nimmagadda Former Professor and Head, Department of General Anatomy and General Histology, Bharti Vidyapeeth Dental College, Navi Mumbai, MS
- Dr Hrishikesh Jadhav Professor and Head, GMERS Medical College, Sola, Ahmadabad, Gujrat
- Dr Indra Kumar Patel Professor and Head, Maharaja Suheldev Autonomous State Medical College, Bahraich, UP
- Dr Jaba Rajguru Professor, Parul Institute of Medical Science and Research, Vadodra, Gujrat
- Dr Jagriti Agrawal Professor and Head, Pt. Jawahrlal Nehru Memorial Medical College, Raipur, CG
- Dr Jami Sagar Prusty Professor and Head, MKCG Medical College, Berhampur, Odisha
- Dr Jasmeen Shaikh Professor, Apollo Institute of Medical Science and Research, Hyderabad, Telangana
- Dr Jaswinder Kaur Professor and Head, MM College of Medical Sciences and Research, Ambala, Haryana
- Dr Jaya Prakash Professor and Head Government Medical College, Kamareddy, Telangana
- Dr Jaya Prakash Professor and Head, Prathima Relief Medical College, Warangal, Telangana
- Dr Jayasree K Former Professor and Head, Government Medical College, Kozhikode, Kerala
- Dr Jessy Rose George Professor Government Medical College, Kozhikode, Kerala
- Dr Jeyanthi G Professor and Head, Government Thirunelveli Medical College, Thirunelveli, TN
- Dr Jitendra Patel Professor and Head, NHL Medical College, Ahmedabad, Gujrat
- Dr Jwalant Waghmare Professor and Head, Mahatma Gandhi Institute of Medical Sciences, Sevagram
- Dr Jyoti Ramling Gaikwad Professor and Head, MGM Medical College, Sanpada, MS
- Dr K K Thakur Professor and Head, Government Medical College, Doda, J&K
- Dr K Udhaya Professor and Head, Swamy Vivekanandha Medical College Hospital and Research Institute, Tiruchengode, TN
- Dr Kalpana Ramachandran Professor and Head, Sri Ramachandra Medical College, Chennai, TN
- Dr Kalyan Bhattacharya Professor and Head, Medical College, Kolkata, WB
- Dr Kanchan Kapoor Professor and Head, Government Medical College, Chandigarh
- Dr Kavita Nanda Professor and Head, Dr. Radhakrishnan Government Medical College Hamirpur, HP
- Dr KK Agarwal Former Professor and Head, Veer Chandra Singh Garhwali Govt. Medical Sciences and Research Institute, Srinagar, Uttarakhand
- Dr Komala B Professor and Head, BGS Global Institute of Medical Sciences, Bengaluru
- Dr Krishnaiah M Professor and Head, Government Medical College, Suryapet, Telangana
- Dr L Hema Professor, Narayana Medical College, Nellore, AP
- Dr Lakshmikantha Former Professor, DM WIMS Medical College, Meppadi, Wayanad, Kerala
- Dr Lalatendu Swain Professor and Head, Shree Jagannath Medical College, Puri, Odisha
- Dr Lola Das Professor and Head, Amala Medical College, Thrissur, Kerala
- Dr M Prasad Professor and Head, Patliputra Medical College, Dhanbad, Jharkhand
- Dr MA Doshi Professor and Head, Krishna Institute of Medical Science, Karad, MS
- Dr Madhusmita Panda Professor and Head, Fakir Mohan Medical College, Balasore, Odisha
- Dr Mahendra Kumar Pant Professor and Head, Government Medical College, Dehradun, Uttarakhand
- Dr Mahesh GM Professor, Basaveshwara Medical College and Hospital, Chitradurga, Karnataka
- Dr Mahesh Ugale Professor and Head, MIMSR Medical College, Latur, MS
- Dr Mahita Bojja Professor and Head, Government Medical College, Nagarkurnool, Telangana.
- Dr Malamoni Dutta Professor and Head, Kokrajhar Medical College and Hospital, Kokrajhar, Assam
- Dr Mamata Sar Professor and Head, Veer Surendra Sai Institute of Medical Sciences and Research, Burla, Odisha
- Dr Mani Kathapillai Professor, Shree Sathya Sai Medical College and Research Institute, Chengalpattu, TN
- Dr Manish Patil Professor and Head, RD Gardi Medical College, Ujjain, MP
- Dr Manisha Nakhate Professor and Head, Dr DY Patil Medical College, Hospital and Research Centre, Navi Mumbai, MS
- Dr Manisha Upadhyay Professor and Head, Government Medical College, Azamgarh, UP
- Dr Manjunath V Motagi Professor and Head, SAIMS Medical College, Indore, MP
- Dr Maria Kala Professor and Head, RVM Institute of Medical Sciences and Research Center, Telangana
- Dr Martin Lucas A Professor and Head, Dr Chandramma Dayananda Sagar Institute of Medical Education and Research, Bengaluru
- Dr Meenakshi Parthsarathy Professor and Head, Shri Atal Bihari Vajpayee Medical College and Research Institution, Bengaluru
- Dr Meghana Mishra Professor and Head, Shyam Shah Medical College, Reva, MP
- Dr Mehandi V Mahajan Professor, Indira Medical College and Research Institute, Thiruvallur, TN
- Dr Mehera Bhoir Professor and Head, HHSBT Medical College and Dr Rustom Narsi Cooper Municipal General Hospital, Mumbai, MS
- Dr MG Puranik Professor, Bharthi Vidyapeeth Medical College, Pune, MS
- Dr Mini Kariappa Professor, Amala Institute of Medical Sciences, Thrissur
- Dr Mrityunjay Pandey Professor and Head, Maharshi Devraha Baba Autonomous State Medical College, Deoria, UP
- Dr Mukul Sarma Professor and Head, Nagaon Government Medical College, Nagaon, Assam
- Dr N Bhanu Sudha Parimala Professor and Head, NRI'S Medical College, Mangalagiri, AP
- Dr Namdeo Y Kamdi Professor and Head, Government Medical College, Chandrapur, MS
- Dr Nandita Dutta Professor and Head, Jalpaiguri Govt Medical College, Jalpaiguri, WB
- Dr Natwar Agrawal Professor and Head, NSC Bose Medical College, Jabalpur, MP
- Dr Neeta Chhabra Professor and Head, Al-Falah School of Medical Science and Research Centre, Faridabad, Haryana
- Dr Neetu Arora Professor and Head, Saheed Hasan Khan Government Medical College, Nalhar, Nuh, Haryana
- Dr Neha Rai Professor, LN Medical College, Bhopal, MP
- Dr Nilesh Rakate Professor, RKDF Medical College, Bhopal, MP
- Dr Nirmaladevi M Professor and Head, Karpagam Medical College, Coimbatore, TN
- Dr Nirupama Gupta Professor and Head, Sharda Medical College, Gr Noida, UP
- Dr Nitin R Mudiraj Professor and Head, Bharti Vidyapeeth Medical College and Hspital, Sangali, MS
- Dr Nivedita Pandey Professor and Head, NC Medical College, and Hospital, Israna, Panipat, Haryana
- Dr Nusrat Jabeen Professor, Government Medical College, Jammu, J&K
- Dr P Bapuji Professor and Head, Alluri Sitaramaraju Academy of Medical Sciences, Eluru, AP
- Dr P Sasikala Professor, Swamy Vivekanandha Medical College Hospital and Research Institute, Tiruchengode, TN
- Dr PV Satya Kumar Professor, NIMRA Medical College, Vijayawada, AP
- Dr Padmasini S Professor Madha Medical College and Hospital, Chennai, TN
- Dr Pankaj Maheria Professor and Head, GMERS Medical College, Valsad, Gujrat
- Dr Patil Shrish Professor and Head, Basaveshwara Medical College and Hospital, Chitradurga, Karnataka
- Dr PG Khanwalkar Professor, Chirayu Medical College, Bhopal, MP
- Dr PK Ramakrishnan Professor and Head, PK Das Institute of Medical Sciences, Palakkad, Kerala
- Dr Poonam Delmotra Professor and Head, Aadesh Medical College and Hospital, Shahbad, Haryana
- Dr PP Kulkarni Professor, Prakash Institute of Medical Science and Research, Islampur, MS
- Dr Prabhakaran K Professor and Head, Nootan Medical College, Ahmedabad, Gujrat
- Dr Prafulla Pralhadrao Nikam Professor, Jawaharlal Nehru Medical College, Wardha, MS
- Dr Prajakta Kishve Professor and Head, Employees State Insurance Coporation Medical College, Hyderabad, Telangana
- Dr Prakash Baburao Hosmani Professor and Head, Dr VM Government Medical College, Solapur, MS
- Dr Prasanna MB Former Professor, Government Medical College, Ernakulam, Kerala
- Dr Praveen B Iyer Additional Professor, Seth GS Medical College, Mumbai, MS
- Dr Praveen Singh Professor and Head, Pramukhswami Medical College, Karamsad, Gujrat
- Dr Prerna Gupta Professor and Head, TS Mishra Medical College and Hospital, Amausi, Lucknow, UP
- Dr Pritha S Bhuiyan Former Professor and Head, Seth GS Medical College, Mumbai, MS

- Dr Priti Sinha Professor and Head, LLRM Medical College, Meerut, UP
- Dr Priya Ranganath Professor and Head, Bangalore Medical College, Bengaluru
- Dr PS Chitra Professor and Head, Government Medical College Hospital, Ariyalur, TN
- Dr Pulipati Anil Kumar Professor and Head, Maharaja Institute of Medical Science, Vizianagaram, AP
- Dr Purushotam Rao Professor and Head, Mahavir Institute of Medical Science, Vikarabad, Telangana
- Dr R Manoranjitham Professor and Head, Dhanalakshmi Srinivasan Medical College and Hospital, Perambalur, TN
- Dr Rajasri Chunder Professor and Head, Jagannath Gupta Institute of Medical Sciences and Hospital, Budge, Kolkata, WB
- Dr Rajendra Prasad Professor and Head, Anugrah Narayan Magadh Medical College, Gaya, Bihar
- Dr Rajendrakumar D Virupaxi Professor and Head, KLE JGMM Medical College, Hubballi, Karnataka
- Dr Rajendrakumar D Virupaxi Professor, JN Medical College, Belagavi, Karnataka
- Dr Rajkumar KR Professor and Head, Gulbarga Institute of Medical Sciences, Gulbarga, Karnataka
- Dr Rajlaxmi Panda Professor, MKCG Medical College, Berhampur, Odisha
- Dr Rajveer Singh Chourasia Professor and Head, SRM Medical College and Hospital, Bhawanipatna, Odisha
- Dr Rakesh Kumar Verma Additional Professor, KGMU, Lucknow, UP
- Dr Rakesh Mishra Reader and Head, Sardar Patel Postgraduate Institute of Dental and Medical Sciences, Lucknow, UP
- Dr Randhir S Chauhan Professor and Head, Maharishi Markendeshwar Medical College, Solan, HP
- Dr Rashmi Deopujari Professor and Head, ABV Medical College, Vidisha, MP
- Dr Rashmi Prasad Professor and Head, Nalanda Medical College, Patna, Bihar
- Dr Rashmoni Jana Professor, Vardhman Mahavir Medical College and Safdarjung Hospital, Delhi
- Dr Raviendra Marathe Professor and Head, RR Kambe Dental College, Akola, MS
- Dr Renuka Ahankari Professor, Smt. Kashibai Navale Medical College and General Hospital, Pune, MS
- Dr Ritesh Shah Professor, GCS Medical College, Ahmadabad, Gujrat
- Dr Ritu Saloi Professor and Head, Diphu Medical College, Diphu, Assam
- Dr Rohini Karambelkar Professor and Head, Prakash Institute of Medical Science, Islampur, MS
- Dr Romi S Professor, Azeezia Medical College Hospital, Kollam, Kerala
- Dr RS Bulagouda Professor and Head, Shri BM Patil Medical College Hospital and Research Centre BLDE (Deemed to be University), Vijayapura, Karnataka
- Dr Rubi Saikia Professor and Head, Jorhat Medical College, Jorhat, Assam
- Dr Rup Sekhar Deka Professor and Head, Nalbari Medical College, Nalbari, Assam
- Dr Rupa Chaparrwal Professor, Sri Aurobindo Medical College and Postgraduate Institute, Indore, MP
- Dr S Babu Rao Professor and Head, Malla Reddy Medical college for Women, Hyderabad, Telangana
- Dr S Bharathi Rani Professor Government Sivagangai Medical College, Sivagangai, TN
- Dr S Karthick Selvaraj Professor and Head, Meenakshi Medical College Kanchipuram, TN
- Dr S Naveen Kumar Professor, Malla Reddy Institute of Medical Sciences, Hyderabad, Telangana
- Dr S Satishkumar Professor and Head, Government Kalakurichi Medical College, Kalakurichi, TN
- Dr S Sundarapandian Professor and Head, SRM Medical College and Hospital, Chengalpattu, TN
- Dr SVV Nagarajamannar Professor and Head, Government Medical College, Rajahmundry, AP
- Dr Sadakat Ali Professor and Head, SGRR Medical College, Dehradun, Uttarakhand
- Dr Samatha Roshini Padala Professor and Head, Surabhi Institute of Medical Science, Siddipet, Telangana
- Dr Sandeep K Sharma Professor and Head, MRA Medical College, Ambedkar Nagar, UP
- Dr Sandhya Kurup Professor and Head, MOSC Medical College, Kolanchery, Kerala
- Dr Sangeeta Gupta Professor and Head, Government Medical College, Jammu, J&K
- Dr Sangeeta M Professor and Head, MVJ Medical College and Research Hospital, Bengaluru
- Dr Sanjeev Kolagi Professor and Head, S. Nijalingappa Medical College and HSK Hospital and Research Centre, Bagalkot, Karnataka
- Dr Santhini Arulselvi Professor and Head, Vinayaka Missions Medical College and Hospital, Karaikal, Puducherry
- Dr Sarada Devi Professor, Bhaskar Medical College, Moinabad, Telangana
- Dr Saritha S Former Professor and Head, Kamineni Academy of Medical Sciences and Research Center, Hyderabad, Telangana
- Dr Satheesha KS Professor, Srinivas Institute of Medical Sciences and Research Center, Mangaluru, Karnataka
- Dr Satyashree Ray Professor and Head, SCB Medical College, Cuttack, Odisha
- Dr Saurjya Ranjan Das Professor, IMS and SUM Hospital, Bhubaneswar, Odisha
- Dr Savithri Krishnan Former Professor and Head, Government Medical College, Kollam, Kerala
- Dr Seema Sharma Professor and Head, Government Medical College, and Associated Hospital, Rajouri, J&K
- Dr Seema SR Professor and Head, ESI Postgraduate Institute of Medical Sciences and Research, Bengaluru
- Dr Shaifaly Madan Rustagi Professor and Head, Army Medical College, Delhi
- Dr Shailaja Shetty Professor and Head, Department of Anatomy, MS Ramaiah Medical College, Bengaluru
- Dr Shantanu Nandy Professor and Head, Bankura Sammilani Medical College & Hospital, Bankura, WB
- Dr Shashi Munjal Professor and Head, Mayo Medical College, Barabanki, UP
- Dr Sheela Sivan Professor and Head, MES Medical College, Perinthalmanna, Malappuram, Kerala
- Dr Shema Nair Professor, LN Medical College, Bhopal, MP
- Dr Shilpa Bhimalli Professor and Head, JN Medical College, Belagavi, Karnataka
- Dr Shobha Ramnarayan Professor and Head, Malankara Orthodox Syrian Church Medical Mission Hospital, Kolenchery, Ernakulum, Kerala
- Dr Shruthi BN Professor and Head, Raja Rajeshwari Medical College, Bengaluru
- Dr Shubhangi Bhagwat Ghule Professor, Dr Ulhas Patil Medica College, Jalgaon, MS
- Dr Simmi Soni Professor, Dr VRK Womens Medical College, Aziznagar, Telangana
- Dr SK Chavan Professor, Maharashtra Institute of Medical Education and Research, Pune, MS
- Dr SM Belsare Professor, MIMER Medical College, Talgaon, Pune, MS
- Dr Smruti Rekha Mohanty Professor and Head, KIMS, Bhubaneswar, Odisha
- Dr SS Saiyad Professor and Head, Dr ND Desai Faculty of Medical Science, Nadiad, Gujrat
- Dr Subhash K Deshpande Professor, SDM Medical College, Dharwad, Karnataka
- Dr Suchetra Chaudhary Professor and Head, BJ Medical College and Hospital, Ahmadabad, Gujrat
- Dr Sudha R Professor and Head, Annapoorana Medical College and Hospital, Salem, TN
- Dr Sujata K Professor, PES Medical College, Kuppam, AP
- Dr Sukhinder Baidwain Professor and Head, Dr YS Parmar Government Medical College, Nahan, HP
- Dr Suman Yadav Professor and Head, Dr. Rajendra Prasad Government Medical College Kangra at Tanda, HP
- Dr Sumedha Anjankar Professor and Head, Shree Balaji Medical College, Raipur, CG
- Dr Sundar Lal Jethani Chief Medical Superintendent and Professor, Himalayan Institute of Medical Sciences, Dehradun, Uttarakhand
- Dr Sunita Gupta Former Professor and Head, AMC Met Medical College, Ahmedabad, Gujrat
- Dr Suresh Kumar Professor and Head, Government Vellore Medical College, Vellore, TN
- Dr Susan Varghese Professor and Head, Government Medical College, Kollam, Kerala
- Dr Susheela Rana Professor and Head, Shri Lal Bahadur Shastri Government Medical College, Mandi, HP
- Dr Swapan Bhattacharjee Professor and Head, Santiniketan Medical College and Hospital, Bolpur, WB
- Dr Sweta Singh Professor and Head, Hind Institute of Medical Sciences, Barabanki, UP
- Dr T Anitha Professor and Head, Government Villupuram Medical College, Villupurum, TN
- Dr T Sreekanth Professor and Head, Shadan Institute of Medical Sciences, Research Centre and Teaching Hospital, Peerancheru, Telangana
- Dr Tapan Kumar Jana Professor and Head, Murshidabad Medical College and Hospitals, Murshidabad, WB
- Dr TC Singel Professor, Zydus Medcal College and Hospital, Dahod, Gujrat
- Dr Tejaswi HL Professor and Head, Adichunchanagiri Institute of Medical Sciences, Mandya, Karnataka
- Dr Tridib Kumar Sett Professor and Head, Tamralipto Government Medical College & Hospital, Tamluk, WB
- Dr Trupti Balwir Professor, Datta Meghe Medical College, Nagpur, MS
- Dr UK Kulkarni Professor and Head, Belagavi Institute of Medical Sciences, Belagavi, Karnataka
- Dr Usha KK Professor and Head, Government Medical College, Manjeri, Kerala
- Dr V Anandhi Professor and Head, K P Viswanathan Government Medical College, Trichy, TN
- Dr V Rajapriya Professor and Head, Government Omandurar Medical College, Omandurar, TN
- Dr V Ravi Kumar Professor and Head, Subbaiah Institute of Medical Sciences, Shimoga, Karnataka
- Dr V Subhashini Professor and Head, Konaseema Institute of Medical Science, Amalapuram, AP
- Dr Vaishali Inamdar Professor and Head, Dr Shankarrao Chavan Government Medical College and Hospital, Nanded, MS
- Dr Vandana Mehta Director and Professor, Vardhman Mahavir Medical College and Safdarjung Hospital, New Delhi
- Dr Vanita Gupta Professor and Head, Government Medical College, Udhampur, J&K
- Dr Varsha Mokhasi Professor and Head, Vydehi Institute of Medical Sciences and Research Centre, Bengaluru
- Dr Vasant Vaniya Former Professor, Medical College and SSG Hospital, Vadodra, Gujrat
- Dr Venkateshwar Reddy Professor and Head, SVS Medical College, Mehboobnagar, Telangana
- Dr Vijay Anand S Nagdeve Professor and Head, RIIMS, Raipur, CG

- Dr Vijayamma KN Professor, Believers Medical College, Kottayam, Former Professor and Head, Kottayam Medical College, Kerala
- Dr Vijisha Phalgunan Professor and Head, Sri Lakshmi Narayana Institute of Medical Sciences, Pondicherry
- Dr Vinay Kumar Professor and Head, Sheikh-Ul-Hind-Maulana Mehmood Govt Medical College, Saharanpur, UP
- Dr Vineet Gohiya Professor and Head, Government Medical College, Khandwa, MP
- Dr Vinodini Professor and Head, Gandhi Medical College, Secunderabad, Telangana
- Dr Vinoth S Professor and Head, Madha Medical College, Chennai, TN
- Dr Vishnu Gupta Professor and Head, Muzaffarnagar Medical College, Muzaffarnagar, UP
- Dr VK Chimurkar Professor and Head, Jawaharlal Nehru Medical College, Wardha, MS
- Dr VP Rukhmode Professor and Head, Government Medical College, Gondia, MS
- Dr X Chandra Philip Professor, Mahatma Gandhi Medical College and Research Institute, Puducherry
- Dr Zeenat Akhtar Professor and Head, Acharya Shri Chander College of Medical Sciences, Jammu, J&K
- Dr Zuberi Hussain Riyaz Professor and Head, JIIU's Indian Institute of Medical Science and Research, Badnapur, Jalna, MS
- Rt. Brig (Dr) Sushil Kumar Professor and Head, Amrita School of Medicine, Faridabad, Haryana
- Dr Amit Kumar Associate Professor, Chhattisgarh Institute of Medical Sciences, Bilaspur, CG
- Dr Amol Durgkar Associate Professor, Chindwana Institute of Medical Sciences, Chindwada, MP
- Dr Amol Shinde Associate Professor, Dr DY Patil Medical College, Hospital and Research Center, Pune, MS
- Dr Amrutha Roopa Ramagalla Associate Professor, Government Medical College, Siddipet, Telangana
- Dr Anil Agrawal Associate Professor, Triveni Institute of Dental Science, Bilaspur, CG
- Dr Anil Kumar Dwivedi Associate Professor, VCSG Govt Medical College, Srinagar, Uttarakhand
- Dr Anwar Unisa Sabry Associate Professor, Government Medical College, Siricilla, Telangana
- Dr Aparna Muraleedharan Associate Professor, Pondicherry Institute of Medical Sciences, Puducherry
- Dr Archana Kalyankar Associate Professor, Government Medical College and Hospital, Aurangabad, MS
- Dr Archana Kannamwar Associate Professor, Shri Vasant Rao Naik Government Medical College, Yavatmal, MS
- Dr Ashok Kumar Singh Associate Professor, Bhagwan Mahaveer Institute of Medical Sciences, Pawapuri, Nalanda, Bihar
- Dr Ashwani K Sharma Associate Professor, Government Medical College, Jammu, J&K
- Dr Badal Singh Associate Professor, Motilal Nehru Medical College, Prayagraj, UP
- Dr Banani Kundu Associate Professor, Sarat Chandra Chattopadhyay Govt. Medical College & Hospital, Uluberia, WB
- Dr Bhavik Doshi Associate Professor, GMERS Mediacl College, Sola, Ahmadabad, Gujrat
- Dr Binod Kumar Former Associate Professor and Head, Shri Krishna Medical College, Muzzafarpur, Bihar
- Dr Charulata A Satpute Associate Professor, Indira Gandhi Medical College, Nagpur, MS
- Dr Dibyendu Dutta Associate Professor, College of Medicine and Sagore Dutta Hospital Kolkata, WB
- Dr Dipti Gautam Associate Professor, GMC, Mahasamund, CG
- Dr G Sundar Associate Professor Government Vellore Medical College, Vellore, TN
- Dr I Gowri Associate Professor, Dr Patnam Mahender Reddy Institute of Medical Sciences, Chevella, Telangana
- Dr J Sreevidya Associate Professor, Stanley Medical College, Chennai, TN
- Dr Jaita Chowdhury Associate Professor, Icare Institute of Medical Science and BC Roy Hospital Haldia, WB
- Dr Jolly Agarwal Associate Professor, Government Medical College, Dehradun, Uttarakhand
- Dr K Shanmuganathan Associate Professor, Indira Gandhi Medical College and Research Institute, Puducherry
- Dr K Manivanan Associate Professor, PES Medical College, Kuppam, AP
- Dr Kanan Shah Associate Professor, NHL Medical College, Ahmadabad, Gujrat
- Dr Kiran V Padeyappanavar Associate Professor, Belagavi Institute of Medical Sciences, Belagavi, Karnataka
- Dr Kirti Nemade Associate Professor, Government Medical College, Nagpur, MS
- Dr KKP Singh Associate Professor, Rajendra Institute of Medical Sciences, Ranchi, Jharkhand
- Dr Kunal Chawla Associate Professor, Indira Gandhi Medical College, Shimla, HP
- Dr Lency Davis Associate Professor, Government Medical College, Thrissur, Kerala
- Dr Mangesh Selukar Associate Professor, Deputy Dean, Vilasrao Deshmukh Government Institute of Medial Sciences, Latur, MS
- Dr Manjusha Tabhane Associate Professor, NKP Salve Institute of Medical Sciences and Research Centre and Lata Mangeshkar Hospital, Nagpur, MS
- Dr Manjusha Tabhane, Associate Professor, NKP Salve Medical College, Nagpur, MS
- Dr Meenakshi Borkar Associate Professor, Hindu Hruday Samrat Balasaheb Thackarey Medical College and Dr Rustom Narsi Cooper Municipal General Hospital, Mumbai, MS
- Dr Meetu Agarwal Associate Professor, Amrita School of Medicine, Faridabad, Haryana
- Dr Mohammad Mujahid Ansari Associate Professor, Government Medical College, Shahdol, MP
- Dr MS Arathi Associate Professor, Chettinad Hospital and Research Institute, Chennai, TN
- Dr Mukesh Mittal Associate Professor, Government Medical College, Shivpuri, MP
- Dr Nagraj S Associate Professor, SVS Medical College, Mahabubnagar, Telangana
- Dr Naina Wakode Associate Professor, ABV Medical College, Vidisha, MP
- Dr Nirmal Kumar K Associate Professor Mahavir Institute of Medical Science, Vikarabad, Telangana
- Dr Nirmalya Saha Associate Professor In-charge, Tripura Medical College, Agartala, Tripura
- Dr Nita Gathe Associate Professor, Government Medical College, Gondia, MS
- Dr P David Anand Kumar Associate Professor Government Medical College Wanaparthy, Telangana
- Dr Phalguni Srimani Associate Professor, Calcutta National Medical College and Hospital, Kolkata, WB
- Dr PN Panshewdikar Associate Professor, Vedanta institute of Medical Sciences, Palghar, MS
- Dr Pradeep Bokariya Associate Professor, Mahatma Gandhi Institute of Medical Sciences, Sevagram, MS
- Dr Pranab Deb Barma, Associate Professor and In-charge Head, Agartala Govt Medical College and Hospital, Tripura
- Dr Priya P Roy Associate Professor, Krishna Institute of Medical Sciences, Karad, MS
- Dr R Azhagiri Associate Professor, ESIC Medical College and PGIMSR, Chennai, TN
- Dr Rajashree S Raut Associate Professor, RCSM Government Medical College, Kolhapur, MS
- Dr Rajesh Dehankar Associate Professor, NKP Salve Medical College, Nagpur, MS
- Dr Rani Raphael M Associate Professor, Government TD Medical College, Alappuzha, Kerala
- Dr Rupali Kavitake Associate Professor, Government Medical College, Alibagh, MS
- Dr Ruta Bapat Associate Professor, Dr DY Patil Medical College, Hospital and Research Centre, Navi Mumbai, MS
- Dr S Archana Associate Professor, Government Chengalpattu Medical College, Chengalpattu, TN
- Dr S Satish Kumar Associate Professor, Government Dharmapuri Medical College, Dharmapuri, TN
- Dr Sajey PS Associate Professor, Government T D Medical College, Alappuzha, Kerala
- Dr Sandeep S Mohite Associate Professor, Krishna Institute of Medical Sciences, Karad, MS
- Dr Santoshkumar A Dope Associate Professor, Medical Superintendent, Vilasrao Deshmukh Government Institute of Medial Sciences, Latur, MS
- Dr Sashi Bhushan Associate Professor, PES Medical College, Kuppam, AP
- Dr Saurabh Kulkarni Associate Professor, Government Medical College, Aurangabad, MS
- Dr Sayantan Das Associate Professor, Mata Gujri Memorial Medical College, Kishanganj, Bihar
- Dr Shalini Kumar Associate Professor, Hamdard Institute of Medical Sciences and Research, Hamdard University, New Delhi
- Dr Shanthini S Associate Professor, Pondicherry Institute of Medical Sciences, Puducherry
- Dr Shilpa Sonare Associate Professor, Government Medical College, Nagpur, MS
- Dr Shrikant Verma Associate Professor, Raipur Institute of Medical Sciences, Raipur, CG
- Dr Shruti Mamidwar Associate Professor, Government Medical College, Chandrapur, MS
- Dr Sreevidya J Associate Professor, Institute of Anatomy, MMC, Chennai, TN
- Dr Subhash Gujar Associate Professor, GMERS Medical College, Vadnagar, Gujrat
- Dr Subhasis Chakraborty Associate Professor and Head, College of Medicine and Sagore Dutta Hospital, Kolkata, WB
- Dr Subodh Kumar Associate Professor and Head, Nalanda Medical College, Patna, Bihar
- Dr Sumedha Anjankar Associate Professor, Datta Meghe Medical College, Nagpur, MS
- Dr Sunita Bharti Associate Professor, Dr DY Patil Medical College, Hospital and Research Centre, Navi Mumbai, MS
- Dr Surekha W Meshram Associate Professor, Government Medical College, Gondia, MS
- Dr Sushil Jiwane Associate Professor, Gandhi Medical College, Bhopal, MP
- Dr Tarkeshwar Golghate Associate Professor, Government Medical College, Nagpur, MS
- Dr V Dharani Associate Professor, Government Villupuram Medical College, Villupuram, TN
- Dr Vandana Tiwari Associate Professor, Dr. Sushila Tiwari Govt Medical College, Haldwani, Uttarakhand
- Dr Varsha Dahiphale Associate Professor, Swami Ramanand Tirth Rural Government Medical College, Ambajogai, MS
- Dr Vishal Bhadkaria Associate Professor, Bundelkhand Medical College, Sagar, MP
- Dr Yogesh Diwan Associate Professor, Indira Gandhi Medical College, Shimla, HP
- Dr Abhinav Kumar Mishra Assistant Professor, Hind Institute of Medical Sciences, Sitapur, UP
- Dr Abid Ali Assistant Professor, Bhaskar Medical College, Yenkapally, Telangana
- Dr Ajay Rathva Assistant Professor, GMERS Medical College, Vadodara, Gujrat
- Dr Alok Saxena Assistant Professor, Gautam Budha Chikitsa Mahavidhyalaya Medical College, Dehradun, Uttarakhand

Acknowledgements

- Dr Amarappa S Nagalikar Assistant Professor, Belagavi Institute of Medical Sciences, Belagavi, Karnataka
- Dr Amrita Kumari Assistant Professor, Patna Medical College, Patna, Bihar
- Dr Anjali Prasad Assistant Professor, Shri Krishna Medical College, Muzzafarpur, Bihar
- Dr Aparna Dixit Assistant Professor, Saraswati Medial College, Unnao, UP
- Dr BS Patil Assistant Professor, Shri BM Patil Medical College, Hospital and Research Centre BLDE (Deemed to be University), Vijayapura, Karnataka
- Dr Chandan Kumar Yadav Assistant Professor, Chandra Dental College and Hospital, Lucknow, UP
- Dr Chetan Sahni Assistant Professor, IMS-BHU, Varanasi, UP
- Dr Deepanshu Shukla Assistant Professor, Career Institute of Medical Sciences and Hospital, Lucknow, UP
- Dr Dipti Nimje Assistant Professor, Government Medical College, Nagpur, MS
- Dr Faizal Mohammad Former Assistant Professor, Government Medical College, Siddipet, Telangana
- Dr Gajanan L Maske Assistant Professor, Shri Vasant Rao Naik Government Medical College, Yavatmal, MS
- Dr Gouri Shankar Jha Assistant Professor, Darbhanga Medical College and Hospital, Laheriasarai, Darbhanga, Bihar
- Dr Gyanraj Singh Assistant Professor, Kalinga Institute of Medical Sciences, Bhubaneswar, Odisha
- Dr Harsh Chawre Assistant Professor, Government Medical College, Datia, MP
- Dr Harsh Mishrikoti P Assistant Professor, Belagavi Institute of Medical Sciences, Belagavi, Karnataka
- Dr Hemlata Ambade Assistant Professor, Government Medical College, Nagpur, MS
- Dr Indushri Assistant Professor, Government Medical College, Kannauj, UP
- Dr Israr Ahmed Khan Assistant Professor, Government Medical College, Shahdol, MP
- Dr Jayasree Reddy Assistant Professor, Surabhi Institute of Medical Sciences, Siddipet, Telangana
- Dr Kiran Kalloor Assistant Professor, Karuna Medical College, Palakkad, Kerala
- Dr Lenin S Assistant Professor, Kanyakumari Government Medial College, Kanyakumari, TN
- Dr M Siva Kumar Assistant Professor, Government Thiruvannamalai Medical College, Thiruvannamalai, TN
- Dr Mamta Kumari Assistant Professor, Bhagwan Mahaveer Institute of Medical Sciences, Pawapuri, Nalanda, Bihar
- Dr Mangesh Lone Assistant Professor, LTMMC and Sion Hospital, Mumbai, MS
- Dr Md Jawed Akhtar Associate Professor, Indira Gandhi Institute of Medical Sciences, Patna, Bihar
- Dr MM Peerzade Assistant Professor, Dr VM Government Medical College, Solapur, MS
- Dr Mohd Ajmal Assistant Professor, Madhav Prasad Tripathi Medical College, Siddharthnagar, UP
- Dr Mohd Ajmal Assistant Professor, Madhav Prasad Tripathi Medical College, Siddharthnagar, UP
- Dr MP Sultana Assistant Professor, Siddhartha Medical College, Nellore, AP
- Dr Mubeen Rashid Assistant Professor, In-charge, Head of the Department, Government Medical College, Kathua, J&K
- Dr Nishigandha Sadamate Assistant Professor, Dr Kiran C Patel Medical College and Research Institute, Bharuch, Vadodara, Gujrat
- Dr Niyati Airen Assistant Professor, VCSG Govt Medical College, Srinagar, Uttarakhand
- Dr P Ashok Assistant Professor, Deccan College of Medical Sciences, Hyderabad, Telangana
- Dr Payal Kasat Assistant Professor, Dr BC Roy Institute of Medical Sciences & Research, Kharagpur, WB
- Dr Piyush Kumar Assistant Professor, SGRR Medical College, Dehradun, Uttarakhand
- Dr Prashant Munjamkar Former Assistant Professor, All India Institute of Medical Sciences, Bibi Nagar, Hyderabad
- Dr Pratibha Shakya Assistant Professor, KGMU, Lucknow, UP
- Dr Praveen Kurrey Assistant Professor, Pt. Jawahrlal Nehru Memorial Medical College, Raipur, CG
- Dr Priti Nemade Assistant Professor, Indira Gandhi Medical College and Hospital, Nagpur, MS
- Dr Rajeev Panwar Assistant Professor, SIC Medical College and PGIMSR, KK Nagar, Chennai, TN
- Dr Rakesh Shukla Assistant Professor, Maa Vindhyawasini Autonomous State Medical College, Mirzapur, UP
- Dr Rashmi S Sinha Assistant Professor, Grant Medical College and Hospital, Mumbai, MS
- Dr Rimpi Gupta Assistant Professor, Kalpana Chawla Government Medical College, Karnal, Haryana
- Dr Ritika Gaddewar Assistant Professor, Indira Gandhi Medical College and Hospital, Nagpur, MS
- Dr Ritu Slathia Assistant Professor and I/c HOD, Government Medical College, Rajouri, J&K
- Dr Roli Joshi Assistant Professor, Saraswati Medical College, Unnao, UP
- Dr S Diwya Lakshmi Assistant Professor, Government Medical College, Virudhunagar, TN
- Dr Sabin Malik Assistant Professor, Sree Narayana Institute of Medical Sciences, Ernakulam, Kerala
- Dr Sagun Shukla Assistant professor, Varun Medical College, Shahjanpur, UP
- Dr Saikat Roy Assistant Professor, College of Medicine and JNM Hospital, Kalyani, Nadia, WB
- Dr Samta Gaur Assistant Professor, Government Medical College, Pali, Rajasthan
- Dr Saleena N Ali Assistant Professor, Government Medical College, Alappuzha, Kerala
- Dr Shailendra Singh Assistant Professor, Rani Durgavati Medical College, Banda, UP
- Dr Shibanee Jena Assistant Professor, Shri Jagannath Medical College and Hospital, Puri, Odisha
- Dr Shubhpreet Sodhi Assistant Professor, Dr YS Parmar Govt Medical College, Nahan, HP
- Dr Sindhu Chaudhary Assistant Professor, Soban Singh Jeena Govt Medical College, Almora, Uttarakhand
- Dr Sonali Thomas Assistant Professor, Dr. Sushila Tiwari Govt Medical College, Haldwani, Uttarakhand
- Dr Suchit Kumar Assistant Professor, Gautam Budha Chikitsa Mahavidhyalaya Medical College, Dehradun, Uttarakhand
- Dr Sudha Rani Assistant Professor and Head, Hazaribagh Medical College, Hazaribagh, Jharkhand
- Dr Sujithaa N Assistant Professor, Government Medical College, Villupurum, TN
- Dr Sumita Agrawal Assistant Professor, Government Doon Medical College, Dehradun, Uttarakhand
- Dr Sumita Shukla Assistant Professor, Rajarshi Dashrath Autonomous Government Medical College, Ayodhya, UP
- Dr Swati Saxena Assistant Professor, Government Doon Medical College, Dehradun, Uttarakhand
- Dr Taqiuddin Mohammed Assistant Professor, Apollo Institute of Medical Sciences and Research, Hyderabad, Telangana
- Dr Tom J Nallikuzhy Assistant Professor, Government Medical College, Idukki, Kerala
- Dr Upendra M Assistant Professor, Mahavir Institute of Medical Sciences, Vikarabad, Telangana
- Dr Yogendra Singh Assistant Professor, Baba Raghav Das Medical College, Gorakhpur, UP
- Dr Yogesh Shridhar Ganorkar Assistant Professor, BJ Medical College and Sassoon Hospital, Pune, MS
- Dr Zeba Alam Assistant Professor, Nalanda Medical College, Patna, Bihar
- Dr Nimisha Madhu Tutor Anugrah Narayan Magadh Medical College, Gaya, Bihar
- Dr Pankaj Soni Tutor, Shri Lal Bahadur Shastri Government Medical College, Mandi, HP
- Dr Rajesh Maurya Tutor, Government Doon Medical College, Dehradun, Uttarakhand
- Dr Thuslima M Tutor, Government Medical College, Omandurar Medical College, Chennai, TN
- Pulkit Jain Christian Medical College, Ludhiana, Punjab

I am thankful to the following students for their support and suggestions: Bankura: Gouranga Rajak, Soujonnyo Chakraborty; Berhampore: Safin Ali; Bolpur: SK Rintu; Burdwan: Projjal Saha; Coochbehar: Glory Mochari; Joka: Shobhit Kumar Majhi; Kolkata: Aktarul Islam, Argadeep Dey, Debmallo Ghosh, Md Ali Mallick, Prabhat Patawari, Sayantan Mallick, Shirol Islam, Subhodip Ghosh, Supriyo Rana; Malda: Md Tahahait, Subhajit Sen; Midnapore: Prajjal Agarwal, Sayed Anowar, Tathagata Das, Tousif Ali; Raiganj: Papan Ghosh, Samir Das; Siliguri: Krishnendu Das; Patna: Swapnil Shyambuj, Raushan Kumar; Dhanbad: Akshay Shankar, Dr Raghunandan Ramanathan (Chennai).

Yogesh Sontakke

eSmartQuiz – Online MCQ Test
Are you ready for the "*eSmartQuiz* – Online MCQ test"?

After attending the class, students should go through the "*eSmartQuiz* – Online MCQ test" for the following reasons:

- *Reinforcement of Learning*: The "*eSmartQuiz* – Online MCQ test" provide an opportunity to reinforce learning after attending a class or reading a book. It helps to assess understanding and retention of concepts, to solidify knowledge and identify areas that need further revision or clarification.
- *Assessment of Comprehension*: The "*eSmartQuiz* – Online MCQ test" is an effective tool to assess comprehension of the subject matter and to demonstrate the ability to apply the concepts learned in the class.
- *Enhancement of attention and critical thinking*: The "*eSmartQuiz* – Online MCQ test" will help to make students attentive for the class and to enhance critical thinking skills by selecting the most appropriate answer among the given options.

Each *eSmartQuiz* test consists of 10 MCQs, mostly image-based, and the student can see their scores at the end of each test. These questions will be modified after a certain interval. Use the given links or scan the QR code (given in corresponding chapters) for the test. One student can solve each test only one time.

Chapter	Google from link
1. Introduction	https://forms.gle/QBTgnJKmNNkNPrpXA
2. Menstrual Cycle	https://forms.gle/6rJ5gMAzMAbcbySn8
3. Gametogenesis	https://forms.gle/3rWPwYunN8iBD5VK8
4. First Week of Development	https://forms.gle/ShUGM3f9A9jYMS6a6
5. Assisted Reproduction Technology	https://forms.gle/ZELjPxTKv2aQp4oX6
6. Second Week of Development: Bilaminar Germ Disc	https://forms.gle/TBcy62oTQjfPawAz6
7. Third Week of Development: Trilaminar Germ Disc	https://forms.gle/1wNzKxr4nWFCLHJp7
8. Further Development of Embryo	https://forms.gle/cAQSkX7eHVCEtYcX7
9. Placenta and Umbilical Cord	https://forms.gle/pF96exEiu4g9ioyE9
10. Integumentary System: Skin, its Appendages, and Mammary Gland	https://forms.gle/kT113Vj9qAS7fzwJ7
11. Pharyngeal Apparatus	https://forms.gle/Sr7Tu3ukW6yfDDP49
12. Alimentary Tract I: Development of Face, Nose and Palate	https://forms.gle/u2WWRz5YnZHhZiYm9
13. Alimentary Tract II: Development of Teeth, Pharynx, Tongue and Salivary Glands	https://forms.gle/tS3SjZf51wG9bgfx8
14. Alimentary Tract III: Development of Intestine	https://forms.gle/qZonZerNdBrmbLD88
15. Alimentary Tract IV: Development of Liver, Gallbladder, Pancreas and Spleen	https://forms.gle/mhzVGSx2QvZAWs1g9
16. Respiratory System	https://forms.gle/WKxaqNdvyBXhcxkQ7
17. Development of Body Cavities and Diaphragm	https://forms.gle/kNG7M4h9gUpydKpj7
18. Cardiovascular System I: Development of Heart	https://forms.gle/VzRX73BNY3w4DDPa9
19. Cardiovascular System II: Blood Vessels and Fetal Circulation	https://forms.gle/hfz3M6QXDFB4n8yJ6
20. Urinary System: Kidney, Ureter, Urinary Bladder, Urethra	https://forms.gle/ob1t5KASRgZv4DaFA
21. Reproductive System: Male and Female Reproductive Organs	https://forms.gle/egW3L7eowxV4AmMi9
22. Nervous System	https://forms.gle/Rkifk1HsD2t1Nk3C6
23. Development of Eye	https://forms.gle/9eMHc5E1MUNkryhA8
24. Development of Ear	https://forms.gle/XUd4mAj8Auvrzp3M6
25. Endocrine System	https://forms.gle/uxhq96AHHZKo2VD37
26 to 30. Miscellaneous	https://forms.gle/gued6ZHG2aBifsgE8

Contents

Preface to the Second Edition — *v*
Preface to the First Edition — *vii*

1. **Introduction** — 1
   Reviewer: Dr Prashant Chaware   *Competencies*: AN76.1, AN76.2

2. **Menstrual Cycle** — 7
   Reviewer: Dr Deepti Shastri   *Competencies*: AN77.1, AN77.2

3. **Gametogenesis** — 15
   Reviewer: Dr C Kishan Reddy, Dr Priya S Patil   *Competency*: AN77.3

4. **First Week of Development** — 25
   Reviewer: Jaideo Manohar Ughade   *Competencies*: AN77.4, AN78.1, AN78.3

5. **Assisted Reproduction Technology** — 35
   In vitro Fertilization and Intracytoplasmic Sperm Injection
   Reviewer: Dr Keshav Malhotra

6. **Second Week of Development: Bilaminar Germ Disc** — 40
   Reviewer: Dr Harsha Pratap   *Competencies*: AN78.2, AN78.4

7. **Third Week of Development: Trilaminar Germ Disc** — 48
   Reviewer: Dr Aparna Muralidharan   *Competencies*: AN79.1, AN79.2, AN79.3

8. **Further Development of Embryo** — 60
   Reviewer: Dr Rohini Motwani   *Competencies*: AN79.4, AN52.4

9. **Placenta and Umbilical Cord** — 73
   Reviewer: Dr Saleena N Ali   *Competencies*: AN80.1, AN80.2, AN80.3, AN80.5, AN80.7, AN78.5

10. **Integumentary System: Skin, its Appendages, and Mammary Gland** — 87
    Reviewer: Dr Rupa Chaparrwal   *Competencies*: AN9.3, AN72.1

11. **Pharyngeal Apparatus** — 96
    Reviewer: Dr Ravi Kant, Dr Ujwala Bhanarkar   *Competency*: AN43.4

12. **Alimentary Tract I: Development of Face, Nose and Palate** — 109
    Reviewer: Dr Gayatri Muthiyan   *Competency*: AN43.4

13. **Alimentary Tract II: Development of Teeth, Pharynx, Tongue and Salivary Glands** — 117
    Reviewer: Dr R Sarah   *Competencies*: AN43.4, AN39.1

14. **Alimentary Tract III: Development of Intestine** — 126
    Reviewer: Dr Nagaraj S   *Competency*: AN52.6

15. **Alimentary Tract IV: Development of Liver, Gallbladder, Pancreas and Spleen** — 141
    Reviewer: Dr Payal Kasat   *Competency*: AN52.6

16. **Respiratory System** — 149
    Reviewer: Dr Hitant Vohra   *Competencies*: AN25.2, AN25.4

17.	**Development of Body Cavities and Diaphragm**	158
	Reviewer: Dr Thuslima M *Competencies*: AN25.2, AN52.5	
18.	**Cardiovascular System I: Development of Heart**	168
	Reviewer: Dr Haritha Nimmagadda *Competencies*: AN25.2, AN25.4	
19.	**Cardiovascular System II: Blood Vessels and Fetal Circulation**	185
	Reviewer: Dr V Dharani *Competencies*: AN25.3, AN25.5, AN25.6	
20.	**Urinary System: Kidney, Ureter, Urinary Bladder, Urethra**	205
	Reviewer: Dr Bertha AD Rathinam, Dr Ujwala Bhanarkar *Competency*: AN52.7	
21.	**Reproductive System: Male and Female Reproductive Organs**	218
	Reviewer: Dr Prajakta Kishve *Competency*: AN52.8	
22.	**Nervous System**	235
	Reviewer: Dr Betty Anna Jose *Competencies*: AN63.2, AN64.2, AN64.3, AN79.3, AN79.5, AN79.6	
23.	**Development of Eye**	259
	Reviewer: Dr Rohit Rao *Competency*: AN43.4	
24.	**Development of Ear**	268
	Reviewer: Dr Nidhi Puri	
25.	**Endocrine System**	275
	Reviewer: Dr Anjali Sabnis *Competency*: AN43.4	
26.	**Skeletal System**	281
	Reviewer: Dr Joti Gaikwad *Competencies*: AN79.4, AN79.5	
27.	**Muscular System**	291
	Reviewer: Dr Anjali Jain	
28.	**Fetal Period: Nine Weeks to Birth**	295
	Reviewer: Dr Sabin Malik	
29.	**Clinical Applications and Ultrasonography in Embryology**	298
	Reviewer: Dr Gunvant Chaudhari	
30.	**Twinning (Multiple Pregnancy)**	303
	Reviewer: Dr Ujwala Bhanarkar *Competency*: AN80.4	

Annexures 309

Reviewer: Dr Jahira Banu T   *Competencies*: AN13.8, AN20.10, AN76.2, AN77.5, AN77.6, AN78.5

   I. Embryonic Remnants
  II. Placenta Previa
 III. Hermaphrodite
 IV. Derivatives of Neural Crest Cells
  V. Miscellaneous: Fetal viability, contraception, teratogenesis, fertility, infertility, sterility, surrogate motherhood, sex ratio, abortion, pregnancy test, development of limbs, development of joints

Index 321

Chapter 1

Introduction

eSmartQuiz

Chapter Outline

- Basic terminology
- Stages of human life
- Trimesters of pregnancy
- Need of embryology
- Descriptive terms in embryology
- Chromosomes
- Cell division
  - Mitosis
  - Meiosis
- Nondisjunction
- Organizer and induction

Competencies:

- AN76.1: Describe the stages of human life.
- AN76.2: Explain the terms – phylogeny, ontogeny, trimester, viability.

BASIC TERMINOLOGY

Embryology
- Embryology is a branch of science that deals with the study of formation and development of an organism before birth (*embryon* = Embryo in Greek).

Reproduction
- Sexual reproduction involves fusion of male and female gametes to produce an offspring.
- It helps in maintenance of species.

Reproductive biology
Reproductive biology is the study of reproduction including study of reproductive systems, endocrinology, sexual development and fertility.

Developmental anatomy
It is the study of structural changes that occur in the body throughout the lifespan (from fertilization to maturity).

Ontogeny
- Ontogeny is a branch of science that deals with complete life cycle (prenatal and postnatal growth and development) of an organism.

Phylogeny
- Phylogeny deals with an evolutionary history and relationship among organisms.
- Phylogenetically, organisms are classified as fishes, amphibians, reptiles, birds, and mammals.
- Mammals are classified as protheria (lay eggs), metatheria (produce extremely young offspring that mature in pouch of mother, marsupials), and eutheria (deliver mature young ones, receive nutrition through placenta till birth).
- Humans are *eutherian* or *placental mammals*.
- During human development, it is found that ontogeny recapitulates phylogeny (Ernst Haeckel, 1866).
- It can be explained by the developing human kidney: Pronephric kidney → mesonephric kidney → metanephric kidney.

Development
- Development of a human from a single-cell stage of life involves growth and differentiation.
- *Development* is a broad term that involves transformation of a simple single cell into a complex multicellular organism.
- *Growth* is a mere increase in the number and size of cells.
- Growth is of three types:
  1. *Multiplicative growth*: It is an increase in cell number by cell division.
  2. *Auxetic growth*: It is an increase in cell size.

3. *Accretionary growth*: It is growth by reserve cells in postembryonic life.
4. *Appositional growth*: Formation of new layers on previously formed one.
- **Differentiation** is a process of cell transformation to acquire specific character and function.
- Zygote divides to form many undifferentiated cells as follows:
  1. *Totipotent cells*: Cells of zygote or morula can form all differentiated cell types of an organism. These are called totipotent cells.
  2. *Pluripotent cells:* For example, inner cell mass of blastocyst can form all types of differentiated cells of an organism except placenta.
  3. *Multipotent cells*: For example, adult stem cells can form more than one cell type.
- Differentiation may involve:
  1. Chemo-differentiation
  2. Histo-differentiation
  3. Organogenesis
  4. Functional differentiation
- **Gametogenesis** is a process of formation of gametes (ovum and sperms) from germ cells.

STAGES OF HUMAN LIFE

- Humans undergo continuous physical changes throughout the life. These progressive, orderly, and predictable changes in human begin at conception and continue till death.
- These changes are influenced by genetic, nutritional, environmental, socioeconomic, and many other factors.
- Developmentally, human life is divided into the following stages or periods (Flowchart 1.1):

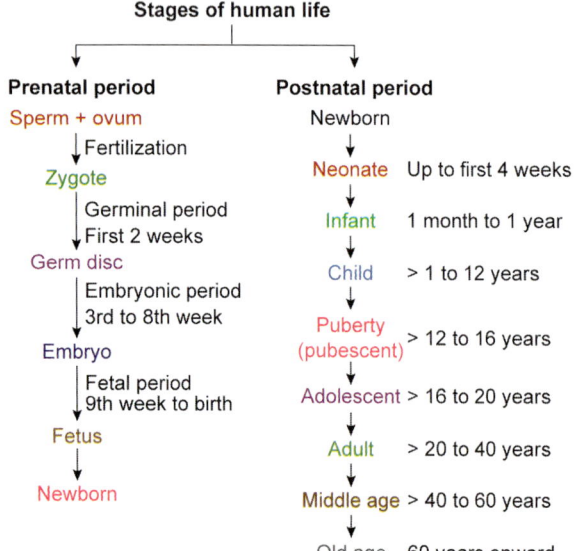

Flowchart 1.1: Stages of human life

1. *Prenatal period:* Most of the clinicians divide human prenatal period into 3 trimesters: First trimester, second trimester, and third trimester. Each trimester consists of a period of 3 months. Embryologically, prenatal period is divided into the following (Fig. 1.1):
   A. *Germinal/ovular period:* First 2 weeks of development after fertilization.
   B. *Embryonic period:* From third to eighth week of development.
   C. *Fetal period:* From third month till the termination of pregnancy.

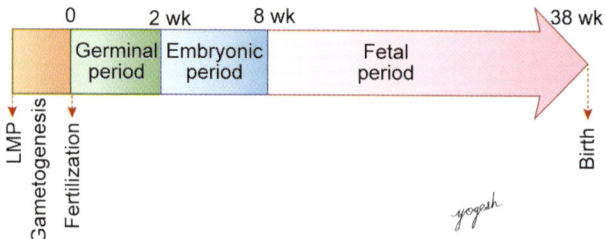

Fig. 1.1: Periods of human embryology. Abbreviations: wk: Week; LMP: Last menstrual period

Period of egg: It extends for 1 week from fertilization to implantation into uterine wall.

Conceptus (product of conception) is also called preimplantation conceptus. In *in vitro* fertilization, *preimplantation conceptus* needs to be transferred to uterus for further growth.

Further, on implantation, conceptus is called *postimplantation conceptus*.

2. *Postnatal period:* It is divided into the following phases:
   A. *Neonatal period:* First 28 days after birth.
   B. *Infancy:* From 1 month till 1 year of age.
   C. *Childhood:* From 1 to 12 years of age.
   D. *Puberty:* After childhood till 16 years of age.
   E. *Adolescence:* After puberty till 20 years of age.
   F. *Adulthood:* From 20 years till 40 years of age.
   G. *Middle age:* From 40 years till 60 years of age.
   H. *Old age:* From 60 years of age till death.
   I. Death.
   The abovementioned periods are overlapping.

Different ages of fetal (embryonic) period:
Gestational or menstrual age
- Gestation age is measured from the beginning of woman's last menstrual period (LMP).
- Gestation age is mostly used by clinician for assessing pregnancy and fetal wellbeing, for calculation of expected date of delivery, and for taking all decisions (amniocentesis, chorionic villus sampling, termination of pregnancy, and so on).

Fertilization or conceptional age
- Fertilization or conceptional age is measured from the time of fertilization.
- Fertilization age is 2 weeks lesser than the gestational age.

Somite age
- Somite age is a triangular mesenchymal mass in the developing embryo.
- In human, 42 to 44 pairs of somites are present.
- First somite appears on 20th day after fertilization. Everyday its number approximately increases by 3 somites. Thus, somites are useful for determination of fetal age from day 20 to 30. (For details, refer Table 8.1).
- Embryologists use somite age to describe the development events.

TRIMESTERS OF PREGNANCY

- Pregnancy lasts for about 40 weeks, beginning from the first day of the last menstrual cycle (ranges from 37 to 42 weeks).
- Clinically, duration of the pregnancy is divided into 3 trimesters as follows:

First Trimester
- It extends from the first day of the last menstrual cycle to 13 weeks.
- It is the most *crucial period* for organ development.
- Most of the miscarriages occur in the first trimester.
- Mothers may have pregnancy symptoms during the first trimester. It includes nausea, vomiting, and so on.
- In the first trimester, exposure to teratogenic agents, smoking, and alcohol may produce fetal anomalies.
- Ultrasound examination is useful for confirmation of pregnancy, presence, size, location, and number of gestational sacs.

Second Trimester
- It extends from 14th to 26th week of gestation.
- Mothers may have varicose veins, backaches, leg cramps, and so on.
- By the 20th week, mothers may feel fetal movements.
- Ultrasound examination by 18th to 22nd week is usually performed for evaluation of fetal wellbeing, volume of amniotic fluid, cardiac activity, placental position, and fetal morphometry.

Third Trimester
- It extends from the 27th week to termination of pregnancy (37–42 weeks).

Expected Date of Delivery (EDD)
- A normal, full-term pregnancy lasts from 37 to 42 weeks.
- Expected date of delivery can be determined by counting 280 days after the first day of last menstrual period (LMP) or 266 days after conception. *Viva*
- *Naegele's formula* [Franz Karl Naegele, German obstetrician, 1801–1851]
  EDD = First day of LMP + 9 months + 7 days = First day of LMP + 280 days

NEED OF EMBRYOLOGY

1. Usually 3–4% of live births children suffer from birth defects. Understanding of this malformation is essential before treatment.
2. All structures in the human body develop from a single cell. Studying embryology will help to understand the gross anatomy and histological structures of body.
3. Deviated growth and development may lead to many diseases. Genes controlling the development may have mutation that results into a disease.
4. In the field of reproductive medicine, embryology helps for better practice for wellbeing of mother and newborn.
5. Knowledge of embryology can be applied in infertility cases (*in vitro* fertilization, intrauterine insemination).
6. Knowledge of embryology is essential for prenatal diagnosis and fetal therapy (amniocentesis, chorionic villus sampling).

Some Interesting Facts
- Aristotle (384–322BC) is the founder of embryology, whereas Karl Ernst von Baer is the father of modern embryology.
- Louise Brown (1978) is the first born test-tube baby.
- Dolly, a female sheep (1996), is the first cloned mammal.
- Y chromosome is acrocentric and smaller in size, whereas X chromosome is large, submetacentric. *NEXT*
- Methods of study of fetal anatomy:
  The following methods are useful to study the fetal anatomy:
  1. Ultrasound examination (USG) (For details, refer Chapter 29)
  2. Fetal magnetic resonance imaging (MRI)
  3. Fetal Doppler

DESCRIPTIVE TERMS IN EMBRYOLOGY

- Ventral: Towards the belly or anterior aspect
- Dorsal: Towards the back or posterior aspect
- Cranial or rostral: Towards the head
- Caudal: Towards the tail or coccyx
- Proximal: Close to the root of the structure or towards the trunk
- Distal: Away from the root of the structure or away from the trunk
- Invagination: Projection inside
- Evagination: Projection outside
- Differentiation: An increase in complexity and organization of cells and tissues during development

- Gamete: Sperm or ovum
- Genotype: Genetic makeup of an individual
- Mesenchyme: Loose cellular tissue that arises from mesoderm
- Phenotype: Observable characteristic of an individual
- Teratogen: Substance that may cause birth defect.

Box 1.1: Chromosomes

- Each human cell has 46 chromosomes except ovum (22 + X chromosomes) and sperms (22 + X or 22 + Y chromosomes).
- Out of 46 human chromosomes, 22 pairs are *autosomes* and one pair is *sex chromosomes* (X and Y chromosome).
- Sex chromosomes determine sex characteristics of an individual.
- *Structure* (Fig. 1.2)
  - Each chromosome consists of deoxyribonucleic acid (DNA) tightly coiled around histone proteins.
  - Each chromosome has sister chromatids connected at centromere.
  - Chromosome shows two arms: Short arm (p arm, p for *petit* means small) and long arm (q arm).
  - This typical structure of chromosome appears only during cell division.
  - In interphase, chromosomes form a thin thread-like structure called *chromatin*.

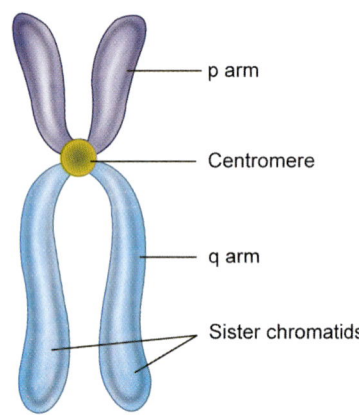

Fig. 1.2: Structure of chromosome

CELL DIVISION

- Cell division is a process of cell multiplication.
- It is of two types: Mitosis and meiosis.

Mitosis

- Mitosis is a cell division that maintains constant number of chromosomes in parent and offspring cells.
- Mitosis is always preceded by S phase where DNA duplicates.

Phases of Mitosis (Fig. 1.3, Flowchart 1.2)

1. *Prophase:* Events – chromosomes condense and become visible; spindle fibres emerge from centrosomes, nuclear envelope breaks down, and centrosome moves toward the opposite pole.
2. *Prometaphase:* Events – continued condensation of chromosomes, centromeres and sister chromatids becomes visible, attachment of microtubules to the centromere.
3. *Metaphase:* Events – chromosomes arranged at metaphase plate, attachment of each centromere to spindle fibres from the opposite pole.
4. *Anaphase:* Events – centromeres split in two, chromatids are pulled towards the opposite poles.
5. *Telophase:* Events – chromosomes arrive at the opposite poles; mitotic spindle breaks, nuclear membrane starts forming.
6. *Cytokinesis:* Event – cleavage furrow appears to separate daughter cells.
   - At the end of one mitotic cycle, two cells are formed from a single cell.

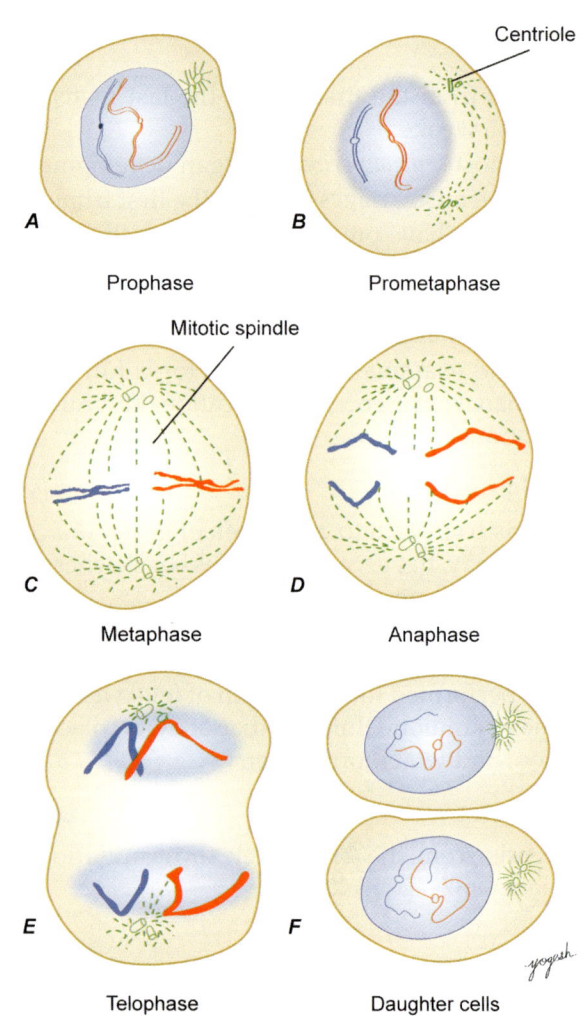

Fig. 1.3: Stages of mitosis

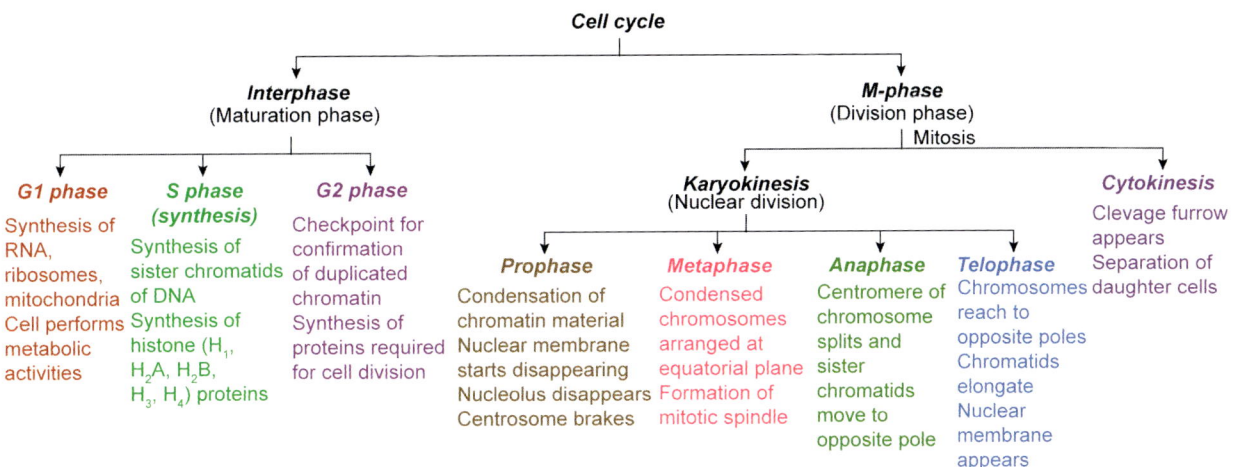

Flowchart 1.2: Cell cycle and mitosis

Significance of Mitosis

- It helps in development and growth of an organism.
- It helps in replacing the damaged body cells.
- It contributes to replace old body cells.
- It produces two daughter cells that are genetically identical to the parent cells.

Meiosis

- Meiosis is the cell division that helps in the formation of gametes with haploid number of chromosomes.
- Meiosis consists of two cell divisions as first meiotic and second meiotic divisions.
- The first meiotic division has prophase I, metaphase I, anaphase I and telophase I, whereas second meiotic division has prophase II, metaphase II, anaphase II and telophase II.

Prophase I

- It is a prolonged phase and consists of the following phases (Fig. 1.4): *NEXT*
  1. **Leptotene:** Events – chromosome becomes visible and condensed, sister chromatids of each chromosome are closely placed.
  2. **Zygotene:** Events – synapsis or conjugation (pairing of homologous chromosomes), paired chromosomes are called **bivalent** or **tetrad chromosomes**.*MCQ*
  3. **Pachytene:** Events – crossing over (there is an exchange of chromatin material in between approximated chromatids of homologous bivalent chromosomes). The point of contact of chromatids during crossing over is called **chiasmata**.*MCQ*
  4. **Diplotene:** Events – homologous chromosomes separate apart from each other.
- Diplotene phase is followed by metaphase I, anaphase I and telophase I. In anaphase I, there is no division of centromere.

Differences between Mitosis and Meiosis

Q. Write the differences between mitosis and meiosis.

Table 1.1	Differences between mitosis and meiosis	
Event	Mitosis	Meiosis
Occurrence	All cells of body	Only in germ cells
Process	It is an *equational* division	It is a reductional division
Prophase	No crossover of genetic material No synapsis	Crossover of genetic material takes place Synapsis occurs in zygotene phase
Metaphase	No chiasmata formation Chromosomes arrange at the equator	Chiasmata formation Homologous chromosome arranges on either side of equator
Anaphase	Centromere divides Chromatids move to the opposite pole	No division of centromere Whole chromosome moves to the opposite pole
Telophase	Daughter cells with the same number of chromosomes (46)	Daughter cells with a haploid number of chromosomes (23)
Number of daughter cells	Two	Four

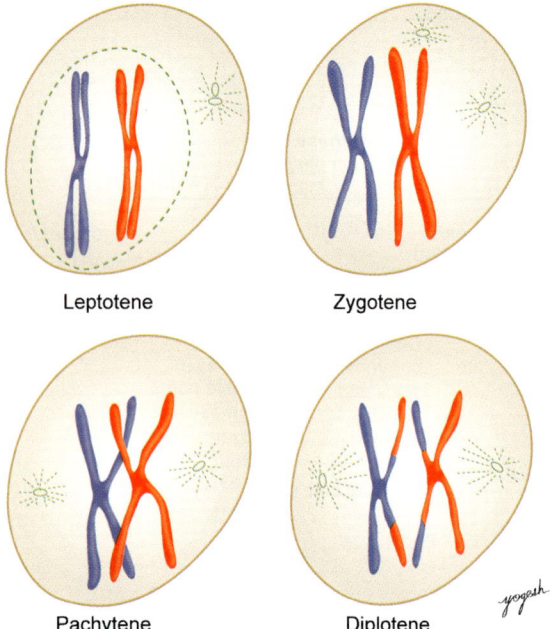

Fig. 1.4: Stages of prophase of first meiotic division

- Homologous chromosome moves towards opposite poles. Hence, resultant daughter cells receive only haploid number of chromosomes.
- The second meiotic division is equivalent of mitosis and just form two cells.
- Thus, at the end of meiosis, four daughter cells with haploid number of chromosomes are produced.

Significance of Meiosis

1. Formation of gametes is the prime aim of meiosis.
2. Meiosis helps to maintain constant chromosome number during sexual reproduction.
3. Exchange of maternal and paternal genes that are carried by homologous chromosomes takes place.
4. Meiosis (crossing over) helps to maintain genetic diversity and mixing of characters.

Box 1.2: Nondisjunction

Nondisjunction
- Usual separation of chromosomes in first meiotic division or sister chromatids in second meiotic division is called disjunction. *MCQ*
- If segregation is not normal, it is called *nondisjunction*.
- On nondisjunction, the resultant cells may receive less number of chromosomes or extra chromosomes.
- Cells of nondisjunction on fertilization may form fetus with an abnormal number of chromosomes (trisomy or monosomy).
- *Examples:*
  – Down syndrome: Trisomy of chromosome 21.
  – Klinefelter syndrome: Extra X chromosome in males (phenotypically male case).
  – Turner syndrome: Lack of Y chromosome (phenotypically female case).

Box 1.3: Organizer and induction

- Organizer is a cluster of cells in developing embryo that can determine differentiation of other regions.
- Primary organizer is a dorsal lip of blastopore that is self-differentiating and its removal results in total failure of embryonic development. *MCQ*
- Influence of an organizer on another area of development is called **induction**.
- Inductors are substances that exert the same effects as that of organizer.
- Hans Spemann was awarded the Nobel Prize in 1935 for his discovery of embryonic induction.

For example:
1. Optic vesicle acts as an organizer and it induces formation of lens on overlying skin.
2. Primary organizer – dorsal lip of primitive streak
   Secondary organizer – notochord
   Tertiary organizer – neutral tube

Some Interesting Facts

Phases of Cell Life (Fig. 1.5, Flowchart 1.2)

- *G1 phase:* It follows M phase. Events – Cytoplasm increases in volume; damaged DNA gets repaired.
- *S phase:* It follows G1 phase. Events – DNA gets replicated to form two sister chromatids of each arm of the chromosome. Each cell contains 4n (double 2n) number of chromosomes.
- *G2 phase:* It follows S phase. Event – it is a check point before mitosis or meiosis for the confirmation of duplicated chromatin.
- *G0 phase:* It is a nondividing phase of cell cycle.
- *M phase:* It is the cell division phase.

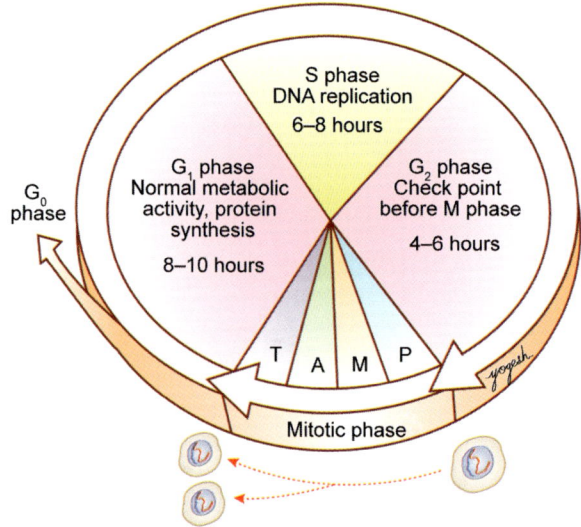

Fig. 1.5: Phases of cell division. *Abbreviations:* P: Prophase; M: Metaphase; A: Anaphase; T: Telophase

Chapter 2

Menstrual Cycle

eSmartQuiz

Chapter Outline

- Duration of menstrual cycle
- Phases of menstrual cycle
  - Follicular phase
  - Luteal phase
- Endometrium
- Uterine changes
- Ovarian changes
- Mechanism of menstrual bleeding
- Hormonal synchronization in menstrual cycle
  - Estrogen
  - Progesterone
  - Luteinizing hormone
- Disorders of menstrual cycle
- Amenorrhea

Competencies:
- AN77.1: Describe the uterine changes occurring during the menstrual cycle.
- AN77.2: Describe the synchrony between ovarian and menstrual cycle.

INTRODUCTION

- Reproductive system in females consists of pair of ovaries, uterine tubes, uterus, vagina and external genitalia.
- *Fertile period* of the female extends from the age of puberty to menopause.
- *Puberty* is a period of adolescence in which a female reaches sexual maturity and becomes capable of reproduction. It occurs by the age of 11–14 years.
- *Menopause* is the absence of menstrual cycle for a period of 12 months or more in the later life of a female and by then she is no longer able for reproduction. It occurs between 49 and 52 years of age.
- A fertile female shows monthly periodic changes in the ovary and uterus from puberty till menopause.
- The periodic structural and functional changes of female reproductive organs are under the control of hormones of the pituitary gland (hypothalamo–pituitary–ovarian axis).
- These periodic changes are grouped as follows:
  a. *Ovarian cycle*: Rhythmic changes in the ovary involves formation and maturation of ovarian follicles, release of gamete (ovum) and secretion of ovarian hormones.
  b. *Uterine cycle* or *menstrual cycle*: It consists of the periodic changes in the endometrium of uterus. It is mainly targeted towards the preparation of uterus for implantation, to nourish fertilized gametes after implantation and shedding of endometrium in absence of fertilization.*Viva*
- Ovarian cycle and ovulation are covered in Chapter 3. This chapter deals with the uterine or menstrual cycle.

MENSTRUAL/UTERINE CYCLE

Definition

- *Menstrual cycle* is a rhythmic change in uterus starting from puberty until menopause.
- *Menstruation* is a cyclic bleeding that occurs due to the shedding of endometrium in the absence of fertilization.
- Menstrual cycle is studied as follows:
  1. Duration of cycle
  2. Phases of menstrual cycle
  3. Changes in reproductive organs

4. Mechanism of menstrual bleeding
5. Hormonal changes
6. Disorders of menstrual cycle

DURATION OF MENSTRUAL CYCLE

- Each menstrual cycle extends from the first day of beginning of the menstrual bleeding up to the first day of beginning of the next menstrual bleeding.
- Length of menstrual cycle varies from female to female. Even in one female, it is not always the same.
- Usually, average menstrual cycle consists of 28 days. Menstrual means lunar month of 28 days in Latin (Flowchart 2.1, Fig. 2.1).
- Factors affecting the duration of menstrual cycle:
  – Emotional status
  – Nutritional status
  – Psychological and social aspects
  – Environmental factors
  – Hormonal status
  – Near menopause
- The normal range of menstrual cycle: 21–35 days.
- Because of hormonal influence, menstrual cycles are absent during pregnancy and lactation. *Clinical fact*

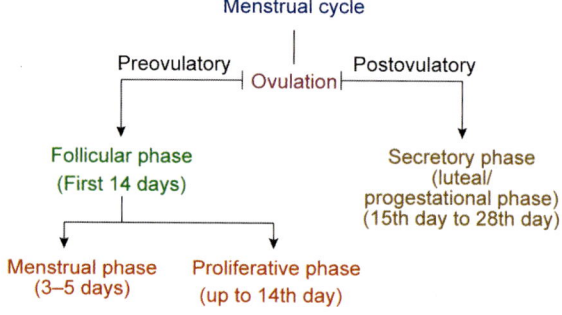

Flowchart 2.1: Phases of menstrual cycle

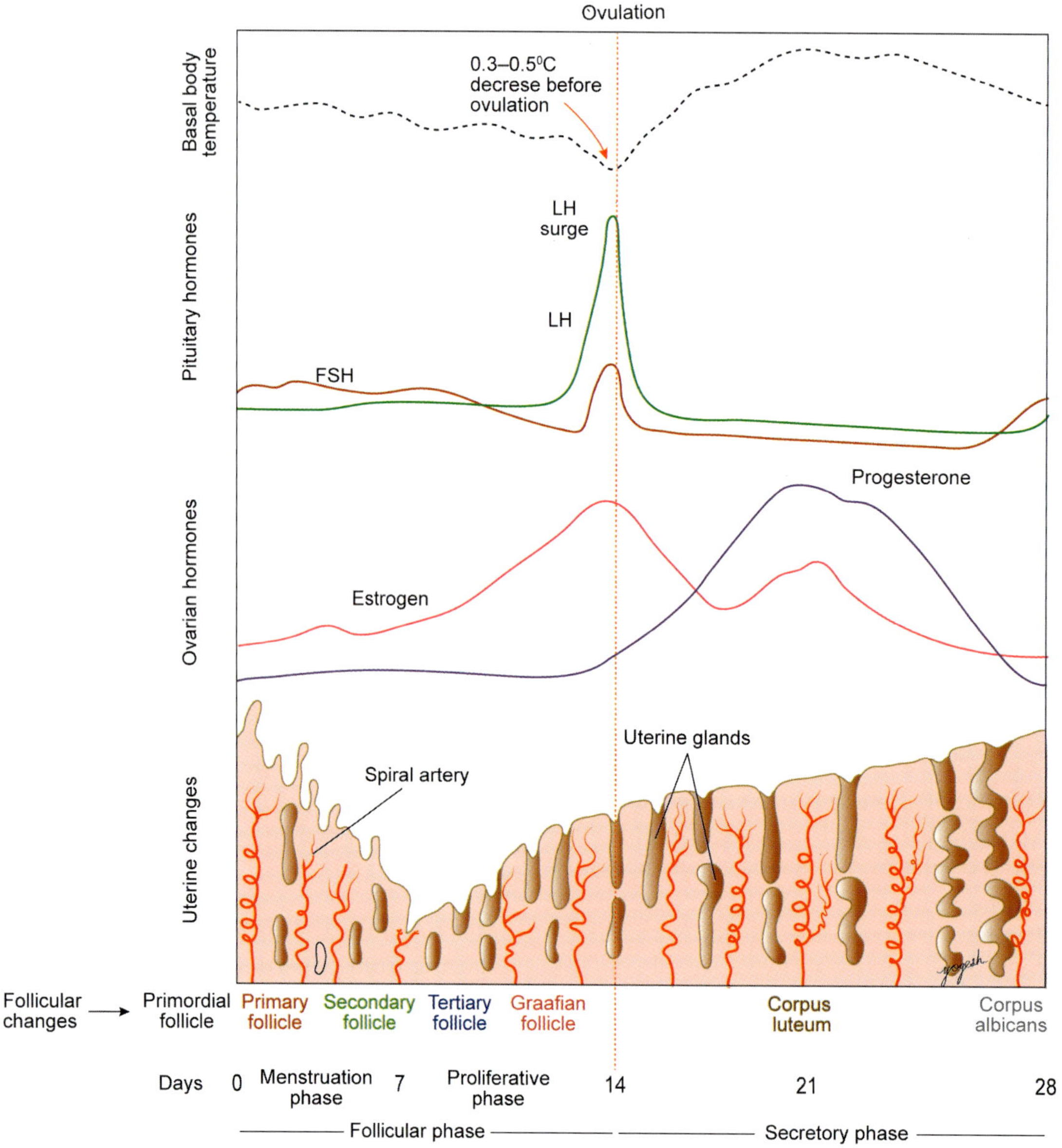

Fig. 2.1: Synchrony between ovarian and menstrual cycle. Hormonal and uterine changes in the menstrual cycle
Abbreviations: FSH: Follicle-stimulating hormone; LH: Luteinizing hormone

Box 2.1: Endometrium

Q. Write a short note on endometrium.

- *Uterine endometrium* shows cyclic changes during menstrual cycle.
- Uterus has three layers: Endometrium, myometrium and perimetrium (inside outwards) (Fig. 2.2, Flowchart 2.2).
- *Myometrium* is very thick and consists of smooth muscles. *Perimetrium* is the outer connective tissue layer covered by visceral peritoneum.
- *Endometrium* is the inner mucous membrane. It is a functional layer of the uterus.
- It consists of columnar epithelium, connective tissue stroma and simple tubular uterine glands.
- The stroma of endometrium contains spiral arteries.
- Endometrium shows three strata as follows:
  a. *Stratum compactum*: Superficial layer containing necks of uterine glands.
  b. *Stratum spongiosum*: Middle layer, consists of loose areolar tissue.
  c. *Stratum basale*: Deep layer, lies adjacent to myometrium. Stratum basale contains fundi of uterine glands.
- During the phase of menstrual bleeding, stratum basale do not shed off, only stratum functionale (stratum compactum and stratum spongiosum) shed off.
- Stratum basale is supplied by straight arteries that are the branches of arcuate artery, whereas stratum spongiosum and compactum are supplied by spiral arteries.

Some Interesting Facts

- Stratum functionale = Stratum compactum + Stratum spongiosum. Basal body temperature falls by 0.3–0.5°C just before ovulation and increases slightly thereafter (Fig. 2.1).
- Length of secretory phase remains constant (14 days). Thus, irrespective of length of the menstrual cycle, ovulation takes place 14 days prior to next menstrual bleeding. *Clinical fact*

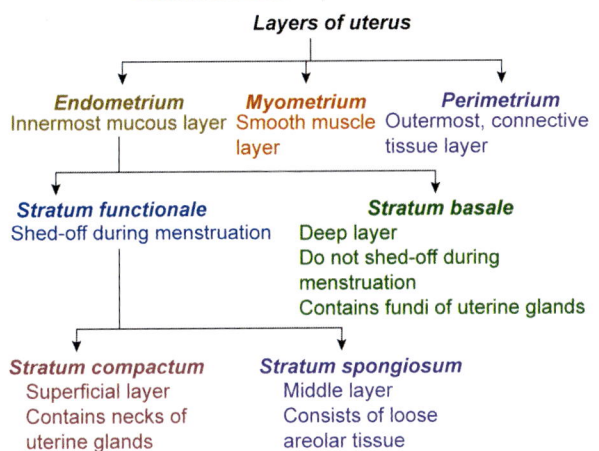

Flowchart 2.2: Layers of uterus

PHASES OF MENSTRUAL CYCLE

Q. Write a short note on the phases of menstrual cycle.

- Menstrual cycle shows 4 phase:
  – Follicular (postmenstrual) phase
  – Proliferative phase
  – Secretory phase
  – Menstrual phase (Flowchart 2.3).
- Recent concept: Menstrual cycle is divided into two phases: Follicular phase (it includes menstrual and proliferative phases) and luteal/secretory phase. These two phases are separated by ovulation.

Follicular Phase (Preovulatory)

- Developing ovarian follicle secretes estrogen that controls the changes in uterus. Hence, this phase of menstrual cycle is called *follicular phase*.
- Follicular phase shows
  i. Menstrual phase
  ii. Proliferative phase
- Follicular phase lasts up to ovulation.
- In initial few days of follicular phase, the superficial parts of the thickened endometrium (stratum compactum and stratum spongiosum) are shed off. It constitutes *menstrual bleeding* that lasts for 3–5 days. This part of follicular phase is also known as *menstrual phase*.
- In remaining part of the follicular phase, uterine endometrium proliferates, hence called *proliferative phase*.

Luteal/Secretory Phase (Postovulatory)

- Following the ovulation, corpus luteum secretes progesterone that influences uterine changes. Hence, this phase is *luteal phase* or *progestational phase*.
- Uterine endometrium becomes secretory in the luteal phase; hence, this phase is also called *secretory phase*.

UTERINE CHANGES IN MENSTRUAL CYCLE

Q. Write a short note on uterine changes in menstrual cycle.

- During menstrual cycle, ovary and uterus show cyclic changes specific to phases of the cycle (Figs 2.1, 2.3, Flowchart 2.3).

Changes in Follicular Phase

- The uterine changes in follicular phase can be grouped into *menstrual phase* and *proliferative phase* (Fig. 2.4).

Menstrual phase

- Degeneration of corpus luteum at the end of the previous menstrual cycle results in stoppage of secretion of progesterone and estrogen.

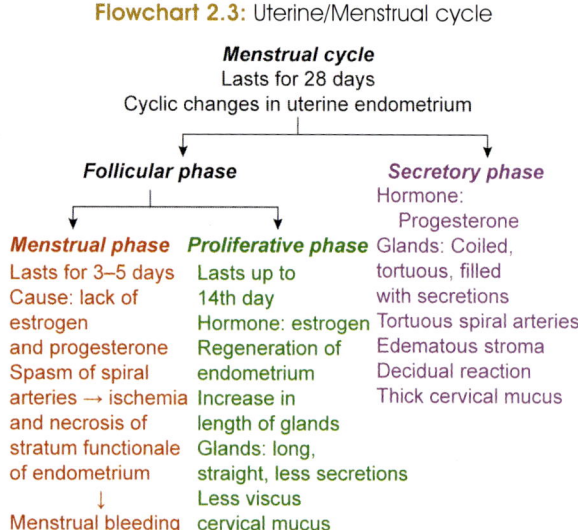

Flowchart 2.3: Uterine/Menstrual cycle

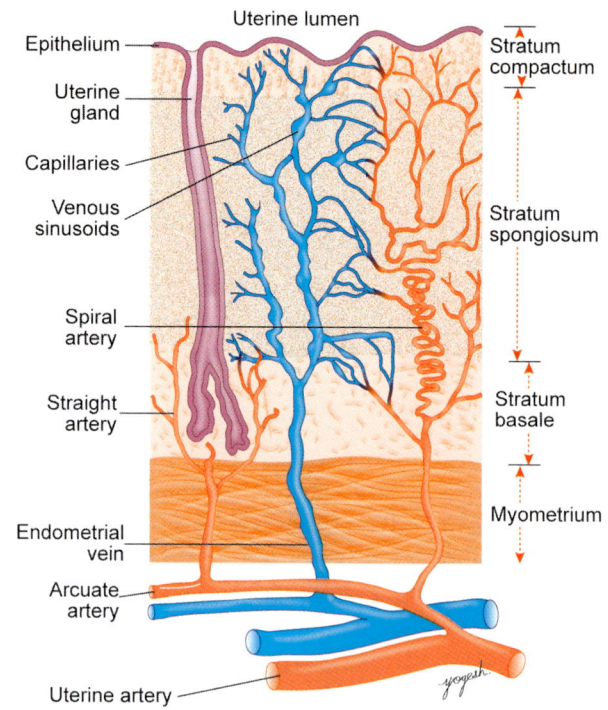

Fig. 2.2: Layers of uterine endometrium during proliferative phase of the menstrual cycle, and blood supply of endometrium

- Absence of these hormones causes temporary spasm (contraction) of spiral arteries. It results in ischemia and necrosis of stratum compactum and spongiosum (superficial 2/3rds of endometrium) (Fig. 2.2, Flowchart 2.4).
- Stratum basale has not been supplied by spiral arteries (but by straight arteries); hence, it does not shed off (Fig. 2.2).
- Average duration: 3–5 days.
- Menstrual blood does not clot due to the presence of proteolytic enzymes. *Clinical fact, MCQ*

Proliferative phase (estrogenic phase)

- On 5th day onward, under the influence of estrogen, the thickness of endometrium starts increasing due to regeneration.
- Uterine endometrium undergoes hypertrophy and hyperplasia.
- The length of uterine gland increases (Fig. 2.4).
- Uterine glands become straight, long, widely separated and they have scanty secretions.
- Number of spiral arteries increases and it enhances blood supply to the endometrium (Fig. 2.4).
- Under the influence of estrogen, the volume, alkalinity and elasticity of cervical mucous increases.

It makes cervical mucous favorable for the passage of sperms through cervix of the uterus.

OVARIAN CHANGES IN MENSTRUAL CYCLE

During menstrual cycle, ovary show cyclic changes specific to phases of the cycle (Figs 2.1, 2.3, Flowchart 2.5).

Changes in Follicular Phase

- In each ovarian cycle, one of the follicles reaches up to the stage of Graafian follicle.
- Some of the important changes occurring in the ovary are as follows (Fig. 2.3):
  1. Primary oocyte undergoes maturation and gets surrounded by follicular cells and subsequently forms primary, secondary and tertiary follicles.

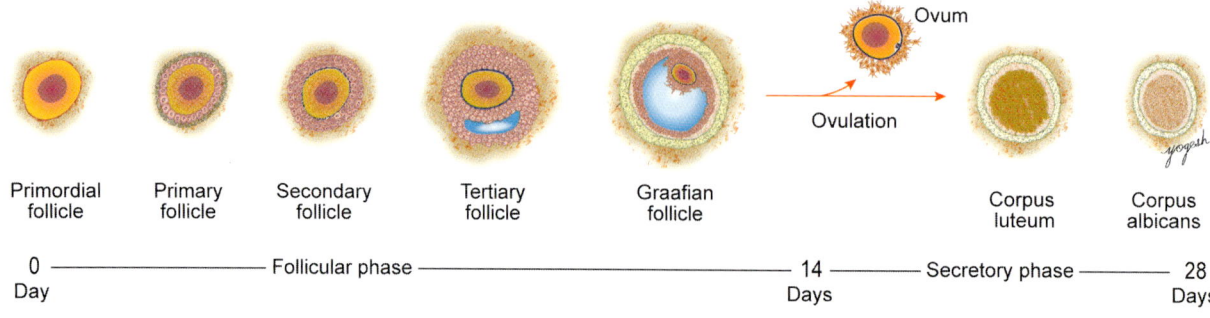

Fig. 2.3: Ovarian changes during the menstrual cycle

Flowchart 2.4: Mechanism of menstrual bleeding

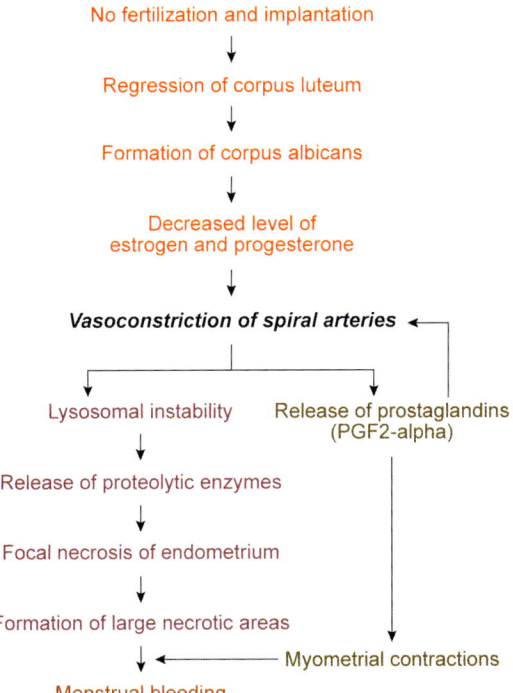

Note: Overproduction of prostaglandins causes excessive uterine contractions and produce dysmenorrhea (painful menstruation).

2. Liquor folliculi separates follicular (granulosa) cells into inner cumulus oophoricus and outer stratum granulosum.
3. Stromal cells condense to form theca interna and theca externa.
4. Granulosa cells secrete estrogen that influences uterine changes.
5. Primary oocyte completes first meiotic division and forms secondary oocyte and first polar body.
6. At the end of follicular phase, secondary oocyte undergoes ovulation.

Flowchart 2.5: Ovarian cycle

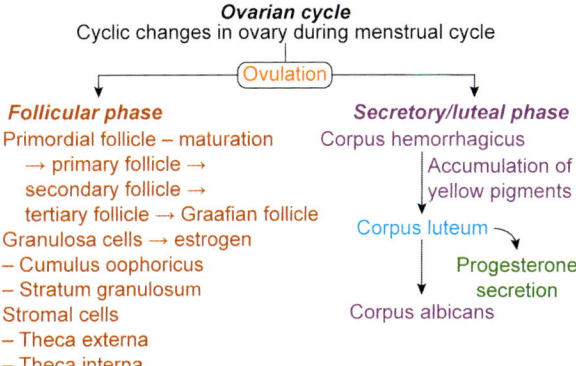

Changes in Luteal (Progestational) Phase

- Luteal phase starts after ovulation.
- Soon after the ovulation, ovarian follicle is filled with blood, hence called corpus hemorrhagicus.
- Granulosa cells start accumulating a yellow pigment (lutein), hence luteal phase. This process is luteinization of granulosa and theca cells.
- Luteal cells secrete progesterone and estrogen.
- If fertilization does not occur, then corpus luteum degenerates by the 26th or 28th day.
- Corpus luteum undergoes luteolysis to form a scar tissue called corpus albicans.

During luteal phase, high level of progesterone enhances the growth of endometrium and induces the following changes:

1. Changes in glands
- Uterine glands become more coiled and tortuous (produces sawtooth appearance).
- Glandular epithelium starts accumulating glycogen. Glands secrete carbohydrate-rich fluid.

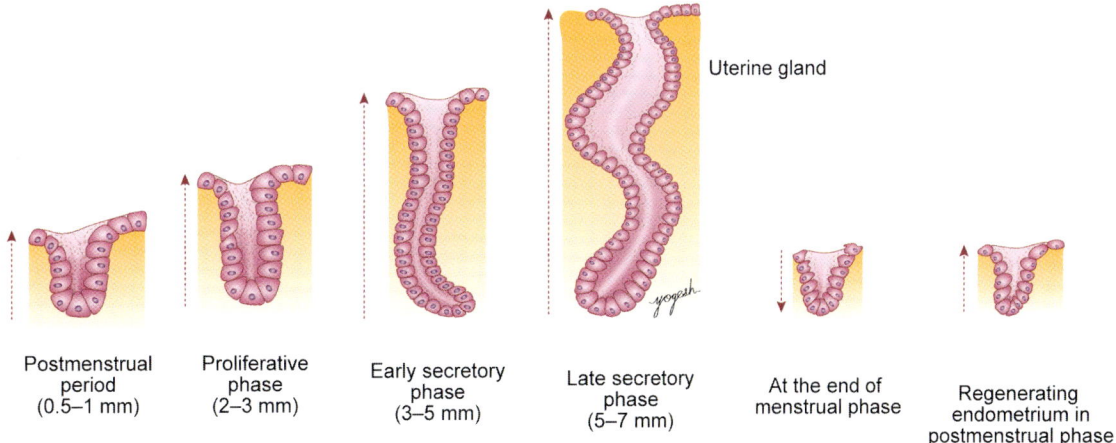

Fig. 2.4: Changes in the uterine endometrium during the menstrual cycle

2. Changes in stroma
- Spiral arteries become more tortuous.
- Vascularity of endometrium enhances.
- Uterine fluid starts accumulating in stroma and makes it oedematous and thick.
- Stromal cells accumulate glycogen and lipid droplets in their cytoplasm. This is called *decidual reaction* (For details, read Chapter 9, Box 9.2).
- In the later part of the luteal phase, due to the absence of progesterone, vasospasm of spiral arteries begins to produce focal necrotic changes in endometrium. At the end of the luteal phase, menstruation begins in the absence of implantation.

3. Cervical mucus changes
- Under influence of progesterone, cervical mucus becomes thick and less elastic. These changes prevent entry of sperms through cervix.

MECHANISM OF MENSTRUAL BLEEDING

Q. Write a short note on mechanism of menstrual bleeding.

- In absence of pregnancy, steroid hormone levels begin to fall due to the degeneration of corpus luteum (Flowchart 2.4).
- Decreased steroid hormone levels cause increased coiling of spiral arteries and constriction. It results in decreased blood supply (ischemia) to endometrium.
- Ischemia of endometrium causes
  1. Destabilization of lysosomal membranes and release of proteolytic enzymes from lysosomes.
  2. Release of prostaglandins, mainly PGF2α.^{MCQ}
- Loss of blood supply and action of proteolytic enzymes initially produce focal areas of necrosis that later fuse to form large necrotic areas in the endometrium.
- Prostaglandins induce smooth muscle (myometrium) contractions and it results into the beginning of menstrual bleeding.
- Because of the presence of proteolytic enzymes, menstrual blood does not form clots.
- Normal amount of menstrual bleed: 30–130 ml.

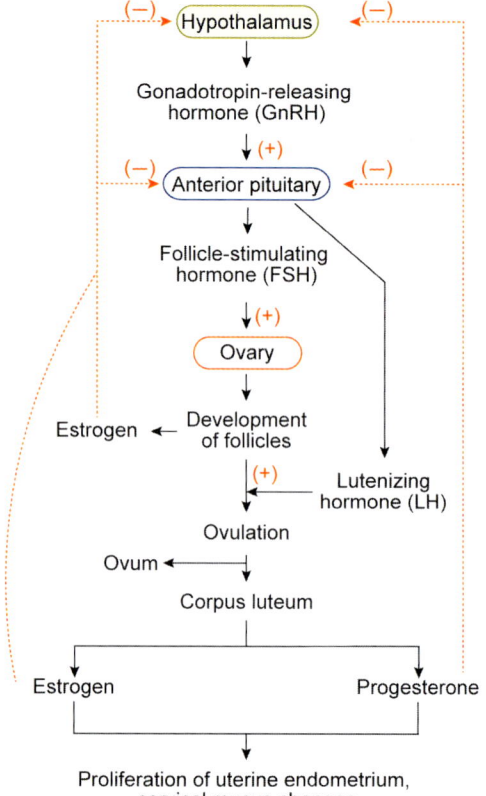

Flowchart 2.6: Hormonal synchronization in menstrual and ovarian cycles

HORMONAL SYNCHRONIZATION IN MENSTRUAL AND OVARIAN CYCLES

Q. Write a short note on hormonal control of menstrual cycle.

- Menstruation in female is under the influence of *hypothalamo – pituitary – ovarian axis* (HPO axis) (Flowchart 2.6).
- Pituitary gland secretes follicle-stimulating hormone (FSH) and luteinizing hormone (LH) (Fig. 2.1).
- Ovaries produce two steroid hormones, estrogen and progesterone under influence of the LH and FSH.
- Secretion of LH and FSH by anterior pituitary is under the control of gonadotropin-releasing hormone (GnRH) of hypothalamus (Table 2.1).

Table 2.1 Hormones in menstrual and ovarian cycles

Endocrine gland	Hormone	Major functions
Anterior pituitary	FSH	• Stimulates follicular growth in ovaries • Stimulates follicles for estrogen secretion
	LH	• LH surge causes ovulation • LH surge, on ovulation, forms corpus luteum
Ovaries	Estrogen	• Stimulates endometrial proliferation • Inhibits secretion of GnRH, FSH and LH
	Progesterone	• Increases thickness of uterine endometrium and makes it suitable for implantation • Inhibits GnRH, FSH and LH secretion
	Inhibin	• Inhibits secretion of FSH by anterior pituitary

Estrogen

- Estrogen hormone is involved in the uterine cycle as well as maintenance of secondary sexual characters.
- Estrogen has two peaks in the menstrual cycle (Fig. 2.1).
  1. First peak: It occurs about 48 hours before ovulation that cause LH surge.
  2. Second peak: It occurs in the middle of the luteal phase.
- Estrogen level continuously rises during development of ovarian follicles. It decreases suddenly after ovulation.
- About 2 days after ovulation, estrogen concentration starts increasing in the luteal phase and reaches again at high in middle luteal phase.

Progesterone

- Progesterone is the hormone of luteal phase and is secreted by corpus luteum. Hence, concentration of progesterone is less in proliferative phase and increases in luteal phase (Fig. 2.1).
- Progesterone rises after ovulation and reaches to peak within 4–5 days after ovulation.
- At the end of luteal phase, progesterone level decreases due to lysis of corpus luteum.

Luteinizing Hormone (LH)

- Luteinizing hormone concentration increases a day prior to ovulation.
- This LH peak is *LH surge* that occurs typically 34–36 hours before ovulation.
- LH levels reach its usual level within 24–48 hours after ovulation.
- High levels of estrogen concentration in the later part of follicular phase induce *LH surge.*^MCQ
- LH surge induces ovulation with help of the following changes:^Viva
  1. Increases prostaglandins and bradykinin secretion that increase blood flow to the developing follicle.
  2. Increased blood flow enhances accumulation of intercellular fluid and increases volume of antral fluid.
  3. Increased antral fluid enhances intrafollicular pressure.
  4. LH induces proteolytic activity by enhancing production of plasminogen activation (secreted by theca cells).
- All the abovementioned changes (1–4) cause rupture of follicular wall and release of an ovum (ovulation).
- For tests/indicators of ovulation, refer to Chapter 3.

DISORDERS OF MENSTRUAL CYCLE

Q. List the disorders of menstrual cycle.
Q. Define amenorrhea, oligomenorrhea, dysmenorrhea, menorrhagia and anovulation.

Disorders of menstrual cycle are grouped as

1. Disorders of flow: Amenorrhea, hypomenorrhea, oligomenorrhea
2. Painful menstruation: Dysmenorrhea, premenstrual syndrome
3. Disorders of timing: Menometrorrhagia, menorrhagia, metrorrhagia
4. Disorders of ovulation: Oligoovulation, anovulation

Definitions

- *Amenorrhea* is the absence of menstrual cycle.
- *Hypomenorrhea* is short or scanty periods (extremely light menstrual flow).
- *Oligomenorrhea* is infrequent menstruation that occurs at intervals of greater than 35 days (only 4–9 menstruations/year).
- *Dysmenorrhea* is painful menstruation. It involves sharp, intermittent pain or dull aching abdominal pain associated with the beginning of menstruation.
- *Premenstrual syndrome* (PMS) are nonspecific symptoms that develop a week before onset of menstrual bleeding. It includes painful or swollen breast, depression, irritability, headache and so on. These symptoms disappear 1–3 days after the menstruation starts.
- *Menorrhagia* is excessive menstrual bleeding.
- *Metrorrhagia* is uterine bleeding that occurs at irregular intervals.
- *Menometrorrhagia* is excessive uterine bleeding at frequent and irregular intervals.
- *Anovulation* is the absence of ovulation.
- *Oligoovulation* is an irregular ovulation, usually if menstrual cycle is more than 36 days.
- *Polymenorrhea* is frequent menstruation (cycle of less than 21 days).

Box 2.2: Amenorrhea

Q. Write a short note on amenorrhea.
Q. Write a short note on primary amenorrhea.

Definition: Amenorrhea is the absence of menstruation in a menstrual cycle in a woman of reproductive age (Flowchart 2.7).

Classification

- Amenorrhea is classified as primary and secondary. It may be physiological or pathological.

Contd.

Contd.

Primary amenorrhea
- Primary amenorrhea is an absence of menstruation since birth of a woman. It can be physiological or pathological.

Physiological primary amenorrhea
- It is normally occurring primary amenorrhea due to physiological reasons.
- Causes
  1. Before puberty: Normally menstruations begin by the age of 12–14 years.
  2. Constitutional amenorrhea is delayed onset of menstruation even up to the age of 18 years without any reason.

Pathological primary amenorrhea
- In pathological primary amenorrhea, menstruation does not start until the age of 18 years.
- Causes
  1. Congenital genetic disorders such as Turner syndrome (45,X).
  2. Congenital anomalies of reproductive tract such as imperforate hymen, absence of uterus, vaginal atresia.

Secondary amenorrhea
- It occurs when menstrual cycle stops in a woman who had menstruation before. It can be physiological or pathological.

Physiological secondary amenorrhea
- Causes
  1. Pregnancy
  2. Lactational amenorrhea: Prolactin secreted during lactation inhibits release of gonadotropin-releasing hormone (GnRH) and prevents ovulation and menstruation.
  3. Menopause (ceasing of menstruation by the age of 45–50 years).
  4. Emotional and environmental factors, such as stress, exposure to extreme climates and so on.

Pathological secondary amenorrhea
- Causes
  1. Hypothalamic disorders causing failure of GnRH release.
  2. Pituitary disorders causing failure of LH and FSH production.
  3. Ovarian diseases causing failure of production of estrogen and progesterone.
  4. Uterine diseases.
  5. Systemic diseases.
  6. Drugs and medication (contraceptive pills).

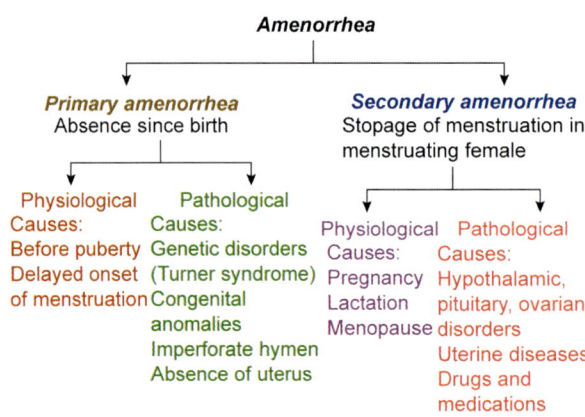

Flowchart 2.7: Amenorrhea

Chapter 3

Gametogenesis

eSmartQuiz

Chapter Outline

- Primordial germ cells
- Teratoma
- Gametogenesis
- Spermatogenesis
- Capacitation of spermatozoa
- Structure of spermatozoa
- Abnormal spermatozoa and their counts
- Oogenesis
- Ovulation
- Tests for ovulation
- Disorders of ovulation
- Structure of ovum

Competency:
- **AN77.3:** Describe spermatogenesis and oogenesis along with diagrams.

INTRODUCTION

Primordial Germ Cells

- Primordial germ cells (PGC) give rise to sperm in males and ovum in females.
- PGC reside in yolk sac (extraembryonic membrane) and can be identified by fourth week of gestation (Fig. 3.1).^{MCQ}
- PGC are derived from epiblast (previous concept: PGC are derived from endoderm of yolk sac).^{NEXT}
- PGC migrate with amoeboid movement from yolk sac to wall of gut from fourth to sixth weeks.
- Later, these cells migrate through mesentery of gut to dorsal body wall and colonize to form gonadal ridge (primitive gonads).
- Cells of the gonadal ridge are invaded by somatic supporting cells from coelomic epithelium.
- Migration of PGC and invasion of coelomic epithelium are essential in the formation of gonads.

GAMETOGENESIS

- Gametogenesis is a process of formation of gametes (sperms in male and ovum in female) from germ cells by cell division.

Box 3.1: Teratoma

- Teratoma is a tumor that consists of tissues derived from all germ layers.
- Sacrococcygeal teratoma is the commonest solid tumor in newborns (1 in 20,000–70,000 births). It arises from primordial germ cells.^{NEXT}
- It occurs more frequently in females than in males.
- It constitutes 3% of childhood malignancies.
- Gonadal teratomas occur due to the capability of germ cells to form many cell types (pluripotency).
- Teratoma shows the presence of hairs, teeth, bone and so on.

- In men, PGCs remain dormant from sixth week of intrauterine life till puberty.
- At puberty, primordial germ cells undergo maturation to form *spermatogonia* that on meiosis form *spermatozoa* until death.
- In females, PGCs differentiate to form *oogonia*. By *fifth month* of intrauterine life, all oogonia enter in meiosis and get arrested in prophase of the first meiotic division to form primary oocytes.^{MCQ}
- Primary oocytes undergo dormancy until puberty.^{MCQ}
- After puberty, each month few primary oocytes form ovarian follicles out of which the only one completes first meiotic division to form *secondary oocyte* and gets ovulated.

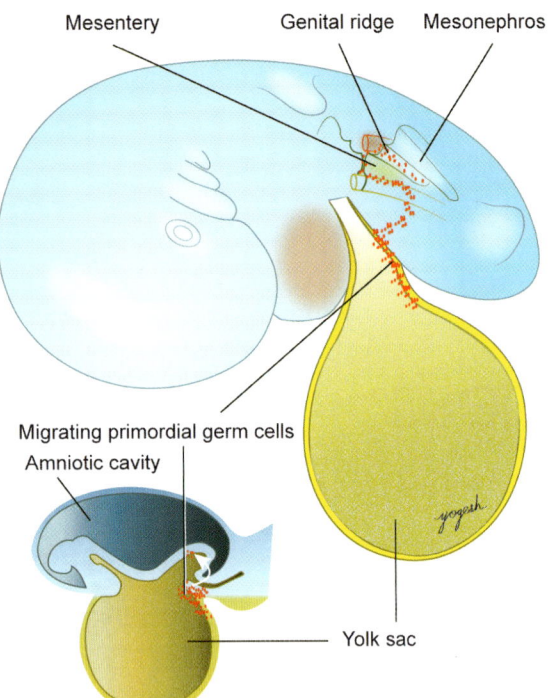

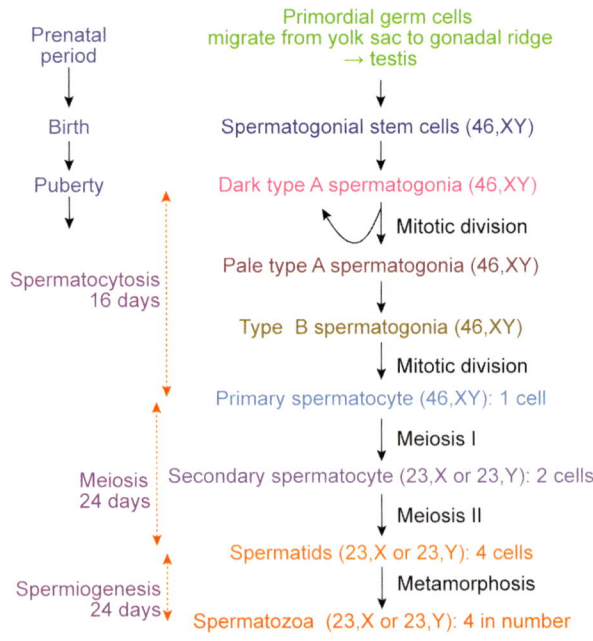

Flowchart 3.1: Stages in spermatogenesis

Fig. 3.1: Primordial germ cells (PGC) and formation of gonads. PGC resides in the yolk sac and migrates to the wall of the gut during fourth to sixth weeks. Later these cells migrate through mesentery of the gut to the dorsal body wall and colonize to form gonadal ridge and subsequently gonads (testis or ovaries)

- Only after fertilization, the second meiotic division can be completed.^{MCQ} These cycles continue until menopause (45–50 years of age).
- Meiosis of PGCs is essential to half the number of chromosomes in gametes.

SPERMATOGENESIS

Q. Write a short note on spermatogenesis.

- *Definition*: Spermatogenesis is a process of formation of sperms (male gametes) from spermatogonia in seminiferous tubules of testis.
- *Site*: Seminiferous tubules of testis
- *Time*: Occurs after puberty and continues even in old age.
- *Duration*: 64–74 days.^{Viva}
- *Responsible hormone*: Testosterone

Process

- It occurs in three steps as follows (Flowchart 3.1, Fig. 3.2):
- **Spermatocytosis**
  - It is a conversion of *spermatogonia → primary spermatocyte*.
  - At puberty, testosterone stimulates spermatogonial stem cells to develop and differentiate into *spermatogonia* (type A dark).
  - Spermatogonia are located immediately under the basement membrane.

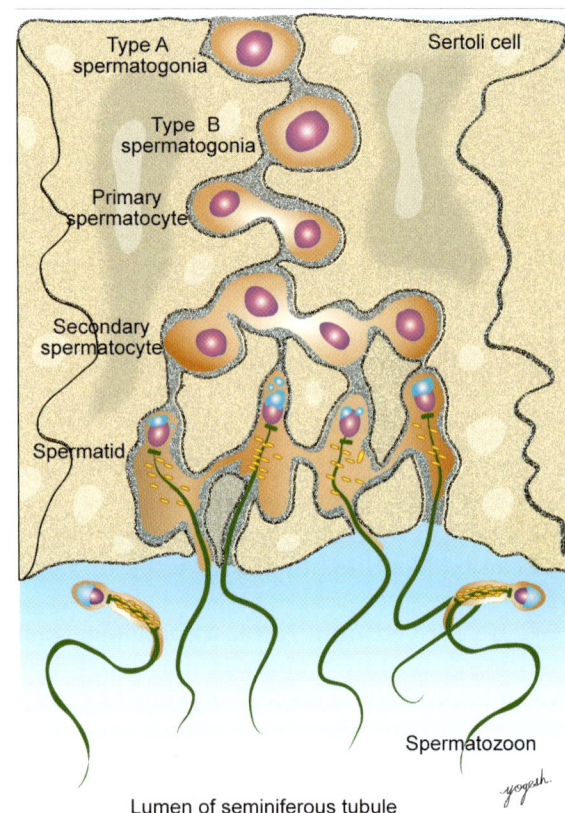

Fig. 3.2: Process of spermatogenesis. Sertoli cells support developing spermatogonia and other cells and finally phagocytose residual bodies

  - Spermatogonia are supported by Sertoli cells.
  - Dark type A spermatogonia undergo *mitosis* to form *pale type A spermatogonia*.^{NEXT}
  - Further pale type A spermatogonia on *mitosis* form *type B spermatogonia* (46,XY).^{NEXT}

- Type B spermatogonia undergo mitosis to form *primary spermatocyte* (46,XY). It is the largest germ cell in the seminiferous tubule.
- **Meiotic division**
  - It is the conversion of *primary spermatocyte* (46, XY) → *spermatids* (23,X and 23,Y).
  - Each primary spermatocyte (46,XY) undergoes first *meiotic* division to form *secondary* spermatocyte (23,X and 23,Y) that later undergoes to form four *spermatids* (23,X; 23,X; 23,Y; 23,Y).^{NEXT}

Spermiogenesis

Q. Write a short note on spermiogenesis.

- *Definition:* Spermiogenesis is the process of **metamorphosis** of spermatids by which they get converted into a *spermatozoon*.^{MCQ, Viva}

Spermatid —Metamorphosis→ Spermatozoon

- Metamorphosis is the change in the form of the cell.
- **Process of spermiogenesis** (Fig. 3.3, Practice Fig. 3.1)
  - *Nucleus:* It condenses and move towards one pole.
  - *Golgi apparatus:* It forms an acrosomal cap and covers two-thirds of the nucleus.
  - *Centromere:* It divides into proximal centriole and distal centriole comes to lie near nucleus (in the neck of sperm) and gives rise to axial filament.
    Distal centriole lies at the junction of the middle piece with tail.

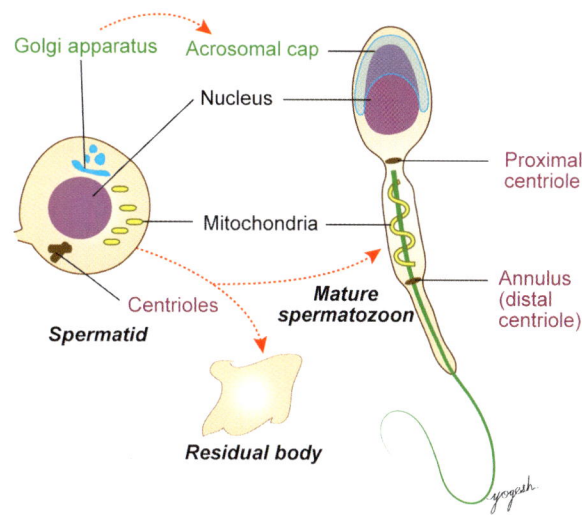

Practice Fig. 3.1: Process of spermiogenesis

- *Mitochondria:* They sheath around axial filament to form a middle piece of sperm.
- *Cytoplasm:* Most of the cytoplasm of spermatid is shaded as *Renaud's residual body*. [Sertoli cells phagocytose residual bodies].^{MCQ}
- *Release of spermatozoa:* Finally, spermatozoa are released into lumen of seminiferous tubules. This is *spermiation*.^{MCQ}
- Spermatogenesis of one sperm: 64 days (70–75 days also given by some authors).^{MCQ}
- It includes mitoses – 16 days, meiosis I – 8 days, meiosis II – 16 days and spermiogenesis – 24 days.^{MCQ}

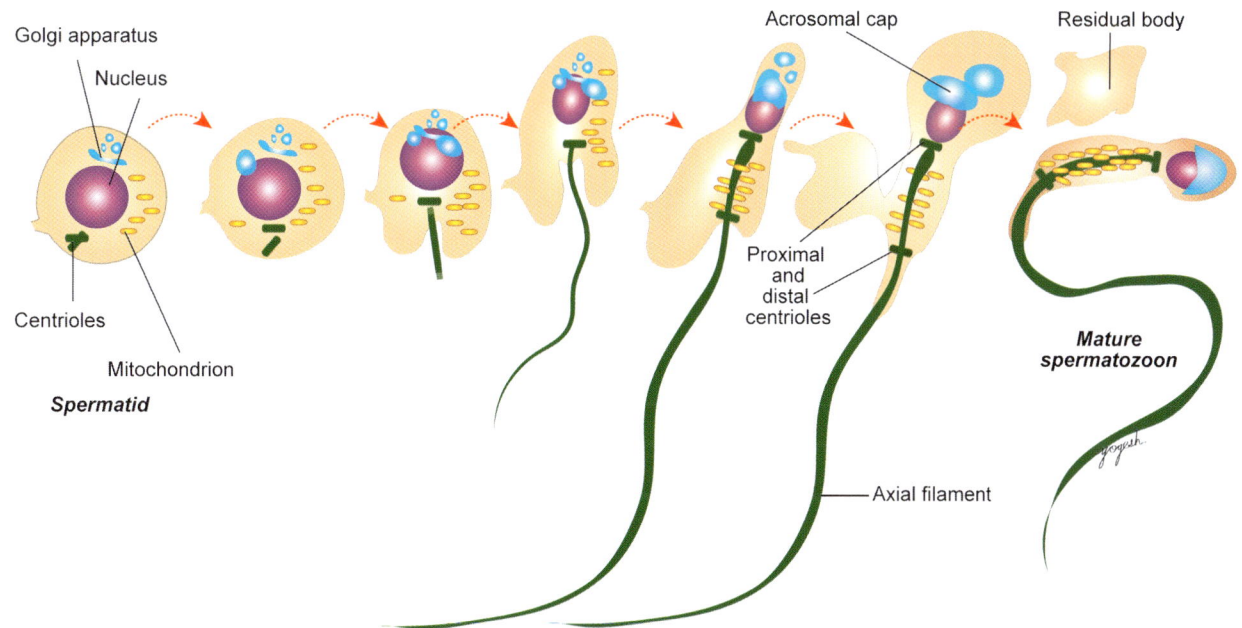

Fig. 3.3: Process of spermiogenesis

Some Interesting Facts

- Spermatogenesis occurs in a continual wave throughout seminiferous tubules.
- During spermatogenesis, because of incomplete cytokinesis, daughter cells produced by mitosis or meiosis are connected with each other by slender cytoplasmic bridges.
- Secretion of fluid in seminiferous tubules pushes immature spermatozoa towards epididymis. Sperms get stored in epididymis and sperms head get coated with glycoproteins.
- Sperm start motility in epididymis.^{NEXT} Sperm acquires full motility only on ejaculation with the help of prostatic and seminal secretions.
- Reduction division (meiosis I) or independent assortment of chromosomes occurs in spermatogenesis during conversion of primary to secondary spermatocyte; hence, secondary spermatocyte onward haploid number of chromosomes are seen.^{NEXT}
- Spermatogonia and primary spermatocytes have diploid number of chromosomes (46,XY). Secondary spermatocytes, spermatids and sperms have haploid number of chromosomes.^{NEXT}
- Spermatogenesis requires temperature that is ~2°C below body temperature.^{NEXT}
- Differences between spermatid and spermatozoon are listed in Table 3.1.

Box 3.2: Capacitation of spermatozoa

Q. Write a short note on capacitation.

- Capacitation is a process of conversion of immature spermatozoa to mature spermatozoa.

Immature spermatozoa $\xrightarrow{\text{Capacitation}}$ Mature spermatozoa

- Capacitation is discovered by Chang and Austin (1951).
- Site: Female reproductive tract (uterus and uterine tubes).^{NEXT,Viva}
- Capacitation involves the following events:
  - Removal of acrosomal membrane
  - Alteration of glycoprotein coat over head of sperm
  - Removal of seminal proteins from head of sperm
- Effect of capacitation:
  - Increases sperm motility
  - Destabilises acrosomal membrane and allows it to penetrate outer layer of egg.

STRUCTURE OF SPERMATOZOA

Q. Write a short note on the structure of spermatozoa or sperm.
Q. Draw a well-labelled diagram of sperm.

- Matured spermatozoa have head, neck, middle piece and tail.

Q. List the differences between spermatid and spermatozoon.

Table 3.1 Differences between spermatid and spermatozoon

Spermatid	Spermatozoon
It is immature male gamete.	It is mature male gamete.
Nucleus: Big, central.	Nucleus: Condensed, lies in head portion.
Golgi apparatus is not fused to form acrosomal cap.	Golgi apparatus fuse to form acrosomal cap.
It has dispersed mitochondria in the cytoplasm.	Mitochondria are arranged spirally in the middle piece.
It does not have tail or axial filament.	It has tail and axial filament.
It has abundant cytoplasm.	It has scanty cytoplasm.

Some Interesting Facts

- Spermatozoa are artificially capacitated and used for *in vitro* fertilization (IVF).
- In assisted reproduction technology (ART) for a patient with defective acrosome, spermatozoon is injected directly into oocyte.
- Sperm with Y chromosome swims faster due to smaller size of Y chromosome.^{NEXT}
- Sperms are stored in seminiferous tubules after formation.^{NEXT}

- Length: 50–60 μm.
- Count: In a single ejaculation, 200–300 million sperms are emitted in a volume of 2–5 ml semen.

Parts of Spermatozoa (Fig. 3.4, Practice Fig. 3.2)

- It has the following parts (Flowchart 3.2):

Head

- Shape: Pyriform
- Length: 4 μm
- Contains haploid condensed nucleus (23,X or 23,Y chromosomes).
- *Acrosomal cap* (galea capitis) covers two-thirds of nucleus (derived from Golgi apparatus).
- Acrosome contains digestive enzymes (hyaluronidase and acrosine) that help to break the outer wall of the ovum.^{MCQ}

Neck

- Length: 0.3 μm
- Contains proximal centriole with transverse and longitudinal cylinders.
- The longitudinal cylinder (basal body) has nine thick filaments that are continuous with axial filaments of body and tail of spermatozoon.

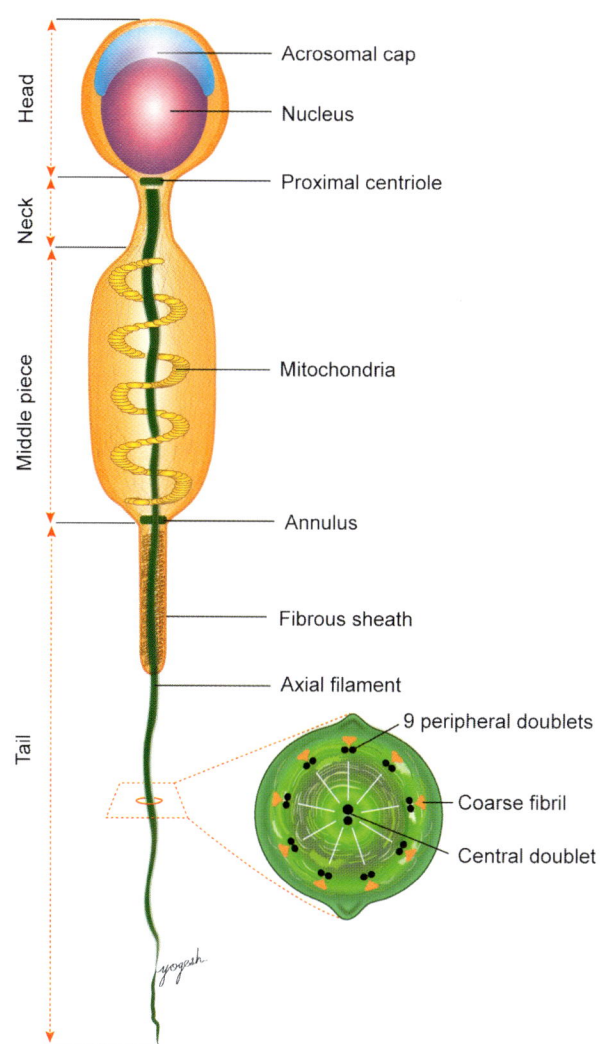

Fig. 3.4: Structure of sperm

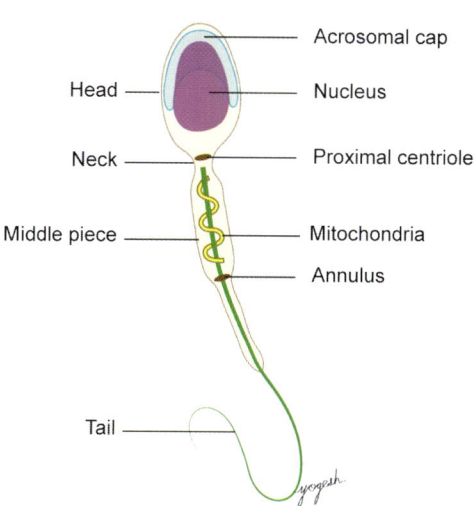

Practice Fig. 3.2: Structure of sperm

Middle Piece/Body

- Length: 4 µm.
- Axial filament passes from neck into middle piece and tail.
- At the junction of a middle piece with tail, distal centriole is present in the form of an *annulus* (ring-like structure).
- The axial filament is surrounded spirally by mitochondrion.
- Axial filament is made up of central doublet of fibril surrounded by nine doublets of fibrils. Each peripheral doublet is associated with coarser, petal-shaped fibril.

Tail

- Length: 40 µm.
- Parts:
  - In *principal piece*, axial filament is surrounded by fibrous sheath and the plasma membrane.
  - In *end piece*, the fibrous sheath is absent.

Life

- Usual period of viability after ejaculation is 48 hours, but may survive up to 4 days in female genital tract.

Box 3.3: Abnormal spermatozoa and their counts (Fig. 3.5)^MCQ,Viva

- *Oligozoospermia*: Sperm count <15 millions/ml of semen is called oligozoospermia (WHO).
- *Azoospermia*: It is the absence of sperms in semen. It affects about 1% of male population and 20% of male infertility cases.
- *Aspermia*: It is the complete lack of semen. It may be due to retrograde ejaculation, prostatectomy, ejaculatory duct obstruction.
- *Asthenozoospermia*: It is reduced sperm motility.
- *Hyperspermia* is large semen volume and *hypospermia* is small semen volume.
- *Teratozoospermia*: It is the abnormal morphology of sperms that affects fertility in males. It includes giant or dwarf sperms, double head or body of sperm. Even during semen analysis of healthy individuals, 10% of abnormal spermatozoa have been observed.

Flowchart 3.2: Structure of spermatozoa

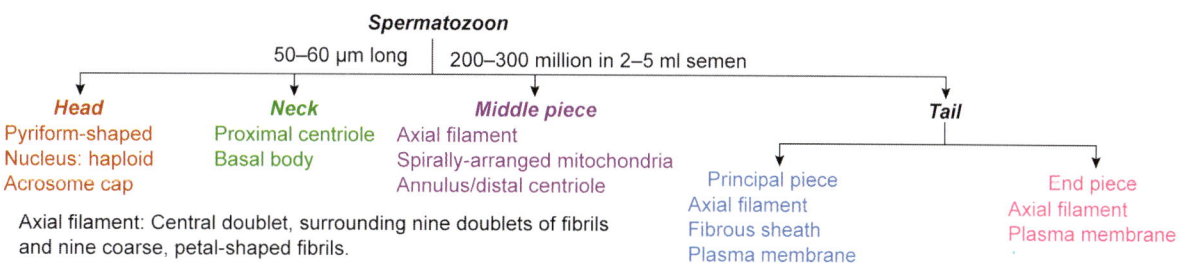

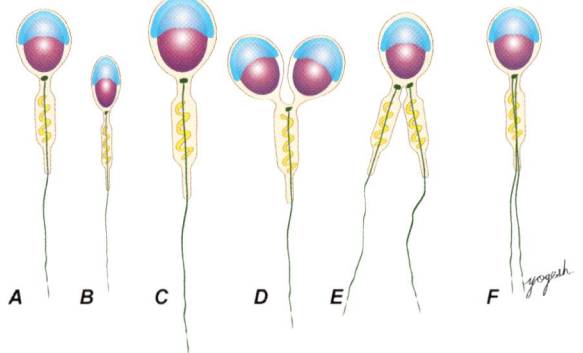

Fig. 3.5: Morphology of sperms: (A) Normal sperm; (B) Microsperm; (C) Giant sperm; (D) Double-headed sperm; (E) Sperm with double body; (F) Sperm with double tail

OOGENESIS

Q. Write a short note on oogenesis.

- **Definition:** Oogenesis is a process of formation of a mature ovum from primordial germ cells.
- **Location:** Ovarian cortex.
- Folliculogenesis is the process of maturation of ovarian follicle.

Process of Oogenesis (Flowchart 3.3, Practice Fig. 3.3)

- It takes in three phases – before birth, after puberty, after fertilization.

Before birth

- Before third month of IUL, the PGCs undergo mitosis to form *oogonia*.

Flowchart 3.3: Stages in oogenesis

```
Before birth       Primordial germ cells
              migrate from yolk sac to gonadal ridge → ovary
                            ↓ Mitotic division
                     Oogonia (46,XX)
                            ↓
                   Primary oocyte (46,XX)
                            ↓ Prophase I
                Arrest in dictyotene stage (46,XX)
                            ↓
After puberty    Primordial follicle (46,XX)
                            ↓
                 Primary ovarian follicle (46,XX)
                            ↓
                 Secondary ovarian follicle (46,XX)
                            ↓
                 Tertiary ovarian follicle (46,XX)
                            ↓
                   Graafian follicle (46,XX)
                            ↓ Meiosis I
              Secondary oocyte (23,X) + 1st polar body
After fertilization         ↓ Meiosis II
              Secondary oocyte (23,X) + 2nd polar body
```

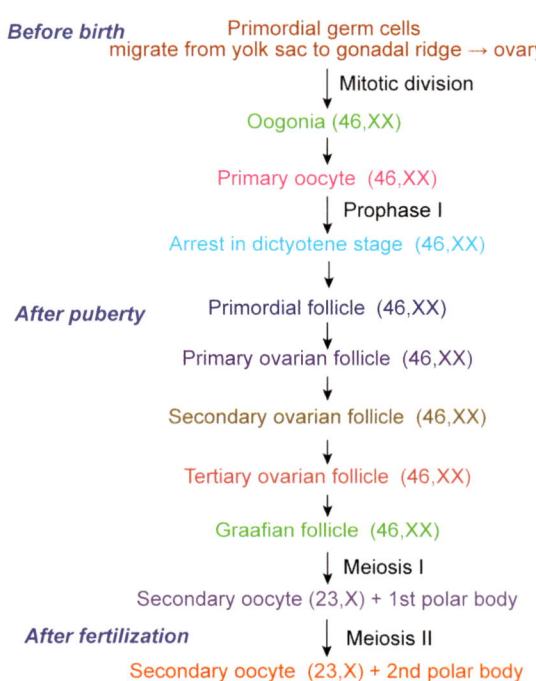

Practice Fig. 3.3: Developing ovarian follicles

- Before 7th month of IUL, oogonia multiply *mitotically* and enlarge to form **primary oocytes** that get surrounded by epithelial cells.[NEXT]
- Seventh month to birth, **primary oocytes** complete prophase I of meiotic division and get arrested at **dictyotene (diplotene) stage** at birth by *oocyte maturation inhibitor* (OMI) factor till puberty.[NEXT]
- *Primordial follicle:* Primary oocyte gets surrounded by single layer of flattened stromal cells of ovary to form primordial follicle. These flat cells are called follicular cells (Fig. 3.6A)
- Out of 6 to 8 lakhs primary oocytes at birth (primordial follicles), 40,000 persist up to puberty and less than 500 ovulate.[NEXT]
- From birth to puberty follicles remain in dormant phase.

After puberty (Fig. 3.6)

- Due to hormonal changes, ovary shows cyclic changes called *ovarian cycle*.
- Primary oocyte (46,XX) undergoes maturation and increase in size.
- *Primary follicle:* Surrounding flattened follicular cells mature and become cuboid cells to form *primary follicle* (Fig. 3.6B)
- *Secondary follicle:* Follicular cells multiply to form multilayered *granulosa layer*. Then, this follicle is called *secondary follicle* (Fig. 3.6C).
- Fluid-filled cavity (follicular antrum) appears in the follicular cells and forms *tertiary/antral follicle* and fluid is called *liquor folliculi* (Fig. 3.6D).
- Antrum folliculi separates granulosa cells as outer *granulos* and inner *cumulus ovaricus* layers that surround primary oocyte.[NEXT] The connecting cells between oocyte and follicular wall form discus proligerus.
- *Graafian follicle:* Finally, stromal cells surround the follicle and condense to form vascular inner layer

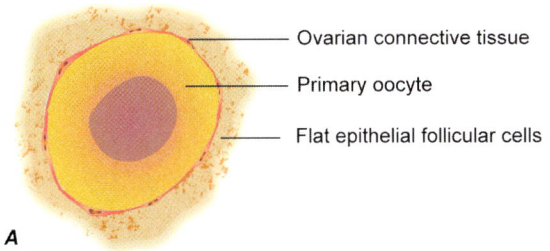

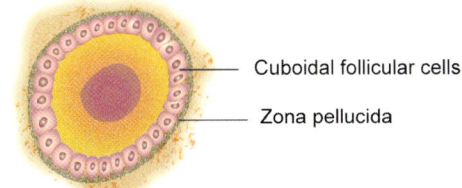

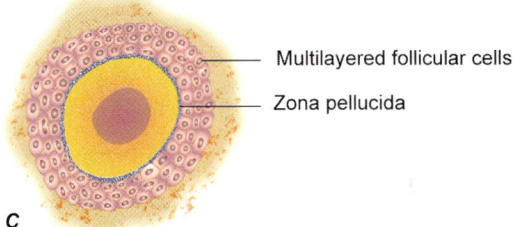

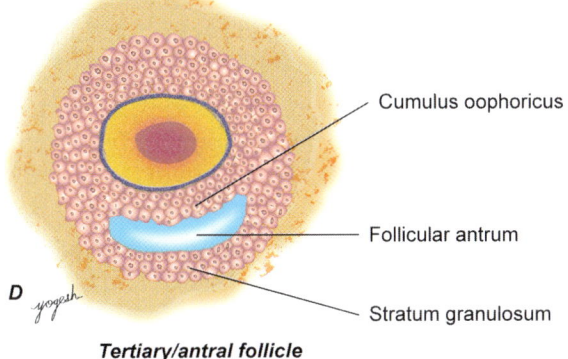

Fig. 3.6: Follicular development

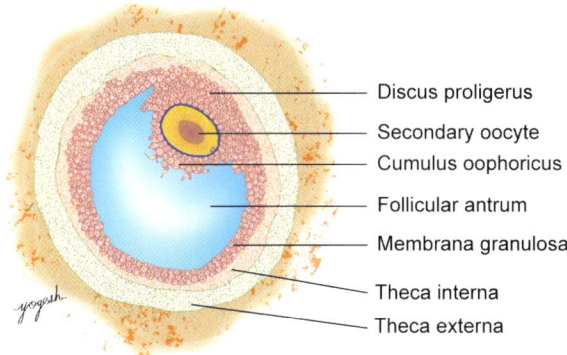

Fig. 3.7: Graafian follicle

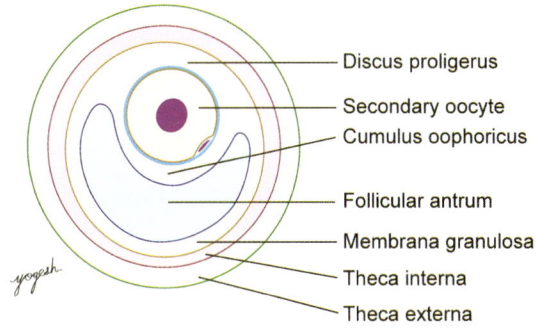

Practice Fig. 3.4: Graafian follicle

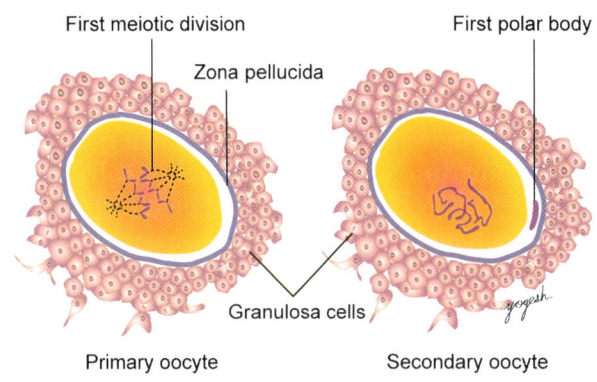

Fig. 3.8: Maturation of oocyte. Primary oocyte completes first meiotic division to form secondary oocyte and first polar body

theca interna (theca = membrane) and outer fibrous layer, *theca externa*. Then this follicle is called *matured Graafian* follicle (named after the Dutch anatomist R. de Graaf, 1641–73) (Fig. 3.7, Practice Fig. 3.4).

- Theca interna secretes estrogen hormone.
- *Zona pellucida*: Accumulated amorphous *glycoprotein* forms a layer between the primary oocyte and follicular cells called zona pellucida.^{MCQ}
- Primary oocyte completes first meiotic division without cytoplasmic division. Primary oocyte retains one nucleus (23,X) and expels another nucleus (23,X) as a *first polar body* in perivitelline space.

- Thus, the primary oocyte is converted into *secondary oocyte*. Secondary oocyte enters in second meiotic division and gets arrested at metaphase untill fertilization (Fig. 3.8).
- Graafian follicle ovulates secondary oocyte.^{MCQ}

After fertilization
- If ovum gets fertilized, secondary oocyte completes second meiotic division.
- During second meiosis, secondary oocyte retains cytoplasm and one nucleus (23,X) and expels another nucleus as a *second polar body* in perivitelline space.
- If fertilization does not occur, secondary oocyte does not complete second meiotic division and undergoes degeneration within *24 hours* after ovulation.^{MCQ}
- After ovulation Graafian follicle collapses and forms *corpus luteum*.

Flowchart 3.4: Features of ovarian follicles

```
                          Ovarian follicles
   ┌──────────────┬──────────────┬──────────────┬──────────────┐
Primordial      Primary       Secondary      Tertiary       Graafian
 follicle       follicle       follicle       follicle       follicle
```

Primordial follicle	Primary follicle	Secondary follicle	Tertiary follicle	Graafian follicle
Primary oocyte	Zona pellucida	Multilayered follicular cells	Follicular cavity	Secondary oocyte + 1st polar body
Flat follicular cell layer	Cuboidal follicular cell layer	↓ Granulosa cells	Granulosa cell layer: a. Discus proligerus b. Cumulus oophoricus c. Membrana granulosa	Zona pellucida Granulosa cells Follicular antrum Theca interna and theca externa

Some Interesting Facts

- In females, formation of gametes occurs at puberty (10–14 years of age) to 45–50 years of age (menopause).
- In males, formation of gametes continues up to old age.
- In each menstrual cycle, 5–30 primary oocytes mature but only one ovulates and other denaturates.
- Polar bodies are formed during oogenesis (not in spermatogenesis).^{NEXT}

Some Interesting Facts

- After fertilization, first polar body also undergoes a second meiotic division.
- Why do only a few follicles develop during menstrual cycle?
  Explanation: Some follicles become progressively sensitive to the effect of FSH and develop earlier than other follicles.
- Ovulation occurs about 38 hours after beginning of LH and FSH surge.
- First polar body is extruded 24 hours prior to the ovulation.^{NEXT}
- Differences between spermatogenesis and oogenesis are listed in Table 3.2.

OVULATION

Q. Write a short note on ovulation.

- **Definition:** Ovulation is a process of *release of ovum* from Graafian follicle.
- **Time:** 14 days prior to onset of next menstrual bleeding.^{MCQ}

Responsible Factors

1. *LH surge:* High concentration of luteinizing hormone (LH) prior to ovulation → increase collagenase activity → digestion of collagen fibers surrounding Graafian follicle.
2. *Prostaglandins:* Increased concentration of prostaglandins → causes contraction of smooth muscles of wall of ovary.
3. *Follicular fluid:* Increased amount of follicular fluid → increased follicular pressure.

Events in ovulation (Flowchart 3.5)

Flowchart 3.5: Events in ovulation

High FSH level and LH surge
↓
Increased follicular fluid
↓
Loosening of cumulus cells
↓
Formation of stigmata (avascular area) over the follicle
↓
Cumulus expansion: Cumulus cells secrete extra cellular matrix containing hyaluronic acid
↓
Digestion of collagen fibres surrounding follicle
↓
Rupture of follicle
↓
Shedding of secondary oocyte with corona radiata (cells of cumulus oophorus)
↓
Entry of ovum in fallopian tube

Box 3.4: Tests for ovulation^{MCQ, Viva}

The following methods are useful for detection of ovulation:

1. *Calendar method:* Ovulation occurs 14 days prior to onset of next menstrual cycle.
2. *Raise in basal body temperature:* Record the temperature every day in the morning. Temperature increases 0.3°–0.5°C during ovulation due to thermogenic effect of the progesterone.
3. *Spinnbarkeit cervical mucus method (Billings method):* Cervical mucus is watery and sticky at the time of ovulation and it shows a fern pattern. A drop of the cervical mucus can be stretched about 10 cm or more like a thread at the time of ovulation. This elastic nature of cervical mucus is called *spinnbarkeit*. Elasticity is less before and after this period.
4. *Hormonal estimation:* Increased LH and estrogen with a decrease in FSH at the time of ovulation. Ovulation kits (ELISA strips, similar to pregnancy test kits) help in the detection of LH surge.
5. *Ultrasonography* monitoring contributes to keep follow-up of ovulation.
6. *Endometrial biopsy* (nowadays, it is not done routinely.)
7. *Mittelschmerz* (short-lived lower abdominal pain): It occurs due to peritoneal irritation by small amount of blood that escapes from follicles during ovulation.
8. *Vaginal discharge or spotting:* There is transient increase in vaginal discharge during ovulation.

Q. *List the differences between spermatogenesis and oogenesis.*

Table 3.2	Differences between spermatogenesis and oogenesis
Spermatogenesis	Oogenesis
It is the process of formation of male gametes (sperms).	It is the process of formation of female gamete (ovum).
Site: Seminiferous tubules in testis.	Site: Cortex of ovary.
It continues from puberty till death.	It continues from puberty till menopause.
It starts only after puberty.	It starts during intrauterine life.
In spermatogenesis, one spermatocyte forms four gametes (sperm).^NEXT	In oogenesis, one primary oocyte forms only one gamete (ovum).^NEXT
Fertilization is not required for second meiotic division.	Fertilization is required for completion of second meiotic division.
Most of the cytoplasm is shed from spermatozoon as residual body.	Cytoplasm is conserved in ovum for nutritional need after fertilization.
Number of gametes release: 200–300 millions per ejaculation.	400–500 in life time of a female.
Occurs at temperature lower than core body temperature	Occurs at core body temperature

Box 3.5: Disorders of ovulation^MCQ

- *Anovulation:* It is absence of ovulation. It may be due to menopausal or due to hormonal imbalance.
- *Oligo-ovulation:* It is infrequent or irregular ovulation.
- *Induced ovulation:* In assisted reproductive technology, *clomiphene citrate* and a low dose of *human chorionic gonadotropin* are used for induced ovulation.
- *Suppressed ovulation:* Contraceptive hormonal pills suppress folliculogenesis and ovulation.

STRUCTURE OF OVUM

Q. *Write a short note on structure of ovum.*

- Ovum is also called the *secondary oocyte.*
- Size: 140 μm.

Structure (Fig. 3.9, Practice Fig. 3.5)

- It consists of a meiotic spindle, ooplasm, vitelline membrane, zona pellucida and corona radiata.

Meiotic spindle

- Nucleus of ovum is not visible. It is represented by spindle of meiosis II.
- It contains 23,X chromosomes.^MCQ

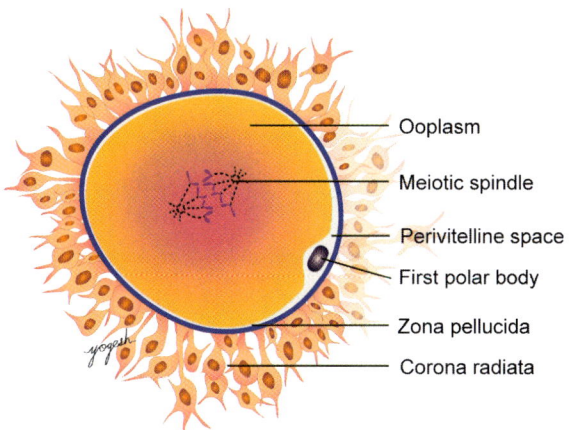

Fig. 3.9: Ovum

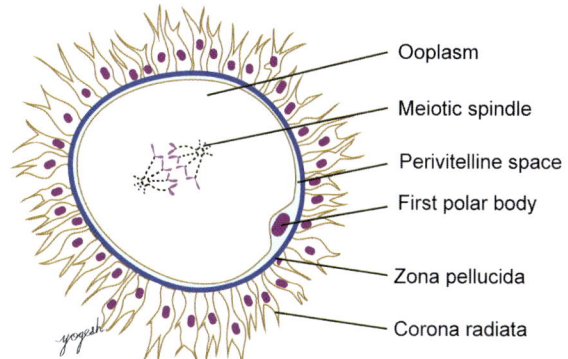

Practice Fig. 3.5: Structure of ovum

Ooplasm/cytoplasm/yolk

- Ooplasm contains droplets of **lecithin-like** substances that forms **deutoplasm**.^MCQ

Vitelline membrane

- It is a cell membrane that is surrounded by *perivitelline space*.
- First polar body lies within the perivitelline space.

Zona pellucida

- It is a glycoprotein coat that surrounds vitelline membrane. Barrier in zona pellucida is provided by fertilin.^NEXT
- Zona pellucida glycoprotein (ZP3) facilitates binding of sperms and induces an acrosomal reaction.^MCQ
- Zona pellucida prevents implantation. Zona pellucida disappears on the fifth or sixth day after fertilization to permit implantation.^MCQ,Viva

Corona radiata

- A few cells of cumulus oophorous remain attached to outer surface of ovum that forms corona radiata.
- Acrosomal enzyme (hyaluronidase) disintegrates corona radiata cells during fertilization.

Some Interesting Facts

- Zona pellucida prevents implantation.
- Deutoplasm provides nutrition to developing embryo in early stages.
- Human ovum is *microlecithal,* as it has scanty amount of deutoplasm.^MCQ
- Eggs of birds are *macrolecithal,* as they contains large amount of deutoplasm.
- Differences between sperm and ovum are listed in Table 3.3.

POSTOVULATORY FATE OF OVARIAN FOLLICLE

- In postovulatory phase, the ovarian follicle undergoes the following changes:

Corpus hemorrhagicus → *Corpus luteum* → *corpus albicans* → *atretic follicle* → *Scar tissue*

Corpus Hemorrhagicus

- Immediately after ovulation, the ovarian follicle collapses, and gets filled with blood to form *corpus hemorrhagicus.*
- The blood clot soon gets absorbed and the follicle gets converted to *corpus luteum.*

Corpus Luteum

- Corpus luteum is yellow-colored structure (*luteum* = yellow, in Latin).
- It is responsible for the luteal phase of menstrual cycle.
- Size: 2–5 cm in diameter.
- *Lutein* is carotenoid (yellow-colored pigment).
- *Luteinization*
  – In luteinization, the follicular cells accumulate the intracellular assembly for the synthesis of steroid hormone.
  – Theca cells form small-sized *theca lutein cells* → secrete progesterone, androgens.
  – Granulosa cells form large-sized *granulosa lutein cells* → secrete progesterone, estrogen and inhibin A.

Q. List the differences between sperm and ovum.

- *Functions*
  Synthesis of progesterone → cause decidualization of endometrium.
- Fate of corpus luteum:
  1. If the ovum is fertilized:
     Implanted embryo secretes human chorionic gonadotropin (hCG) → that stimulates the formation of *corpus luteum of pregnancy* (*corpus luteum graviditatis*) → continue secretion of progesterone till placenta takes over the function.
  2. If the ovum is not fertilized:
     Corpus luteum undergo degradation by 10th day after ovulation → to form *corpus albicans* → fibrous scar.
- Note: The hCG hormone inhibits leutolysis.

Corpus Albicans

- If fertilization does not occur, by 10th day after ovulation, corpus luteum gets converted to corpus albicans. It is also called *atretic corpus luteum* or *corpus candicans* (*albicans* = white body in Latin).
- *Luteolysis*: During the formation of corpus albicans, the cells of corpus luteum are removed by macrophages and fibroblast lay down collagen fibers (white-colored). This process is called luteolysis. Finally, corpus luteum shrinks and results in scar formation.

Clinical Embryology

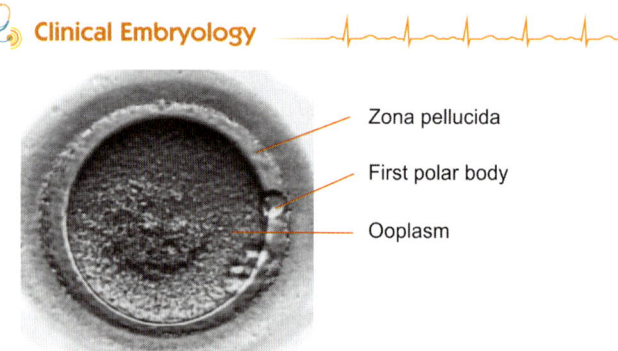

Clinical image 3.1: Human ovum (secondary oocyte) is collected for *in vitro* fertilization. It consists of a nucleus, ooplasm, thin vitelline membrane, thick zona pellucida and first polar body (Image courtesy: *Dr Keshav Malhotra*)

Table 3.3	Differences between sperm and ovum
Sperm	Ovum
It is a male gamete.	It is a female gamete.
It has less width (2 μm) than ovum.	It has more width (120 μm) than sperm.
It is motile.	It is immotile.
It has very less cytoplasm.	It has abundant cytoplasm.
It has X or Y chromosome.	It has only X chromosome.
It undergoes capacitation.	It does not undergo capacitation.
It does not undergo second meiotic division after fertilization.	It undergoes second meiotic division after fertilization.
It is not surrounded by any cell layer.	It is surrounded by corona radiata cells.
It has acrosome cap, spirally arranged mitochondrion, axial filament and tail.	It has zona pellucida.

Chapter 4

First Week of Development

eSmartQuiz

Chapter Outline

- Fertilization
  - Stages of fertilization
    - Approximation of gametes
    - Contact and fusion of gametes
    - Consequences of fertilization
- Parthenogenesis
- Cleavage
- Hydatidiform mole
- Functions of zona pellucida
- Implantation
  - Site of implantation
  - Process of implantation
  - Abnormal implantation
- Changes in trophoblast during implantation

Competencies:
- **AN77.4:** Describe the stages and consequences of fertilization.
- **AN78.1:** Describe cleavage and formation of blastocyst.
- **AN78.3:** Describe the process of implantation and common abnormal sites of implantation.

INTRODUCTION

- A period of first week of development starts with fertilization (fusion of an ovum and a spermatozoon) and ends with implantation (process of penetration of product of conceptus into uterine endometrium).
- Major events of the first week of human development are listed in Table 4.1 and Fig. 4.1.

Table 4.1 Events in the first week of development

Day	Event
Day 0	Approximation of ovum and sperms
	Fertilization of ovum
Day 1	2-cell stage
Day 2	4-cell stage
Day 3	8-cell stage
Day 4	Formation of morula
Day 5	Formation of blastocyst
Day 6	Beginning of implantation

FERTILIZATION

Q. Write a short note on fertilization.

- **Definition**
  Fertilization is the process of fusion of two mature germ cells, an ovum and a spermatozoon (haploid cells) to form a single cell, ***zygote*** (diploid cell).
- Fertilization is a process of fusion or antithesis of cell division.^{MCQ} Haploid gametes fuse to form a diploid undifferentiated zygote.
- Usual site of fertilization: Ampulla of uterine (fallopian) tube.^{NEXT,Viva}

Stages of Fertilization (Practice Fig. 4.1)

- Fertilization involves three basic steps events:
  1. Approximation of gametes
  2. Contact and fusion of gametes
  3. Consequences or effects of fertilization.

1. Approximation of Gametes (Fig. 4.2, Fig. 4.3A)

- It involves transport of spermatozoa and ovum in female genital tract towards the ampulla of uterine tube (usual site of fertilization) (Flowchart 4.1).
- Spermatozoa transport is affected by the following factors:

25

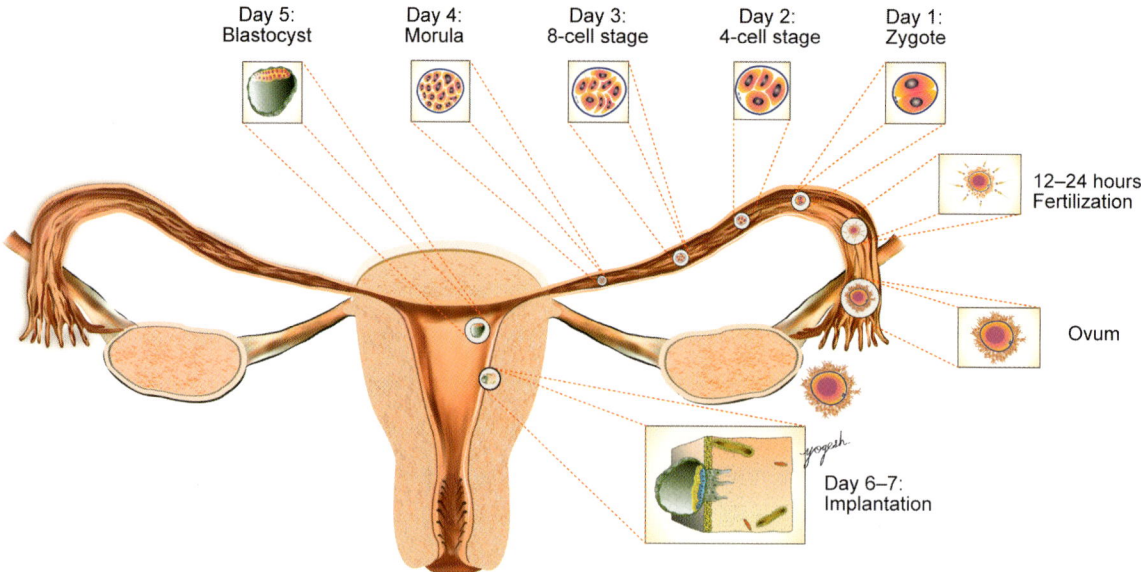

Fig. 4.1: Events in the first week of development

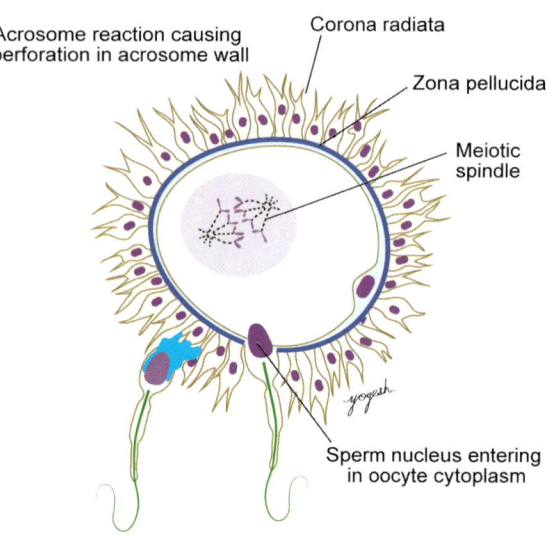

Practice Fig. 4.1: Fertilization

- *Liquefaction of semen*: Semen contains fibrinolysin that liquefies semen within 30 minutes after ejaculation.
- *Contractions of uterine muscles:* Prostaglandins of semen stimulate peristaltic contractions in the female genital tract.
- *Effect of oxytocin:* Sexual intercourse stimulates secretion of oxytocin from neurohypophysis that also produces uterine contractions.
- *Aspiration of sperms:* Repeated uterine contractions generates vacuum (syringe-like action) that aspirates sperm into uterine cavity and later into uterine tube.
- *Chemotaxis:* Sperm is attracted towards ovum by chemicals secreted by corona radiata cells that surround the ovum.

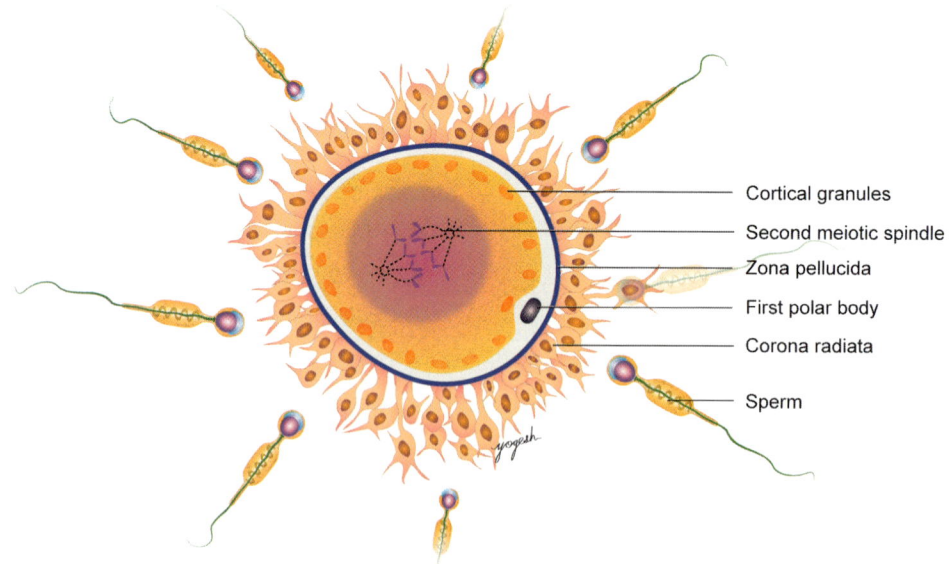

Fig. 4.2: Fertilization. Phase of approximation of gametes

- Only 1% of deposited sperms in vagina enter the uterine cervix and only 300–500 sperms reach the fallopian tube (at the site of fertilization).^MCQ,
- Sperms require 2–7 hours for transport from cervix to fallopian tube.
- *Lifespan of sperm*: After ejaculation, sperms are viable for 24–48 hours in female reproductive tract (maximum up to 4 days).^NEXT,Viva
- Transport of ovum
  - Ovum enters the fimbriated part of fallopian tube due to ciliary beats and rhythmic contractions of uterine tube musculature. Sweeping movements of fimbria also helps in oocyte transport.
  - Transcoelomic migration: Ovum released by an ovary aspirated into fallopian tube by transcoelomic migration. Even ovum may enter the fallopian tube of opposite side.
  - Duration: Ovum takes 25 minutes to reach ampulla of uterine tube.
- *Lifespan of ovum:* Ovum is viable for 24–48 hours after ovulation (Flowchart 4.1).^NEXT,Viva

Flowchart 4.1: Approximation of gametes

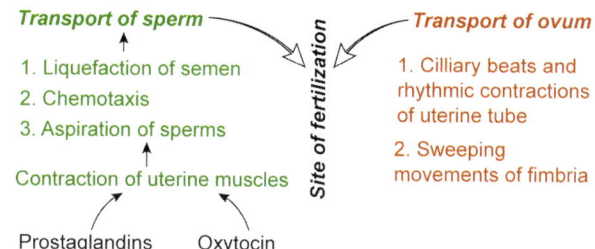

Some Interesting Facts
Clinical Facts
- Nonsteroidal anti-inflammatory drugs (like aspirin) have antiprostaglandin effects. Their regular intake by female reduces sperm transport in female reproductive tract and may impart reduced fertility.

2. Contact and Fusion of Gametes (Fig. 4.3, Flowcharts 4.2, 4.3)

- *Three barriers:* Sperm must break three barriers (corona radiata, zona pellucida and vitelline membrane) of secondary oocyte for fertilization.^MCQ,Viva

Flowchart 4.2: Contact and fusion of gametes

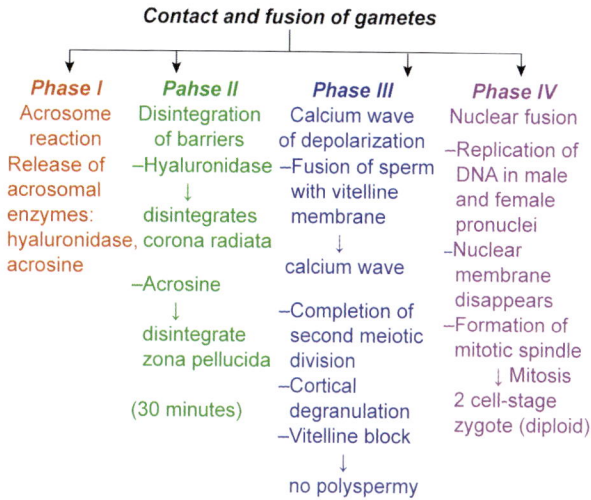

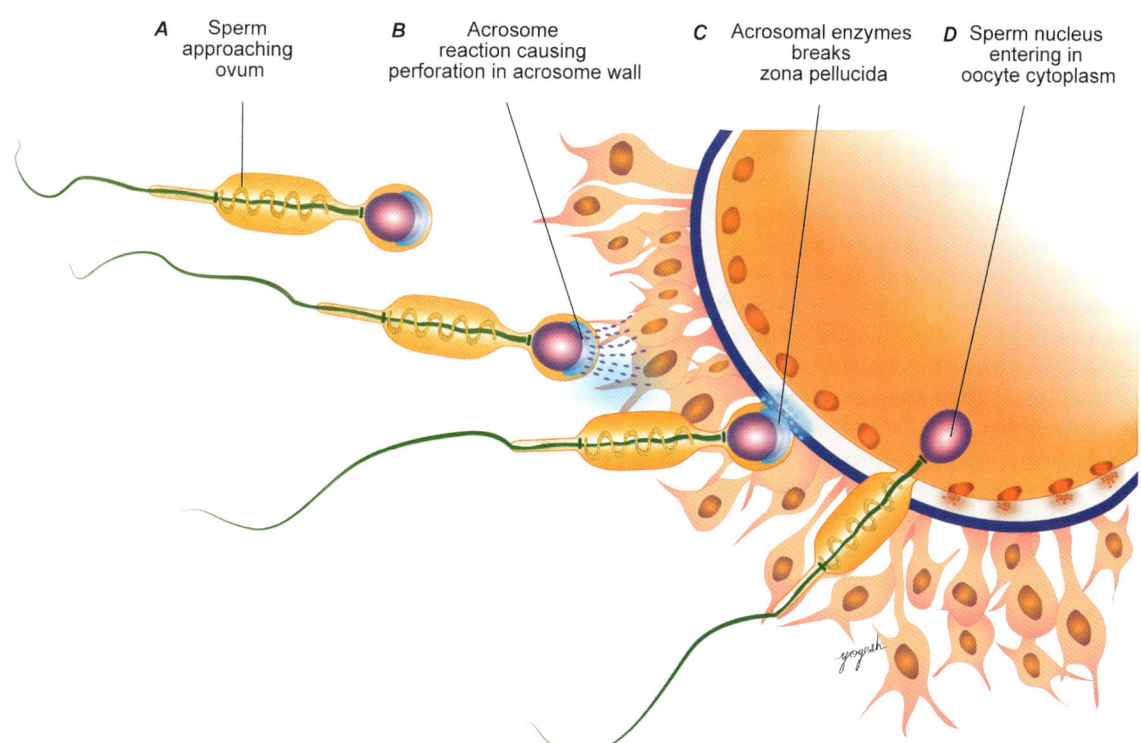

Fig. 4.3: Fertilization. Phase of sperm penetration through coverings of the ovum

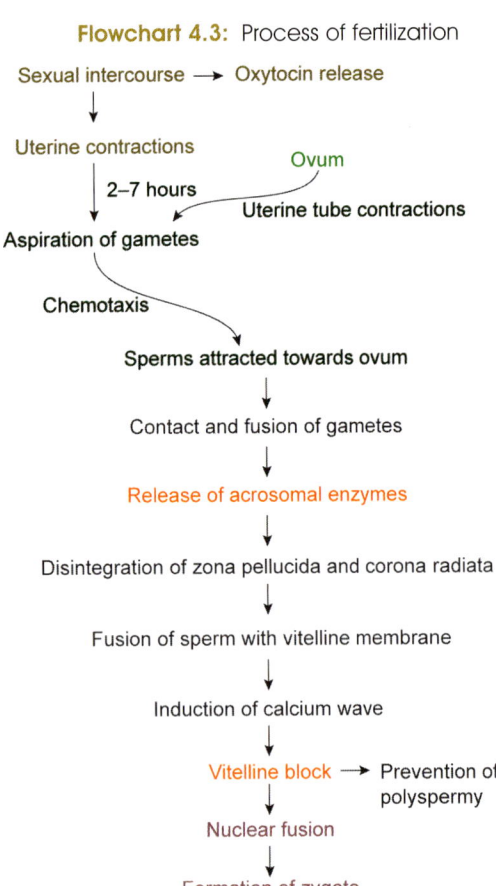

Flowchart 4.3: Process of fertilization

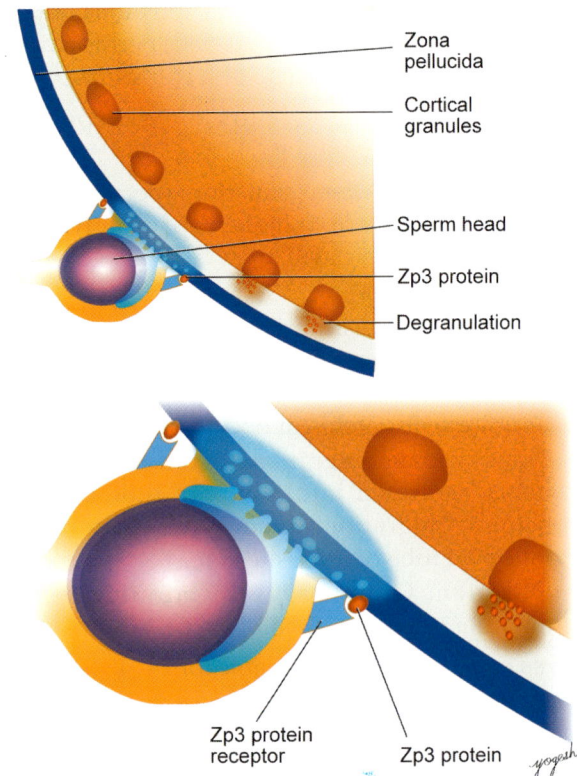

Fig. 4.4: Role of Zp3 proteins. Zp3 proteins of zona pellucida bind with Zp3 receptors of sperm

- *Capacitation:* During transport of sperm in female reproductive tract, they undergo capacitation. It is a process of conditioning or maturation of spermatozoa. During capacitation, coat of glycoproteins and seminal plasma proteins from head of spermatozoa is removed to enhance sperm motility. Capacitation requires 7 hours.$^{MCQ, Viva}$
- Four phases are involved in the penetration of sperm into ovum as follows:^{NEXT}

Phase I: Acrosome reaction

- Acrosome cap establishes multiple contacts with plasma membrane of sperm head and releases acrosomal enzymes.
- Acrosome enzymes include hyaluronidase, acrosine (protease enzyme and acid phosphatase).^{MCQ,,Viva}

Phase II: Disintegration of barriers (Figs 4.3, 4.4)

- Hyaluronidase (acrosomal enzyme) disintegrates corona radiata (Fig. 4.3B).
- Sperm head binds with Zp2 and Zp3 receptor proteins of zona pellucida (Zp = zona pellucida).
- Acrosine (protease enzyme from acrosome) disintegrates zona pellucida (Fig. 4.3C).
- Disintegrin peptides of sperms and integrin of vitelline membrane of ovum help in fusion of sperm plasma membrane with vitelline membrane (Fig. 4.3D).
- Phase II takes about 30 minutes to complete.

Phase III: Calcium wave for the depolarization of oocyte

- Sperm fusion with vitelline membrane of oocyte induces calcium wave and depolarizes vitelline membrane.
- Calcium wave is responsible for the following changes:
  i. Secondary oocyte completes second meiotic division and one set of chromosomes as a female pronucleus, whereas expel another set as a *second polar body* in perivitelline space.
  ii. *Calcium* wave triggers release of cortical granules (lysosomal enzymes) to form oocyte that hydrolyses Zp3 receptors on zona pellucida (called zona reaction) and prevents further binding of sperms.^{NEXT}
  iii. Release of cortical granules alters the vitelline membrane and induces *vitelline block* that prevents *polyspermy* (entry of multiple sperms in ovum).^{NEXT}

Phase IV: Nuclear fusion (Fig. 4.5)

- Only nucleus and tail of sperm enter into the cytoplasm of oocyte (ooplasm) leaving behind body and cytoplasm.
- Male pronucleus (sperm nucleus) approaches towards the female pronucleus. Tail of the sperm degenerates (Fig. 4.5A, Flowchart 4.2).
- Both male and female pronuclei replicate their DNA and lose their nuclear membrane (Fig. 4.5B).
- DNA condenses to form mitotic spindle and later with longitudinal splitting at centromere, sister chromatids move towards the opposite poles (Fig. 4.5C).

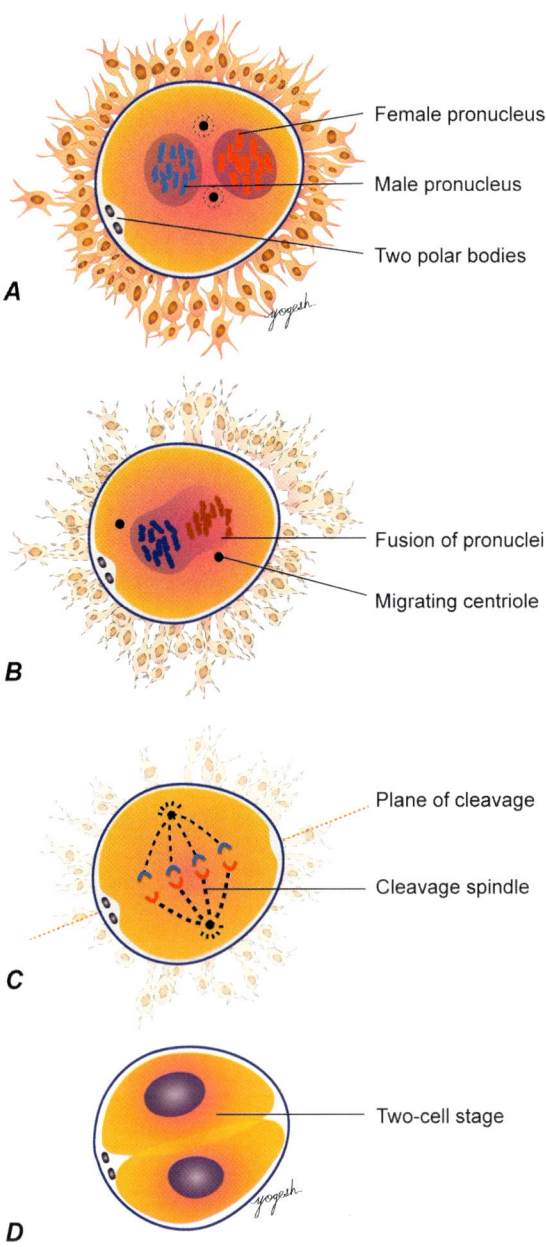

Fig. 4.5: Formation of zygote

Formation of zygote: Finally, cytoplasm divides to form two cells with a diploid number of chromosomes. It is called *zygote* (*zugotos* = *yolked*, in Greek).

3. Consequences or effects of Fertilization

Q. List the effects (consequences or results) of fertilization.

Fertilization has the following results (Flowchart 4.4): *Viva*

1. Completion of second meiotic division of secondary oocyte (female gamete).
2. Restoration of a diploid number of chromosomes (46). Haploid male (23) and haploid female (23) pronuclei fuse to form a diploid zygote (46).
3. Determination of chromosomal sex: If a fertilizing sperm carries X chromosome, the resultant zygote forms a female fetus and if a fertilizing sperm carries *Y chromosome*, the resultant zygote forms a male fetus.
4. Initiation of cleavage: Fertilization provides energy for repetitive cell divisions of zygote.

Some Interesting Facts

1. Embryo receives mitochondria from ooplasm (mother) only. Sperm does not contribute any mitochondria. Hence, abnormal mitochondrial DNA shows *maternal inheritance*. *MCQ*
2. Sex determination entirely depends on sex chromosome of sperm (male partner) only.
3. Fallopian tubes are lined by ciliated columnar epithelium. *NEXT*
4. Secondary oocyte has haploid number of chromosomes (2N). *NEXT*
5. Fertilization takes place within 1–2 days after ovulation. *NEXT*
6. In *in vitro* fertilization, the fertilization is considered as complete on the appearance of second polar body. *NEXT*
7. *Mosaics and chimera* are the individuals that have more than one genetically distinct population of cells. All cell lines arise from single zygote in mosaic, whereas from more than one zygote in chimeras. *NEXT*

Box 4.1: Parthenogenesis

Definition

- Parthenogenesis is a method of asexual reproduction that involves development of embryo by cleavage division of female gamete without fertilization.
- *Parthenas* means *virgin* and *genesis* means *creation* in Greek.
- Parthenogenesis occurs in many plants, some invertebrate animals and a few vertebrates (some fish and reptiles).
- In human, parthenogenesis may occur as an ovarian teratoma, but a complete viable fetus cannot be formed.

Flowchart 4.4: Consequences/effects of fertilization

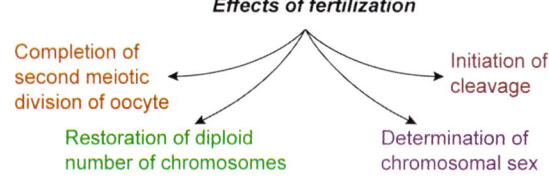

CLEAVAGE

Q. Write a short note on cleavage.
Q. Write a short note on morula.

- *Definition*
  Cleavage is a process of repeated mitotic segmentation of zygote within zona pellucida to give rise to small cells called *blastomeres*. *Viva*

- In a cleavage, fertilized ovum is divided to form 2-cell, 3-cell, 4-cell stage and so on.
- *Duration*: Up to 6–7 days after fertilization till implantation.
- *Site*: It continues from the ampulla of fallopian tube till conceptus reaches the site of implantation in uterus.

Events or Stages (Fig. 4.6, Practice Fig. 4.2)

- In each division of cleavage, zygote divides the cytoplasm unequally to form one large and another small cell. Larger cell divides first followed by a smaller one (Flowchart 4.5).
- Cleavage aims at formation of morula and later blastocyst.

A. Formation of morula

- Zygote continues divisions one after another to form various stages as follows:

  1st cleavage: 2-cell stage (24–30 hours after fertilization) (Fig. 4.6A)

  2nd cleavage: 4-cell stage (40–50 hours after fertilization) (Fig. 4.6B)

  3rd cleavage: 8-cell stage (66 hours after fertilization) (Fig. 4.6C)

  Compaction: After third cleavage, blastomeres maximize contact with each other to form a compact ball of cells. During compaction, blastomeres segregates into inner cell mass and outer trophoblasts (wide below).

  4th cleavage: 16-cell stage (96 hours after fertilization) (Fig. 4.6D)

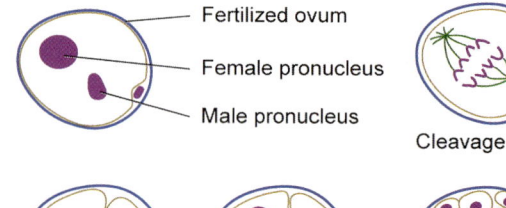
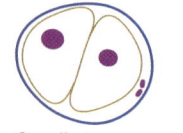
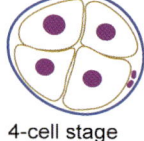
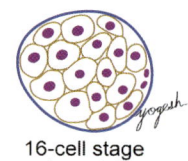

Practice Fig. 4.2: Cleavage and formation of morula

Flowchart 4.5: Cleavage and formation of morula

Cleavage
– Repeated mitotic segmentation of zygote → blastomeres
– Lasts for 6–7 days after fertilization

Diploid zygote
1st cleavage ↓ 30 hours after fertilization
2-cell stage
2nd cleavage ↓ 40–50 hours after fertilization
4-cell stage
3rd cleavage / Compaction ↓ 72 hours after fertilization
8-cell stage
4th cleavage ↓ 96 hours after fertilization
16-cell stage (morula)
↓ ↓
Inner embryoblast   Outer trophoblast
↓ ↓
Embryo   Placenta

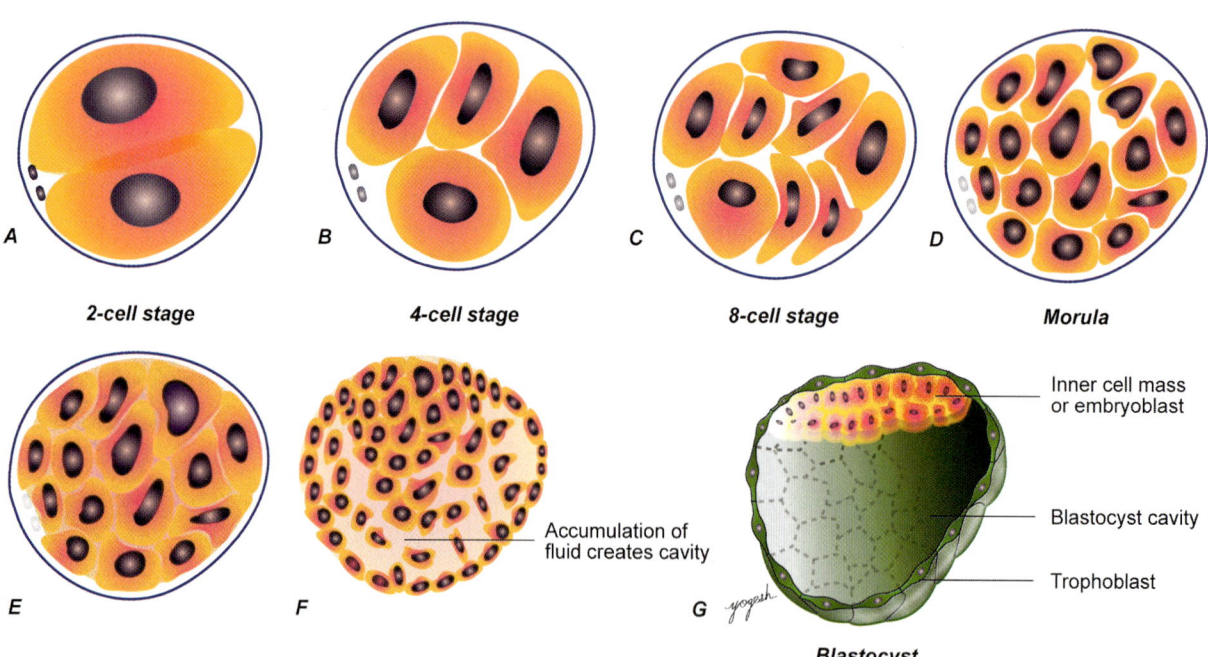

Fig. 4.6: Formation of morula and blastocyst

- *Morula*
  - 16-cell stage looks similar to mulberry; hence, called *morula*.^{NEXT}
  - Morula consists of
    - *Inner cell mass* or *embryoblast* that forms future embryo. These cells communicate with each other by gap junctions.
    - Outer *trophoblast* that forms covering of embryo.^{NEXT} Trophoblast is also called **trophectoderm** (Gray's Anatomy, 41st Ed).^{NEXT}
    - Morula is covered by zona pellucida.^{NEXT}

B. **Formation of blastocyst** (Figs 4.6, 4.7, Practice Fig. 4.3, Flowchart 4.6)

Q. Write a short note on formation of blastocyst.
- Cells of morula continue to divide and form 32–64-cell stage (Fig. 4.6E).
- Uterine fluid slowly diffuses through zona pellucida and gets accumulated in intercellular spaces of morula (Fig. 4.6F).
- Accumulated fluid increases intercellular spaces, forms cavities that fuse to form a single cavity called *blastocoel* (Fig. 4.6G).
- Outer flattened lining cells of blastocoel form a *trophoblast* and the inner cell mass forms *embryoblast*.

Flowchart 4.6: Formation of blastocyst

Morula
↓ Cellular divisions
32–64 Cell stage
↓ Diffusion of uterine fluid
Increased intercellular spaces
↓
Fusion of intercellular spaces
↓
Formation of blastocoel (cavity)
↓   ↓
Outer trophoblast   Inner embryoblast
↓
Formation of blastocyst

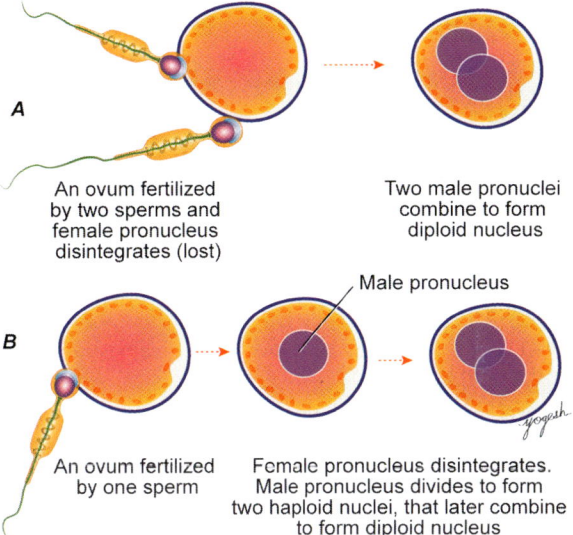

Fig. 4.8: Formation of complete hydatidiform mole

- Thus, embryoblast with blastocoel and trophoblast form *blastocyst*.
- Side of the embryoblast attachment with the trophoblast is *embryonic* or *animal pole*, whereas the opposite side is an *abembryonic pole* (Practice Fig. 4.3).
- Trophoblast in contact with embryoblast is *polar trophoblast*, whereas the rest is *mural* trophoblast.
- Transport during cleavage:
  - Zygote gradually migrates away from fertilization site towards uterine cavity.
  - This migration is assisted by *ciliary beats* and contraction of musculature of fallopian tube.^{NEXT}
- Fate of blastocyst
  - Embryoblasts – embryo
  - Trophoblasts – placenta (*trophe* = nutrition, in Greek)
  - Blastocoel – yolk sac

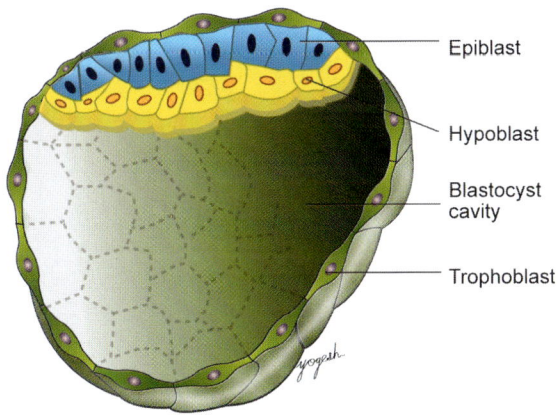

Fig. 4.7: Blastocyst. Differentiation of inner cell mass into epiblast and hypoblast

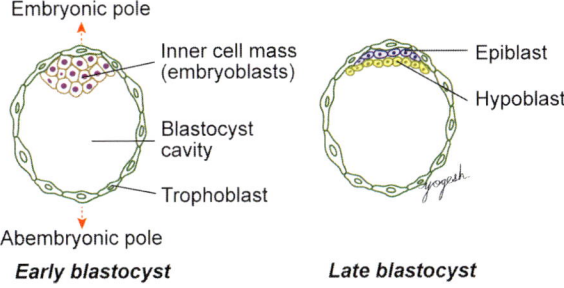

Practice Fig. 4.3: Blastocyst

Box 4.2: Hydatidiform mole

- Hydatidiform mole is also called *molar pregnancy* in which a nonviable fertilized ovum implants in the uterus.^{MCQ}
- Pathology:
  - Complete mole: During fertilization, female pronucleus disintegrates, and male chromosomes duplicate. Later, such fertilized egg having only paternal chromosomes can form only trophoblasts and fail to form an embryo (Fig. 4.8A, B).
  - Partial mole: Duplicated paternal chromosomes fuse with female pronucleus to form triploidy (69,XXY or 69,XYY) chromosomes (Fig. 4.9).^{MCQ}
- The differences between complete and partial hydatidiform mole are listed in Table 4.2.

Table 4.2	Difference between complete and partial hydatidiform mole	
Difference	Complete mole	Partial mole
Karyotype	46,XX or 46,XY	Triploid (69,XXY or 69,XYY)
Embryo	Absent	Present
Swelling of chorionic villi	Diffuse	Focal
Human chorionic gonadotropin	Very high levels	Elevated levels
Choriocarcinoma conversion	2% chance	rare
Pathology	2 sperms + empty egg	2 sperms + egg

Note: Choriocarcinoma is an invasive trophoblastic tumor.

IMPLANTATION

Q. Write a short note on implantation.

- **Definition**

  Implantation is a process of penetration of product of conceptus (blastocyst) into the uterine endometrium (Fig. 4.9).

- *Time*: Implantation begins on 6th or 7th day after fertilization and completes by the 12th day (20th–22nd day of the menstrual cycle).^{NEXT}

- *Note*: Implantation begins at the end of first week (at the stage of blastocyst), hence it is included in this chapter.

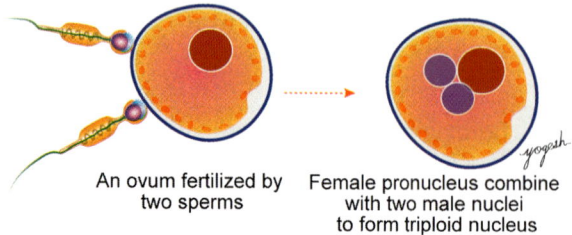

Fig. 4.9: Formation of partial hydatidiform mole

Box 4.3: Functions of Zona Pellucida^{Viva}

Q. Write a short note on functions of zona pellucida.

Zona pellucida is the acellular layer that surrounds ovum, zygote, morula and disappears on hatching of blastocyst in 4–7 days after fertilization.^{NEXT}

1. Prevents implantation: Zona pellucida prevents trophoblast from sticking with uterine epithelium.
2. Zp3 proteins of zona pellucida help in sperm binding.
3. Zona pellucida glycoproteins induce acrosomal reaction.
4. On penetration of sperm, it undergoes zona reaction to prevent polyspermy (entry of multiple sperms.)
5. Allows diffusion of uterine secretion for nourishment of blastomeres and formation of blastocyst cavity.
6. Disappearance of zona pellucida only on 6–7 days of fertilization facilitates implantation in uterus and prevents ectopic pregnancy.

Site of Implantation (Fig. 4.10)

- Usually, implantation occurs in the upper part of body of the uterus in mid-sagittal plane.^{MCQ, Viva}
- Mostly, it happens on the posterior uterine wall (55%) or anterior uterine wall (45%).
- In human, as blastocyst implants in endometrium, it is called *interstitial implantation*.^{MCQ, Viva}

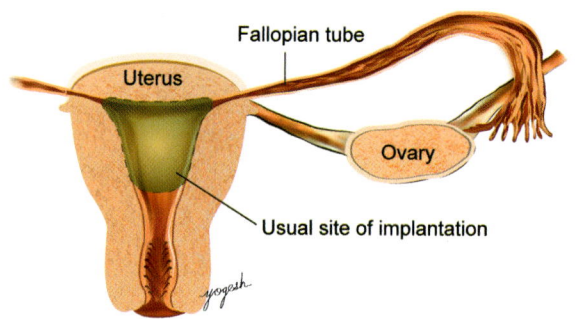

Fig. 4.10: Normal site of implantation. On seventh day after fertilization, blastocyst usually implants in endometrium of uterus at the posterior wall of superior part of uterus (the site of implantation is shown by shaded region)

Process of Implantation (Fig. 4.11, Practice Fig. 4.4, Flowchart 4.7)

- *Hatching of blastocyst:* Zona pellucida prevents implantation. By the sixth day of fertilization, zona pellucida disintegrates by the enzymes releasesd from trophoblast.^{NEXT}
- Polar trophoblast adheres with the uterine epithelium.
- Trophoblast secretes proteolytic enzymes that erode endometrium to make passage for blastocyst.
- Blastocyst burrows deep till it completely come to lie within the endometrium.

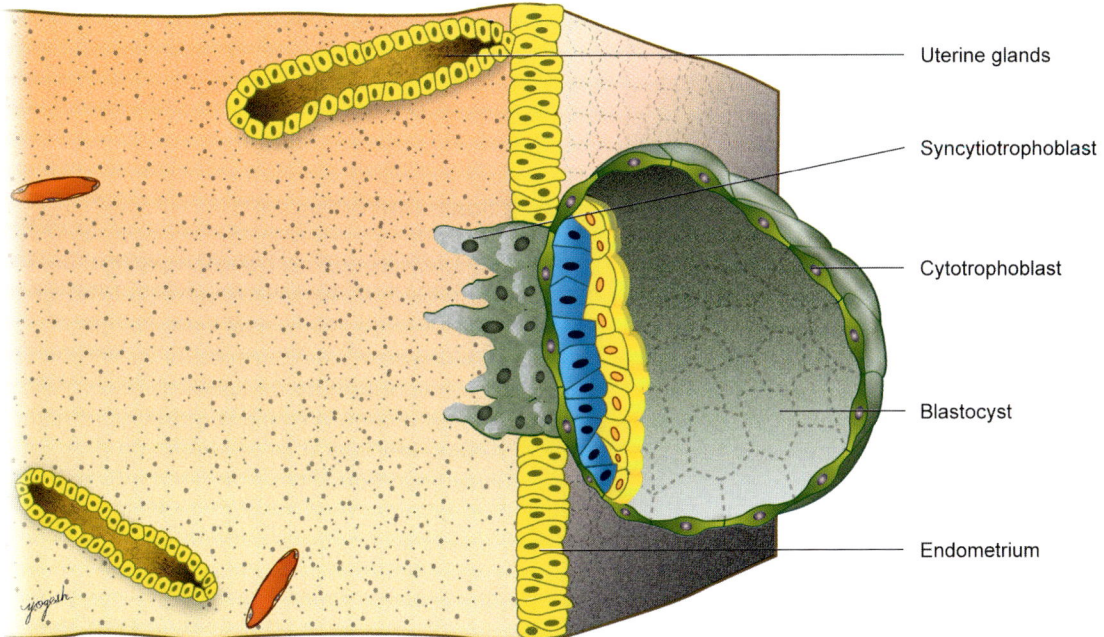

Fig. 4.11: Implantation – trophoblastic invasion. Trophoblastic cells start invading endometrium

- *Note:* Binding of trophoblast is assisted by an interaction between the pentasaccharide-lato-*N*-fucopentose-1 of epithelial surface and its receptor on trophoblast. L-selectin of trophoblast cells binds with carbohydrate receptors of uterine endometrium.
- Closure of penetration defect by surface epithelium takes place by 9th day after fertilization with the formation of fibrin plug.

Abnormal Implantation (Fig. 4.11)^Viva

Q. List the abnormal sites of implantation.

- If conceptus does not implant at the usual site, that is, upper part of body of uterus in endometrium, it is called abnormal or ectopic implantation and it results in *ectopic pregnancy*.
- Ectopic pregnancy or implantation are classified according to their site of implantation as follows:

  A. Uterine abnormal implantation:
  - *Placenta previa (cervical):* It is an implantation in lower uterine segment in which placenta overlaps internal os.^MCQ
  - *Intramural implantation:* The conceptus lies within the myometrium.

  B. Tubal implantation: It is an implantation in uterine tube. It is the most common extrauterine implantation.^MCQ,

  C. Abdominal implantation: It is a rare ectopic implantation. It usually occurs in the ovary or mesentery (Fig. 4.12).

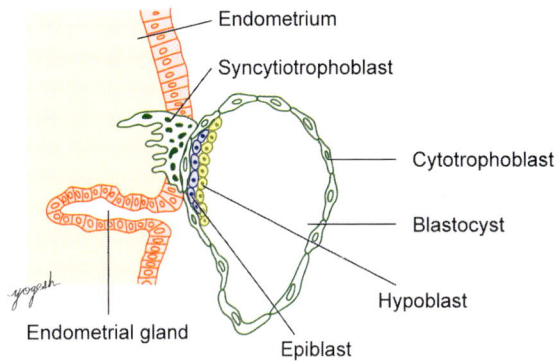

Practice Fig. 4.4: Implantation

Flowchart 4.7: Process of implantation

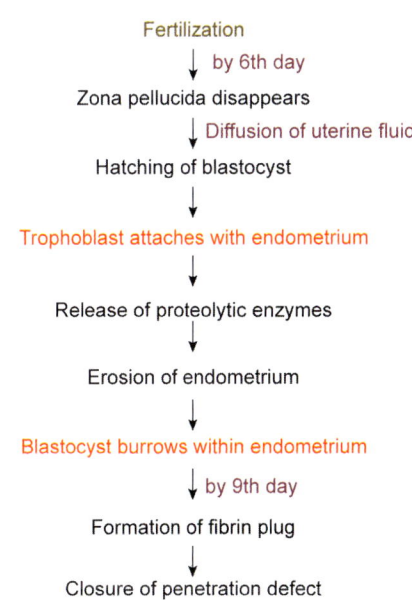

• First Week of Development

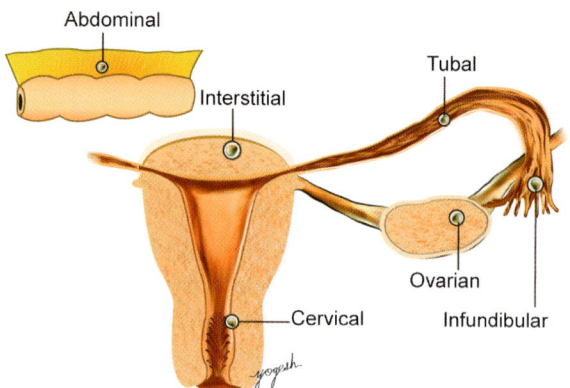

Fig. 4.12: Abnormal sites of implantation. Ovarian, tubal, infundibular, cervical, interstitial, abdominal

CHANGES IN TROPHOBLAST DURING IMPLANTATION

- As soon as polar trophoblast attaches to uterine endometrium, trophoblasts start differentiating into two layers on 6–8 days after fertilization (Fig. 4.9).*NEXT*
  - Cytotrophoblast forms inner cell layer.*NEXT*
  - Syncytiotrophoblast forms outer layer. Cells of syncytiotrophoblast form multinucleated protoplasmic mass without distinct cell boundaries.
  - Finger-like processes of syncytiotrophoblast help to invade endometrium.

Some Interesting Facts

- Humans are *viviparous animals*. Embryos of viviparous animals receive nutrition from mothers and retain scanty egg yolk.
- Continuous expression of *Oct4* and *Nanog* transcription factor converts blastomeres into inner cell mass and repression (decreased expression) of these factors by eomesodermin convert blastomere into trophoblasts.
- Fertilized ovum reaches the uterus in 4–5 days (at 32-cell stage).*NEXT*
- *Decidual reaction* is a change in uterine endometrium that occurs in secretory phase of menstrual cycle. These changes make endometrium favorable for implantation of blastocyst.
- Blastocyst makes contact with endometrium on 5–7 days (1–2 days prior to the implantation).*NEXT*

Clinical Embryology

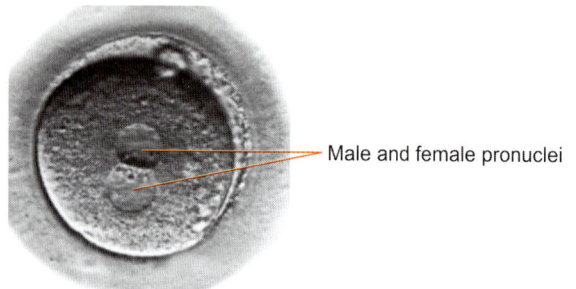

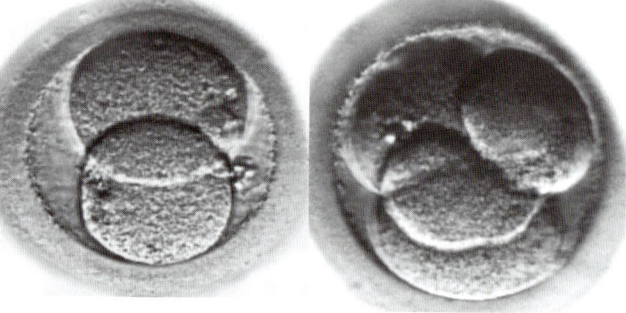

2-cell stage   4-cell stage

Clinical image 4.1: Human zygote. In fertilization, fusion of two mature germ cells, an ovum and a spermatozoon (haploid cells) form a single cell, zygote (diploid cell) (Image courtesy: Dr Keshav Malhotra)

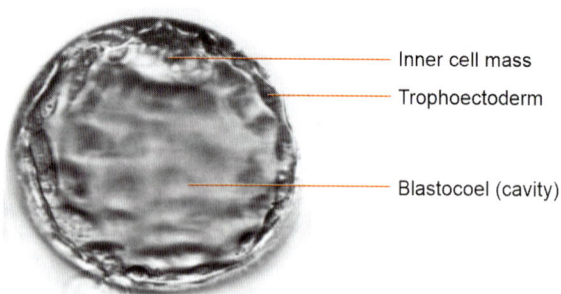

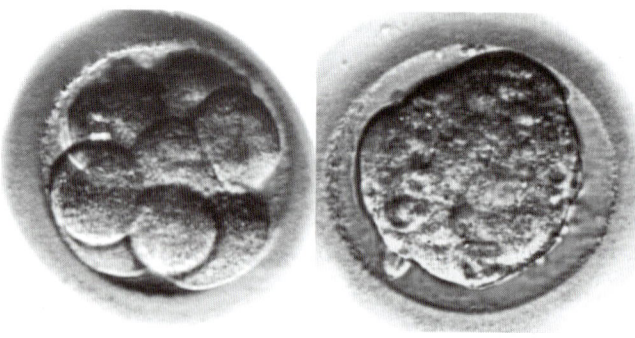

8-cell stage   Morula

Clinical image 4.2: Cells of morula continue to divide and form 32–64 cell stage. Accumulated fluid increases intercellular spaces, form a cavity called blastocoel. Outer flattened lining cells of blastocoel form trophoblast and inner cell mass forms embryoblast. Embryoblast with blastocoel and trophoblast form blastocyst (115–120 hours after fertilization). (Image courtesy: Dr Keshav Malhotra)

Clinical image 4.3: Human zygote continues division one after another. 1st cleavage: 2-cell stage (24–30 hours after fertilization), 2nd cleavage: 4-cell stage (40–50 hours after fertilization), 3rd cleavage: 8-cell stage (66 hours after fertilization) and 4th cleavage: 16-cell stage (90–96 hours after fertilization). The 16-cell stage looks similar to mulberry; hence, called morula (Image courtesy: Dr Keshav Malhotra)

Assisted Reproduction Technology
In vitro Fertilization and Intracytoplasmic Sperm Injection

Chapter 5

Chapter Outline

- *In vitro* fertilization
  - Uses of *in vitro* fertilization
  - Stages of IVF
- Ovarian hyperstimulation syndrome
- Success rate in ART
- Surgical sperm extraction
- Intracytoplasmic sperm injection (ICSI)
  - Indications
  - Protocol
- Artificial insemination
- Gamete intrafallopian transfer
- Zygote intrafallopian transfer
- Egg freezing (oocyte cryopreservation)

INTRODUCTION

- Having a child is always a great gift of nature to human beings.
- About 1 in 6 couples have difficulty in conceiving naturally.
- About 90% of infertile couples can conceive with medical intervention.
- Assisted reproductive technology is used to support the infertile patients.
- Table 5.1 lists various assisted reproductive techniques.

Table 5.1 Methods of assisted reproductive technology

1. Counselling for reproduction
2. Fertility medications that help to form ovarian follicles. For example, gonadotropins and gonadotropin-releasing hormone.
3. *In vitro* fertilization (IVF): It involves fertilization of ovum outside the female body.
4. Gamete intrafallopian transfer (GIFT): It involves the direct transfer of sperms and ovum in the fallopian tube.
5. Zygote intrafallopian transfer (ZIFT): It involves the direct transfer of zygote in the fallopian tube.
6. Surgical approach: It involves surgical treatment of fallopian tube obstruction and vas deferens obstruction.

IN VITRO FERTILIZATION

- *Definition: In vitro* fertilization is a process of fertilizing ovum outside the body.
- The first baby born by *in vitro* fertilization was *Louise Brown* on 25th July 1978. Kanupriya Agarwal (Durga) is world's second and India's first IVF baby born on 3rd October 1978.
- Founders of IVF are Robert Edward (The Noble Prize, 2010) and Patrick Steptoe.
- IVF is also known as *test-tube baby*.

Uses (Indications) of IVF

- *In vitro* fertilization is useful in the following conditions:
  1. Blockage of fallopian tube
  2. Problem with ovulation
  3. Endometriosis
  4. Polycystic ovarian syndrome
  5. Cervical problems
  6. Male infertility factors

Stages of IVF

The basic steps involved in IVF are as follows (Flowchart 5.1, Fig. 5.1):

Stage 1: Ovarian stimulation and monitoring
Stage 2: Oocyte retrieval

Flowchart 5.1: Stages of *in vitro* fertilization

Stage 1: Ovarian stimulation
Injectable GnRH, FSH, LH
↓
Stage 2: Oocyte retrieval
hCG → induction of ovulation
USG guided aspiration
↓
Stage 3: In vitro fertilization
↓
Stage 4: Development of embryo
Fertilized ovum is incubated at 37°C till the stage of blastocyst
↓
Stage 5: Transfer of embryo
Embryo transfer through vaginal route using a catheter
↓
Stage 6: Luteal phase support
Injectable progesterone to maintain pregnancy

Abbreviations: GnRH: Gonadotropin-releasing hormone; FSH: Follicle stimulating hormone; LH: Luteinizing hormone; hCG: Human chorionic gonadotropin; USG: Ultrasonography

Stage 3: Fertilization
Stage 4: Embryo development
Stage 5: Embryo transfer
Stage 6: Luteal phase support

Stage 1: Ovarian Stimulation and Monitoring

- During each menstrual cycle, the following hormones play important roles:
  i. Gonadotropin-releasing hormone (GnRH): It is secreted by hypothalamus (part of a brain) and stimulates pituitary gland to release follicle stimulating hormone.
  ii. Follicle stimulating hormone (FSH): It is secreted by pituitary on GnRH stimulus and promotes maturation of ovarian follicles and prepares endometrium for implantation.
  iii. Luteinizing hormone (LH): It is secreted by pituitary gland and induces ovulation.

- *Medicine for follicle development:*
  – In assisted reproductive technology, injectable hormones are given to induce follicle development and ovulation. In each cycle, 5–10 secondary oocytes are collected.
  – For this purpose, the following treatments may be given:
    a. FSH (gonadotropin): It is given in injectable form for the development of follicles.
    b. GnRH: It is given in injectable form on a daily basis for the first 2 weeks to prevent premature ovulation. It makes multiple eggs available for IVF.
    c. Nafarelin acetate: It has same effects similar to GnRH. It is given on a daily basis (morning and night) as a nasal spray.
    d. Leuprorelin: It has same effects similar to GnRH. It is given as subcutaneous injections.
    e. Cetrorelix and ganirelix: These are injectable GnRH antagonists and prevent premature ovulation.
    f. Luteinizing hormone (LH): LH induces ovulation. In IVF, naturally occurring LH surge (that usually induces ovulation) needs to be avoided by suppressing pituitary gland's LH and FSH secretion. It is called *pituitary suppression* or *down regulation*.

    Protocol 1: It is achieved with the help of nafarelin or leuprorelin given for first 10 days of the cycle.

    Protocol 2: It can also be achieved with the help of GnRH antagonists (cetrorelix or ganirelix) given from fifth or sixth day after commencement of FSH injections and continued till ovulation induction.

Monitoring:
- Ultrasound examinations are used for monitoring follicle growth in ovaries.
- Estrogen or estradiol (E2) blood levels can be monitored. These hormones are produced by developing follicle in response to FSH treatment.
- Monitoring is required to determine the timing for induction of ovulation.

Stage 2: Oocyte Retrieval

- It is also called egg retrieval or egg pickup.
- Induction of ovulation: Injectable human chorionic gonadotropin or luteinizing hormone is given 36 hours before preplanned egg pickup.
- Methods of egg pickup:
  1. Ultrasound-guided aspiration: Under mild sedation and local anesthesia, eggs are aspirated with the ultrasound-guided fine needle. The needle is passed through the vaginal wall into mature follicle to collect egg.
  2. Laparoscopy assisted aspiration: If ovaries are not readily available via transvaginal approach due to disorders, such as uterine fibroid, laparoscopy is used. Under general anesthesia, eggs are aspirated with gentle suction from matured follicles.
- Collected fluid is examined microscopically for eggs.
- Collected eggs are placed in an incubator.

Box 5.1: Ovarian hyperstimulation syndrome (OHSS)

- Stimulation of ovary by various fertility medicines may produce OHSS.
- Ovaries enlarge and produce a large quantity of fluids.
- Symptoms: Pain and blotting in abdomen.

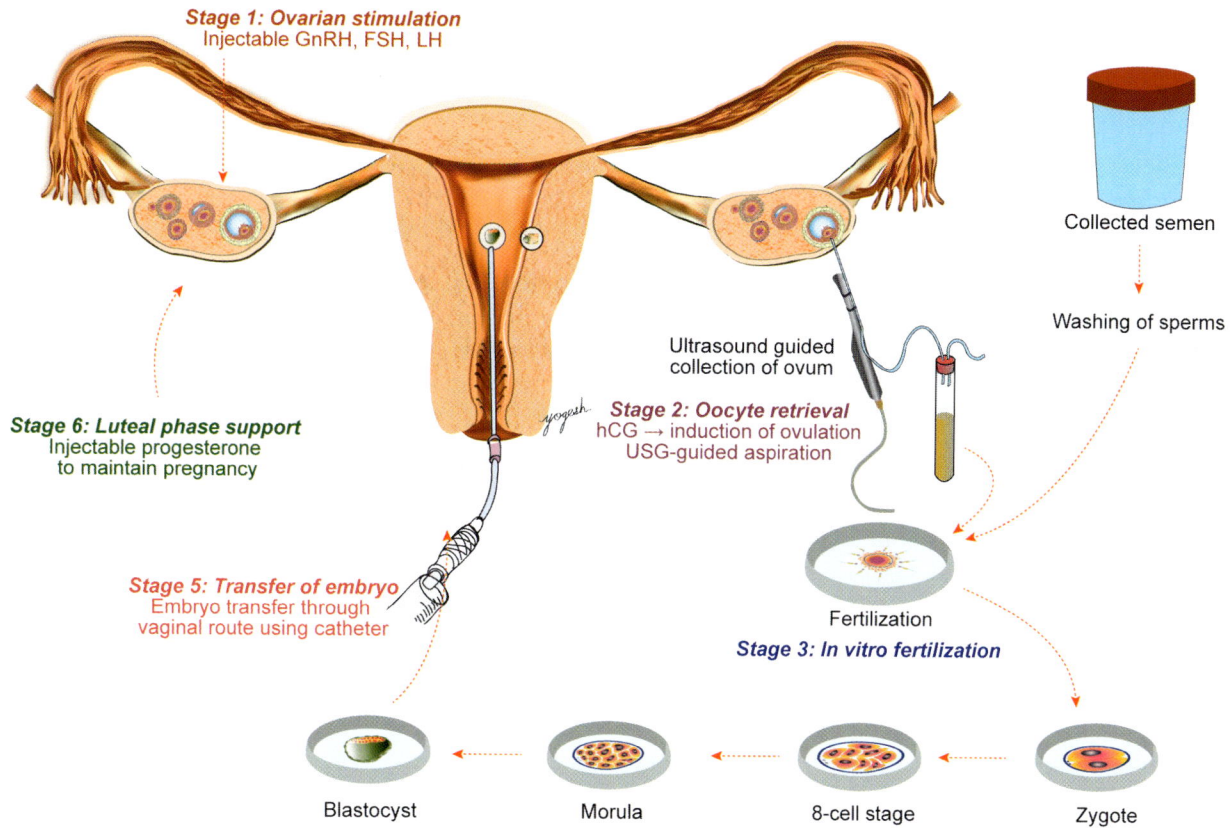

Fig. 5.1: *In vitro* fertilization. It involves six stages as follows: Stage 1, ovarian stimulation and monitoring; Stage 2, oocyte retrieval; Stage 3, fertilization; Stage 4, embryo development; Stage 5, embryo transfer; Stage 6, luteal phase support. Abbreviations: GnRH: Gonadotropin-releasing hormone; FSH: Follicle-stimulating hormone; LH: Luteinizing hormone; hCG: Human chorionic gonadotropin; USG: Ultrasonography

Stage 3: Fertilization

- Collection of sperms: Sperms are collected at clinics 2–3 hours before egg collection.
- Sperm washing: It is a process to remove seminal plasma and nonmotile sperms from semen to improve the chances of fertilization.
- Procedure: Sperms are washed by density gradient centrifugation or direct swim-up technique. Washed sperm are kept in media at 37°C.
- IVF: Sperms and egg are incubated at 37°C for overnight. Next day (16 hours post insemination), eggs are examined microscopically to confirm fertilization.

Stage 4: Embryo Development

- Fertilized ovum is nothing but a cell and it can be grown in a culture media at 37°C.
- *In vitro*, in culture media, zygote starts cleavage.
- A zygote is transferred on or before the day of development, at the stage of the blastocyst. Only one or two fertilized embryos are transferred to uterus for implantation and the remaining are stored with cryopreservation for future use.

Stage 5: Embryo Transfer

- Fertilized embryo or blastocyst is transferred to the uterus using a catheter via vaginal route.
- In one cycle, one or two blastocysts are transferred, whereas remaining is stored with cryopreservation for future.

Stage 6: Luteal Phase Support

- In ART, a collection of ovum results in improper formation of corpus luteum. Hence, there will be lack of sufficient estrogen and progesterone hormone.
- Hence, in IVF pregnancy should be supported at least for first 2 weeks after ovum collection with progesterone.
- Pregnancy can be confirmed by detection of hCG hormone in maternal blood or ultrasonography after 2 weeks of fertilization date.

Success Rate in ART

- Numerous meta analysis have shown live birth rates with ART is to the tune of 30%, clinical pregnancy rate could be 40–50%.
- The success rate is influenced by many factors, such as maternal age, cause of infertility, sperm quality and so on.

> **Box 5.2: Surgical sperm extraction**
>
> - In assisted reproductive technology, if male partner does not have sperms in semen, then it can be collected surgically from epididymis or testis.
>
> *Conditions requiring surgical sperm extractions:*
> 1. Blockage in the ejaculatory duct or vas deferens
> 2. Vasectomy patients

Some Interesting Facts

1. **Assisted hatching**: Disintegration of zona pellucida (hatching) is essential for implantation. In case of repeated IVF failures, older females or cryopreserved egg, assisted hatching may be required. It is done with the help of LASER.
2. **Preimplantation genetic diagnosis (PGD)**: In IVF, PGD can be performed to identify the genetic disorder. Before the transfer of blastocyst on day five to the uterus, one or more cells are collected from the blastocyst. DNA from these cells is analyzed for genetic disorders such as Down syndrome, hemophilia A and so on.

INTRACYTOPLASMIC SPERM INJECTION (ICSI)

- *Definition*: ICSI is a procedure that involves a direct transfer of a single sperm into a cytoplasm of oocyte.
- ICSI technique is developed by G Palermo (1991).

Indications for ICSI

1. Teratozoospermia: Abnormal sperm morphology
2. Poor sperm motility
3. Low sperm count
4. Vasectomy cases or obstruction in passage sperm
5. Antisperm antibodies in male that inhibit sperm functions
6. Obstructive azoosperm

Protocol

- ICSI involves six steps as follows:
  - Stage 1: Ovarian stimulation and monitoring
  - Stage 2: Oocyte retrieval
  - Stage 3: Fertilization
  - Stage 4: Embryo development
  - Stage 5: Embryo transfer
  - Stage 6: Luteal phase support
- All the abovementioned steps are similar to the steps involved in IVF.
- In step 3: Fertilization is carried out with the help of micromanipulator using fine glass micropipettes.
- A glass tool or pipette tip is used to hold the egg in place.
- A sperm is aspirated in a tiny microinjection needle and it is inserted in the cytoplasm of ovum under microscopic view.
- Fertilized egg is incubated overnight at 37°C and observed on next day for fertilization. Later, embryo is transferred to the uterus on fifth day at blastocyst stage.

ARTIFICIAL INSEMINATION

- Artificial insemination is a method of assisted reproductive technology.
- *Definition*: Artificial insemination is the deliberate introduction of sperm into uterus or cervix by means other than sexual intercourse.
- Artificial insemination is of two types:
  1. *Intrauterine insemination* (IUI), and
  2. *Intracervical insemination* (ICI).

Indications

Artificial insemination is preferred in the following conditions:
1. Sperm donation
2. Male infertility
3. Failure of reproduction on natural course

Technique

- Artificial insemination involves the following steps:
  1. Collection of sperms
  2. Transfer of sperms either into cervix (unwashed sperms) or into uterus (washed sperms) using a catheter.
- Female is asked to rest on the table for 15 minutes to increase the pregnancy rate.

Success rate

- The success rate for ICI is 10–15% per menstrual cycle and for IUI is 15–20% per cycle.
- In IUI about 60–70% females achieve pregnancy in 6 cycles.

Table 5.2 lists the indications for commonly used methods of assisted reproductive techniques.

> **Box 5.3: Gamete Intrafallopian Transfer (GIFT)**
>
> - In assisted reproductive technology, collected eggs and sperms are transferred into the fallopian tube using a laparoscope. This technique is currently not in use.
>
> Indications:
> 1. Ovary and at least one of the fallopian tubes of the female should be normal.
> 2. GIFT is preferred in cases of sperm dysfunction or couple with unknown cause of infertility.
> 3. Success rate: Approximately 25–30%.

> **Box 5.4: Zygote Intrafallopian Transfer (ZIFT)**
>
> - In ART, *in vitro* fertilized egg is transferred to fallopian tube using a laparoscope.
> - Success rate: 64.8%. This technique is currently not in use.

Table 5.2	Commonly used methods of assisted reproductive techniques and their indications
Method	Indications
***In vitro* fertilization:** It is a process of fertilizing ovum outside the body.	• Blockage of fallopian tube • Problem with ovulation • Endometriosis • Polycystic ovarian syndrome • Cervical problems
Intracytoplasmic sperm injection (ICSI): It is a procedure that involves the direct transfer of a single sperm into a cytoplasm of oocyte.	• Teratozoospermia • Poor sperm motility • Low sperm count • Vasectomy cases or obstruction in passage of sperm • Antisperm antibodies in male
Artificial insemination: It is a method of assisted reproductive technology.	• Sperm donation • Male infertility • Failure of reproduction on natural course
Gamete intrafallopian transfer (GIFT): It is transfer of collected eggs and sperms into fallopian tube (redundant technique).	• Ovary and at least one of the fallopian tube should be normal. • Sperm dysfunction or couple with unknown cause of infertility.
Zygote intrafallopian transfer (ZIFT): It is zygote transfer to fallopian tube using a laparoscope (redundant technique).	

Box 5.5: Egg freezing (oocyte cryopreservation)

- Human oocyte cryopreservation or egg freezing is a procedure to preserve an ovum.
- Procedure:
  – Ovum are extracted from a female same as in IVF.
  – The extracted ova are frozen and stored in liquid nitrogen at −196°C.
- In the future, ova will be thawed, fertilized and transferred to the uterus as embryos to facilitate a pregnancy.
- Indications: As germ cell deteriorate but uterus remains active till middle age, egg freezing can be used to postpone maternity until suitable situations (to set carrier or medical conditions that require chemotherapy).
- Success rate:
  – Varies with the age of woman at the time of egg retrieval.
  – It ranges from 14.8 to 31.5%.

Clinical Embryology

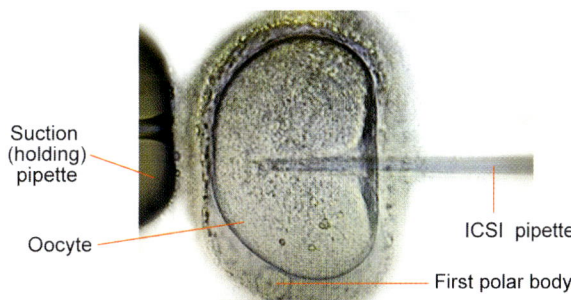

Clinical image 5.1: Intracytoplasmic sperm injection (ICSI) is a procedure that involves a direct transfer of a single spermatozoon into a cytoplasm of oocyte. Oocyte is held with a suction pipette and ICSI pipette, containing a single spermatozoon, is used to penetrate the zona pellucida and oocyte. After pressure injection of the spermatozoon, the ICSI pipette is withdrawn (Image courtesy: *Dr Keshav Malhotra*)

Chapter 6

Second Week of Development: Bilaminar Germ Disc

eSmartQuiz

Chapter Outline

- Day 8
  - Changes in trophoblasts
  - Changes in embryoblast
- Day 9–10
  - Changes in trophoblasts
  - Changes in embryoblast
- Day 11–12
  - Changes in trophoblasts
  - Changes in embryoblast
- Day 13–14
  - Changes in trophoblasts
  - Changes in embryoblast
- Endometrial changes
- Yolk sac
- Fetus as graft
- Genomic imprinting
- X chromosome inactivation

Competencies:
- **AN78.2:** Describe the development of trophoblast.
- **AN78.4:** Describe the formation of extraembryonic mesoderm and coelom, bilaminar disc, and prochordal plate.

INTRODUCTION

- Process of implantation that begins in the first week gets completed in the second week.
- During implantation, blastocyst sinks in the endometrium due to the invading capacity of trophoblasts.
- Blastocyst completely embeds in the endometrial stroma by the 12th day of development.^{MCQ}
- Site of penetration is initially sealed by fibrin and coagulation plug and is later healed by the lining epithelial of endometrium.
- Developmental changes in the second week can be grouped as follows:
  1. Changes in the trophoblast
  2. Changes in the embryoblast
  3. Changes in the endometrium
- For study purpose, day by day changes in the second week are described in this chapter.

DAY 8 (Fig. 6.1)

Changes in Trophoblasts

- The blastocyst partially sinks in the endometrium.
- Trophoblast differentiates into two layers.^{Viva}
  1. Inner cytotrophoblast
  2. Outer syncytiotrophoblast (produces human chorionic gonadotropin hormone)
- Cytotrophoblast on mitosis migrates outwards to form the syncytiotrophoblast.

Changes in Embryoblast

Q. Write a short note on bilaminar germ disc or bilaminar blastocyst.

- Embryoblast (inner cell mass) differentiates into the following two layers:
  1. *Hypoblast:* It is a flat (squamous or low cuboidal) cell layer facing towards the blastocele (cavity of blastocyst). Hypoblast is the first germ layer to be formed.
  2. *Epiblast:* Embryoblasts facing towards cytotrophoblast of embryonic pole forms a layer of columnar cells called *epiblast*.
- A cavity forms within the epiblast called the amniotic cavity.
- Epiblast cells that line the roof of the amniotic cavity become flat and are called amnioblasts (amnion),

whereas epiblast cells continue to line the floor of the cavity.
- Upon formation of an amniotic cavity, hypoblasts, and epiblasts form a *bilaminar germ disc*.
- The junction of amnioblast with germ disc is called *amnio-ectodermal junction*.

DAY 9–10 (Fig. 6.1, Practice Fig. 6.1)

Changes in Trophoblasts

- Blastocyst further penetrates endometrium.
- Penetration defect is closed by a fibrin coagulation plug.
- Syncytiotrophoblast develops more rapidly along embryonic pole.
- Cells of syncytiotrophoblast grow rapidly and lose their cell membranes to form a multinucleated protoplasmic mass. *Viva*
- **Lacunar stage of trophoblast** *MCQ, Viva*
  Several small spaces appear within syncytiotrophoblast called lacunar spaces. These lacunar spaces coalesce with each other to form large lacunar spaces.

Changes in Embryoblast

- *Formation of exocelomic or Heuser's membrane:* *MCQ*
  At the abembryonic pole, hypoblast cells proliferate to form flattened mesothelial cells. These mesothelial cells line the inner surface of the cytotrophoblast, (the surface facing the blastocyst cavity) and form the *Heuser's membrane*.
- On formation of exocoelomic membrane, blastocoel cavity modifies to form *primary yolk sac or exocoelomic cavity*.
- Thus, bilaminar germ disc lies between the amniotic cavity and the primary yolk sac.

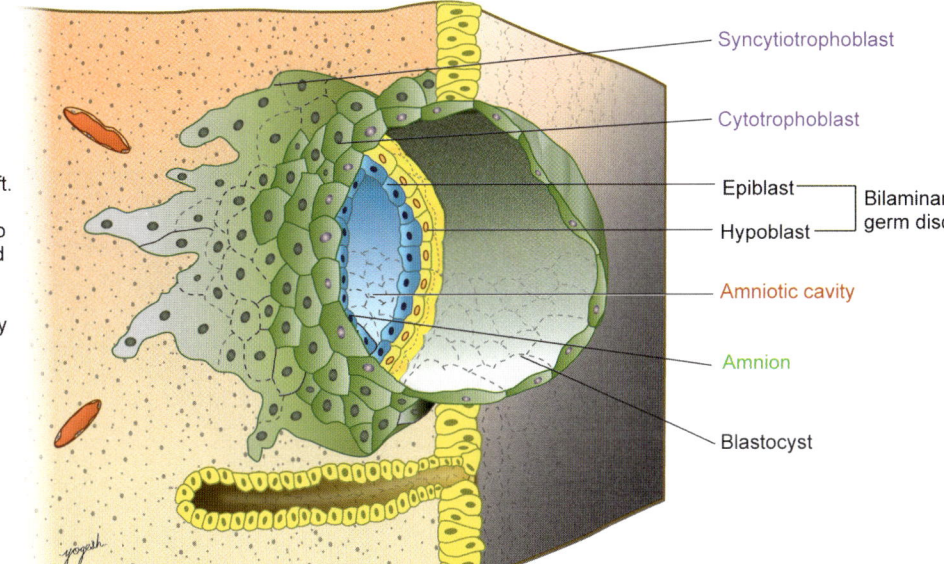

Day 8: Implantation

Formation of amniotic cavity.

Epiblast cells multiply and amniotic cavity appears in between them as a small cleft.

Trophoblast differentiates into outer syncytiotrophoblast and inner cytotrophoblast.

The embryoblast is formed by the epiblast and hypoblast layers.

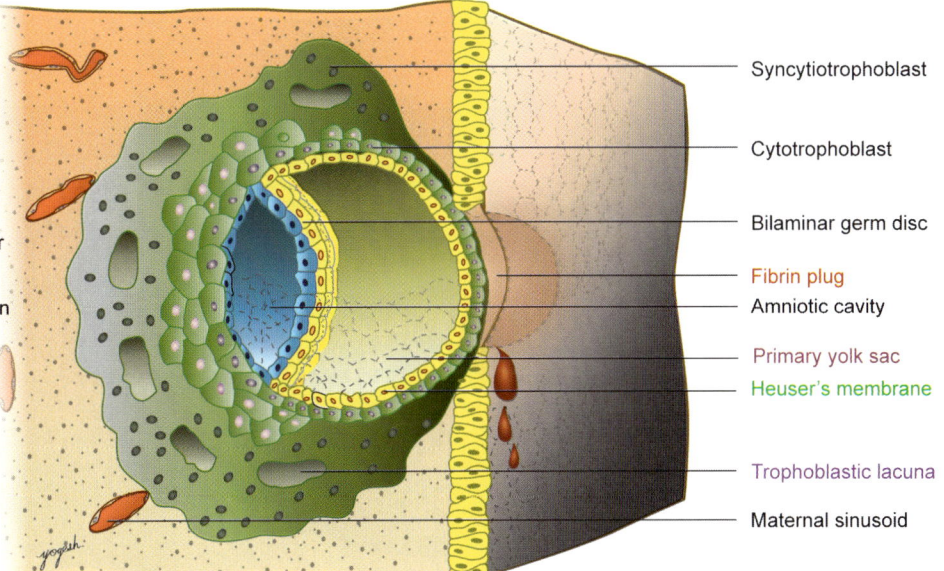

Day 9 embryo

Formation of trophoblastic lacunae.

Small lacunar cavities appear in syncytiotrophoblast.

A layer of columnar epiblast cells and a layer of cuboidal hypoblast cells forms bilaminar germ disc.

The bilaminar disc lies between amniotic cavity and primary yolk sac.

The endometrial surface defect is closed by a fibrin coagulum.

Hypoblast cells multiply to form flat cells layer called Heuser's membrane that lines yolk sac.

Fig. 6.1: Day 8: Implantation and formation of amniotic cavity. Day 9 embryo – formation of trophoblastic lacunae

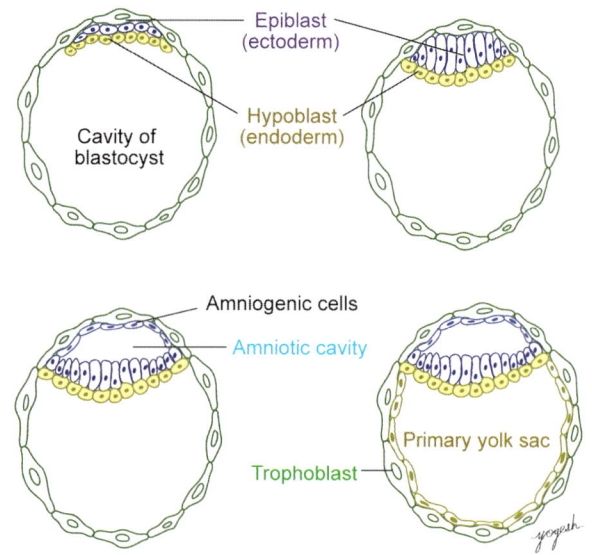

Practice Fig. 6.1: Formation of ectoderm, endoderm, amniotic cavity and primary yolk sac

DAY 11–12 (Fig. 6.2, Practice Fig. 6.2)

Changes in Trophoblasts

- Endometrial epithelium completely heals the defect caused due to implantation.
- Lacunar spaces continue to enlarge and communicate with each other. This change is more prominent along the embryonic pole.
- Cords of syncytiotrophoblasts form the trabeculae.
- Development of uteroplacental circulation

Syncytiotrophoblast erodes maternal capillaries and other vessels; hence, lacunar spaces are filled with maternal blood.

Erosion of maternal veins takes place earlier than the maternal arteries. *MCQ*

Filling of lacunar spaces with maternal blood establishes ***uteroplacental circulation***.

Day 10–11

Formation of extraembryonic mesoderm.

Establishment of communication between maternal blood vessels and trophoblastic lacunae.

The trophoblastic lacunae get filled with maternal blood.

The extraembryonic mesodermal cells separates Heuser's membrane from cytotrophoblast.

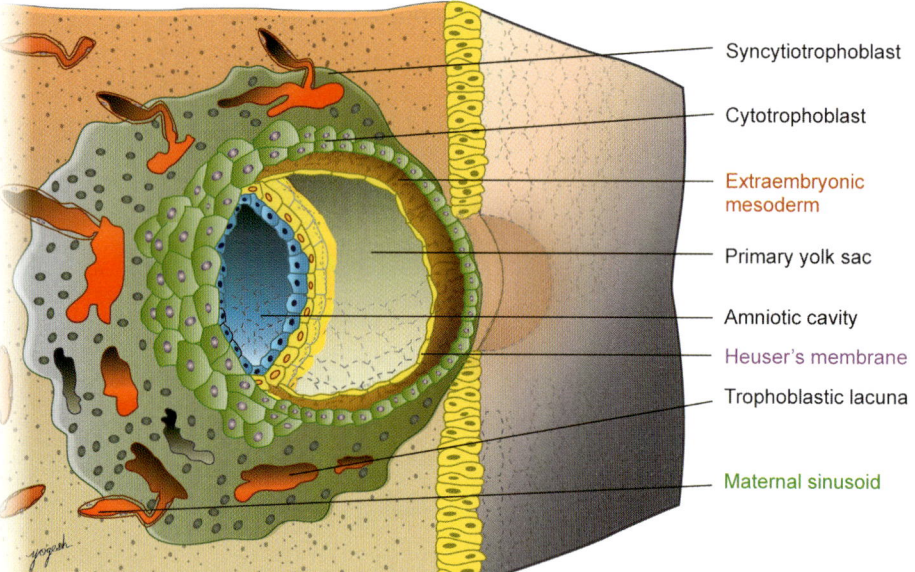

Day 12

Formation of extraembryonic coelom.

Extraembryonic coelomic cavities appear in extraembryonic mesoderm.

The trophoblastic lacunae at the embryonic pole develop communication with maternal vessels.

Extraembryonic mesoderm proliferates and separates bilaminar germ disc, amniotic cavity and yolk sac with exocoelomic membrane from trophoblastic shell.

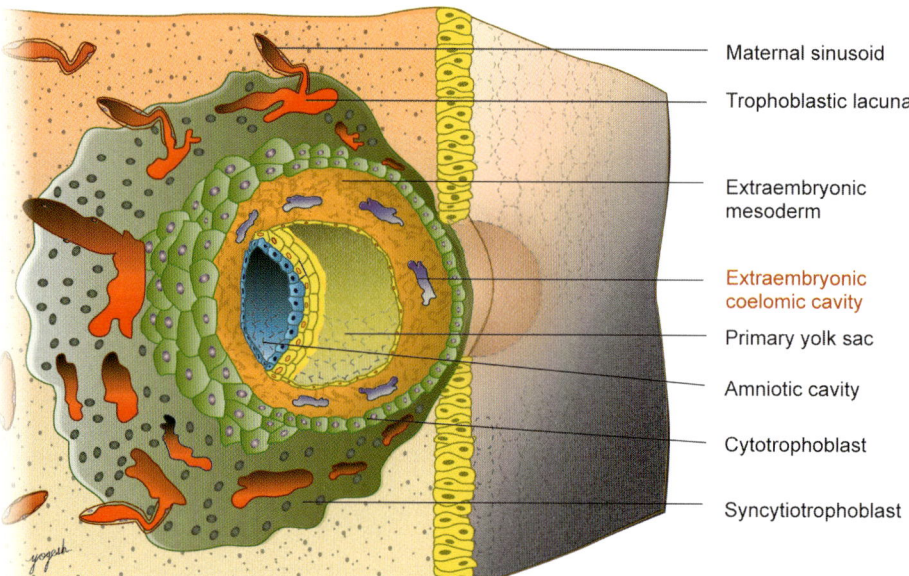

Fig. 6.2: Day 10–11: Formation of extraembryonic mesoderm. Day 12 – Formation of extraembryonic coelom

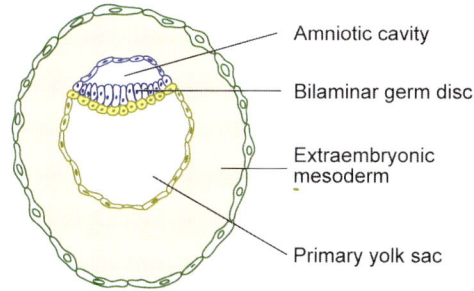

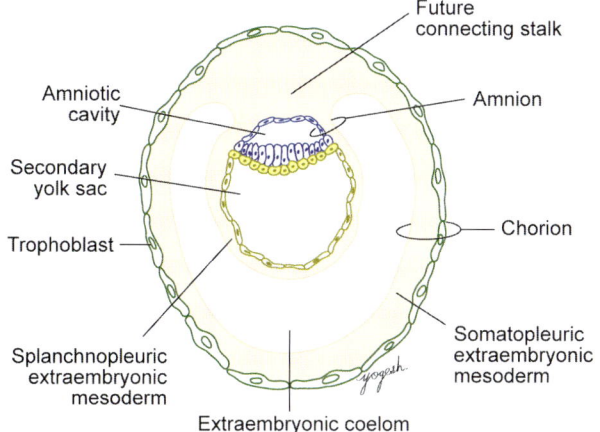

Practice Fig. 6.2: Formation of extraembryonic mesoderm, extraembryonic coelom, amnion and chorion

Changes in Embryoblast

- *Formation of extraembryonic mesoderm:* Cells of yolk sac multiply to form a layer of loosely arranged connective tissue around the amnion and the exocoelomic membrane called *extraembryonic mesoderm.*^NEXT Extraembryonic mesoderm forms structures that do not contribute to future body of embryo.^NEXT
- Extraembryonic mesoderm spreads underneath the cytotrophoblast.
- Spreading of the extraembryonic mesoderm separates the germ disc, amniotic cavity and yolk sac from the cytotrophoblast.
- *Formation of chorionic cavity:* Cavities start appearing in the growing extraembryonic mesoderm. These cavities soon fuse to form an *extraembryonic coelom or cavity.*
- *Formation of connecting stalk:* Continue increase in extraembryonic coelom isolates the yolk sac and amniotic cavity from the cytotrophoblast except at the caudal end of the germ disc where it forms a *connecting stalk* of extraembryonic mesoderm.
- Connecting stalk ultimately develops into *umbilical cord.*^MCQ
- Exocoelomic cavity divides extraembryonic mesoderm into *somatopleuric* and *splanchnopleuric mesoderm.*^MCQ
- Somatopleuric (somatic) extraembryonic mesoderm lines the amnion and cytotrophoblast, whereas splanchnopleuric extraembryonic mesoderm lines the yolk sac.

Chorion

Q. What is chorion?

- Trophoblast and somatopleuric layer of extraembryonic mesoderm together form the **chorion** and blastocystic cavity called the **chorionic cavity.**^MCQ, Viva

Some Interesting Facts

- *Embryotroph* is a fluid that appears in syncytiotrophoblastic lacunar spaces.
- Embryotroph nourishes bilaminar disc through diffusion before the development of uteroplacental circulation.

DAY 13–14 (Figs 6.3, 6.4, Practice Fig. 6.2)

Changes in Trophoblasts

- Formation of primary villi
- Endometrial surface defect heals completely.

  Syncytiotrophoblast forms column-like structures called *villi*. The villi lie between adjacent lacunar spaces.

  Syncytiotrophoblastic villi are invaded by cytotrophoblastic cells to form *primary stem villi.*^MCQ, Viva (Fig. 6.5)

  Primary stem villi have a central core of cytotrophoblast and peripheral syncytiotrophoblast.

Some Interesting Facts

- Occasional bleeding from the penetration site of the endometrial surface defect may occur due to increased maternal blood to lacunar spaces.
- This bleeding may occur on the 28th day of menstrual cycle and may be confused with usual menstrual bleeding.^MCQ

Changes in Embryoblast

- **Formation of secondary yolk sac**

  A portion of primary yolk sac is pinched off by developing extraembryonic coelom. Thus, the primary yolk sac results in the reduction in size to form smaller *secondary yolk sac*. The pinched off portion of yolk sac form exocoelomic cysts in the chorionic cavity.^MCQ

- A 14-day embryo is a flat, bilaminar germ disc. It is sandwiched between the floor of the amniotic cavity and roof of the yolk sac.
- **Formation of prechordal plate** (Fig. 6.4, Practice Fig. 6.3)

Q. Write a short note on prechordal plate.

  Hypoblast cells become columnar in a small area near cranial end of germ disc (head end). This small circular area is called *prechordal plate* (also called prochordal plate).

Day 12

Formation of extraembryonic splanchnopleuric and somatopleuric mesoderm.

Extraembryonic coelomic cavities fuse and divide extraembryonic mesoderm into two layers – somatopleuric and splanchnopleuric layers.

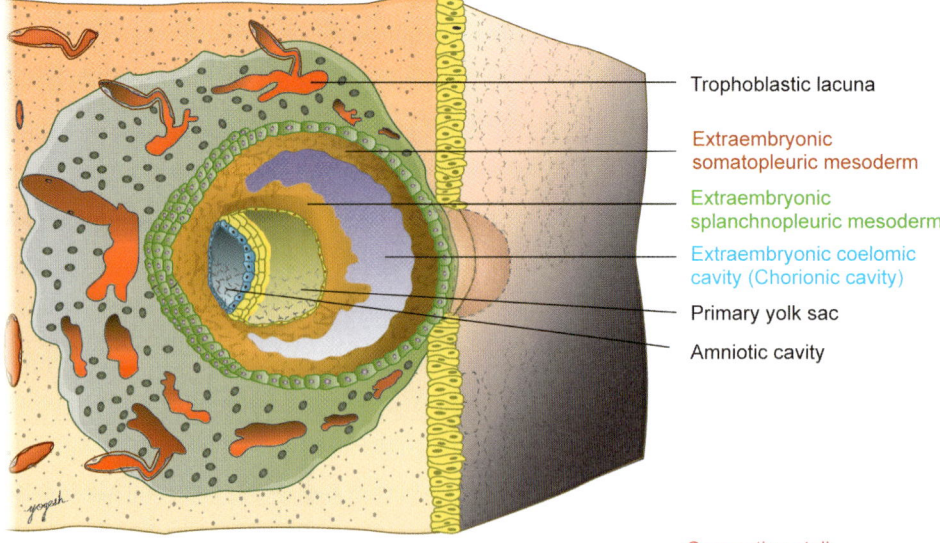

- Trophoblastic lacuna
- Extraembryonic somatopleuric mesoderm
- Extraembryonic splanchnopleuric mesoderm
- Extraembryonic coelomic cavity (Chorionic cavity)
- Primary yolk sac
- Amniotic cavity

Day 13

Development of extraembryonic coelom and formation of secondary yolk sac.

Enlarged cavity of extraembryonic coelom pinch primary yolk sac and forms smaller secondary yolk sac and exocoelomic cyst.

Developing embryo is connected with trophoblast by connecting stalk (future umbilical cord).

Protruding cytotrophoblast forms primary villi.

Cytotrophoblast proliferates into syncytiotroblast to form primary villi.

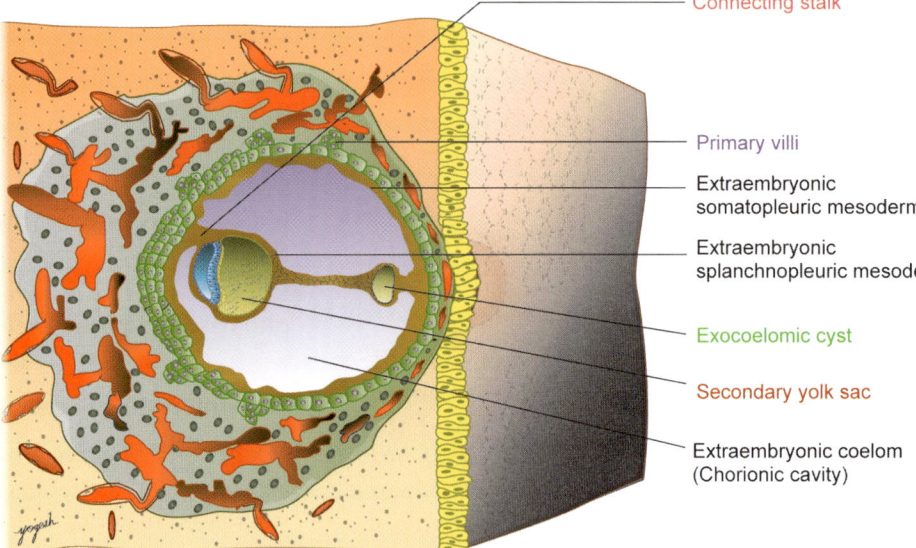

- Connecting stalk
- Primary villi
- Extraembryonic somatopleuric mesoderm
- Extraembryonic splanchnopleuric mesoderm
- Exocoelomic cyst
- Secondary yolk sac
- Extraembryonic coelom (Chorionic cavity)

Day 14

Exocoelomic cavity enlarges and pushes developing germ disc with yolk sac towards embryonic pole.

Exocoelomic cysts break up to a collection of vesicles at the abembryonic end of the chorionic cavity and get absorbed slowly.

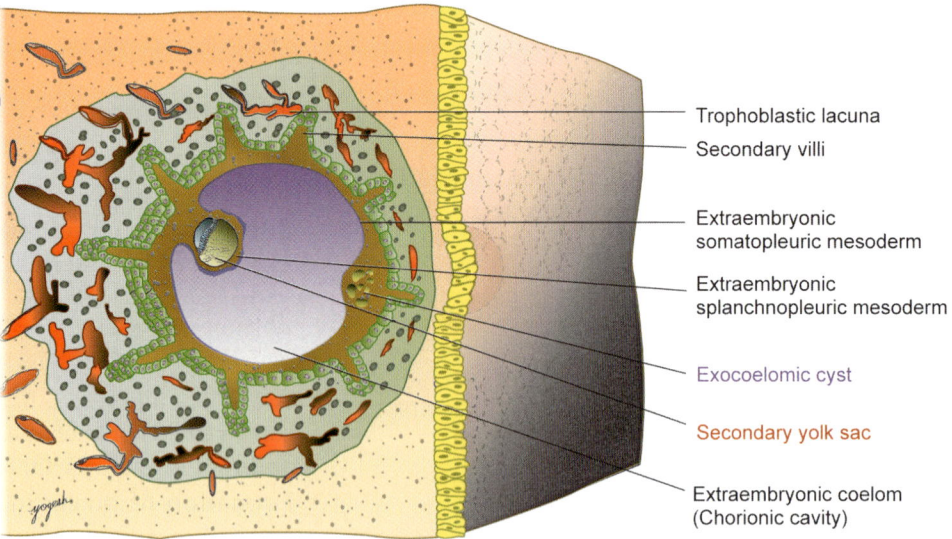

- Trophoblastic lacuna
- Secondary villi
- Extraembryonic somatopleuric mesoderm
- Extraembryonic splanchnopleuric mesoderm
- Exocoelomic cyst
- Secondary yolk sac
- Extraembryonic coelom (Chorionic cavity)

Fig. 6.3: Day 12–14: Developing germ disc with yolk sac

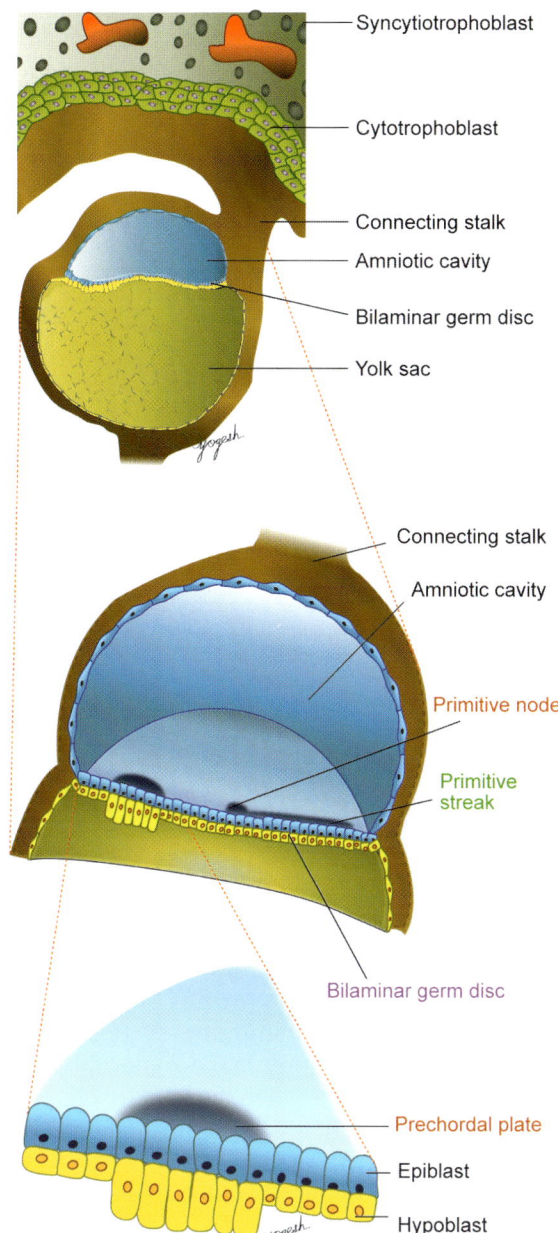

Fig. 6.4: Bilaminar germ disc seen on section through amnion and secondary yolk sac. Hypoblast cells become columnar in a small area near the cranial end of the germ disc (head end). This small circular area is called prechordal plate

Summary of changes in trophoblast and embryoblast is given in Flowcharts 6.1 and 6.2.

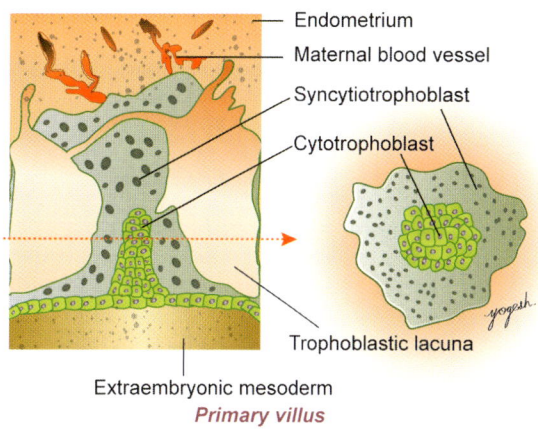

Fig. 6.5: Formation of primary villi. Cytotrophoblast invades syncytiotrophoblastic villi to form primary villi

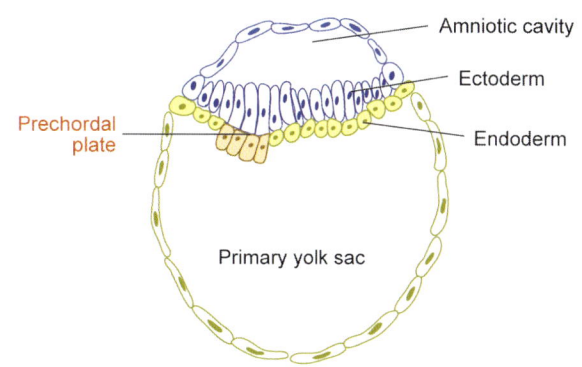

Practice Fig. 6.3: Formation of prechordal plate

- **Significance of prechordal plate** ^{MCQ}
  – It shows the first sign of differentiation.
  – It establishes *cephalocaudal axis* (head and tail ends).
  – It is an important *organizer* of head region.

ENDOMETRIAL CHANGES

- During implantation, blastocyst sinks in the endometrium due to the invading capacity of trophoblasts.
- Blastocyst is completely embedded in the endometrial stroma by 12th day of development.^{MCQ}
- Site of penetration is initially sealed by fibrin and coagulation plug and later healed by lining epithelium of endometrium.
- Blastocyst lies in the stratum compactum of endometrium. Stratum compactum sheds off during child birth; hence, it is called *decidua*. Part of decidua that lies deep to blastocyst is *decidua basalis*, thus trophoblast invades only decidua basalis (*deciduous* = falling, in Latin).^{NEXT}

Some Interesting Facts
• Transvaginal sonography (endovaginal sonography) is useful for measuring the diameter of chorionic sac to evaluate embryonic development.
• Human chorionic gonadotrophin radio immunoassay or ultrasonography can be used for detection of implantation (pregnancy) by the end of second week. ^{MCQ}

Flowchart 6.1: Trophoblastic changes in the second week

Q. List the trophoblastic changes in the second week.

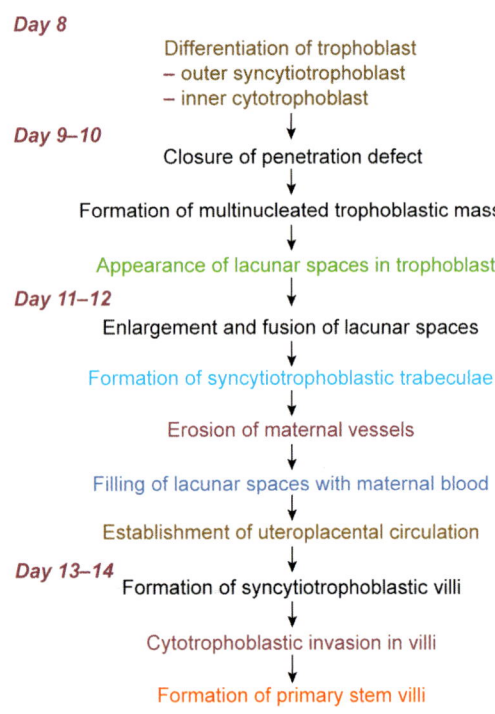

Flowchart 6.2: Changes in embryoblasts in the second week

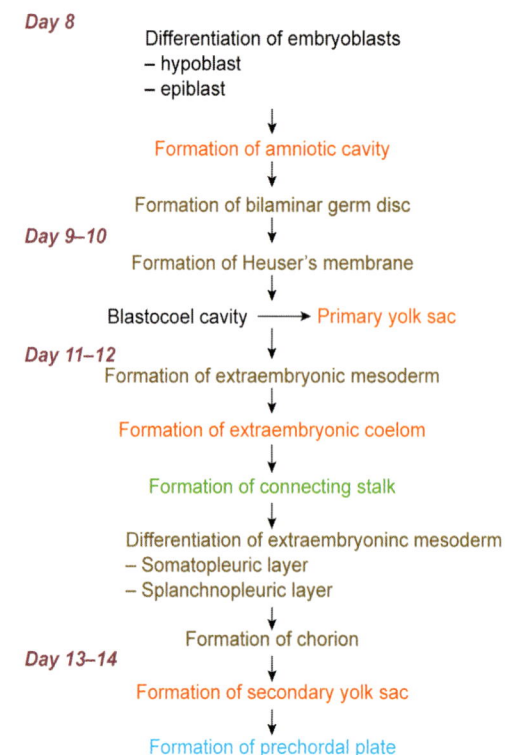

Box 6.1: Yolk sac

- Yolk sac (umbilical vesicle) attains full development and reaches its maximum size by 32nd day of IUL (4–5 weeks) (Practice Fig. 6.3).*NEXT*
- Yolk sac is visible from 5th to 20th week after which it becomes invisible on ultrasonography.
- Yolk sac in human is essential because
  1. It gives nutrition to embryo in 2nd and 3rd weeks.*NEXT*
  2. It is a source for primordial germ cells.*NEXT*
  3. It is the first organ for hematopoietic germ cells.*NEXT*
  4. Incorporated part of the yolk sac forms gut tube endoderm and it gives rise to lung buds (trachea, bronchi, parenchyma of lungs) and gastro-intestinal duct.*NEXT*

Box 6.2: Fetus as graft

Q. Explain 'why conceptus is not rejected by its mother'?^{Viva}

- Allograft is the transfer of tissue from one member of species to another member of species. Here, fetus is the allograft for mother (human to human).
- Mother accepts the fetus (conceptus) without inducing any immune reactions.
- Antigens (from conceptus) bound to the major histocompatibility complex (MHC) molecules that induce immune reaction on exposure to host's (mother) T cells, but there is no such response during pregnancy.

- Probable reasons (Medawar, 1953): (Fig. 6.6)
  1. **Physical separation:** Trophoblast separates fetus from mother. Trophoblast poorly expresses MHC molecules.
  2. **Tolerant maternal immune system:** Specific hormonal conditions make maternal immune system nonresponsive to the fetal tissue, even for a few fetal circulating cells in maternal blood. Mother during pregnancy is not having suppressed immunity for infections.
  3. **Antigenically immature conceptus:** Conceptus is not antigenically mature. Hence, conceptus cannot induce an antigenic reaction.
  4. **Apoptosis of activated maternal T cells:** Trophoblast produces a tumor necrotic factor (TNF) that induces apoptosis in maternal activated T cells.

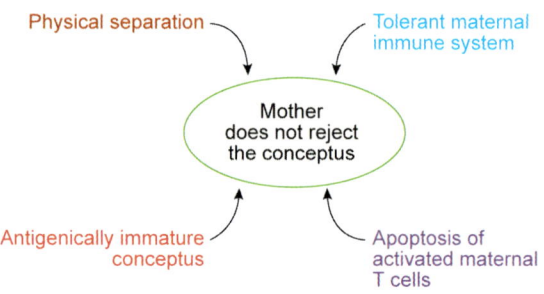

Fig. 6.6: Reasons for nonrejection of fetus by mother

GENOMIC IMPRINTING

Q. Write a short note on genomic imprinting.

- In experimental studies, zygote containing two male pronuclei gives rise to only the trophoblastic mass (similar to hydatidiform mole), whereas zygote containing two female pronuclei gives rise to only nonsurviving embryoblast. This fact indicates that genomic contribution of both the parents is essential for healthy fetal development.^Viva

- **Cause**
  - Genomic imprinting is a phenomenon that involves expression of a gene depending on its maternal or paternal origin. (*Source*: Clinical Genetics, Yogesh Sontakke, 2nd edn.).
  - Basis of genomic imprinting is methylation of DNA that leads to gene silencing or activation.
  - DNA of female germline is more methylated than DNA of male germ lines.
  - In primordial germ cells, imprints (methylation) are erased and they again get established during gametogenesis. Hence, during spermatogenesis male-specific patterns and oogenesis female-specific patterns (methylation) are formed.

- Genomic imprinting affects inheritance of congenital disease.

- For example, deletion of long arm of chromosome 15 (15q11.2–q13) results in Prader-Willi syndrome if inherited from the father, whereas Angelman syndrome is inherited from the mother (*Source*: Clinical Genetics, Yogesh Sontakke, 2nd edn.).^MCQ, Viva

- *Decidual reaction:* ^Viva

  Q. Explain decidual reaction.

  It involves the following changes:
  - Increased hormonal levels during pregnancy increase glycogen and lipids deposited in decidual cells (endometrial cells).^MCQ
  - Intracellular substances also increase.
  - Decidua becomes edematous.
  - Tortuosity of endometrial gland increases.

Box 6.3: X chromosome inactivation

Q. Write a short note on X chromosome inactivation.

- In female embryoblast, one of the two X chromosomes is inactivated irrespective of its parental source; however, in trophoblast of female blastocyst, paternal X chromosome is inactivated.

- **Process:** Inactivation of X chromosome involves expression of a particular X chromosome locus *Xist* (X inactive specific transcript gene) that produces methylation of X chromosome.^MCQ

- Inactivated X chromosome lacks histone H4 acetylation and it results in the condensation of X chromosome to form *Barr body*.

- Inactive X chromosome is reactivated only in the early fetal life and remains dormant throughout the remaining life.

Chapter 7

Third Week of Development: Trilaminar Germ Disc

eSmartQuiz

Chapter Outline

- Gastrulation
- Notochord
- Allantois
- Development of chorionic villi
- Formation of neural tube
- Neural crest

Competencies:
- **AN79.1:** Describe the formation and fate of primitive streak.
- **AN79.2:** Describe the formation and fate of notochord.
- **AN79.3:** Describe the process of neurulation.

INTRODUCTION

Q. Enlist the major events of third week of gestation.
- The third week of development begins after five weeks of onset of the last menstrual period.
- Characteristics of the third week of development are as follows:
  1. Formation of primitive streak^{NEXT}
  2. *Gastrulation*: Formation of three germ layers^{NEXT}
  3. Formation of notochord^{NEXT}
  4. Formation of allantois
  5. Formation of neural plate, neural tube, and neural crest
  6. Development of chorionic villi
  7. Formation of somites
  8. Formation of intraembryonic coelom

GASTRULATION (FORMATION OF GERM LAYERS)

Q. Write a short note on: (a) gastrulation, (b) prochordal, (c) primitive streak.

Definition
- Gastrulation is a process of conversion of *bilaminar* embryonic disc to *trilaminar* disc during the *third week* of development.^{NEXT,Viva}

Steps (Flowchart 7.1)
- Bilaminar embryonic disc of second week continues its development (Figs 7.1 to 7.4, Practice Figs 7.1, 7.2).
- On 15th day, **primitive streak** appears that **induces** gastrulation. Primitive streak is a thickened linear band of **epiblast** in midline **at the caudal end** on the dorsal part of embryonic disc.^{NEXT} Formation of primitive streak is an indicator (the first sign) of the start of gastrulation.^{NEXT}
- Elevated rounded cranial end of primitive streak forms a primitive node (*Hensen's node* or primitive

Flowchart 7.1: Process of gastrulation

Gastrulation = Bilaminar germ disc → trilaminar germ disc

Day 15: Primitive streak
↓
Formation of Hensen's node with blastopore and primitive groove
↓
Migration and invagination of epiblast cells
↓
Formation of
1. Embryonic definitive endoderm
2. Intraembryonic mesoderm
3. Definitive ectoderm

Bilaminar regions of trilaminar germ disc
↓
Germ disc area devoid of mesodermal cells
↓
At cranial end → Buccopharyngeal membrane (break down in 4th week)
At caudal end → Cloacal membrane (break down in 7th week)

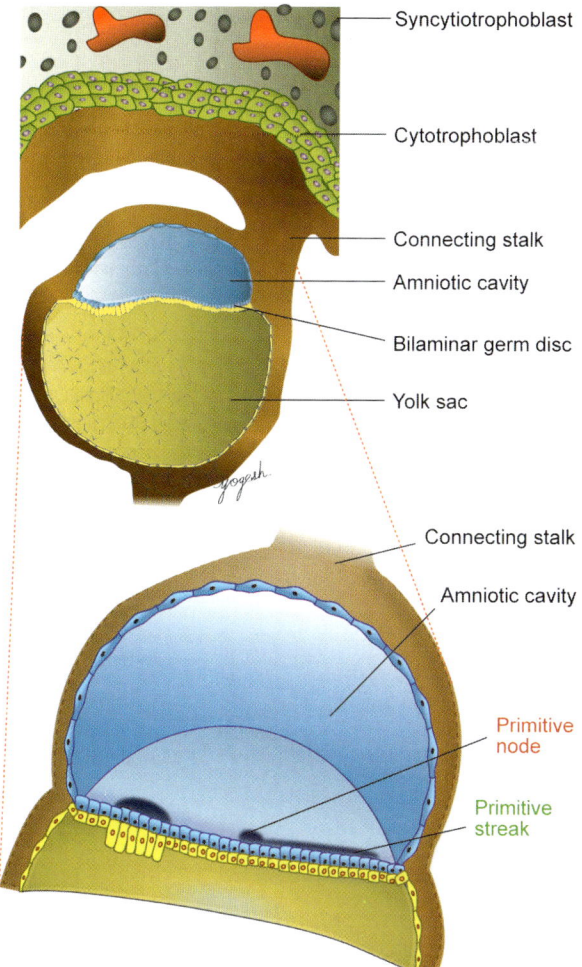

Fig. 7.1: Bilaminar germ disc at the end of second week (longitudinal section). Hypoblast cells become columnar in a small area near the cranial end of the germ disc (head end). This small circular area is called prechordal plate

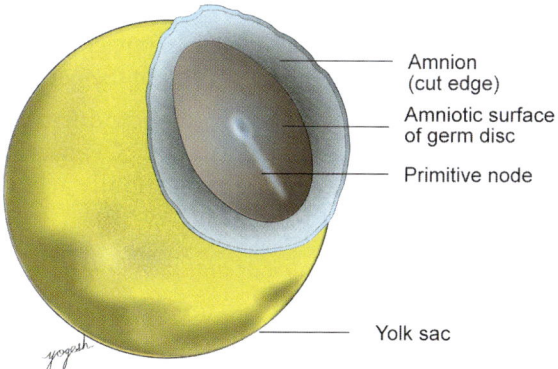

Fig. 7.2: Formation of the primitive streak (Day 16: Dorsolateral view)

knot) that surrounds a depressed pit called primitive pit or **blastopore.**

Axis Formation

Formation of primitive streak defines all the major body axes.

The primitive streak appears caudally in the midline on dorsal surface of bilaminar germ disc. Thus, it

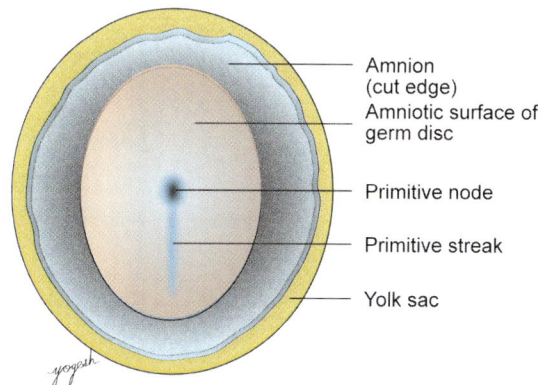

Fig. 7.3: Formation of primitive streak (Day 16: Dorsal view)

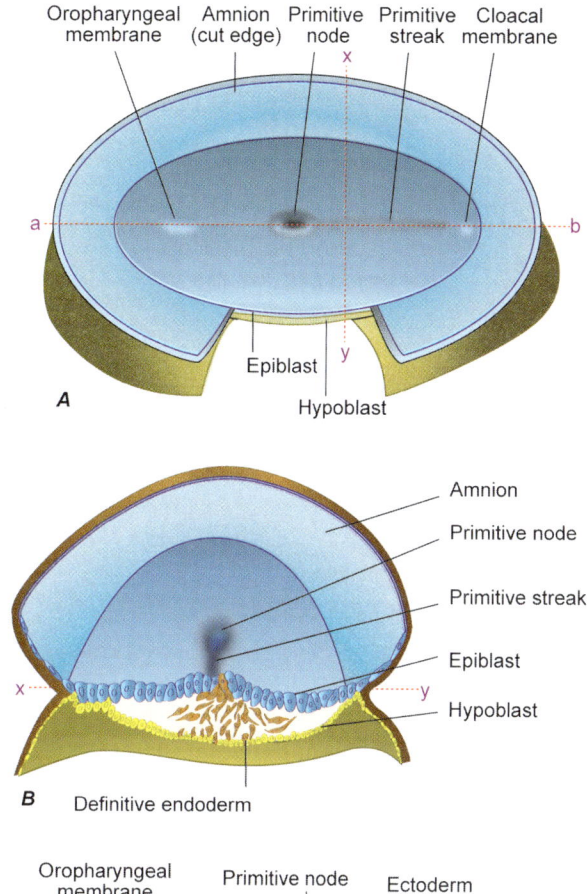

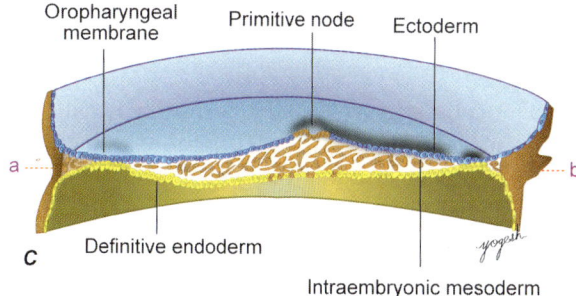

Fig. 7.4: 15–16-day embryo: (A) Gastrulation: Formation of intra-embryonic mesoderm and definitive endoderm. Cells migrate from primitive streak and node to invaginate between hypoblast and epiblast. Migrated cells replace cells of hypoblast to form definitive endoderm and remaining cells form intraembryonic mesoderm; (B) Germ disc is cut along the transverse axis in between primitive node and cloacal membrane; (C) Germ disc is cut along the longitudinal axis

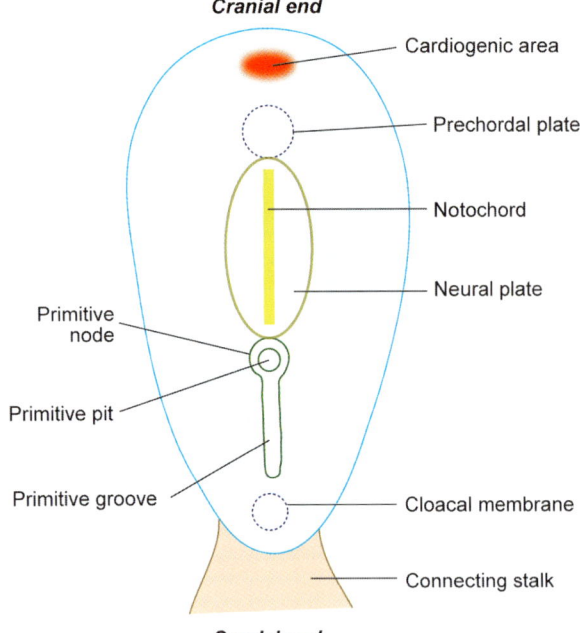

Practice Fig. 7.1: Germ disc showing notochord, primitive pit, primitive knot, primitive groove and cloacal membrane (Dorsal view)

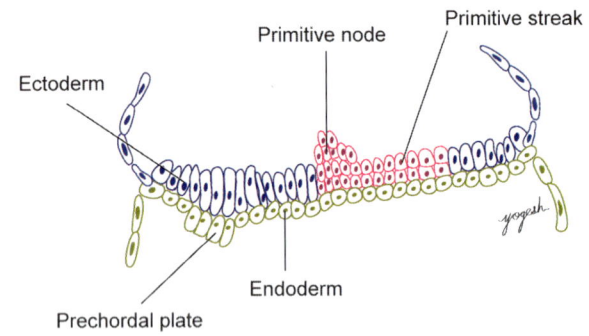

Practice Fig. 7.2: Bilaminar germ disc showing primitive node and primitive streak (longitudinal section)

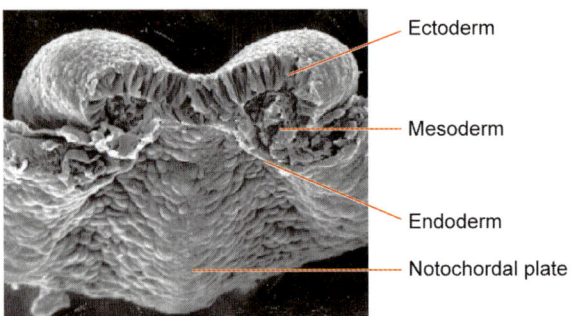

Scanning electron micrograph (SEM) 7.1: SEM showing three germ layers. A cut through anterior end of embryo illustrates three germ layers: Ectoderm, endoderm and intraembryonic mesoderm. The mesoderm in ventral midline is notochordal plate [Species: Mouse, approximate human age: 17 days, ventral view]

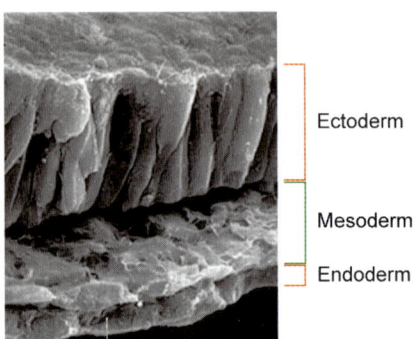

Scanning electron micrograph 7.2: SEM showing three germ layers in high magnification. A cut through the embryo illustrates the three germ layers: Ectoderm, mesoderm, and endoderm [Species: Mouse, approximate human age: 17 days, dorsal view]

defines craniocaudal axis and medial – lateral axes and ventrodorsal axis.

- Germ disc and primitive streak elongate craniocaudally.
- A narrow depressed central area of primitive streak called *primitive groove* develops.
- Epiblast cells *migrate* toward primitive streak. The migrating cells lose epithelial junctions detach from primitive streak and begin invagination.^{Viva}
- Invaginated cells (SEM 7.1, 7.2)
  1. Displace hypoblast cells to form embryonic definitive *endoderm*. This is the first germ layer to be formed.
  2. Form a layer between endoderm and epiblast – known as *intraembryonic mesoderm* by the process of epithelial to mesenchymal transformation (EMT).
- Remaining cells (noninvaginating cells) of epiblast form definitive *ectoderm*.

- *Thus, epiblast forms all three germ layers by gastrulation.*$^{NEXT, Viva}$
- Migrating mesodermal cells establish contact with extraembryonic mesoderm at lateral end of the germ disc.
- Migrating mesoderm separates ectoderm from endoderm except at two places: Cranially at buccopharyngeal membrane and caudally at cloacal membrane (Fig. 7.5, Practice Fig. 7.3^{NEXT}).
- *Buccopharyngeal membrane or oral membrane:*
  – It is a small oval depressed area at cranial end of the germ disc and it appears in prechordal plate.
  – In buccopharyngeal membrane, endodermal cells are firmly adherent with ectodermal cells.
  – It is bilaminar as it is devoid of mesodermal cells.
  – Oropharyngeal membrane breaks down in fourth week to form opening of oral cavity or the stomatodeum.^{MCQ}
- *Cloacal membrane*
  – At caudal end of primitive streak, germ disc remains bilaminar due to firm endodermal attachment with ectoderm. This small circular bilaminar area is called cloacal membrane.

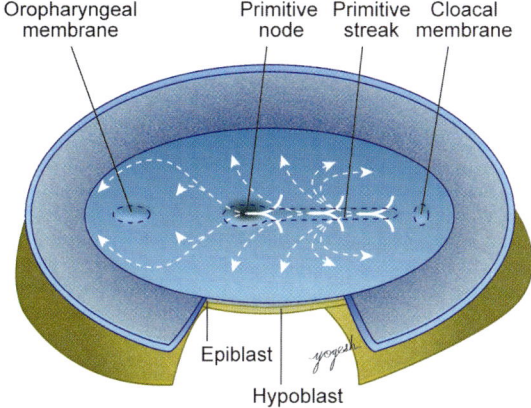

Fig. 7.5: Day 16: Germ disc showing a path for the movement of surface epiblast cells (white solid arrows) through the primitive streak and node and their subsequent migration between the hypoblast and epiblast (white dashed arrows) during gastrulation

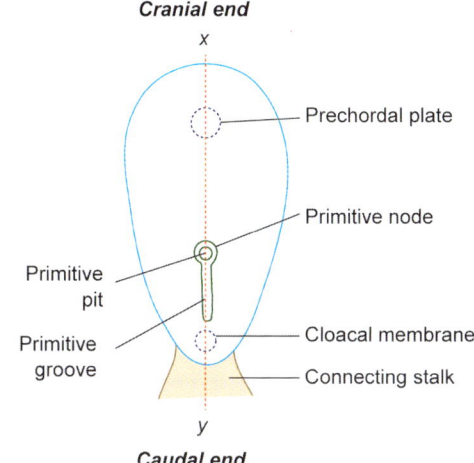

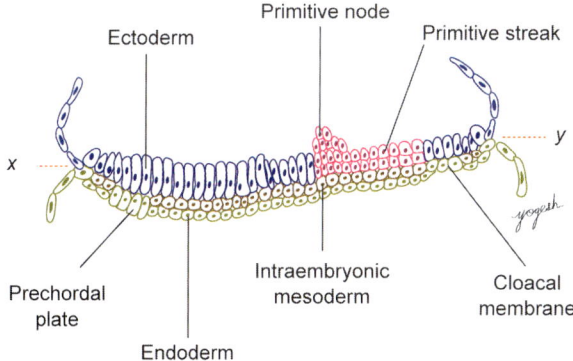

Practice Fig. 7.3: Formation of intraembryonic mesoderm, x-y: longitudinal axis

- Later, on further development, the cloacal membrane divides into anal and urogenital membranes.
- Cloacal membrane disintegrates in 7th week to form opening of anus, urethra and genital tracts.^{MCQ}
- **Pericardial bar**
  - It is midline horseshoe-shaped mesodermal cell condensation that is cranial to the buccopharyngeal membrane.

Box 7.1: Cellular basis of primitive streak formation

- ***Koller's sickle*** or ***Rauber's sickle*** is a local thickening of extraembryonic tissue at the caudal edge of germ disc.^{MCQ}
- Koller's sickle induces adjacent epiblast to form primitive streak by cell–cell interactions at the caudal end of germ disc.
- Cellular basis of primitive streak formation involves four major processes, that is, cell migration, oriented cell division, progressive delamination from epiblast and convergent extension.^{MCQ}
- Primitive streak formation is initiated and maintained by expression of nodal gene.^{NEXT}
- Nodal gene is a member of transforming growth factor β (TGF-β) superfamily. Nodal gene continue to get expressed only on left and it induces expression of transcription Factor Pitx2. Thus, nodal gene and Pitx2 are responsible for right-left asymmetry.^{NEXT}

NOTOCHORD

Q. Write a short note on notochord.

Definition

- Notochord is a midline embryonic structure that develops during **third week** of development from epiblast cells in the region of primitive node.^{NEXT}
- Axial mesoderm (chordamesoderm) is a mesoderm that lies along the central axis and it will give rise to notochord.^{NEXT}

Extent

- From cranial end of primitive streak to prechordal plate.

Formation of Notochord (Fig. 7.6, Flowchart 7.2, Practice Fig. 7.4)

- Formation of primitive pit: Cells of primitive knot proliferate and form depression called ***primitive pit***. In lower animals, primitive pit is also called ***blastopore***.
- Formation of notochordal process: On 17th–18th day, proliferated cells invaginate between ectoderm and endoderm up to prechordal plate to form **solid cord** called **notochordal process** or head process.
- Formation of notochordal canal: Cavity of primitive pit extend into notochordal process to form **notochordal canal.**
- Cells of notochordal canal fuse with endoderm.
- *Formation of neurenteric canal:* The cells of the notochord canal disappear in a craniocaudal direction to form a **communication** between amniotic cavity (via primitive pit) and yolk sac. This communication is called **neurenteric canal.**

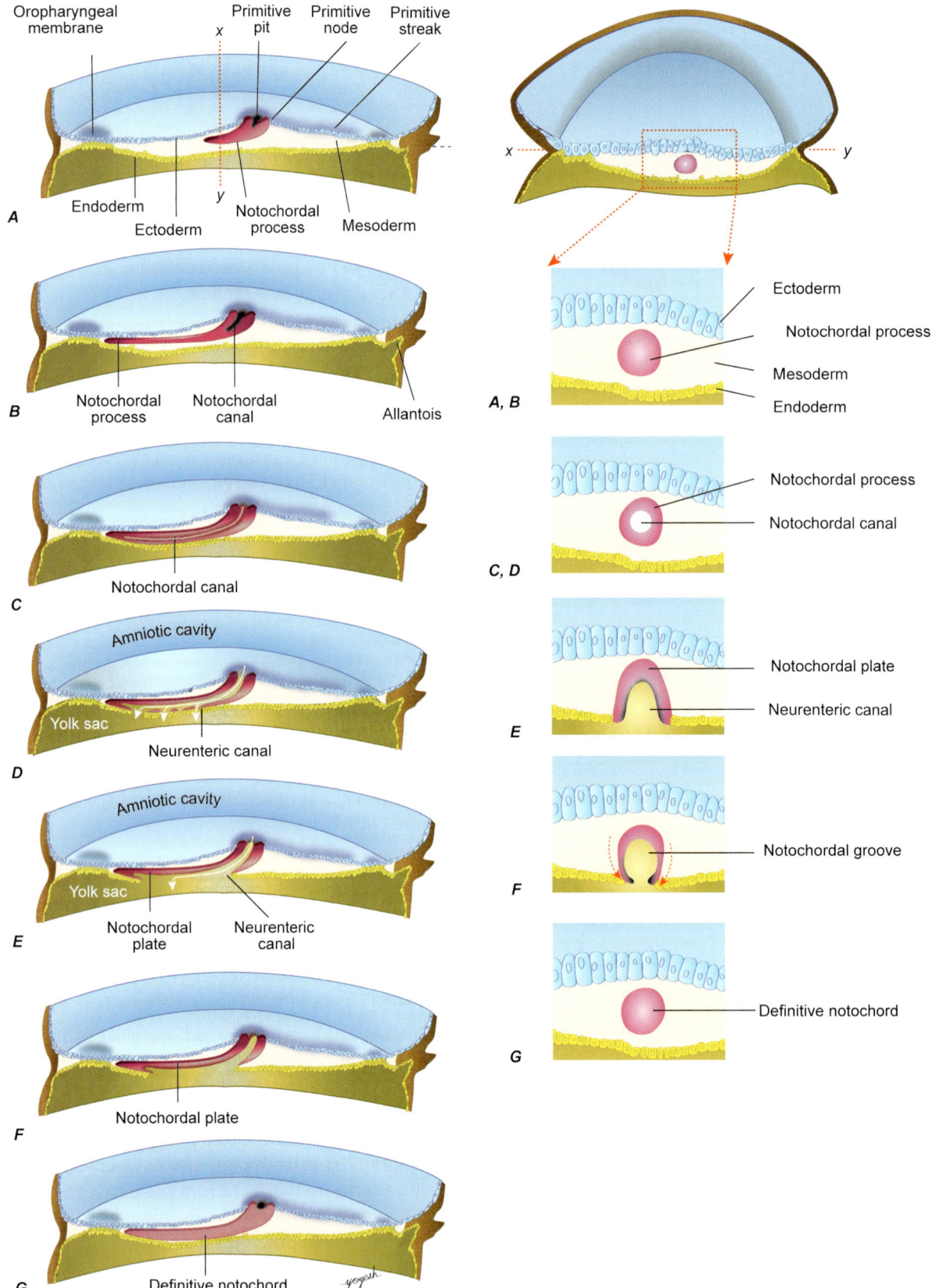

Fig. 7.6: Formation of notochord: (A) At 16th day, cells of primitive node proliferate and form notochordal process; (B) Notochordal process proliferates and extends up to oropharyngeal membrane; (C) Notochordal canal develops in the centre of notochordal process by extension of primitive pit; (D and E) Cells of the floor of notochordal plate and adjoining endodermal cells disappear to form neurenteric canal which connects amniotic cavity to yolk sac through the embryo transiently; (F) Cells of the roof of the neurenteric canal form notochordal plate; (G) Notochordal plate folds to form solid mass of cells *definitive notochord* (x-y: transverse axis of germ disc)

Flowchart 7.2: Notochord

Notochord
– Midline cord-like structure that develops in third week
– Extent: from precordal plate to primitive streak

Formation

Proliferation of cells of **primitive node**
↓
Formation of **primitive pit**
↓
Day 17–18: Formation of **notochordal process**
↓
Formation of **notochordal canal**
↓
Formation of **neurenteric canal**
(Communication: amniotic cavity → yolk sac)
↓
Formation of **notochordal plate**
↓
Formation of **definitive notochord**

Significance
– Feature of phylum chordata
– Defines axis of embryo
– Primary inducer
– Forms nucleus pulposus of intervertebral disc and apical ligament of dens

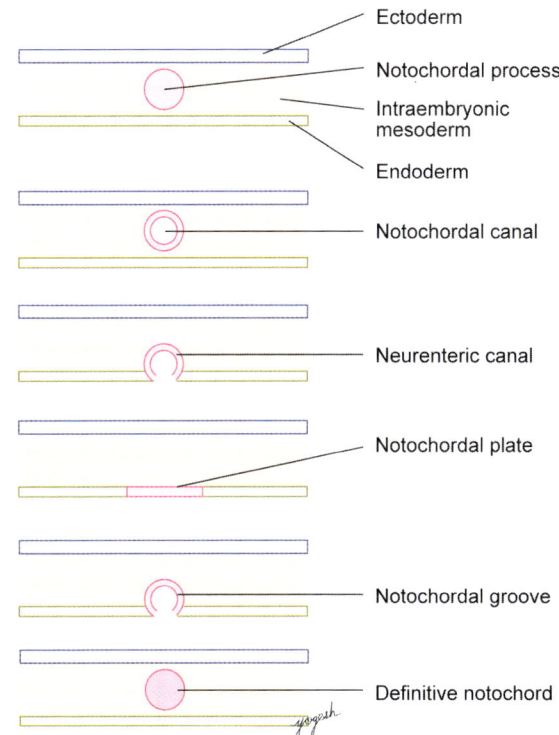

Practice Fig. 7.4: Formation of notochord

Box 7.2: Cellular basis of gastrulation

- During gastrulation, cells undergo morphogenetic movements as follows:
  1. **Epiboly**: Epiboly is spreading of an epithelial sheet.
  2. **Emboly**: Emboly or internalisation is movement of cells into interior of an embryo.
  3. **Convergence**: It is movement of cells toward midline.
  4. **Extension**: It is lengthening in cranial caudal plane.
- Morphogenetic changes include changes in cell shape, size, position, number, cell-to-cell and cell to extracellular matrix adhesion.
- Epithelial to mesenchymal transformation involves changes in cell-to-cell adhesion, cell shape and changes in cytoskeleton.
- **Snail gene** (*zinc finger transcription factor*) expression represses epithelial characteristics in mesenchymal cells.
- Snail gene ceases E-cadherin (cell-to-cell adhesion molecule) and induces expression of vimentin (cytoskeletal proteins) in mesodermal cells.

Establishing medial–lateral subdivisions of mesoderm

- Mesodermal patterning involves interaction between dorsalising factors (proteins of Noggin, Chordin, Nodal, Follistatin and Cerberus genes) and ventralising factors (Bmps and Wnts).
- Low Bmp and Wnt signalling dorsalises mesoderm and induces notochord formation, whereas high expression of Bmp and Wnt signalling ventralises mesoderm and converts it to lateral plate mesoderm.[MCQ]

Some Interesting Facts

1. Embryonic disc remains bilaminar at two places, one at buccopharyngeal membrane (prechordal plate) and another at cloacal membrane.[MCQ]
2. Continuous migration of cells from primitive streak towards cranial region makes disc elongated craniocaudally.
3. Cilia of cells of the primitive node (nodal cilia) may be responsible for right–left visceral side determination. Its abnormality may cause **situs inversus** (major visceral organs are reversed from their normal positions) and may be associated with other anomalies of ciliary movements.
4. Primitive streak regresses by 26th day of intrauterine life. After contributing to the formation of lower abdominal wall. Early regression is associated with ventral body wall defects affecting the lower abdomen. Incomplete regression is associated with sacrococcygeal teratoma.[MCQ, Viva]
5. Anterior visceral endoderm (cells at cranial margin of germ disc) produces certain transcription factors (OTX2, cerebrus). Primitive streak also produces transforming growth factor β, bone morphogenic protein 4, fibroblast growth factor and so on. These factors determine body axes, anteroposterior, right–left, and dorsoventral sides.
6. During epithelial to mesenchymal transformation, epiblast cells often elongate, become flask or bottle shaped, and develop pseudopodia (foot-like processes), filopodia (thinner processes) or lamellipodia (flattened processes), which allow them to migrate through primitive streak into the space between epiblast and hypoblast.

- *Formation of notochordal plate:* Neurentric canal flattens to form **notochordal plate** in the roof of yolk sac.
- Soon, flattening of notochordal plate reverses by folding of notochordal plate to form notochordal groove.
- *Formation of definitive notochord:* Cells of notochordal plate get separated from endoderm to form solid cord of cells called **definitive notochord.**

Significance of Notochord

1. Notochord is a characteristic feature of phylum Chordata animals.
2. Notochord *defines various axes of embryo* (cephalocaudal, anteroposterior, right-left axes)[NEXT] and forms basis for developing axial skeleton, specifically vertebral body.
3. It acts as primary inducer or inductor.[NEXT]
4. In humans, notochord disappears except its remnants in adult represent *nucleus pulposus* of intravertebral discs or *chordomas*[NEXT] (SEM 7.3).

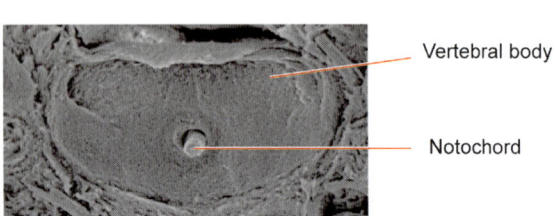

Scanning electron micrograph 7.3: SEM showing intervertebral disc and notochord that forms nucleus pulposus [Species: Mouse, approximate human age: 9 weeks, transverse view]

Box 7.3: Importance of neurentric canal

- Neurentric canal provides nutrition from yolk sac to rapidly differentiating ectoderm as intraembryonic blood circulation is not developed during the third week of development.[MCQ, Viva]

Box 7.4: Role of E-cadherin and FGF8

- E-cadherin is a transmembrane protein that play role in epiblast cell adhesion.
- Fibroblast growth factor 8 (FGF8) is expressed by epiblast cells. FGF8 acts as an '*organizer*' and controls cell migration.
- FGF8 inhibits E-cadherin production and thus, promotes cell migration at primitive streak and node.
- Hence, primitive node is known as *embryonic organizer* or *Spemann organizer* as it promotes formation of three germ layers (discovered by Hans Spemann and Hilda Mangold in 1924).[MCQ]

Box 7.5: Sacrococcygeal teratoma

- *Primitive streak regresses* at the end of third week of development and completely disappears by *26th day* of development.[NEXT]

Cause

- Persistent **remnant** of primitive streak (especially the cells of primordial germ cells) form tumor in coccygeal region of newborn known as *sacrococcygeal teratoma*.

Features

- It is the most common tumor in newborn (1 in 20,000–70,000 births).
- It is usually nonmalignant tumor.
- As it is derived from primitive streak (pluripotent cells), tumor contains incompletely differentiated derivatives of all the three germ layers; for example, hairs, bone, cartilage, muscles and so on.

Treatment

- Surgical removal of tumor.

Teratogenic agents

- Teratogenesis is development of abnormality during germinal period (1–3 weeks of intrauterine life) or embryonic period (4–8 weeks) due to toxicity.
- Teratogenic agent exposure (radiation, infection or rays) between 15th and 18th day of development produces gross malformation.

ALLANTOIS

Q. Write a short note on allantois.

Definition

- Allantois or *allantoenteric diverticulum* is a finger-like outpouching of the yolk sac into the connecting stalk (*allas* = sausage, in Greek).

Development and Fate

- On day 16 of intrauterine life, finger-like outpouching of yolk sac in connecting stalk forms *allantois*.
- On formation of the embryonic tail fold, allantois is connected with cloaca (caudal part of hindgut).
- Part of allantois is absorbed in primitive urinary bladder, whereas the remaining part of allantois forms *urachus*.[MCQ]
- After birth, urachus forms *median umbilical ligament*.[MCQ]

Significance

1. In birds, reptiles and some mammals, allantois acts as a reservoir of urine during embryonic life.
2. In human, allantois remains small as placenta take over its function.
3. Allantoic blood vessels later form umbilical vessels.

Clinical Aspects MCQ, Viva

- During second month of intrauterine life, extraembryonic part of allantois degenerates and intraembryonic portion forms urachus (median umbilical ligament after birth) and part of urinary bladder.
- *Urachal cyst:* It is a remnant of lining epithelium of urachus.
- *Urachal sinus:* It is a remnant of urachus that communicates with urinary bladder or outside the body.
- *Urachal fistula:* It is a persistent urachus that forms a passage from an umbilicus to the urinary bladder.

DEVELOPMENT OF CHORIONIC VILLI

Q. Write a short note on chorionic villi.

Development of Fetoplacental Circulation
(Fig. 7.7, Practice Fig. 7.5)

- *Secondary villi:* In second week of gestation, *primary chorionic villi* (inner cytotrophoblast and outer syncytiotrophoblast) appear.
- In the beginning of the third week, extraembryonic mesodermal cells penetrate in the core of primary villi to form *secondary villi.*
- By the end of the third week, mesodermal cells differentiate to form capillaries. Such villi with capillaries are called *tertiary* or *definitive chorionic villi.*
- *Anchoring villus* extends from chorionic plate to decidua basalis.
- Branches of anchoring villi form *free villi* that floats in trophoblastic lacunar spaces. Free villi are main site for nutrient exchange.^{Viva}
- Development of communication between capillaries of villi, chorionic plate and connecting stalk and intraembryonic vessels form *fetoplacental circulation* (which begins by 17th day).
- Cytotrophoblast cells penetrate syncytiotrophoblast and form *outer cytotrophoblast shell* that helps in the firm attachment with endometrial stroma.

Some Interesting Facts

Holoprosencephaly
- High alcohol consumption during period of gastrulation may result in holoprosencephaly.
- It includes small forebrain, fused lateral ventricles, hypotelorism (closely set eyes).

Sirenomelia/caudal dysgenesis
- It is also known as *mermaid syndrome.*
- Insufficient mesoderm in caudal portion of germ disc results in hypoplasia or fusion of lower limbs, anomalies of vertebrae, kidney and genital organs and imperforated anus. It mostly has one aberrant umbilical artery.

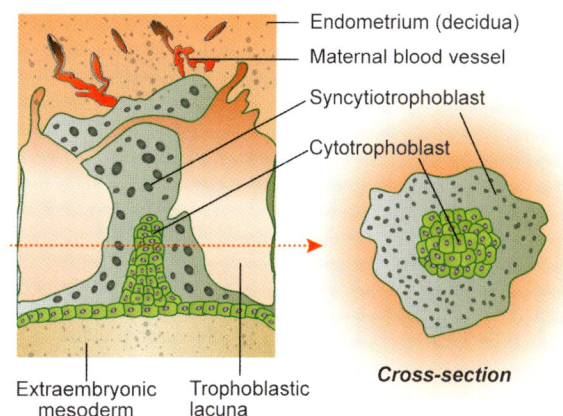

Primary villus

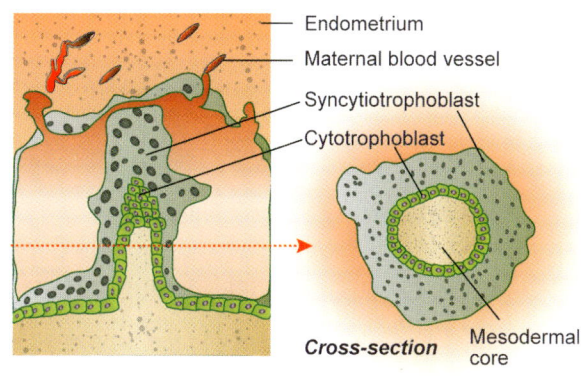

Secondary villus

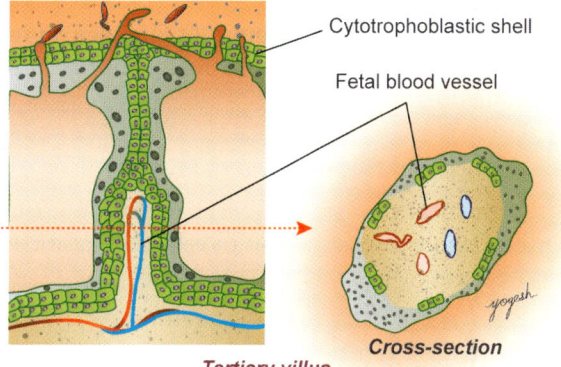

Tertiary villus

Fig. 7.7: Development of chorionic villi. Primary villi have core of cytotrophoblast under cover of syncytiotrophoblast. Secondary villi have core of mesoderm under cover of cytotrophoblast and syncytiotrophoblast. Fetal blood vessels develop in mesodermal core to form tertiary villi

Box 7.6: Fate of the germ layers

- Each of the three germ layers gives rise to specific structures as follows:
  - Ectoderm gives rise to epidermis, central and peripheral nervous system and retina.
  - Endoderm gives rise to epithelial lining of respiratory tract, gastrointestinal tract, glands opening in these tracts, pancreas, liver, and gallbladder.
  - Mesoderm gives rise to musculature, bone, cartilage, cardiovascular, reproductive and excretory system.

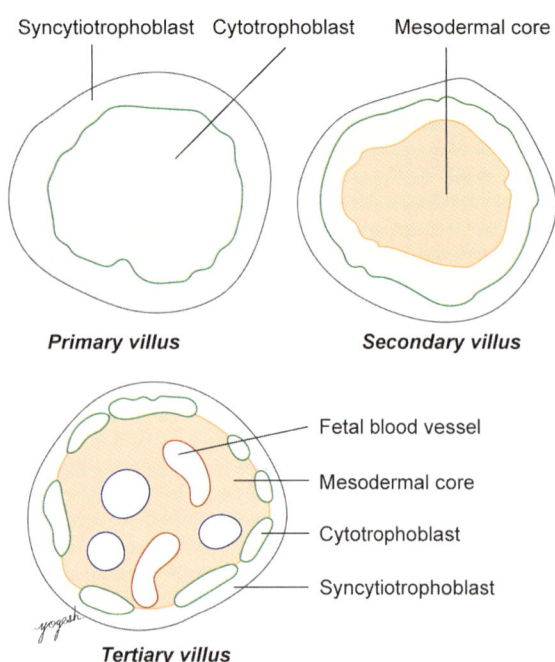

Practice Fig. 7.5: Placental villi

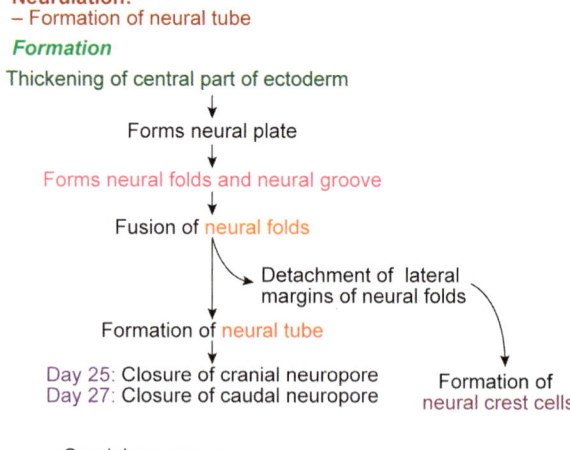

Flowchart 7.3: Process of neurulation

Scanning electron micrograph 7.4: SEM showing neural folding with cranial and caudal neuropores. The developing face is represented by the frontonasal region, and the first pharyngeal (branchial, visceral) arch. [Species: Mouse, approximate human age: 22 days, dorsolateral view]

FORMATION OF NEURAL TUBE/NEURULATION

Q. Define neurulation and list the steps involved in it.

Definition

- A process of formation of neural plate, neural folds and closure of these folds to form neural tube is called *neurulation.*^{Viva}

Process of Neurulation (Fig. 7.8, Flowchart 7.3)

- After gasturation, the ectoderm is divisible into a midline neuroectoderm that overlies the notochord and a surrounding surface ectoderm.
- *Formation of neural plate:* At the beginning of the third week, midline central part of *ectoderm* (in between primitive node and prechordal plate) lying above the developing notochord *thickens*. This thickened part forms *neural plate or medullary plate.*
- *Formation of neural groove:* Elevation of edges of neural plate form peripheral *neural folds* and central depressed part forms *neural groove.*
- Formation of neural tube: Elevation of neural folds continue and start fusion in a future cervical region and then extend in *craniocaudal direction (bidirectional)* to form neural tube. Conversion of neural plate into neural tube is called *neurulation.* Closure of neural tube begins in cervical region at the level of 5th somite.^{NEXT}

Recent concept: Closure of neural tube begins in multiple sites and proceeds simultaneously.

- *Cranial and caudal neuropores* are open ends of neural tube (SEM 7.4).

- On 25th day, cranial neuropore closes, whereas on 27th day, caudal neuropore closes to form closed *neural tube.*^{MCQ,Viva} Closure of cranial neuropore occurs at the 20 somite stage and posterior neuropore at 25 somite stage.^{MCQ, Viva}
- During detachment of neural tube from ectoderm, cells from lateral margins of neural plate/folds separate from both the surface ectoderm and neuroectoderm, and come to lie between neural tube and ectoderm and these detached cells are called **neural crest cells.**^{MCQ, Viva}
- Neural crest cells undergo epithelial to mesenchymal transformation.^{NEXT}
- Neural tube forms central nervous system and neural crest cells form peripheral and autonomic nervous system.
- Prior to closure of neuropores, the amniotic fluid circulates through developing neural tube to provide nutrition.

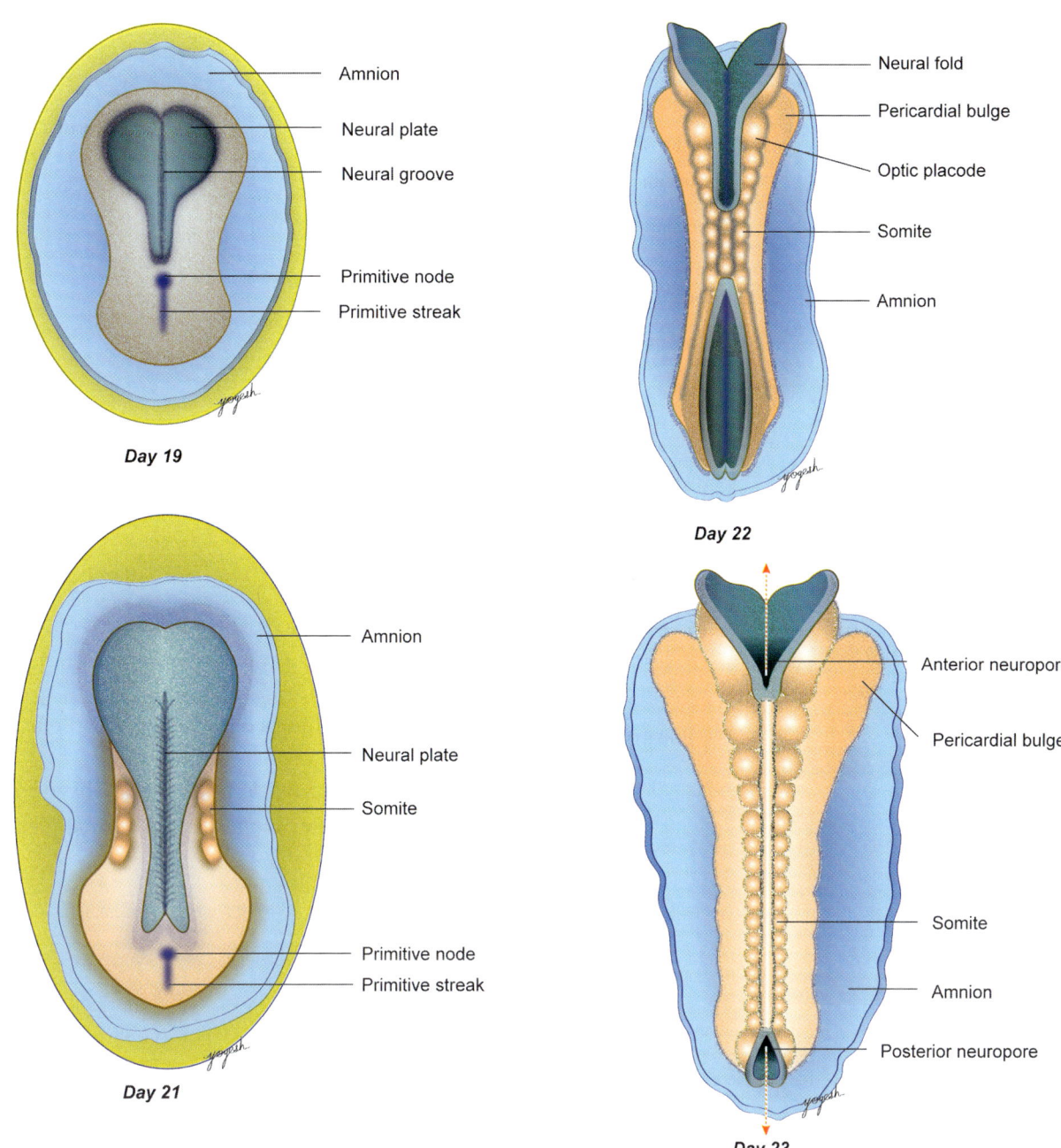

Fig. 7.8: Formation of the neural tube. Neural plate continues its folding to form neural tube

NEURAL CREST

Q. Write a short note on neural crest.

Definition

- Neural crest is a portion of *lateral margins of the neural plate* at its junction with rest of surface ectoderm.

Process of Formation (Fig. 7.9, Practice Fig. 7.6, Flowchart 7.3)

- At the time of separation of neural tube from surface ectoderm, the cells of neural crest also get separated and come to lie between ectoderm and neural tube.
- Thus, neural plate forms neural tube and neural crest cells.
- Neural crest cells further divide to form dorsal mass and ventral mass.
- Neural crest cells give rise to various structures in the body at various locations. Hence, it is also called the fourth germ layer. *Viva*
- For further details about derivatives of neural crest cells, refer Chapter 22 (Nervous System).

FURTHER DEVELOPMENT

- In the third week of IUL, neural tube formation begins and gets completed by 27th day.
- In the third week, mesodermal elements also differentiate to form paraxial mesoderm, intermediate mesoderm and lateral plate mesoderm (SEM 7.5).

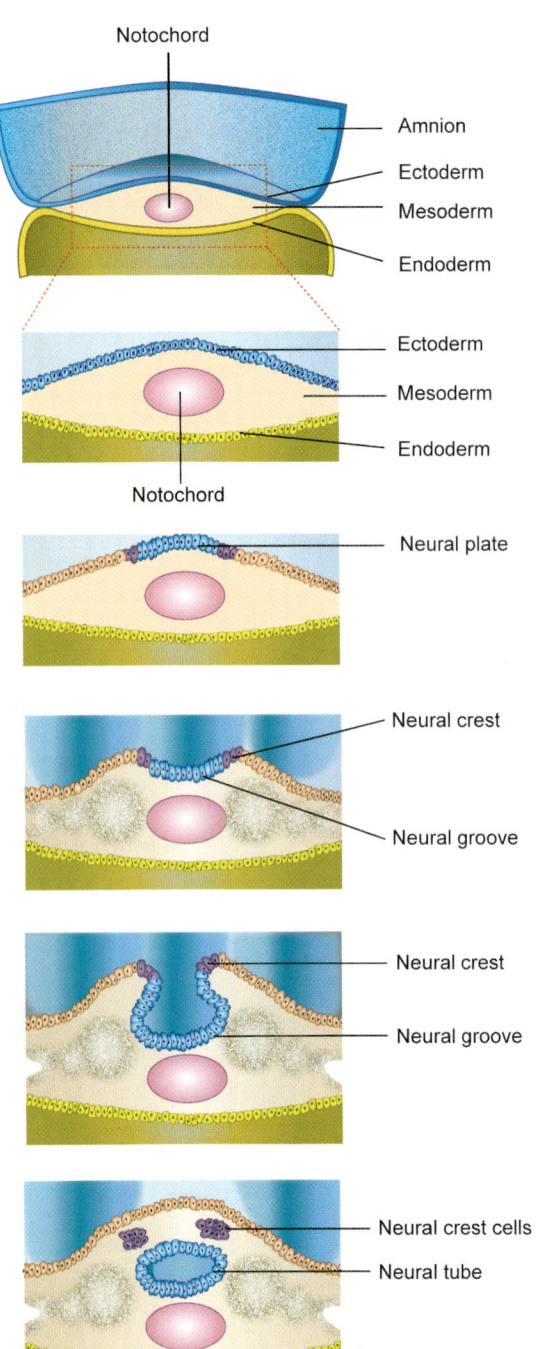

Fig. 7.9: Formation of neural tube and neural crest cells. The neural plate folds on itself to form neural tube. At the time of separation of the neural tube from the surface ectoderm, cells at the margin of the neural plate also separate to form neural crest cells. These cells lie between neural tube and the ectoderm (Transverse section)

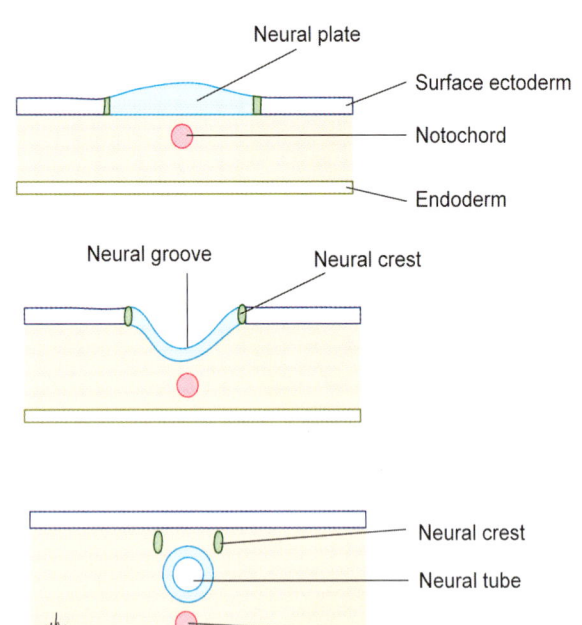

Practice Fig. 7.6: Formation of neural plate and neural crest

- A horseshoe-shaped cavity called intraembryonic coelom appears in mesoderm that divides lateral plate mesoderm into two layers (somatopleuric and splanchnopleuric).
- By the end of third week, folding of embryo begins.
- For detailed development of mesodermal elements and folds of the embryo refer Chapter 8.

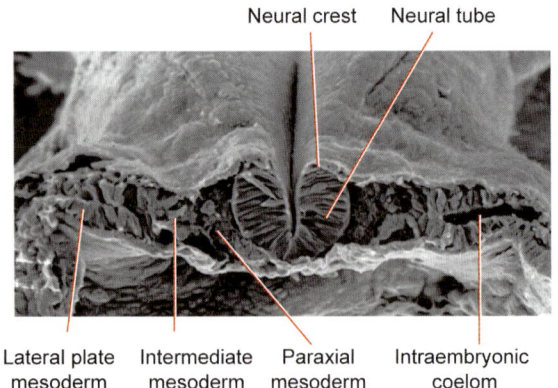

Scanning electron micrograph 7.5: SEM showing differentiation of intraembryonic mesoderm. The intraembryonic mesoderm differentiates into paraxial, intermediate and lateral plate mesoderm [Species: Mouse, approximately human age: 22 days, transverse section]

Clinical Embryology

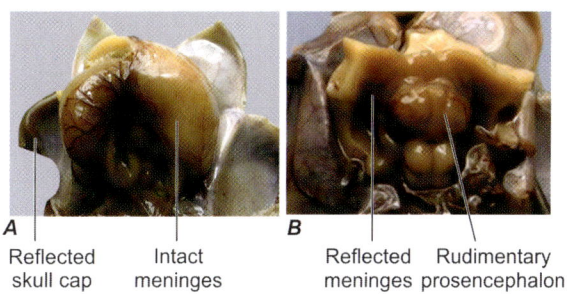

Clinical image 7.1: *Holoprosencephaly (HPE)* is a cephalic disorder with failure of prosencephalon (the forebrain of the embryo) development. Normally, the forebrain is formed and face begins to develop in 5th–6th weeks of intrauterine life: (A) Skull coverings are dissected to show the intact meninges. (B) Meninges are dissected to expose brain–holoprosencephaly (Image courtesy: *Dr Mamatha Gowda*)

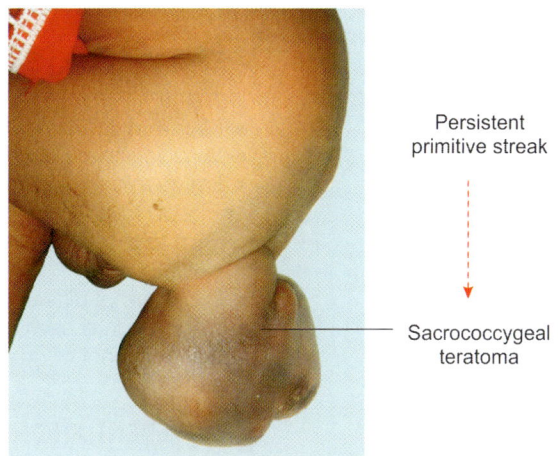

Clinical image 7.2: *Sacrococcygeal teratoma*. Sacrococcygeal teratoma is a tumor derived from primitive streak and it develops at the base of coccyx. Its incidence is 1 in 40,000 live births. Prenatally, it can be diagnosed using sonography. Treatment of choice is the surgical removal. *Note*: Teratoma is a tumor made up of derivatives of all germ layers (ectoderm, endoderm and mesoderm) such as hairs, muscle, bone, tooth, cartilages and so on. Sometime sacrococcygeal teratoma may contain embryonic connective tissue (Image courtesy: *Dr Kumaravel S*)

Chapter 8

Further Development of Embryo

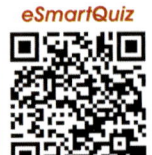
eSmartQuiz

Chapter Outline

- Ectodermal differentiation
  - Neuroectoderm
  - Surface ectoderm
- Mesodermal differentiation
  - Paraxial mesoderm
  - Intermediate mesoderm
  - Lateral plate mesoderm
- Somite
- Midline structures of trilaminar germ disc
- Vasculogenesis and angiogenesis
- Embryonic folding
  - Head fold
  - Tail fold
  - Lateral fold
- Endodermal differentiation
- Changes in embryonic period
- Development of anterior abdominal wall

Competencies:
- **AN79.4:** Describe the development of somites and intra embryonic coelom.
- **AN52.4:** Describe the development of anterior abdominal wall.

INTRODUCTION

- Period of 2nd week to 8th week of development is *embryonic period*.
- During the embryonic period, the germ layers are changing and assigning fate for further development and organ formation. Hence, this period is also called *organogenic period*.^{NEXT}
- During the embryonic period, germ disc gets folded to form identifiable shape of human embryo.
  By the end of the embryonic period, the main organ system have been established, rendering the major features of the external body form recognizable by the end of second month.
- For understanding, the events of embryonic period are grouped under the following headings:
  - Ectodermal differentiation
  - Mesodermal differentiation
  - Embryonic folding
  - Endodermal differentiation
- Teratogens (factor causing embryonic malformation) affect the developing embryo to produce congenital anomalies.

DIFFERENTIATION OF ECTODERM

- At the beginning of the third week, the central part of ectoderm overlying the developing notochord thickens to form a neural plate or *neuroectoderm*.
- Remaining part of the ectoderm is called *surface ectoderm*.
- Ectoderm = Neuroectoderm + Surface ectoderm

Neuroectoderm

- **Neurulation:** Neural plate grows to form peripheral *neural folds* and a central depressed area called *neural groove* (Fig. 8.1).
- Neural folds start fusion in the central (cervical) region. Fusion extends craniocaudally to form *neural tube*.
- Cranial open end of neural tube called *anterior neuropore* closes by the 25th day of IUL (18–20 somite age) (Figs 8.2, 8.3, SEM 8.1).
- Caudal open end of neural tube called *posterior neuropore* closes by the 27th day (25 somite age).
- Cells at the margin of neural plate form the *neural crest*.
- Neural tube gets separated from surface ectoderm, whereas neural crest cells come to lie between ectoderm and neural tube.
- Cephalic part of neural tube shows dilations as forebrain vesicle, midbrain vesicle, and hindbrain vesicle, whereas distal part of neural tube remains

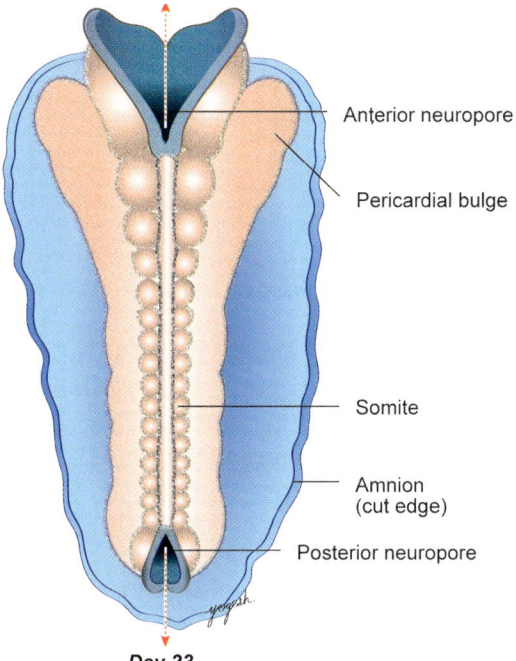

Fig. 8.1: Day 23: Top view of the developing embryo. Anterior and posterior neuropores are open

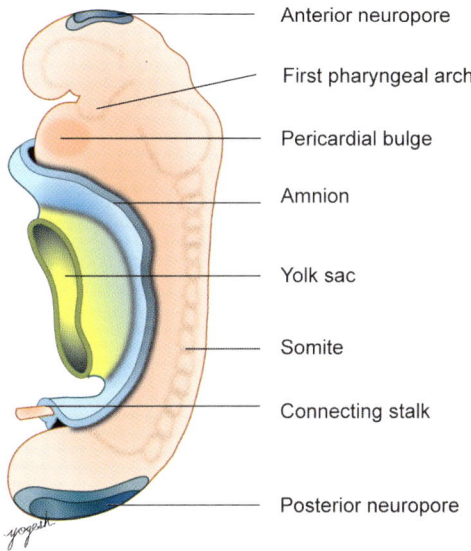

Fig. 8.2: Embryo by day 24: Side view

tubular and forms spinal cord (for details, read Chapter 22, Nervous System).
- Neuroectoderm forms entire central and peripheral nervous system and autonomic ganglia.

Surface Ectoderm

- Surface ectoderm shows depression at *buccopharyngeal membrane* and *cloacal membrane*. At these two depressions, ectoderm is firmly adherent to endoderm. Intraembryonic mesoderm separates ectoderm and endoderm, except at prechordal plate and cloacal membrane.

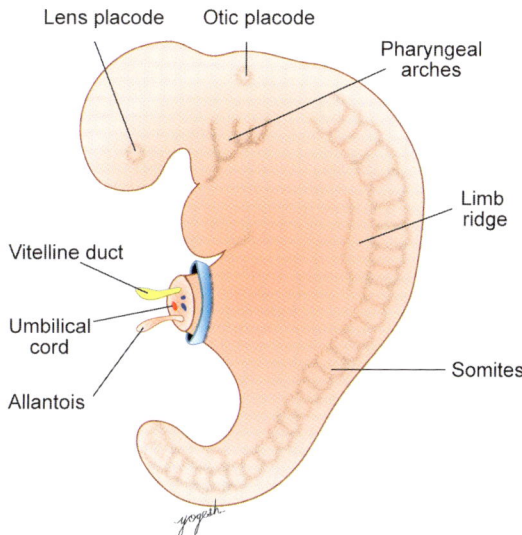

Fig. 8.3: Embryo by day 28: Side view of developing embryo. At the end of the fourth week, first four pharyngeal arches, limb ridge, otic placode and lens placode are seen

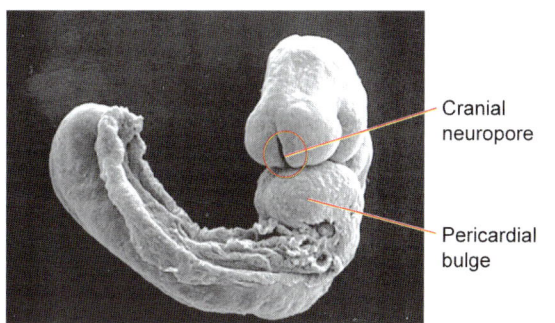

Scanning electron micrograph 8.1: SEM showing embryo at 25th day with closing anterior neuropore [Species: Mouse, approximate human age: 25 days, frontolateral view]

Buccopharyngeal membrane (oropharyngeal membrane)
- In the third week, it lies cranial to the prechordal plate. On development of head fold, prechordal plate comes to lie between forebrain vesicle and pericardial bulging.
- At the beginning of fourth week, buccopharyngeal membrane ruptures to form communication between amniotic cavity and primitive gut.^{MCQ}
- Cloacal membrane divides into anterior urogenital membrane and posterior anal membrane (for details, read Chapter 14).
- Surface ectoderm also forms the following structures:
  1. Epidermis, hair and nail
  2. Sebaceous glands and sweat glands
  3. Olfactory pit (Chapter 23)
  4. Optic vesicle and lens vesicle (Chapter 23)
  5. Otic vesicle (Chapter 24)
  6. Branchial clefts (Chapter 11)
  7. Rathke's pouch
  8. Epithelial lining of cheek, gum, teeth enamel, roof of mouth, nasal cavity and paranasal air sinuses

9. Salivary glands
10. Mammary glands
11. Pituitary glands

Some Interesting Facts

- All the muscles of the body are derived from the mesoderm except muscles of iris and arrectores pilorum of the skin are derived from ectoderm.

MESODERMAL DIFFERENTIATION

- By the end of third week, primitive streak starts regressing.
- Mesodermal cells that are migrated from primitive streak start forming rod-shaped structure on either side of notochord on 17th day of IUL.
- Shallow longitudinal grooves separate condensed mesodermal rods into three parts (Fig. 8.4, SEM 8.2):
  A. *Paraxial mesoderm*: Lies on either side of notochord underneath neural plate.
  B. *Intermediate mesoderm*: Lies lateral to paraxial mesoderm.
  C. *Lateral plate mesoderm*: The lateral most part of mesoderm.

- These components of mesoderm form specific structures in developing embryo.
- Mesoderm = Paraxial mesoderm + Intermediate mesoderm + Lateral plate mesoderm.

Paraxial Mesoderm

- Paraxial mesoderm is situated on either side of notochord.
- *Extent*: It extends from prechordal plate to primitive streak.
- Paraxial mesoderm condenses to form a series of rounded, whorl-like mass called *somitomeres*.
- The somitomeres further develop a discrete block of segmental *paraxial mesoderm* called *somites* or *metameres*.^NEXT

Intermediate Mesoderm

- It lies between the paraxial mesoderm and lateral plate mesoderm.
- On differentiation, intermediate mesoderm forms kidneys and sex glands (ovaries and testis).

Lateral Plate Mesoderm

- Lateral plate mesoderm extends from intermediate mesoderm to extraembryonic mesoderm.

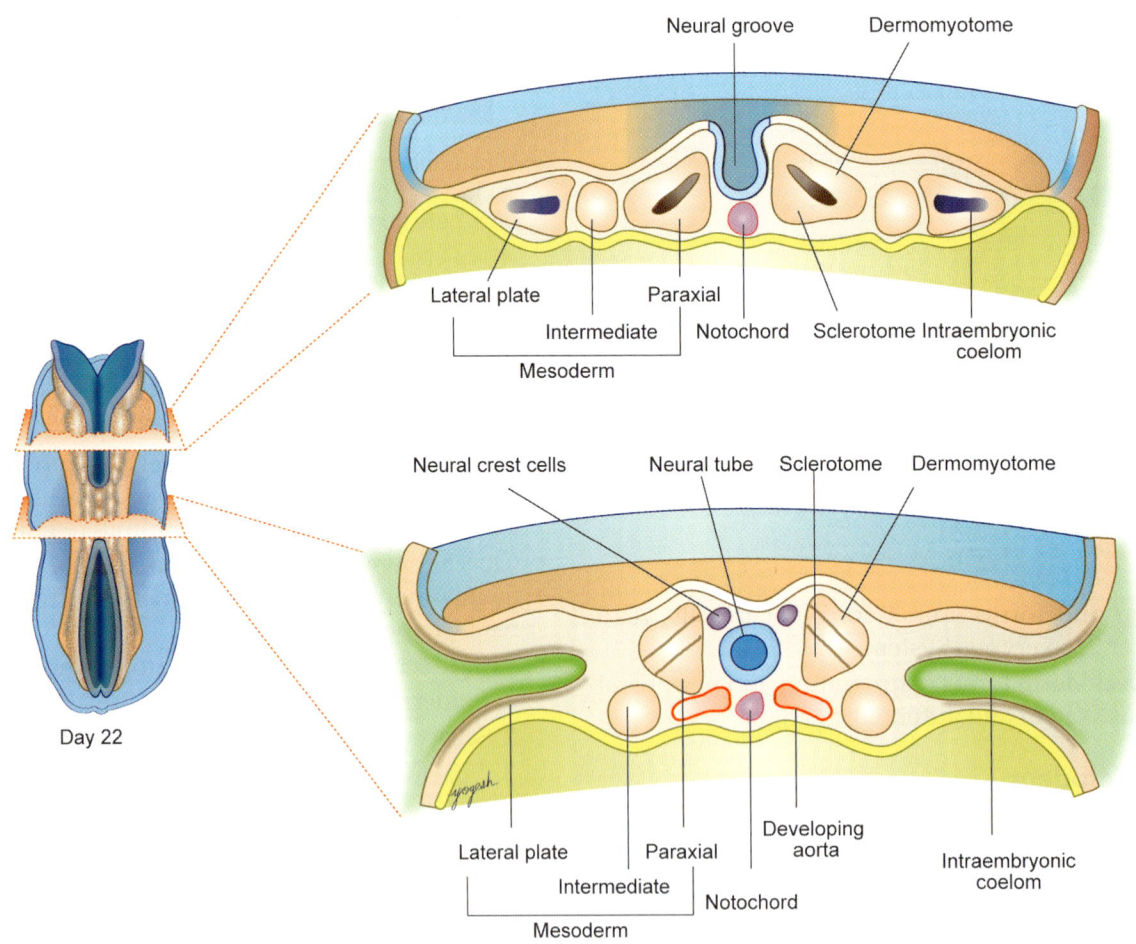

Fig. 8.4: Formation of somites

- Cranially, lateral plate mesoderm is continued with pericardial bar. (*Pericardial bar* is mesodermal condensation, cranial to the buccopharyngeal membrane.)
- Small intercellular cavities appear in the lateral plate mesoderm that fuse to form *intraembryonic coelom*.
- Similar cavity develops in pericardial bar that fuses to form *pericardial sac*.

Formation of Coelomic Cavity

- Pericardial sac communicates with intraembryonic coelom to form inverted U-shaped tubular passage.
- Coelomic cavity forms pericardial, pleural and peritoneal cavities.^{NEXT}

Formation of Layers of Lateral Plate Mesoderm

- Intraembryonic coelom divides lateral plate mesoderm into two layers:
  A. *Somatopleuric layer*: It is a parietal layer that lies in contact with the ectoderm.
  B. *Splanchnopleuric layer*: It is a visceral layer that lies in contact with the endoderm.
- Continuously growing intraembryonic coelom separates somatopleuric and splanchnopleuric layers laterally and develop communication with extraembryonic coelom.

- Communication between intraembryonic and extraembryonic coelomic cavities provides nutrition till the complete development of uteroplacental circulation.
- A cranial mesodermal horseshoe-shaped bar connecting somatopleuric layer with splanchnopleuric layer is called *septum transversum*.
- Septum transversum later participates in the formation of liver (For details refer Chapter 15).

Fate of Lateral Plate Mesoderm

A. Somatopleuric layer
  - It forms
    – Parietal layers of peritoneal, pericardial and pleural cavities
    – Dermis
    – Pectoral and pelvic girdles
    – Skeletal elements of limbs (muscles develop from migrating myotomes)

B. Splanchnopleuric layer
  - It forms
    – Visceral layer of pericardial, peritoneal and pleural cavities
    – Musculature and connective tissue of gut, respiratory tract and heart

SOMITE

Q. Write a short note on somites.

- From prechordal plate to primitive streak, the paraxial mesoderm undergoes condensation to form *somitomeres* (Flowchart 8.1).
- Later, somitomeres undergo segmentation to form *somites*.
- Proximal somitomeres (underlying the developing brain, rostral to the otic vesicle) remain unsegmented and do not form somites. These form striated muscles of face, jaw and throat.^{MCQ}
- *Note*: Prechordal plate mesoderm forms *preoccipital somites* that later form extrinsic muscles of eye.

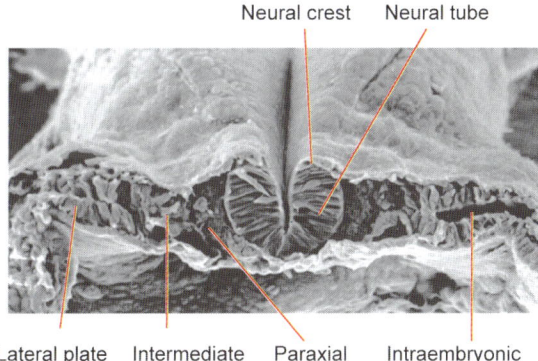

Scanning electron micrograph 8.2: Neural tube formation: SEM showing folding of neural plate and differentiation of intraembryonic mesoderm into paraxial, intermediate and *lateral* plate mesoderm [Species: Mouse, approximately human age: 22 days, transverse cut section]

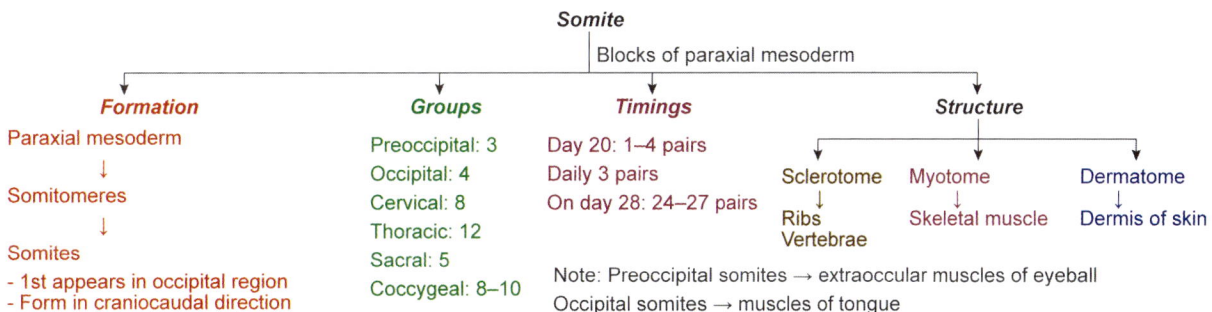

Flowchart 8.1: Somite

- The *first* pair of somites appears on day 20 on each side of the cranial end of the notochord in the occipital region (*cervical level*).[NEXT, Viva]
- Somites continue to appear from day 20 to day 30 in craniocaudal direction.
- In human, 42 to 44 pairs of somites form and they can be grouped as follows:
  - Preoccipital 3 pairs
  - Occipital 4 pairs
  - Cervical 8 pairs
  - Thoracic 12 pairs
  - Sacral 5 pairs
  - Coccygeal 8–10 pairs
- First cervical and last five to seven coccygeal pairs of somites eventually disappear till they reach a final count of 37 pairs of somites. Remaining somites form the axial skeleton.

Counting of Somites

- First somite pair appears on day 20 and further three pairs of somites get segmented each day until the end of the fifth week. Hence, somites give an idea about the fetal age (Table 8.1).[MCQ, Viva]

Structure of Somite

- A somite is a triangular mass of mesenchyme and it is differentiated into three parts as follows (Fig. 8.5):
  1. *Sclerotome*: It is ventromedial part that surrounds the neural tube and forms ribs and vertebrae.
  2. *Myotome*: It is the middle part and forms skeletal muscles. (Hence, paraxial mesoderm forms skeletal muscles through myotomes of somites.[NEXT])
  3. *Dermatome*: It is dorsolateral part and it forms dermis of the skin.
- A small cavity (*myocele*) of somite is obliterated by proliferation of cells.

Table 8.1 The correlation between embryo age with number of somites[MCQ]

Age in days (approximately)	Number of pairs of somites (approximately)
20	1–4
21	4–7
22	7–10
23	10–13
24	13–17
25	17–20
26	20–23
27	23–26
28	26–29
30	34–35
End of 5th week	42–44[NEXT]

- Each somite is supplied by a single spinal nerve. Some authors consider *dermomyotome* instead of separate dermatome and myotome.
- *Note*: Occipital somites and preotic somites participate in the formation of skull base.
- The distribution of sites and their fate is listed in Table 8.2.

Table 8.2 Distribution and fate of somites

Somites	Number (in pairs)	Muscular derivatives	Skeletal derivatives
Preoccipital	3	Extraocular muscles of eyeball	Base of skull
Occipital	4	Muscles of tongue except palatoglossus	
Cervical	8	Skeletal muscles of trunk, limbs and diaphragm	Vertebrae (ribs from thoracic somites)
Thoracic	12		
Lumbar	5		
Sacral	5		
Coccygeal	8–10		

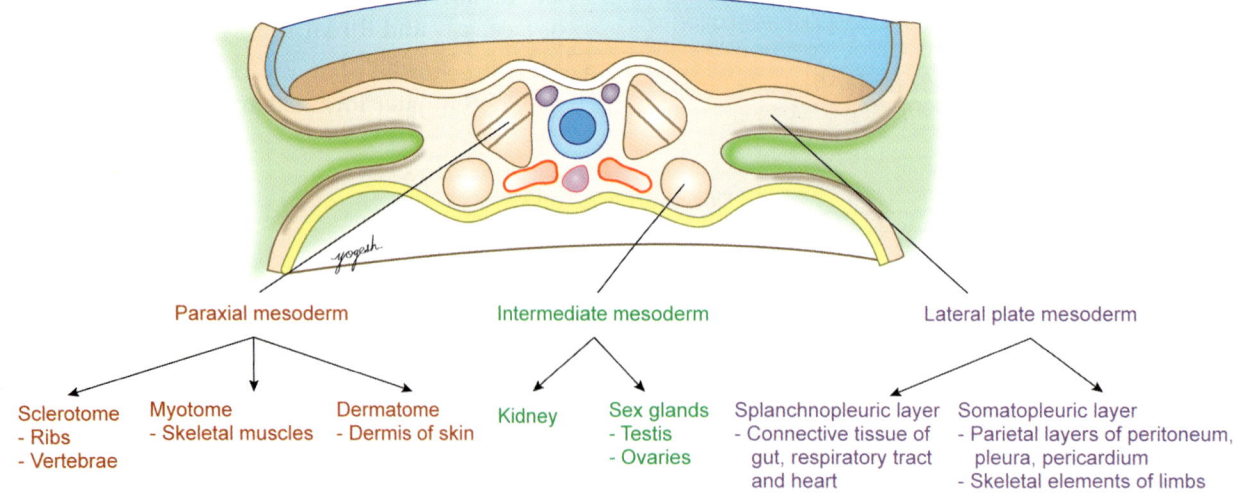

Fig. 8.5: Derivatives of the mesoderm. Intraembryonic mesoderm divides into paraxial, intermediate and lateral plate mesoderm that later give rise to various structures

Box 8.1: Midline structures of trilaminar germ disc

Q. Enlist the midline structures of germ disc.
- Trilaminar germ disc has the following structures in the midline from cranial to caudal direction:
  1. Septum transversum
  2. Pericardial sac
  3. Buccopharyngeal membrane
  4. Notochord, neural tube
  5. Primitive node
  6. Primitive streak
  7. Cloacal membrane
  8. Connecting stalk

Box 8.2: Vasculogenesis and angiogenesis

- Vasculogenesis is formation of a new vessel from mesenchymal tissue in embryo (Flowchart 8.2).
- Angiogenesis is sprouting of vessel into adjacent area by endothelial budding.
- At beginning of the third week, formation of vasculature begins in extraembryonic mesoderm of yolk sac, connecting stalk and chorion.^{MCQ}

Steps of formation of vasculature
- On day 17, mesenchymal cells differentiate into hemangioblasts (first in the splanchnic mesoderm of yolk sac and later in the mesoderm of the connecting stalk and the chorion) (Fig. 8.6).
- Hemangioblasts aggregate to form the cluster of cells called **blood island** (Flowchart 8.2).
- Hemangioblasts differentiate into two cell lineages as follows:
  A. Primitive hematopoietic stem cells (HSC) that on differentiation form erythropoietic cells, megakaryocytes and primitive macrophages.
  B. Endothelial precursor cells (EPC) that form epithelial lining of primitive endothelium.
- Small cavities appear in blood island to form lumen of primitive capillaries.
- Primitive hemangioblastic islands fuse to develop capillary networks (vasculogenesis).
- Endothelial precursor cells sprout into adjacent mesenchyme and fuse with adjacent hemangioblastic island and develop new capillaries (angiogenesis) to expand network.
- By the end of third week, yolk sac, connecting stalk and chorionic villi get completely vascularized.
- *Note:* Yolk sac is the first supplier of blood cells and it continues up to 60 days as hematopoietic organ. Later, liver, spleen, thymus and bone marrow take over the hematopoietic function.^{MCQ}
- Capillary hemangioma (strawberry birthmark): It is a noncancerous tumor produced by abnormal overgrowth of tiny blood vessels. It is present in all about 10% born babies.

Flowchart 8.2: Vasculogenesis

Vasculogenesis: Formation of new blood vessels
Angiogenesis: Sprouting of new blood vessels from existing vessels

Steps
Day 17
Mesenchymal cells of yolk sac →(Differentiation)→ Hemangioblasts

Aggregation of hemangioblasts
- HSC → Erythrocytes, Megakaryocytes, Macrophages
- EPC → Primitive endocardium
- Blood island → Cavities → Lumen of vessels

Note: Sites of hematopoiesis: Yolk sac (up to 60 days), liver, spleen, thymus, bone marrow, HSC: hematopoietic stem cells, EPC: endothelial presursor cells.

FOLDING OF EMBRYO

- In the third week, embryo is in the form of flat trilaminar germ disc (Flowchart 8.3).
- *Reason for foldings of embryo:* Cells in central part of germ disc multiply rapidly than that at periphery. Overgrown central part results in folding of germ disc and forms a primitive cylindrical embryo.
- Due to overgrowing tissue, the embryo shows folding in median plane (cephalocaudal folding) and lateral plane (*lateral foldings*).

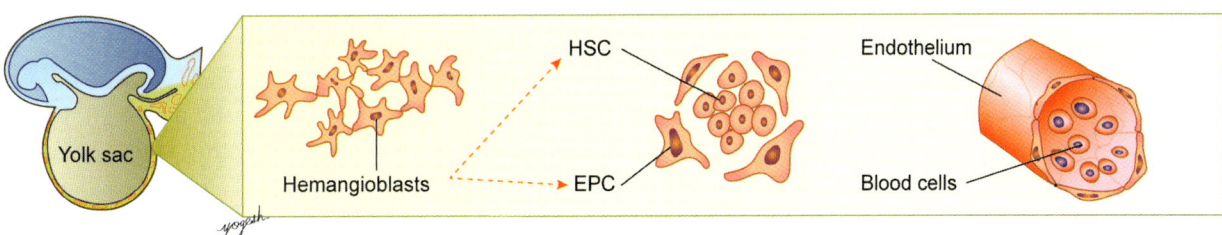

| Vasculogenesis begins in the yolk sac, connecting stalk and extraembryonic mesoderm in tertiary villi | Mesodermal cells form cell masses called blood islands. It consists of hemangioblasts | Hemangioblasts differentiate into primitive hematopoietic stem cells (HSC) and endothelial precursor cells (EPC) | HSC on differentiation forms blood cells, whereas EPC differentiate to form vascular endothelium |

Fig. 8.6: Vasculogenesis

Flowchart 8.3: Foldings of embryo, formation of umbilical cord

```
                    Foldings of embryo
                            ↓
    Reason      Rapid growth of central part of embryo
                            ↓
              4 folds: head fold, tail fold, 2 lateral folds
    Effects
    1. Flat trilaminar germ disc ──→ Cylindrical embryo
    2. Hourglass contraction of yolk sac ──→ Gut tube
                                        ↘ Vitellointestinal duct
                                        ↘ Umbilical vesicle
    3. Formation of connecting stalk ──→ Umbilical cord
```

- Cephalocaudal folding can be studied as cranial *head fold* and caudal *tail fold*.
- Before embryonic folding, septum transversum lies at the cranial most part of the embryo.^{NEXT}

Effects of folding:

1. Folding gives cylindrical shape to the embryo.
2. All folds converge on ventral surface of embryo to produce hourglass constriction of yolk sac.
3. Amniotic cavity enlarges to enclose ventral surface of embryo and amniotic membrane forms a tubular covering around connecting stalk.
4. Part of yolk sac trapped within embryo forms primitive gut and protruding part of yolk sac (extra-embryonic part) forms an *umbilical vesicle*.
5. *Vitellointestinal duct* (omphaloenteric duct) temporarily connects primitive gut with umbilical vesicle. Part of primitive gut cranial to vitello-intestinal duct is *foregut* and caudal to it is *hindgut*, whereas part of gut communicating with vitello-intestinal duct is called *midgut*.

Head Fold

Q. Write a short note on head fold of embryo

- Overgrowing germ disc folds around cranial end of notochord to form a head fold (Figs 8.7 to 8.9, Practice Fig. 8.1, SEM 8.3).
- Head fold produces following changes:
  1. *Foregut*: Trapped part of yolk sac in head fold is called foregut.
  2. *Anterior intestinal portal*: It is a communication between foregut and midgut.
  3. *Ventral relations of foregut*: Buccopharyngeal membrane, pericardial sac septum transversum lie ventral to foregut.
  4. *Dorsal relations of foregut*: Notochord and brain vesicles lie dorsal to the foregut.
  5. *Cranial relation of foregut*: Rapidly growing forebrain vesicle lies cranial to foregut.

Some Interesting Facts

- Due to head fold, the buccopharyngeal membrane comes to lie on ventral surface of embryo and becomes cranial to pericardial sac and septum transversum.
- During the fourth week, buccopharyngeal membrane ruptures.
- Foregut is separated from pericardial sac by a cardiogenic plate (mesenchyme that forms heart).
- Septum transversum is a mesenchymal tissue that lies caudal to the pericardial sac. Septum transversum form fibrous pericardium, and part of ventral mesentery of foregut.
- Microglia and dura mater are mesodermal in origin.^{NEXT}

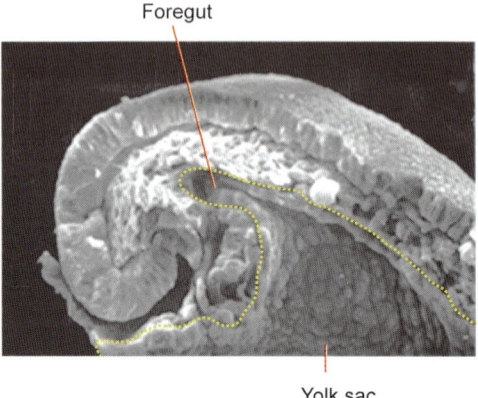

Scanning electron micrograph 8.3: SEM showing the formation of the head fold. Incorporated part of the yolk sac within the embryo can be seen [Species: mouse, approximate human age: 19 days, sagittal cut view]

Tail Fold

Q. Write a short note on tail fold of embryo.

- Overgrowing germ disc also fold ventrally around caudal end of notochord to form a tail fold (Practice Fig. 8.1).
- Tail fold produces the following changes:
  1. *Formation of hindgut*: Trapped part of yolk sac in the tail fold is called *hindgut*.
  2. *Formation of allantoenteric diverticulum*: Allantois communicates with hindgut and comes to lie ventral to hindgut in the form of *allantoenteric diverticulum*.
  3. *Cloacal membrane*: Bilaminar cloacal membrane later divides into urogenital and anal membrane and lies caudal to connecting stalk.
  4. *Dorsal relations of hindgut*: Notochord and neural tube lie dorsal to developing hindgut.
  5. *Caudal relations of hindgut*: Degenerating primitive node and streak lie caudal to developing hindgut.
  6. Allantoenteric diverticulum divides hindgut into preallantoic and postallantoic parts.

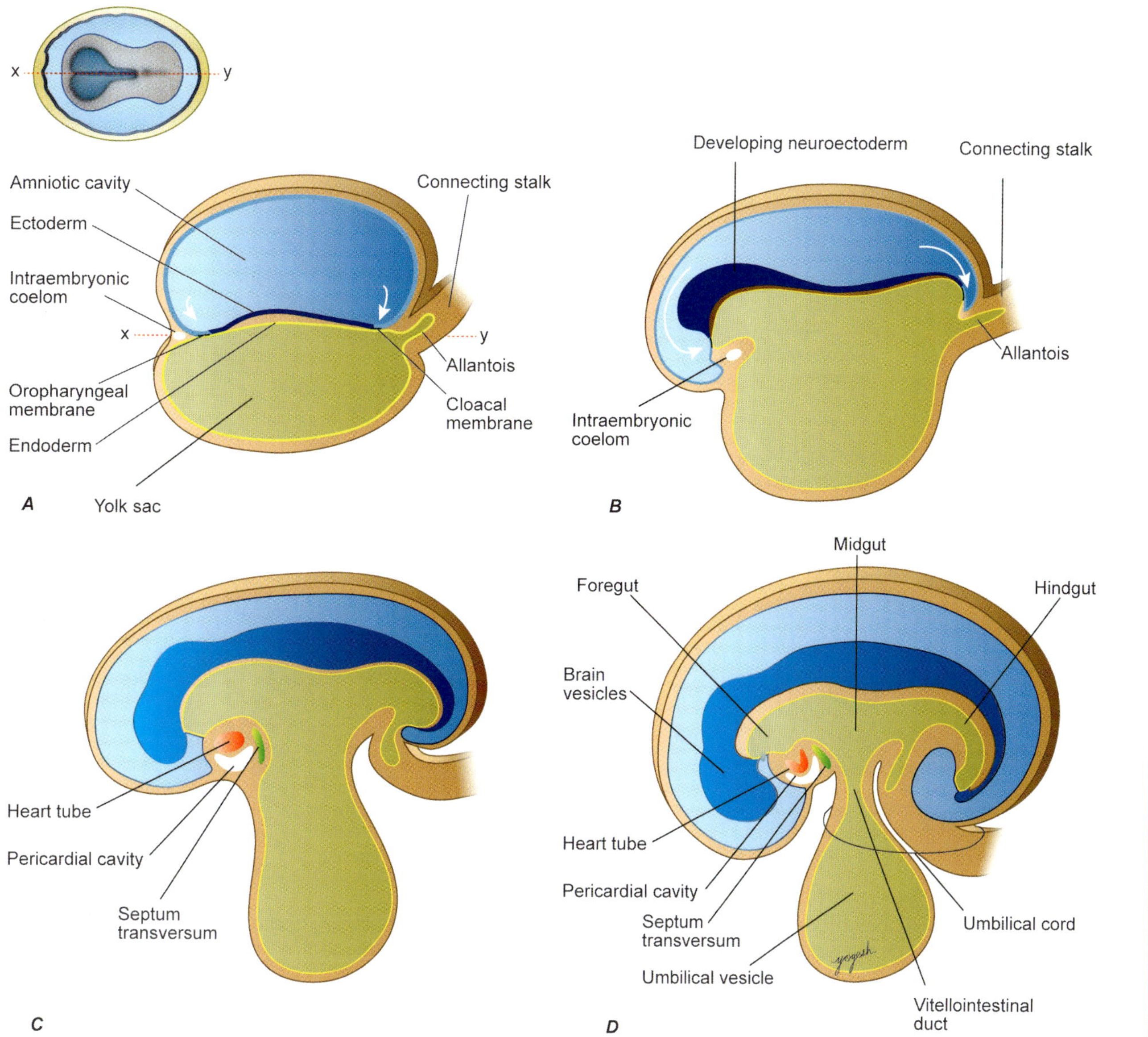

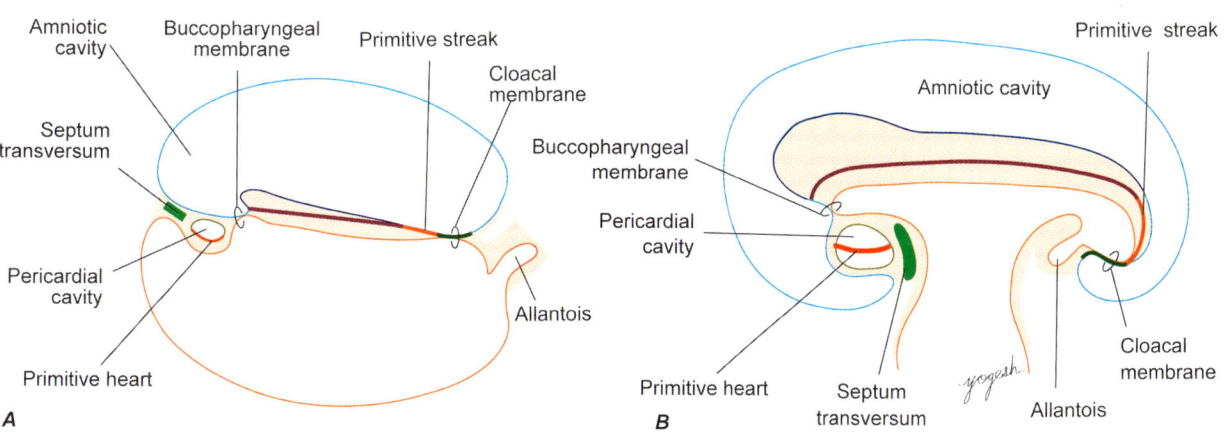

Fig. 8.7: Formation of craniocaudal (head and tail) foldings of the embryo. Progressive midsagittal sections of the developing embryo show craniocaudal foldings: (A) Day 18–19; (B) 22 days; (C) 24 days; (D) 28 days. Amnion is pulled ventrally. Yolk sac lining and endoderm form foregut, midgut, hindgut, vitellointestinal duct and umbilical vesicle

Practice Fig. 8.1: Head and tail folds of embryo

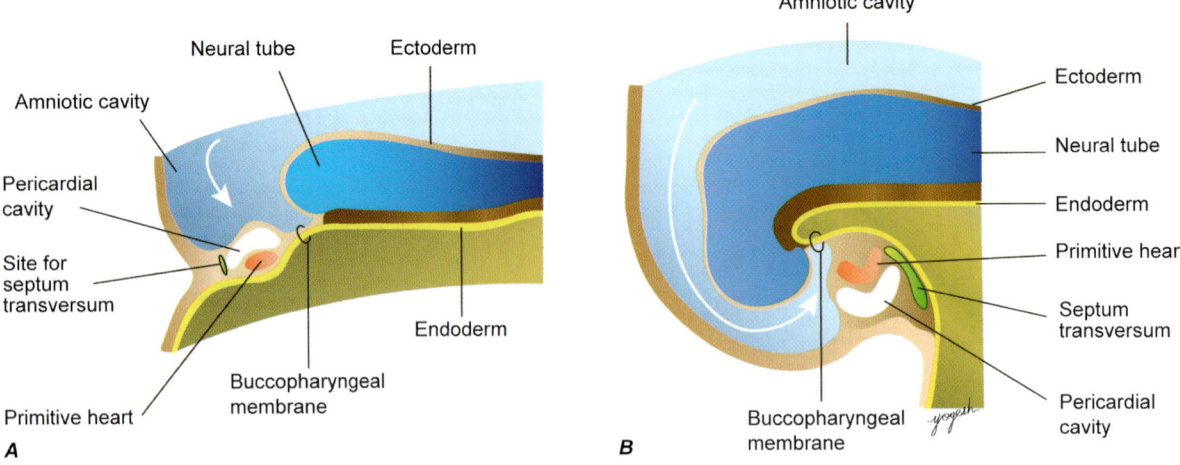

Fig. 8.8: Cranial folding of the embryo. Sagittal section of the embryo at the beginning (A) and at the end of the fourth week (B). Rapidly growing neural tube and change in the positions of the buccopharyngeal membrane, pericardial cavity, primitive heart and septum transversum

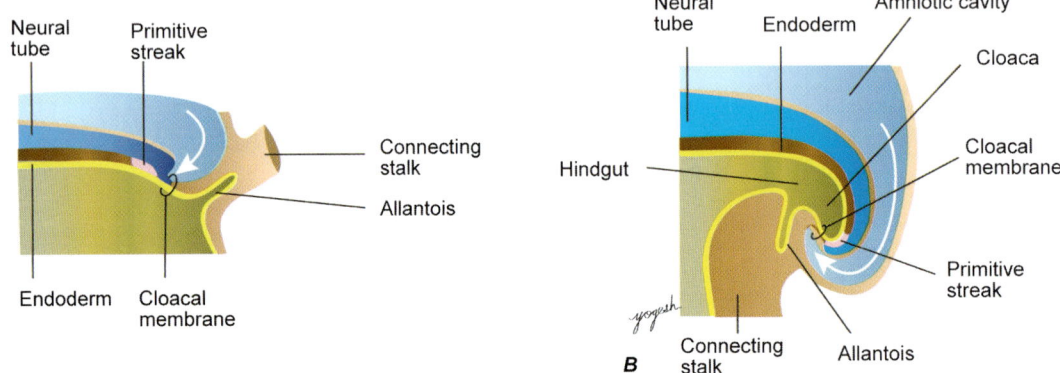

Fig. 8.9: Caudal folding of the embryo. Sagittal section of the embryo at the beginning (A) and at the end of the fourth week (B). Rapidly growing ectoderm and neural tube change the positions of the primitive streak, cloacal membrane, allantois and connecting stalk

7. *Posterior intestinal portal*: It is a communication between midgut and preallantoic part of hindgut.

Lateral Folds

- Overgrowing central part of the germ disc forms two lateral folds (right and left) (Fig. 8.10).
- Lateral folds make the embryo cylindrical on fusion with head and tail fold at the primitive umbilical ring.

Changes due to Formation of Lateral Folds
(Fig. 8.10)

1. *Shifting of amnioectodermal junction*: Amnioectodermal junction comes to lie on umbilical cord (connecting stalk).
2. *Formation of midgut, vitellointestinal duct and umbilical vesicle*: Lateral fold trap part of yolk sac called *midgut*. Midgut communicates through a *vitellointestinal duct* with remaining small part of yolk sac called *umbilical vesicle*.
3. *Formation of dorsal mesentery of gut*: Lateral folds make splanchnopleuric intraembryonic mesodermal layer to cover ventrolateral surface of gut and to reflect dorsally on developing as dorsal mesentery.

Box 8.2: Connecting stalk

- Formation of tail fold moves attachment of connecting stalk form dorsal end of germ disc to ventral aspect of embryo and limits it at umbilical opening.
- Structure of connecting stalk in the fifth week
  It contains following the structures:
  1. Vitellointestinal duct
  2. Remnants of the yolk sac
  3. Extraembryonic mesodermal connective tissue that later forms Wharton's jelly (connective tissue of umbilical cord) and vessels of umbilical cord
- Connecting stalk is a site of amnioectodermal reflection and continuation of intraembryonic and extraembryonic coelom. This coelomic continuation persists up to 10th week.

4. *Formation of peritoneal cavity*: Splanchnopleuric intraembryonic mesoderm (dorsal mesentery) continue with somatopleuric intraembryonic mesoderm via intermediate mesoderm. Somatopleuric intraembryonic mesoderm fuse ventrally in midline and converts intraembryonic coelom to *peritoneal cavity*.

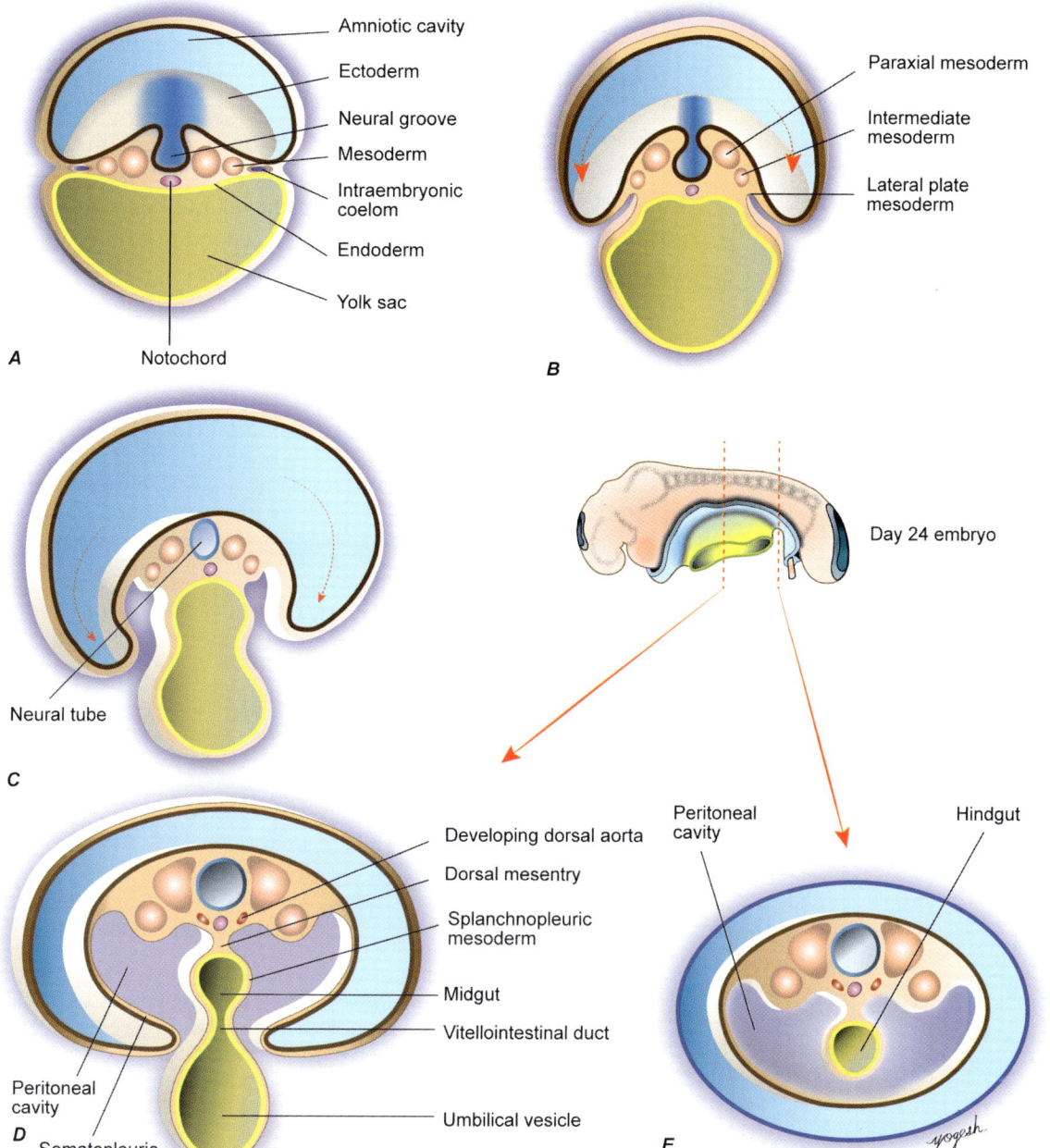

Fig. 8.10: Lateral folding of the developing embryo. Transverse sections through various stages of the embryo. Section D passes through midway between craniocaudal axis, whereas E section passes through caudal part of embryo: (A) At the beginning of the third week, embryo shows neural folds; (B) By 20 days, intraembryonic coelom appears and divides lateral plate mesoderm into splanchnopleuric and somatopleuric layers; (C) By 21 days, intraembryonic coelom communicates with extraembryonic coelom; (D) By 24 days, lateral folds approach ventrally and make hourglass contracture of yolk sac. Midgut communicates with the yolk sac vesicle via vitellointestinal duct; (E) At the end of the fourth week, splanchnopleuric layer forms a double-layered membrane called dorsal mesentery. Dorsal mesentery connects developing gut with developing posterior wall of the embryo

DIFFERENTIATION OF ENDODERM

- Flat endoderm is converted into tubular structure due to formation of embryonic folding (head, tail and lateral folds).
- Endodermal tubular structure is divided into foregut, midgut and hindgut (Fig. 8.11).
- Derivatives of primitive gut are listed in Table 8.3. The detailed development of these structures is described in the Chapters 12–15 on the development of the digestive tract.

MAJOR CHANGES IN 4TH TO 8TH WEEKS

- Changes of 4th to 8th weeks are listed below.
- At the beginning of fourth week, embryonic disc is almost flat and has 4–12 somites.

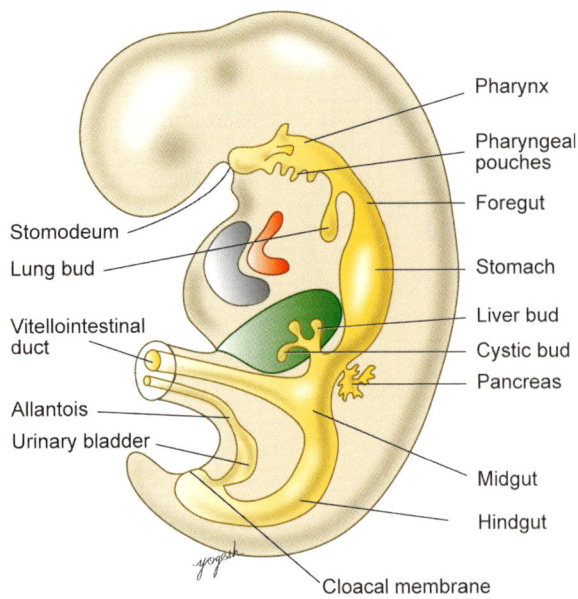

Fig. 8.11: Sagittal section of the embryo showing the derivatives of the endoderm. For understanding, other structures such as neural tube, dorsal aorta are not shown

Table 8.3	Derivatives of primitive gut[MCQ,Viva]
Part of the gut	Derivatives
Foregut	• Lining of epithelium of pharynx, esophagus, stomach, duodenum up to the ampulla of Vater, tongue, floor of mouth
	• Lining epithelium of respiratory system, auditory tube, tympanic cavity
	• Parenchyma of tonsil, thyroid, parathyroid, thymus, liver and pancreas
Midgut	• Lining epithelium of distal part of duodenum, jejunum, ileum, caecum, appendix, ascending colon, right two-thirds of transverse colon
Hindgut	• Lining epithelium of left one-third of transverse colon, descending colon, sigmoid colon, rectum, anal canal up to mucocutaneous junction
	• Lining epithelium of urinary bladder except trigone, urethra (except posterior wall of prostatic part and terminal part of penile urethra), vagina[NEXT]
	• Parenchyma of prostate (except glandular zone), bulbourethral gland[NEXT]

Fourth Week

During fourth week of intrauterine life, the following changes occurs:
- Increase in the somite numbers
- Formation of three brain vesicles from the neural tube
- Formation of head and tail folds
- 21st days and later: Heart starts beating
- 24th day: First pharyngeal arch appears[MCQ]
- 26th day: Three pairs of pharyngeal arches
- 26th–27th day: Rudimentary forelimb bud
- 28th day: Rudimentary hindlimb bud
- Formation of prominence of forebrain vesicle
- Otic pits, lens placodes (ectodermal thickening) appear

Fifth Week

During fifth week of intrauterine life, the following changes occur (SEM 8.4):
- Rapid growth of facial and head prominences
- Rapid growth of a second pharyngeal arch
- Growth of the limb buds
- Formation of alar and basal laminae of the neural tube
- Appearance of olfactory placodes, maxillary and frontonasal process
- Appearance of gonadal ridges

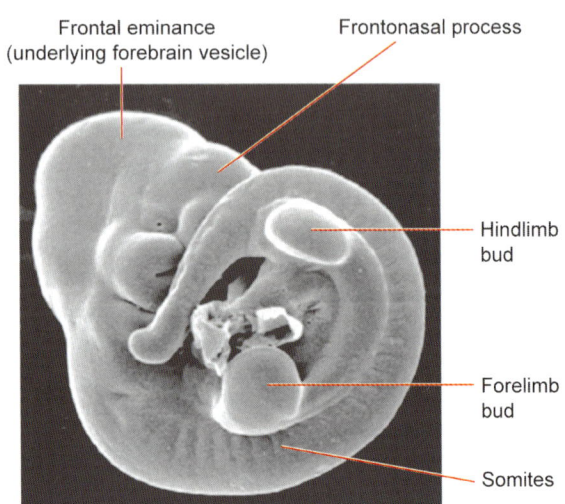

Scanning electron micrograph 8.4: SEM showing embryo of 5th week. Rapidly growing facial processes, head, and limb buds can be noted. The thickened ectoderm at the distal rim of the limb bud is termed the apical ectodermal ridge [Species: Mouse, approximate human age: 33 days, lateral view]

Sixth Week

During sixth week of intrauterine life, the following changes occur:
- Shows spontaneous movements
- Growth of brain vesicles
- Appearance of nasal processes
- Buccopharyngeal membrane ruptures
- Development of appendix, caecum and spleen
- Differentiation of the limb digits begins. Differentiation in lower limb starts 4–5 later than upper limb.
- Umbilical herniation is common.

Seventh and Eighth Weeks

During seventh and eighth weeks of intrauterine life, the following changes occur:
- Development of face, external ear (auricular hillock) and eye

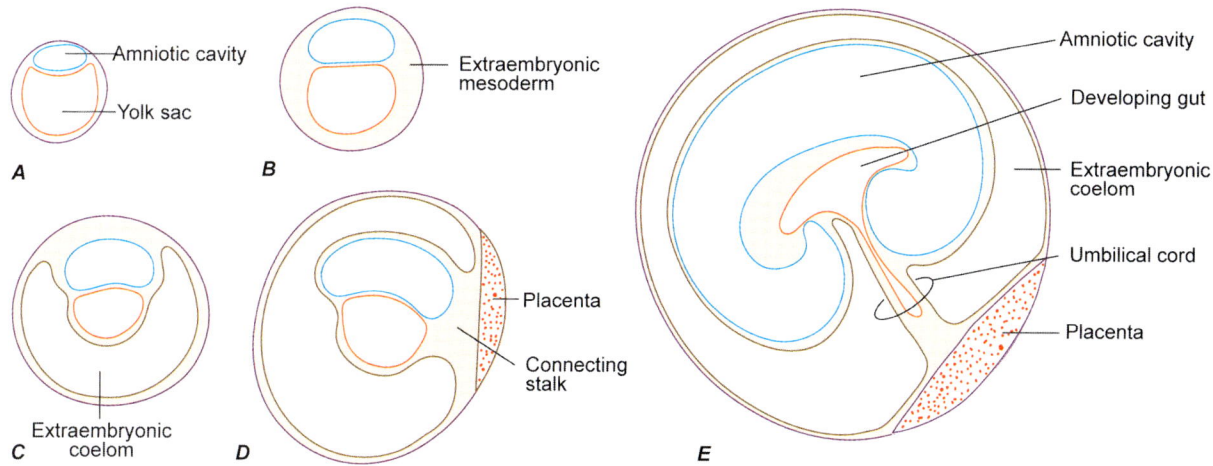

Practice Fig. 8.2: Folding of embryo, formation of umbilical cord

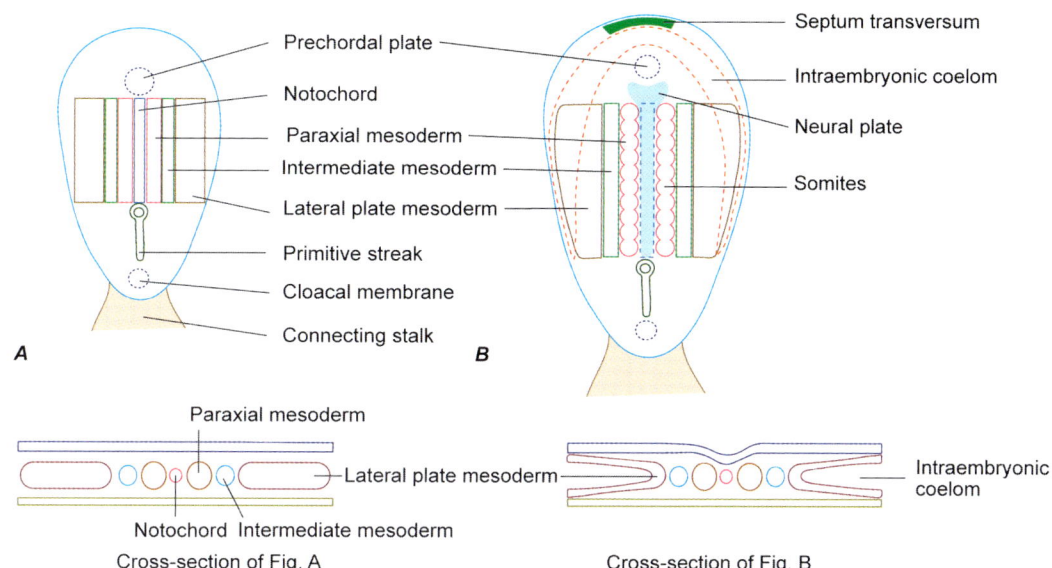

Practice Fig. 8.3: Subdivisions of intraembryonic mesoderm, intraembryonic coelom and somites

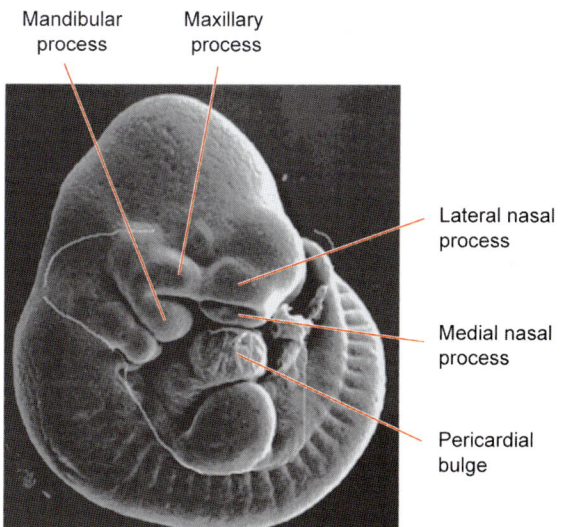

Scanning electron micrograph 8.5: SEM showing 6-week embryo with rapid growth of cranial and facial prominences [Species: Mouse, approximate human age: 6 weeks, lateral view]

- Well-defined limbs and digits
- Development of metanephric kidney
- Development of testis and ovaries
- Differentiation of external genitalia
- During the eighth week, coordinated limb movements occur
- Primary ossification centers start appearing
- Caudal tail-like eminence disappears

Some Interesting Facts

- **Agenesis:** It is the absence of precursor cell of an organ with subsequent complete absence or nondevelopment of the organ.^{NEXT}
- **Aplasia:** It is a partial failure of an organ to develop that result to rudimentary organ.
- **Atresia:** It is a closure or absence of a duct or passage or orifice that is usually present in the body.
- **Atrophy:** It is decrease in a size of an organ due to decrease in number of cells and size.

• Further Development of Embryo

DEVELOPMENT OF ANTERIOR ABDOMINAL WALL

- Anterior abdominal wall consists of the following layers:
  - Skin (epidermis, dermis)
  - Fascia
  - Muscles
  - Parietal peritoneum
  - It encloses peritoneal cavity.

Stages of Development

- Initially, embryo is trilaminar and have
  1. Ectoderm
  2. Mesoderm – Paraxial, intermediate, and lateral plate mesoderm
  3. Endoderm
- The intraembryonic coelome divides lateral plate mesoderm into somatopleuric and splanchnopleuric mesoderm.
- Folding of embryo (Figs 8.7 to 8.9)
  - Folding of embryo begins in the 4th week.
  - There are following four folds:
    - Head fold
    - Tail fold
    - Two lateral folds
  - All folds meet at the umbilicus on the ventral surface of embryo.
- Due to folding of embryo (Fig. 8.10):
  - Part of intraembryonic coelom forms peritoneal cavity.
  - Somatopleuric layers of right and left side fuse in the midline to form connective tissue and muscle layers of anterior abdominal wall.
  - Ectoderm forms epidermis covering anterior wall.
- Unfused portion gives passage to umbilical vessels and form umbilical cord.

Clinical Correlation Defects of Ventral Body Wall

- Ventral body wall defects occur approximately in 1:2000 live births.
- Gastroschisis: It is the condition of defective anterior abdominal wall. Through the defect, coils of intestine and other abdominal viscera protrude outside. There is absence of peritoneal sac covering the contents (Cinical image 14.5).
- Omphalocele: It is a rare abdominal wall defect in which the intestine remains outside the abdominal wall in a peritoneal sac. It occurs because of failure of normal return of intestine into the abdominal cavity (Clinical image 14.1, 14.4).

Chapter 9

Placenta and Umbilical Cord

eSmartQuiz

Chapter Outline

- Placenta
  - Gross features
  - Measurements
  - Structure
  - Development
  - Chorionic villi and their branching pattern
  - Placental barrier
  - Classification
  - Functions
- Umbilical cord
  - Measurements
  - Development
  - Contents
- Amnion
  - Constituents of amniotic fluid
  - Functions of amniotic fluid
  - Volume of amniotic fluid
  - Clinical aspects
- Yolk sac
  - Formation and changes in yolk sac
  - Functions

Competencies:
- **AN80.1:** Describe formation, functions and fate of chorion, amnion, yolk sac, allantois, and decidua.
- **AN80.2:** Describe formation and structure of umbilical cord.
- **AN80.3:** Describe role of placenta, its physiological functions, foetomaternal circulation and placental barrier.
- **AN80.5:** Describe role of placental hormones in uterine growth and parturition.
- **AN80.7:** Describe various types of umbilical cord attachments.
- **AN78.5:** Describe decidual reaction,...

PLACENTA

Q. Describe the placenta. (Long-answer question for postgraduate students)

- Placenta is an organ that performs exchange of nutrients and gases between mother and fetus. Thus, the placenta is a *fetomaternal organ*.
- The placenta is a characteristic feature of eutherian mammals.
- Human placenta is discoid, choriodeciduate organ.
- Placenta has two components
  A. *Maternal component* that is derived from uterine endometrium (decidua).
  B. *Fetal component* that develops from trophoblast and extraembryonic mesoderm (chorion).
- Placenta with fetal membrane is also expelled out of the uterus in 30 minutes after parturition (childbirth).

Gross Features

Q. Draw a well-labelled diagram of the placenta showing maternal and fetal surfaces (Fig. 9.1).

- Full-term placenta is disc-shaped and shows two surfaces: Fetal and maternal (Fig. 9.1).

Fetal Surface

- Fetal surface of the placenta is shiny, grey and translucent.
- Fetal surface of the placenta is smooth and covered by chorionic plate and amnion.^{NEXT}
- It provides attachment to the umbilical cord.
- Radiating umbilical vessels can be easily seen under the translucent amnion.

Maternal Surface

- Maternal surface of the placenta is rough and dark maroon.

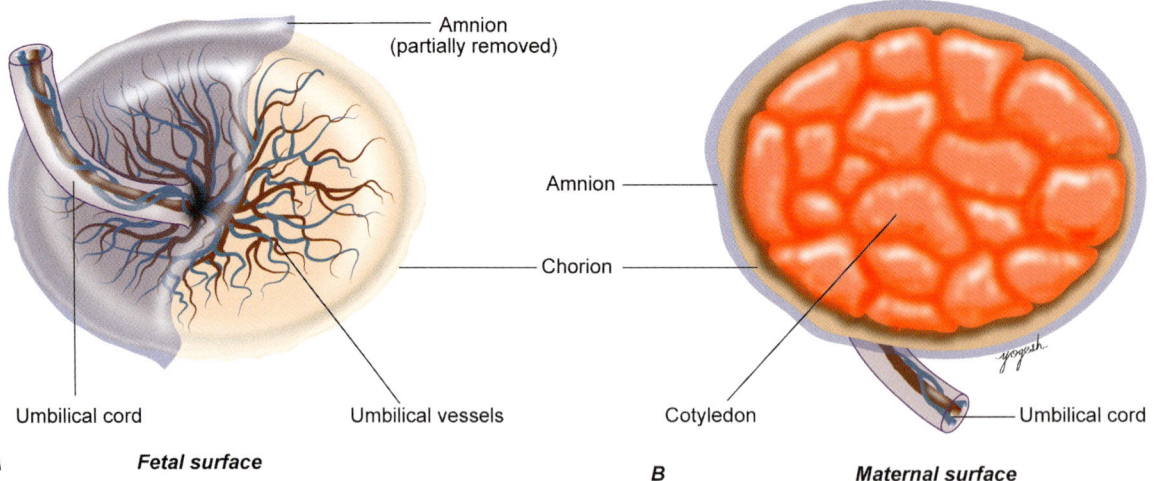

Fig. 9.1: Surfaces of placenta. Placenta has two surfaces: Fetal and maternal. Fetal surface is smooth, covered by translucent layer of amnion and shows attachment of the umbilical cord. Maternal surface shows 15–30 polygonal cotyledons

- It is divided into 15–30 polygonal lobules that are separated from each other by fissures (cobblestone appearance).
- These polygonal lobules are called *cotyledons*.
- Fissures separating cotyledons are occupied by *placental septae*.
- Each cotyledon mostly contains single stem villus and its branches.

Measurements

- The full-term placenta is discoid in shape, 15–25 cm in diameter.
- It is 3 cm thick at the centre.
- It weighs about 500–600 gm.

Structure of Placenta (Flowchart 9.1)

- Placenta consists of
  1. Chorionic plate
  2. Stem villi
  3. Intervillous space with maternal blood
  4. Basal plate
- Placenta shows basal plate on the maternal side and chorionic plate on the fetal side.

Basal Plate

- It consists of
  1. Stratum spongiosum of decidua basalis (Boxes 9.1, 9.2, Fig. 9.2)
  2. Cytotrophoblastic shell
  3. Syncytiotrophoblast layers

Chorionic Plate

- It consists of extraembryonic mesoderm, cytotrophoblast and syncytiotrophoblast.

Development of Placenta

- Trophoblastic proliferation penetrates decidua (endometrium).

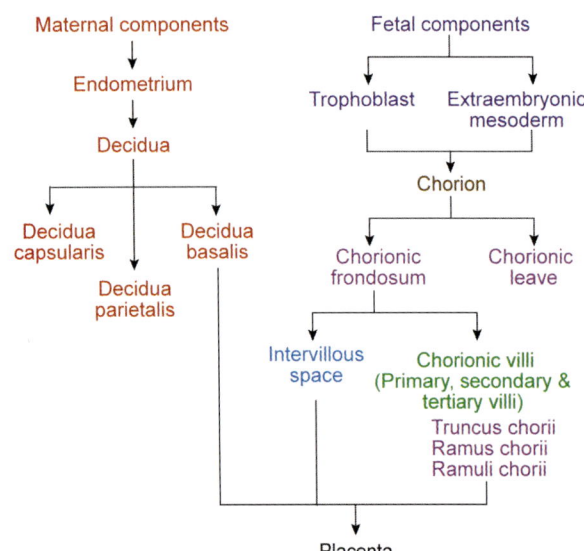

Flowchart 9.1: Structure of the placenta

Box 9.1: Decidua

- Uterine endometrium during pregnancy is called decidua (Fig. 9.2, Practice Figs 9.1, 9.2). *Viva*
- Decidua forms maternal part of the placenta.
- Word *decidus* means *falling off* or *shedding*, in Latin.
- Decidua sheds off during parturition (childbirth).
- There are three regions of the decidua as follows:
  A. *Decidua basalis or serotina*: The part of decidua that lies deep to the blastocyst. Decidua basalis forms the placenta. NEXT
  B. *Decidua capsularis or reflexa*: The part of the decidua that covers the blastocyst.
  C. *Decidua parietalis or vera*: It is the remaining part of the decidua that lines uterine cavity.

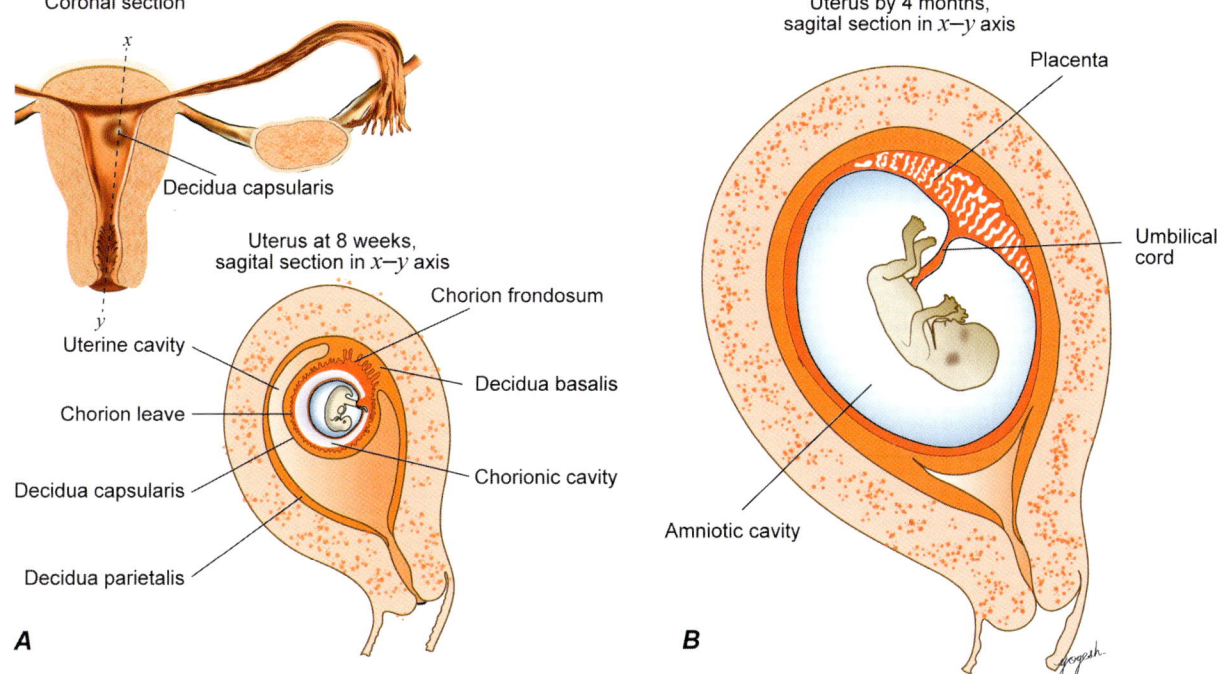

Fig. 9.2: Fusion of the decidua capsularis and parietalis: (A) By the end of the eighth week, decidua shows three zones as decidua basalis, capsularis and parietalis; (B) By the end of third month, decidua basalis is converted into placenta. Owing to the enlarging amniotic cavity, chorionic cavity and uterine cavity become obliterated and decidua capsularis fuses with decidua parietalis

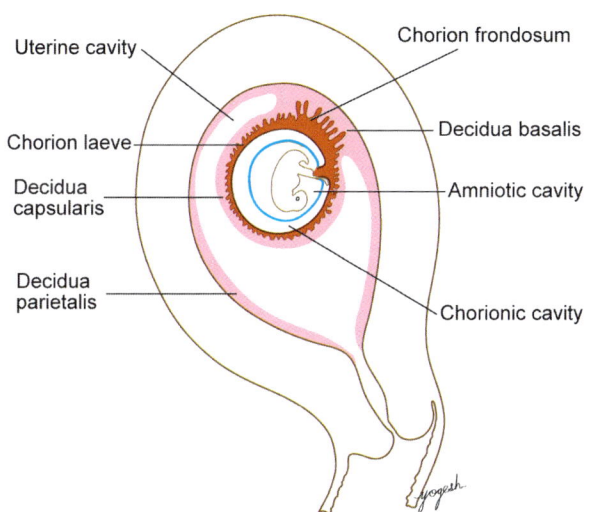

Decidua = Endometrium during pregnancy

Practice Fig. 9.1: Zones of decidua (three zones: Decidua basalis, capsularis and parietalis)

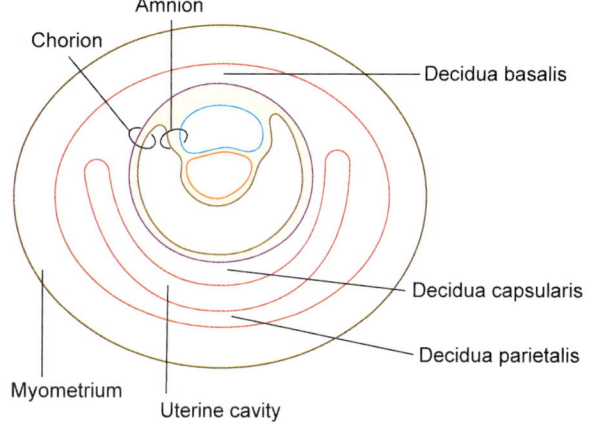

Transverse section of uterus

Practice Fig. 9.2: Subdivisions of decidua, interstitial implantation

---

Box 9.2: Decidual reaction (Fig. 9.3)

- The cellular and vascular changes in the decidua during pregnancy are called *decidual reaction* (Fig. 9.3).
- It includes glycogen and lipid deposition in decidual cells that produces enlarged pale-staining decidual cells.
- A high progesterone level in maternal blood is responsible for the decidual reaction.

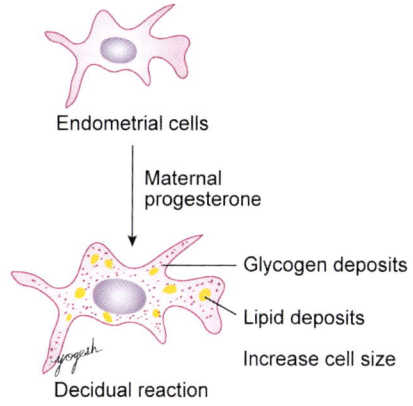

Fig. 9.3: Decidual reaction. During pregnancy, high level of progesterone enhances glycogen and lipid deposition in the decidual cells (cells of endometrium)

• Placenta and Umbilical Cord — 9

- On complete invasion of blastocyst, decidua can be divided into decidua basalis, decidua capsularis and decidua parietalis (Fig. 9.2).
- Trophoblastic layer differentiates into outer syncytiotrophoblast and inner cytotrophoblast (Fig. 9.4).
- Hypoblast cell forms an extraembryonic mesodermal layer.
- The syncytiotrophoblast, cytotrophoblast and extraembryonic mesoderm together form *chorion*.^MCQ
- Lacunar spaces appear in rapidly growing syncytiotrophoblast. These lacunar spaces occur more towards decidua basalis.
- Enlarging spaces communicates with adjacent ones. In between adjacent lacunae, syncytiotrophoblast cells persist as columns called *trabeculae*.
- Expanding syncytiotrophoblast erodes maternal capillaries and maternal blood starts entering the lacunar spaces and induces *uteroplacental circulation* at 17–22 days (in 3rd week).^NEXT
- Columns of syncytiotrophoblastic trabeculae get penetrated by cytotrophoblast to form *primary villi* (Practice Fig. 9.3).
- Mesoderm enters the core of primary villi to form *secondary villi*.

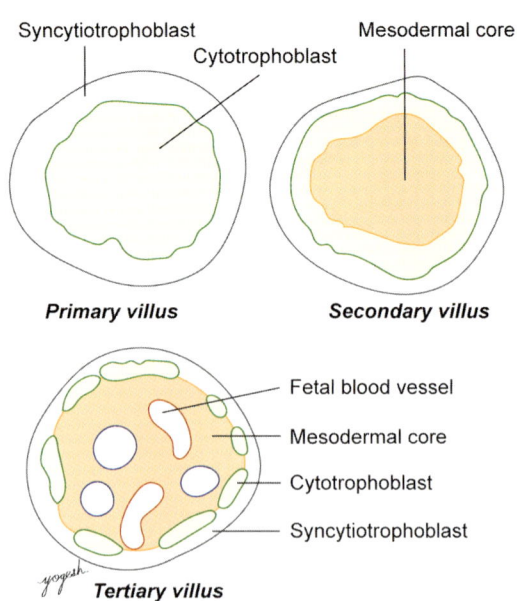

Practice Fig. 9.3: Placental villi

- In third week, capillaries appear in the mesodermal core and the villi are then called *tertiary villi*.^NEXT
- On formation of villi, lacunar spaces are then termed *intervillous spaces* (Fig. 9.4, Box 9.3).

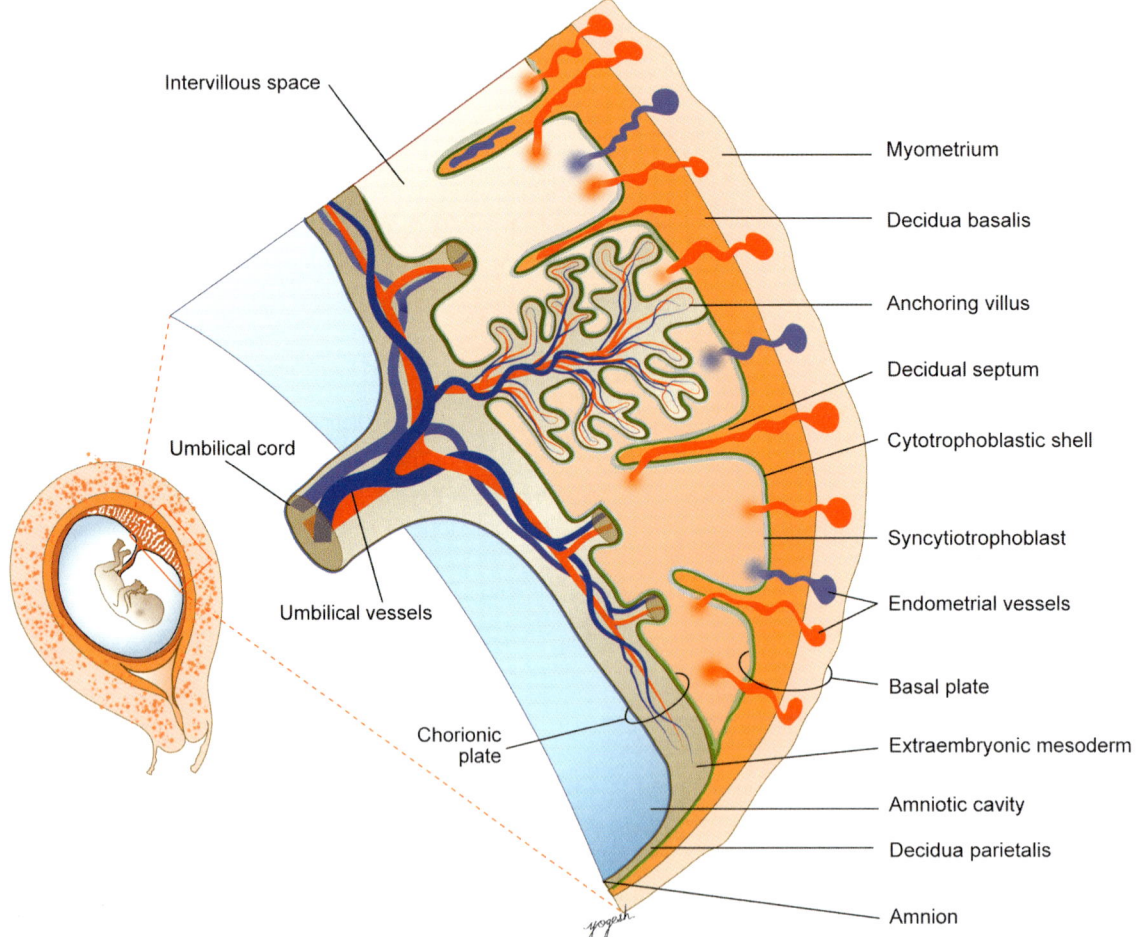

Fig. 9.4: Structure of the placenta. Intervillous spaces are filled with maternal blood. Cotyledons are partially separated by the decidual septa. Anchoring villi extend between basal plate and chorionic plate. Branches of the anchoring villus contain fetal blood vessels. Endometrial arteries bring oxygenated blood to intervillous space and drained by endometrial veins

Box 9.3: Intervillous space

Q. Write a short note on intervillous space in placenta.

- Intervillous space is the placental space that is formed by fusion of lacunar spaces of syncytiotrophoblast.
- These intervillous spaces are partially separated from each other by placental septa as these septa do not reach chorionic plate (fetal surface).
- Maternal blood enters the intervillous space through spiral arteries of the decidua basalis. Intervillous space is drained by endometrial veins.
- The volume of intervillous space is about 150 ml.^{MCQ}
- About 500 ml/minute maternal blood flows through the intervillous space.^{MCQ}

- Cytotrophoblast penetrates the syncytiotrophoblast and forms an outer *cytotrophoblastic shell*.
- Initially chorionic villi are formed all around the embryo. Later, the villi related to the decidua capsularis degenerate and this part of chorion becomes smooth and called *chorion leave*.
- The villi related to the decidua basalis grow considerably and form disc-shaped chorion frondosum, and later placenta (Fig. 9.2, Practice Fig. 9.4).

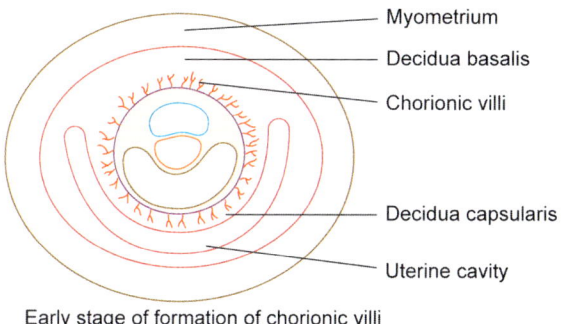

Early stage of formation of chorionic villi

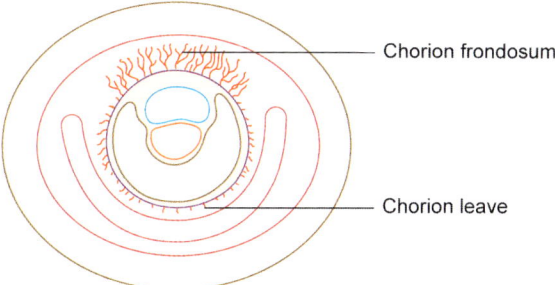

Early stage of formation of chorionic villi

Practice Fig. 9.4: Subdivisions of decidua, interstitial implantation

Chorionic villi and their Branching Pattern

Q. Write a short note on chorionic villi (Figs 9.4, 9.5, Flowchart 9.2).

- Columns of syncytiotrophoblastic trabeculae get penetrated by cytotrophoblast to form *primary villi*.

Box 9.4: Phylogeny of placenta

- Based on the retention of the maternal layers, placentae are classified as follows (Table 9.1):
  A. Epithelio-chorial: Maternal endometrial epithelium remains intact. For example, pig.
  B. Syndesmo-chorial: Endometrial epithelium disappears. For example, bovine placenta.
  C. Endothelio-reticular: Endometrial epithelium and stroma is eroded. Maternal vessels come in direct contact with fetal placental (chorionic) vessels. For example, dog.
  D. Hemo-chorial: Maternal blood vessels are eroded and maternal blood enters intervillous spaces of fetal chorion. For example, human.
  E. Hemo-endothelial: Trophoblastic layers also degenerate and maternal blood makes direct contact with fetal placental (chorionic) blood vessels. For example, rabbit.

Some Interesting Facts

- Fetal chorion frondosum and maternal decidua basalis together form the placenta.^{MCQ}
- By the end of the third month, decidua capsularis fuses with decidua parietalis due to increased size of the fetus.
- Cytotrophoblast shell isolates syncytiotrophoblast from decidua basalis and helps in anchoring the placenta.
- Chorion = Trophoblast + Extraembryonic somatopleuric mesoderm.
- Decidua = Stratum compactum of uterine endometrium during pregnancy.

Mesoderm enters the core of primary villi to form *secondary villi*. Capillaries appear in the mesodermal core and the villi are then called *tertiary villi*.

- The villi towards decidua basalis proliferate rapidly to form *chorion frondosum*, whereas other villi degenerate and disappear. These disappearing villi are called *chorion leave* (Fig. 9.2). Thus, placenta develops from decidua basalis (maternal component) and chorionic frondosum (fetal component).^{NEXT}
- The villi that extend from chorion (fetal side of the placenta) to the decidua basalis (maternal side of the placenta) are called *anchoring villi*.
- Several branches arise from the lateral side of anchoring villi that enter in the intervillous space. These branches are termed as follows (Fig. 9.5, Practice Fig. 9.5):
  A. *Truncus chorii* or stem villus that connects chorion with decidua basalis.
  B. *Rami chorii*: These are branches of stem villi.

Table 9.1	Phylogeny of placenta		
Type	Maternal component	Fetal component	Example
Epithelio-chorial	Intact endometrial epithelium	Trophoblast separates fetal blood vessels	Pig
Syndemso-chorial	Endometrial stroma		Bovine
Endothelio-chorial	Endothelium of maternal vessels		Dog
Hemo-chorial	Erosion of endothelium of maternal vessels	Trophoblast separates maternal blood from fetal vessels	Human
Hemo-endothelial		Trophoblast disappears	Rabbit

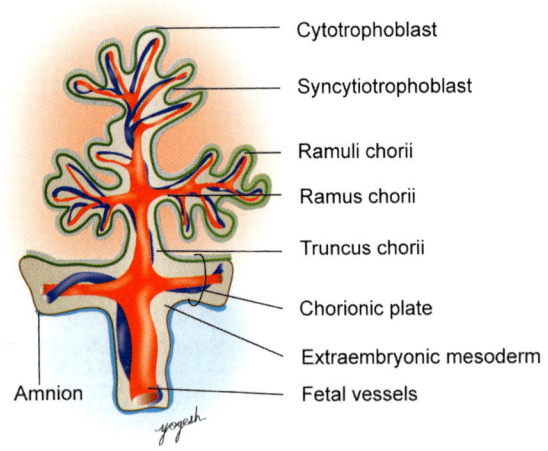

Fig. 9.5: Branching pattern of the villi. Villi are truncus chorii, ramus chorii and ramuli chorii

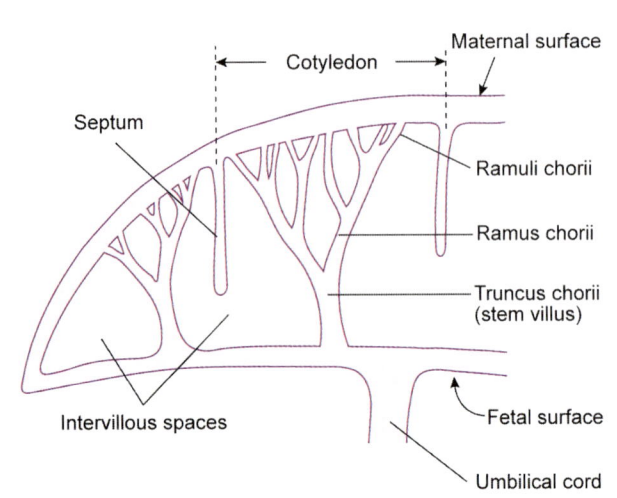

Practice Fig. 9.5: Arrangement of villi

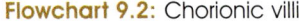

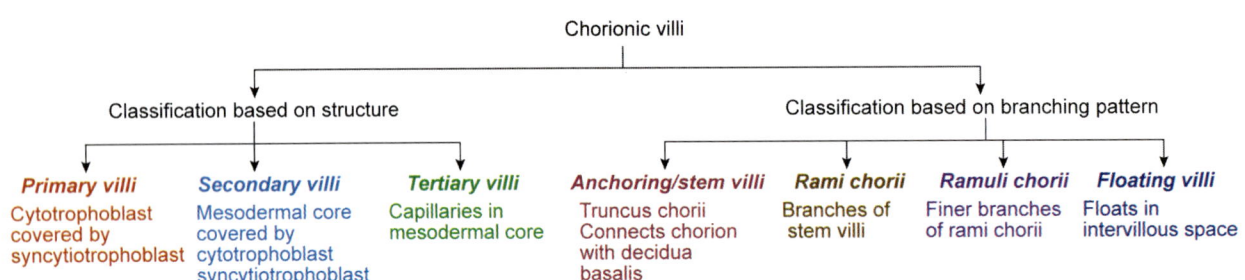

C. *Ramuli chorii*: These are finer branches of rami chorii.

D. *Floating or free villi*: These are numerous villi that freely floats in the intervillous spaces.

- Microvilli of syncytiotrophoblast projects into the intervillous space and increases the surface area (up to 14 square metre) for absorption.^MCQ

- Zones of villi
  - Beta zone: In the beta zones, cytotrophoblast separates syncytiotrophoblast and fetal capillaries.
  - Alpha zone: On the disappearance of cytotrophoblast, syncytiotrophoblast fuse with fetal capillaries in some zones of villi. These zones are called *alpha zones*.
  - Exchange of nutrients takes place more rapidly through alpha zones than beta zones.

Some Interesting Facts

- Tips of the stem villi penetrate deeper in the endometrium (decidua basalis) than any other part of the chorion.
- The projecting stem villi are separated from each other by a portion of decidua. These decidual separation forms placental septa (decidual septa) and projecting stem villi form cotyledons.
- Size of placenta increases parallel to the developing fetus and uterus. Placenta covers approximately 15–30% of the internal surface of the uterus throughout the pregnancy.^MCQ

Placental Barrier

Q. Write a short note on placental barrier.

- In the placenta, maternal blood circulates through intervillous space, whereas fetal blood circulates through blood vessels of chorionic villi. Here, maternal blood is separated from fetal blood by a placental barrier (Flowchart 9.3).

Flowchart 9.3: Placental barrier

Pacental barrier
Separates maternal blood from fetal blood
Componets
1. Synctiotrophoblast
2. Cytotrophoblast — disappear 4th month onward
3. Extraembryonic mesoderm
4. Basement membrane of endothelium
5. Capillary endothelium

Function
Physical isolation
Allows selective transmission iof substances

- Placental barrier allows the exchange of gases, nutrients, fetal waste products between maternal blood and fetal blood.
- During the initial stages of the fetal development, the placental barrier consists of (Fig. 9.6, Practice Fig. 9.6):
  1. Endothelium of fetal blood vessels
  2. Basement membrane of endothelium of fetal blood vessels
  3. Extraembryonic mesoderm
  4. Cytotrophoblast
  5. Syncytiotrophoblast

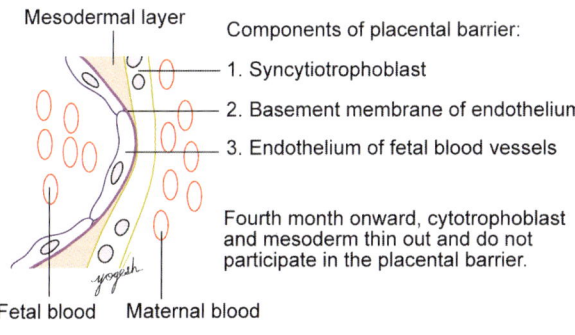

Practice Fig. 9.6: Placental barrier

Some Interesting Facts

Nitabuch's membrane
- Nitabuch's membrane is the fibrinoid deposition over the outer cytotrophoblast shell. It makes a demarcation between maternal and fetal tissue.

Rohr's fibrinoid stria
- Rohr's fibrinoid stria is the fibrinoid deposition on the intervillous surface of the syncytiotrophoblast. It was first described by Wolska (1888).
- These membranes play a major role in the immunological separation of fetal tissue from maternal tissue.

Fetal cotyledons
- Chorionic plate shows 40–60 extensions that extend towards decidua basalis. These extensions are *fetal cotyledons*.
- Each fetal cotyledon consists of stem villus and its ramification.

Langhans layer
- Cytotrophoblast layer is also called *Langhans layer*. Some authors also refer the Langhans layer as a fibrinoid layer separating intervillous space from chorion.

- Fourth month onward, cytotrophoblast and mesoderm thin out and thus, placental barrier is represented only by a thin layer of syncytiotrophoblast and fetal capillary endothelium (Fig. 9.6).

Classification of Placenta (Flowchart 9.4)

According to Shape

Q. List the types of placenta based on its shape.

- According to the shape of the placenta, it can be classified as follows (Fig. 9.7):
  1. Discoid placenta: It is round or disc-shaped.
  2. Bidiscoid placenta: It consists of two discs.
  3. Lobed placenta: It consists of two or more lobes.
  4. Placenta succenturiata: It shows accessory lobe of the placenta.
  5. Placenta membranacea: It is diffuse and thin chorionic villi projecting around entire blastocyst.

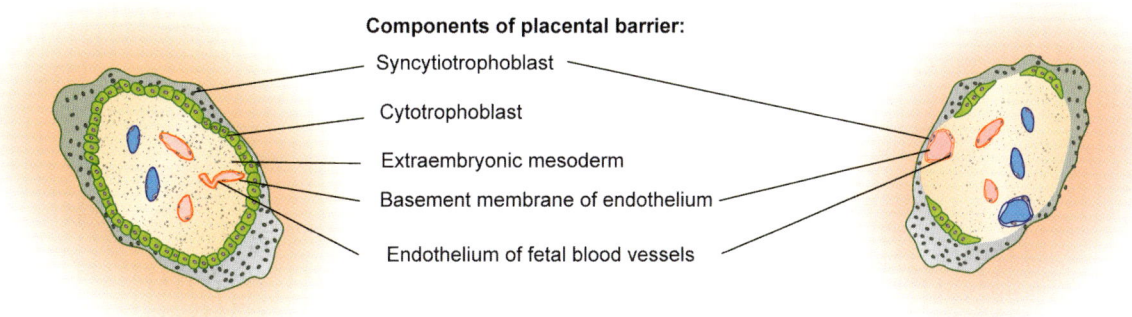

Fig. 9.6: Placental barrier. In early fetal life, placental barrier consists of endothelium of fetal blood vessels, its basement membrane, mesodermal layer, cytotrophoblast, and syncytiotrophoblast. Fourth month onward, cytotrophoblast and mesoderm thin out and thus, placental barrier is represented only by a thin layer of syncytiotrophoblast and fetal capillary endothelium

Flowchart 9.4: Classification of placentae

Placentae

According to shape	*According to attachment of umbilical cord*	*According to degree of adhesion*
1. Discoid: disc-shaped	1. Normal: central umbilical cord	1. Placenta accreta: adhered with decidua basalis
2. Bidiscoid: two discs	2. Battledore placenta: umbilical cord attached to margin	2. Placenta increta: penetrates myometrium
3. Lobed: two or more lobes	3. Velamentous: umbilical cord attached to fetal membranes	3. Placenta percreta: penetrates uterine wall
4. Placenta succenturiata: accessory lobe		
5. Placenta membranacea: diffuse		
6. Circumvallate: circular fold coving peripheral edge		

6. Circumvallate placenta: In the circumvallate placenta, peripheral edge of the placenta is covered by a circular fold of decidua.

According to the Attachment of the Umbilical Cord

- According to the attachment of the umbilical cord, placentae are classified as follows (Fig. 9.8):
  1. Normal placenta: Umbilical cord is attached to the centre of the placenta.^MCQ
  2. Battledore placenta: Umbilical cord is connected to the margin of the placenta.^MCQ
  3. Velamentous placenta: Umbilical cord is attached to fetal membranes near peripheral margin of the placenta.^MCQ

According to Degree of Adhesion

- According to the degree of adhesion, the placentae are classified as follows (Fig. 9.9):
  1. Placenta accreta: It is pathologically adhered placenta with decidua basalis.
  2. Placenta increta: This placenta penetrates the myometrium.
  3. Placenta percreta: This placenta penetrates entire uterine wall.

Functions of Placenta (Fig. 9.10)

Q. Write a short note on functions of placenta.

Q. Write a short note on endocrine functions of placenta or list the hormones secreted by placenta and their roles.

1. *Gaseous exchange:* O_2 and CO_2 exchange takes place across placenta through simple diffusion. Fetal hemoglobin has high affinity for the oxygen and high hemoglobin concentration in fetus facilitates the transfer of oxygen from mother to the fetus.
2. Transport of nutrients such as glucose, fatty acids, amino acids and electrolytes such as sodium, potassium and chloride.
3. Excretion of urea, uric acid and creatinine from the fetal blood into the maternal blood.
4. *Passive immunity:* Maternal antibodies (immunoglobulins) pass placental barrier by pinocytosis of syncytiotrophoblast. These antibodies provide

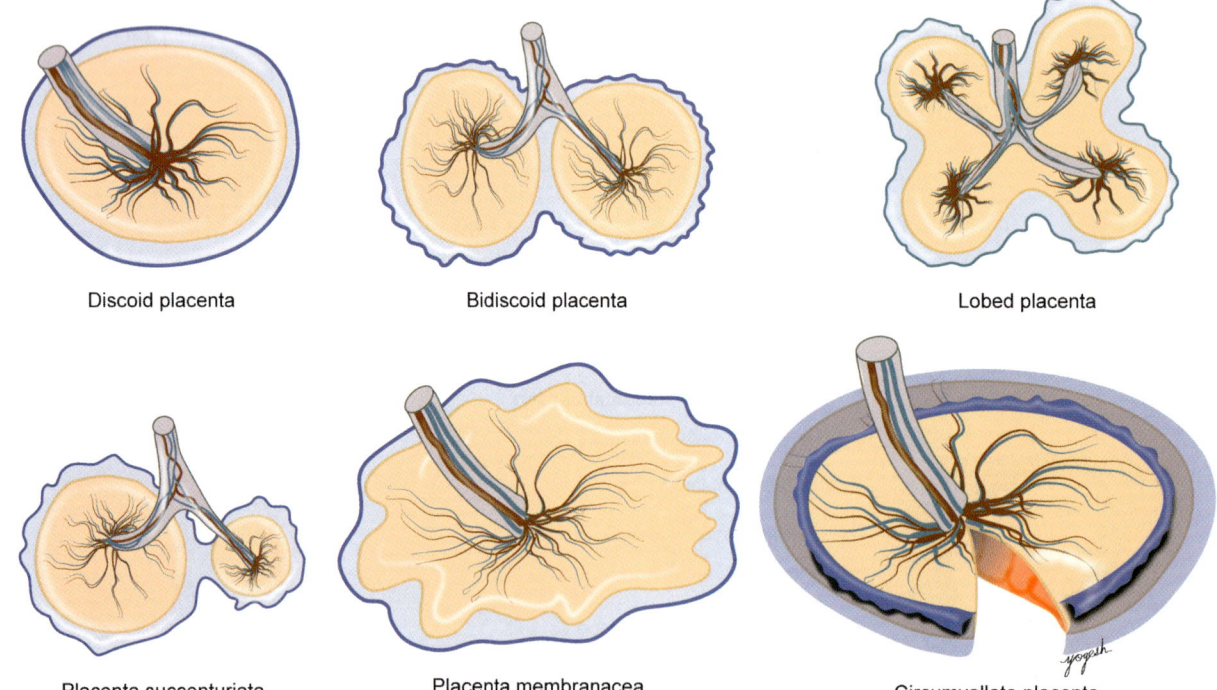

Discoid placenta   Bidiscoid placenta   Lobed placenta

Placenta succenturiata   Placenta membranacea   Circumvallate placenta

Fig. 9.7: Classification of the placenta according to its shape. Placenta can be classified as discoid placenta (round or disc-shaped), bidiscoid placenta (two discs), lobed placenta (two or more lobes), placenta succenturiata (accessory lobe), placenta membranacea (diffuse and thin), circumvallate placenta (peripheral edge of the placenta is covered by a circular fold of decidua)

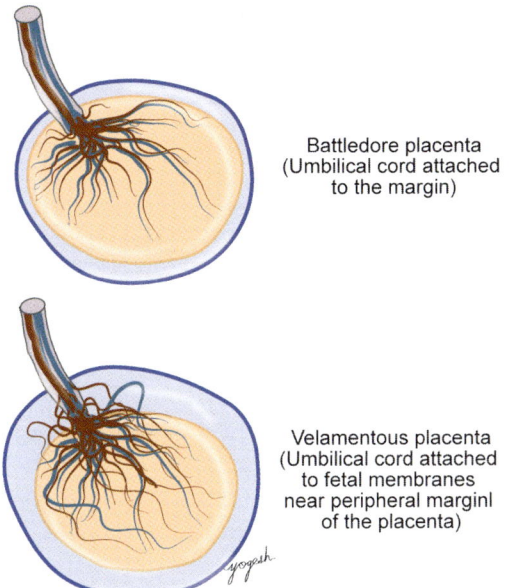

Fig. 9.8: Classification of the placenta according to the attachment of the umbilical cord. Placenta can be classified as battledore placenta and velamentous placenta. In normal placenta, umbilical cord is attached to the centre of the placenta

passive immunity to the fetus against diphtheria, measles, smallpox and so on. Maternal antibodies do not protect from chickenpox and whooping cough.^MCQ

5. Placental barrier: It prevents entry of many drugs and bacteria. But almost all viruses can cross the placental barrier. Some of the fetal blood cells may cross the placental barrier and circulate in the maternal blood.
6. Storage: The placenta stores glycogen, calcium and iron.
7. Endocrine function (Flowchart 9.5):
   Placenta secretes following hormones:
   – Human chorionic gonadotropin
   – Placental oestrogen
   – Placental progesterone
   – Placental lactogen
   – Relaxin

Human chorionic gonadotropin resembles luteinizing hormone and maintains corpus luteum up to three months.^MCQ

Placental estrogen changes the female reproductive tract to make it suitable for growing fetus. These changes include growing size of uterus, relaxation of various pelvic ligaments and so on.

Human placental progesterone helps to supresses contractality of uterine muscles (called progesterone block on myometrium) growth of decidua (maternal endometrium).

Placental lactogen helps in growth of female breasts and makes it ready for lactation.

Relaxin (also produced by corpus luteum) causes relaxation of pelvic ligaments and myometrium.

UMBILICAL CORD

Q. Write a short note on umbilical cord.

- *Definition*
  Umbilical cord is a tubular cord-like structure by which fetus is connected with the placenta.
- The umbilical cord is covered by an amniotic membrane.
- It has two ends:
  – Placental end: It is attached to the centre of the placenta.
  – Fetal end: It is attached to the umbilicus of the fetus.

Measurements of Full-term Umbilical Cord

- Length: 50–55 cm
- Thickness: 2 cm

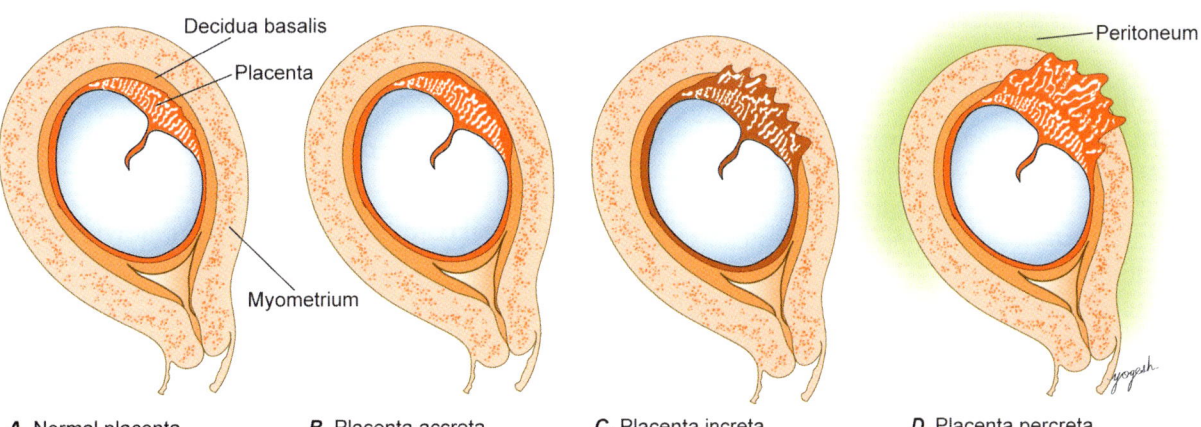

Fig. 9.9: Types of placenta according to the degree of adhesion: (A) Normal placenta; (B) Placenta accreta (placenta adhered with decidua basalis); (C) Placenta increta (placenta penetrates the myometrium); and (D) Placenta percreta (placenta penetrates entire uterine wall and reaches peritoneum). *Note:* Fetus is not shown in the amniotic cavity

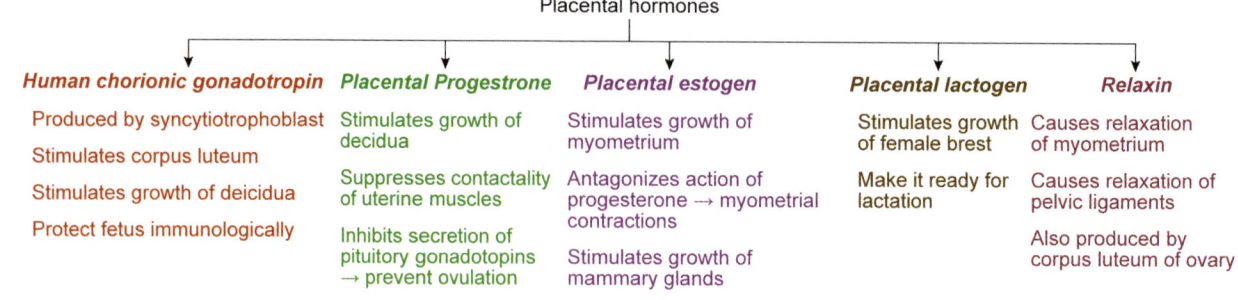

Flowchart 9.5: Placental hormones

Human chorionic gonadotropin	Placental Progestrone	Placental estogen	Placental lactogen	Relaxin
Produced by syncytiotrophoblast	Stimulates growth of decidua	Stimulates growth of myometrium	Stimulates growth of female brest	Causes relaxation of myometrium
Stimulates corpus luteum	Suppresses contactality of uterine muscles	Antagonizes action of progesterone → myometrial contractions	Make it ready for lactation	Causes relaxation of pelvic ligaments
Stimulates growth of deicidua	Inhibits secretion of pituitary gonadotopins → prevent ovulation	Stimulates growth of mammary glands		Also produced by corpus luteum of ovary
Protect fetus immunologically				

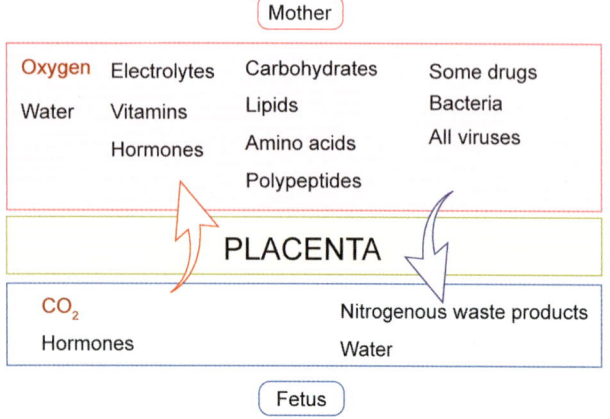

Fig. 9.10: Transport across placenta

Box 9.5: Hofbauer cells

- Hofbauer cells are small eosinophilic cells found in the placenta.
- These cells are named after J. Isfred Isidore Hofbauer (1878–1961).
- These cells are derived from mesoderm (extra-embryonic).
- Function: Hofbauer cells act as *macrophages* and prevent transmission of an infectious agent from mother to fetus.

Box 9.6: Human chorionic gonadotropin (hCG)

Q. Write a short note on human chorionic gonadotropin.

- The hCG is a hormone produced by syncytiotrophoblast of the placenta after implantation.
- The hCG is a polypeptide hormone (237 amino acids) identical to luteinizing hormone (LH) of the anterior pituitary gland.
- It is excreted in the urine of the mother after one week of missed menstrual period.

Functions

1. It stimulates the corpus luteum to secrete progesterone for first three months of the pregnancy. Later, the placenta starts secretion of sufficient progesterone.
2. Through progesterone, hCG stimulates growth of decidua (uterine endometrium).
3. hCG repels maternal immune cells and protects fetus during the first trimester. hCG also induces maternal T cell apoptosis.

Clinical aspects

1. Owing to the similarity between hCG and LH, hCG is used for stimulating ovulation.
2. Chromatographic immunoassay or urine test is used for detection of hCG and confirmation of the pregnancy.
   Positive immunoassay test can be seen after 6–12 days of ovulation.
3. Elevated hCG is seen in hydatidiform moles or molar pregnancy, germ cell tumors in males and teratomas (choriocarcinoma, seminoma).

Development of Umbilical Cord

- On the formation of embryonic folds, the yolk sac and connecting stalk come to lie on ventral surface of the fetus.
- Amnioectodermal junction comes to lie on ventral surface of the fetus and forms *umbilical ring* through which vitellointestinal duct and allantois protrude.
- Extraembryonic mesodermal tissue of the connecting stalk gets vascularised to form two umbilical arteries and two umbilical veins during third and fourth week of development. During later part of pregnancy, *right umbilical vein gets obliterated*.
- Mesodermal connective tissue of connecting stalk forms mucoid tissue called *Wharton's jelly*.

Contents of Umbilical Cord

Q. List the contents of umbilical cord.

Umbilical cord is made up of the following structures (Fig. 9.11, Practice Fig. 9.7, Table 9.2):

1. *Umbilical vessels:*
   - Umbilical cord has *two umbilical arteries and only one (left) umbilical vein*. **Right umbilical vein disappears**.[NEXT]
   - Umbilical arteries carry deoxygenated blood from internal iliac arteries of fetus to the placenta.
   - Umbilical veins are two in number, but the right umbilical vein disappears.[MCQ]

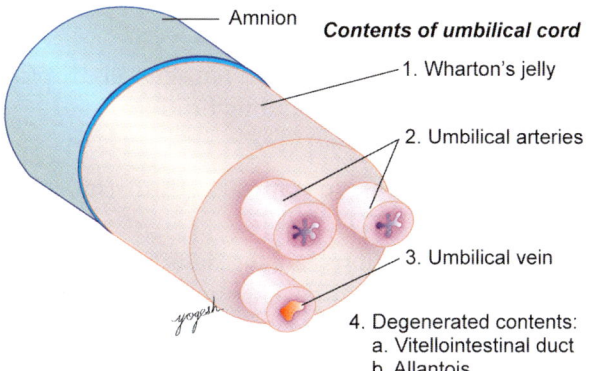

Fig. 9.11: Structure of the umbilical cord. It contains two umbilical arteries and one umbilical vein. Umbilical arteries carry deoxygenated blood from fetus to placenta (mother), whereas umbilical vein carries oxygenated blood from placenta to the fetus. Near the placental end, umbilical cord shows degenerating remnants of vitellointestinal duct and allantois

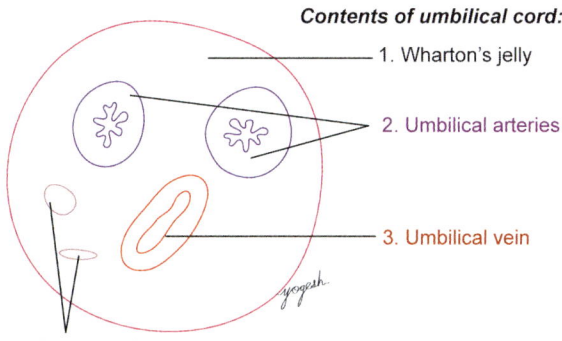

Practice Fig. 9.7: Structure of the umbilical cord

Table 9.2	Contents of umbilical cord^{MCQ, Viva}
1. Two umbilical arteries
2. One umbilical vein
3. Wharton's jelly
4. Part of allantois
5. Vitellointestinal duct and umbilical vesicle

- Left umbilical vein conveys oxygenated blood from placenta to the fetus.^{NEXT}
- Left umbilical vein joins the left branch of the portal vein that conveys blood to inferior vena cava via ductus venosus.^{MCQ}

2. *Wharton's jelly:*
   - Mucoid connective tissue of the umbilical cord is called Wharton's jelly.
   - Twisting of the umbilical vessels produces beaded appearance of umbilical cord.

3. Part of allantoic diverticulum
   - Part of allantoic diverticulum enters in the umbilical cord (earlier connecting stalk) and it undergoes fibrosis to form urachus.

Some Interesting Facts

- Umbilical cord contains two umbilical arteries and only one (left) umbilical vein.^{NEXT}
- Close to the attachment of umbilical cord with placenta, two umbilical arteries are connected by transverse anastomosis called *Hyrtl's anastomosis*.^{NEXT}
- Left umbilical vein gets obliterated after birth and forms *ligamentum teres hepatis*.^{MCQ}
- After the birth, umbilical arteries undergo muscle spasm earlier than umbilical vein and hence, newborn receives blood from placenta and does not give blood to the placenta.

Box 9.7: Physiological umbilical hernia

- Midgut loop communicates with the yolk sac. The midgut loop elongates to form a U-shaped loop that projects into the proximal part of umbilical cord.
- Midgut loop projects from 6th to 10th week.
- This midgut herniation is called physiological hernia. It occurs due to smaller abdominal cavity that is not enough to accommodate enlarged elongated midgut loop.
- After 10th week, hernia decreases owing to increasing availability of the abdominal space.

- Remaining part of allantois forms part of urinary bladder.

4. Vitellointestinal duct and umbilical vesicle
   - Part of the yolk sac communicating with midgut forms vitellointestinal duct.
   - Unabsorbed part of the yolk sac forms umbilical vesicle.
   - In the later part of pregnancy, vitellointestinal duct and umbilical vesicles disappear.

AMNION

- Definition: Amnion is a thin membrane that lines the roof of the amniotic cavity.
- Inner cell mass (embryoblast) of the trophoblast form an amniotic cavity and gets separated from a layer of amniotic cells.
- Amnion forms the roof and bilaminar germ disc forms floor of the amniotic cavity.
- Amnion consists of angiogenic cells that are covered by somatopleuric layers of extraembryonic mesoderm.
- By the end of the 8th week, on the formation of embryonic folding, amnion entirely covers embryo.^{MCQ}
- The amniotic cavity contains amniotic fluid.
- Amniotic fluid is also called *liquor amnii or camerous fluid*.

Constituents of Amniotic Fluid

1. Water, electrolytes
2. Fetal waste including urine

3. Hormones: Human chorionic gonadotropin and human placental lactogen
4. Cells exfoliated from fetus

Functions of Amniotic Fluid

1. Shock absorption: Amniotic fluid provides *water-cushion* that absorbs jerks and protects the fetus.
2. Nutrition: Amniotic fluid provides nutrition to developing neuroectoderm as it passes through anterior and posterior neuropore.
3. Amniotic fluid allows free fetal movements.
4. Fetus excretes urine in amniotic fluid. Fetus swallows and absorbs amniotic fluid through gut into fetal blood. Finally, fetal waste products reach maternal blood through feto-placental circulation.

Volume of Amniotic Fluid

Amniotic fluid volume increases from 10th week to 28th week and then decreases (Table 9.3).

Clinical Aspects

1. Amniocentesis
   - It is a procedure to aspirate 20–30 ml of the amniotic fluid for the analysis.
   - The amniotic fluid analysis involves biochemical analysis (lecithin:sphingomyelin ratio for lung maturity), and chromosomal analysis by karyotyping for genetic disorders.
   - High level of α-fetoprotein in amniotic fluid is an indicator of neural tube defects.^{MCQ}
2. Oligohydramnios
   - It is a condition in pregnancy characterized by low volume of amniotic fluid (less than 400 ml).
   - It can be detected by ultrasonography when largest amniotic liquid pool size becomes less than 2 cm.
3. Amnion nodosum
   - It is a nodule on the fetal surface of amnion (mostly found in oligohydramnios).
   - It is composed of a squamous cell aggregate and is derived from vernix caseosa of the fetal skin.
4. Potter syndrome
   - It is a fetal condition produced by oligohydramnios.
   - It includes pulmonary hypoplasia, limb defects, cranial anomalies and renal defects.
   - Causes: Placental failure, renal agenesis, ruptured amnion leading to amniotic fluid leakage.
5. Polyhydramnios
   - It is the excessive amniotic fluid (more than 2000 ml).
   - Causes: Conditions causing defective swallowing in the fetus such as esophageal atresia, fetal neurological disorders (anencephaly).
   - Due to defective swallowing, amniotic fluid cannot be absorbed by fetal gut.
   - Polyhydramnios is diagnosed by ultrasonography when amniotic fluid index is greater than 24 cm.

Box 9.8: Amniotic fluid index (AFI)

Q. Write a short note on amniotic fluid index.
- AFI is an indicator of amniotic fluid quantity and fetal health.^{Viva}

Method of measurement
- Amniotic cavity is scanned ultrasonically.
- The cavity is divided into four imaginary quadrants.
- Vertical length of each quadrant is measured and added up.
- The quadrant containing loop of umbilical cord is excluded.

Interpretation^{MCQ}

AFI	Interpretation
8–18	Normal
<5	Oligohydramnios
>24	Polyhydramnios

YOLK SAC

Q. Write a short note on yolk sac.
- Yolk sac is a cavity. It develops from the blastocystic cavity (Practice Fig. 9.8, Flowchart 9.6).

Formation and Changes in Yolk Sac

- The yolk sac is formed in the following stages: Primary yolk sac → secondary yolk sac → definitive yolk sac → umbilical vesicle and vitellointestinal duct

Primary yolk sac
- Hypoblast cells multiply and forms a flat cellular lining of the blastocyst cavity. This lining layer is called Heuser membrane and then the blastocystic cavity is called primary yolk sac.

Secondary yolk sac
- On formation of the extraembryonic coelom, part of yolk sac is pinched off and resultant reduced yolk sac cavity is termed *secondary yolk sac*.

Table 9.3	Amniotic fluid volume
Gestational age	*Volume of the amniotic fluid*
10th week	25 ml
20th week	400 ml
28th week	800 ml
36th week	1000 ml (at birth)
42nd week	400 ml

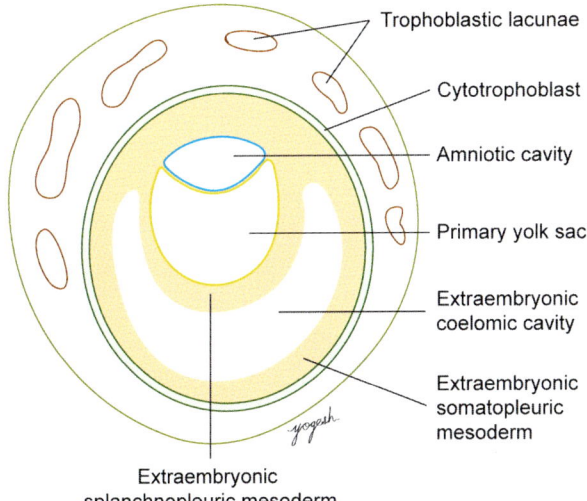

Practice Fig. 9.8: Yolk sac, amniotic cavity and extraembryonic coelomic cavity

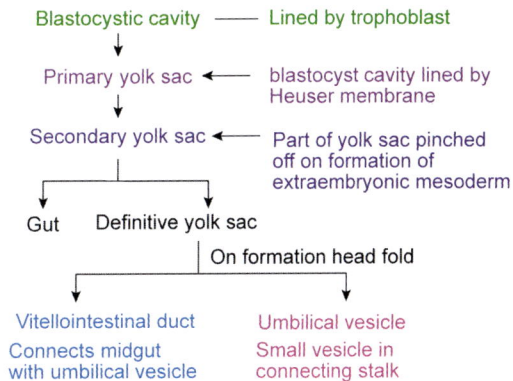

Flowchart 9.6: Yolk sac

Definitive yolk sac
- On formation of the embryonic folding, intraembryonic part of yolk sac forms primitive gut and extraembryonic part forms *definitive yolk sac*.

Umbilical vesicle and vitellointestinal duct
- Extraembryonic part of the yolk sac or definitive yolk sac undergo hourglass contraction due to embryonic folding and it form small umbilical vesicle that communicates with midgut through vitellointestinal duct.

Functions of Yolk Sac
- **Hematopoiesis:** Yolk sac produces blood cells up to sixth week of intrauterine life.
- **Formation of primitive gut:** Part of the yolk sac forms primitive gut.
- **Formation of primordial germ cells:** Primordial germ cells develop in the wall of the yolk sac. These cells migrate and forms gonads (ovary and testis) during fourth week.
- **Allantois:** A small diverticular extension of the yolk sac in the connecting stalk form allantois. Later allantois forms part of the urinary bladder.

Clinical Aspects
Meckel's diverticulum is the remnant of the vitellointestinal duct.

RELATIONSHIP OF AMNIOTIC CAVITY, EXTRAEMBRYONIC COELOM, AND UTERINE CAVITY
- In early developmental stages, there are three cavities in embryo, namely amniotic cavity, extraembryonic coelom (also called chorionic cavity in later stage of development), yolk sac. Due to growth of the amniotic cavity, the yolk sac, extraembryonic coelom, and uterine cavity get obliterated (Fig. 9.2, Practice Fig. 9.9).
- It results in fusion of chorion with amnion and together they form *amniochorionic membrane*.
- Later, decidua capsularis fuses with decidua parietalis and uterine cavity gets obliterated completely.
- The amniotic cavity increases in size due to accumulation of amniotic fluid and it is permitted by increase in uterine size.
- *Fetal membrane:* Clinician term fused amniochorionic membrane along with decidua capsularis as fetal

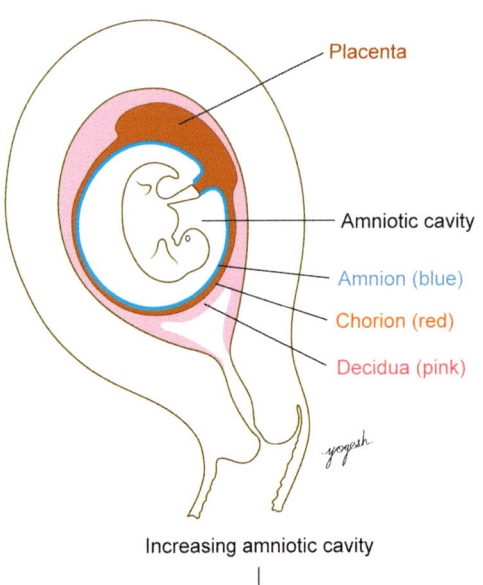

Practice Fig. 9.9: Obliteration of chorionic cavity and uterine cavity

membrane that gets ruptured during parturition (childbirth).
- *Bag of waters*: It is a bulging fetal membrane through cervix just before childbirth.
- Uterine contractions help in the formation of bag of waters and also help in the dilatation of the uterine cervix. Continued rise in pressure leads to rupture of fetal membrane, release of amniotic fluid, and delivery of the baby.

Clinical Embryology

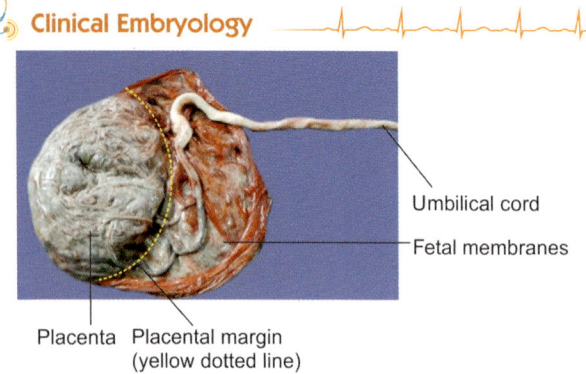

Clinical image 9.1: Velamentous placenta: Umbilical cord is attached to fetal membranes near peripheral/margin of the placenta. (Image courtesy: *Dr Haritha Sagili*)

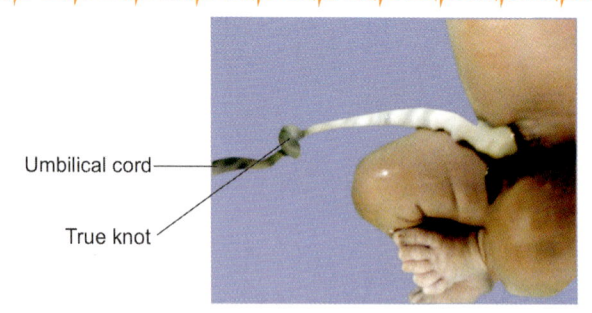

Clinical image 9.2: True knot of umbilical cord. Incidence: 0.3% to 2% of all births. (Image courtesy: *Dr Haritha Sagili*)

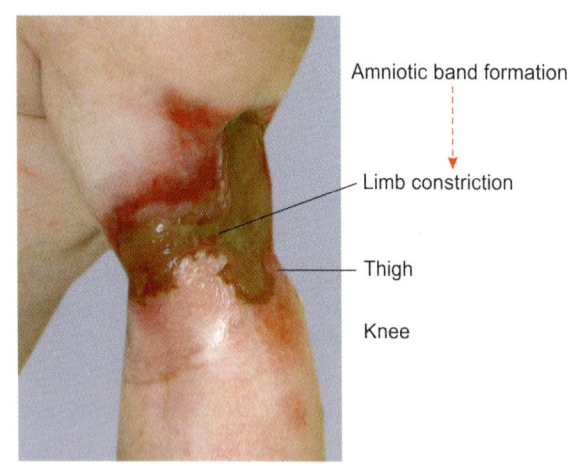

Clinical image 9.3: Limb constriction (soft tissue defect) probably secondary to amniotic band formation following domestic violence in pregnancy (Image courtesy: *Dr Haritha Sagili*)

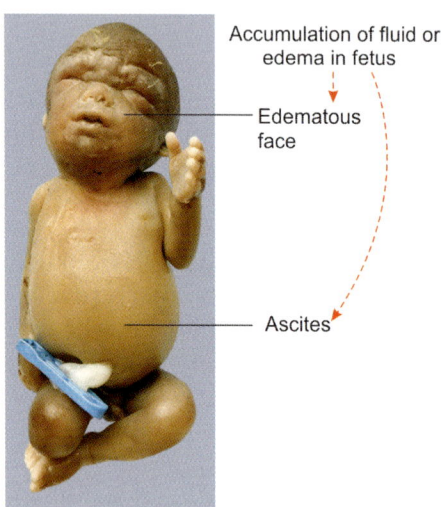

Clinical image 9.4: Hydrops fetalis. It is a condition characterized by accumulation of fluid or edema in fetus. Locations of hydrops fetalis include subcutaneous tissue (scalp), pleural cavity, pericardial cavity and peritoneal cavity. Fetal anemia is the most common cause of hydrops fetalis. In the above image, protruding abdomen (due to ascites) and edematous face are seen (Image courtesy: *Dr Haritha Sagili*)

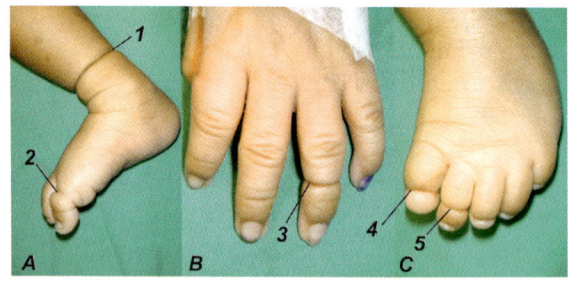

Entrapment of fetal parts
in fibrous amniotic bands while *in utero*

Amniotic band syndrome

Clinical image 9.5: Amniotic band syndrome: (A) Right lower limb showing constriction rings in lower part of leg (1) and at proximal phalanx of great toe (2); (B) Left hand showing constriction ring at middle phalanx of ring finger (3); (C) Left foot showing constriction bands at distal phalanx of great toe with the absence of nail (4) and constriction band at middle phalanx of second toe (5) (Image courtesy: *Dr Kumaravel S*)

Chapter 10

Integumentary System: Skin, its Appendages, and Mammary Gland

eSmartQuiz

Chapter Outline

- Development of skin
  - Stages of development
  - Anomalies of skin and appadages
- Dermatoglyphics
- Development of hair
  - Stages of development
  - Anomalies related to hair
- Sweat glands
  - Eccrine sweat glands
  - Apocrine sweat glands
- Sebaceous glands
  - Development
  - Mode of secretion
- Nails
  - Structure of nail
  - Stages of development
  - Clinical aspects
- Mammary glands
  - Stages of development
  - Malformations

Competencies:
- **AN9.3:** Describe development of breast.
- **AN72.1:** Skin and its appendages.

INTRODUCTION

Skin

- Skin and its appendages such as sebaceous glands, sweat glands, hairs and nails constitute integumentary system.
- Skin is the largest organ of body.
- It consists of two layers
  A. Epidermis – a superficial layer
  B. Dermis – a deep layer
- Epidermis consists of keratinocytes and has five layers as stratum basale (germinativum), stratum-spongiosum, stratum granulosum, stratum lucidum (only in palms and soles) and stratum corneum.
- Epidermis also contains a few melanocytes (produce melanin), Langerhans cells (antigen-presenting immune cells) and Merkel cells (mechanoreceptors for tactile/light-touch sensation).
- Dermis is a connective tissue layer that has a superficial papillary and a deep reticular layer.

DEVELOPMENT OF SKIN

Summary (Examination Guide)

- Epidermis develops from the surface ectoderm (Fig. 10.1, Table 10.1, Flowchart 10.1).
- Melanocytes and Merkel cells are derived from neural crest cells, whereas Langerhans cells from bone marrow (mesoderm).
- Dermis develops from the somatopleuric mesoderm.
- Appendages of skin (sebaceous glands, sweat glands and nails) are derived from the epidermis.

Table 10.1 Development of skin

Component of skin	Embryonic source
Epidermis	Surface ectoderm
Melanocyte (dendritic cells), Merkel cells	Neural crest cells
Langerhans cells	Mesoderm (bone marrow)
Dermis	Somatopleuric mesoderm, dermatomes
Sweat glands, sebaceous glands, nails, hairs	Surface ectoderm (epidermis)

87

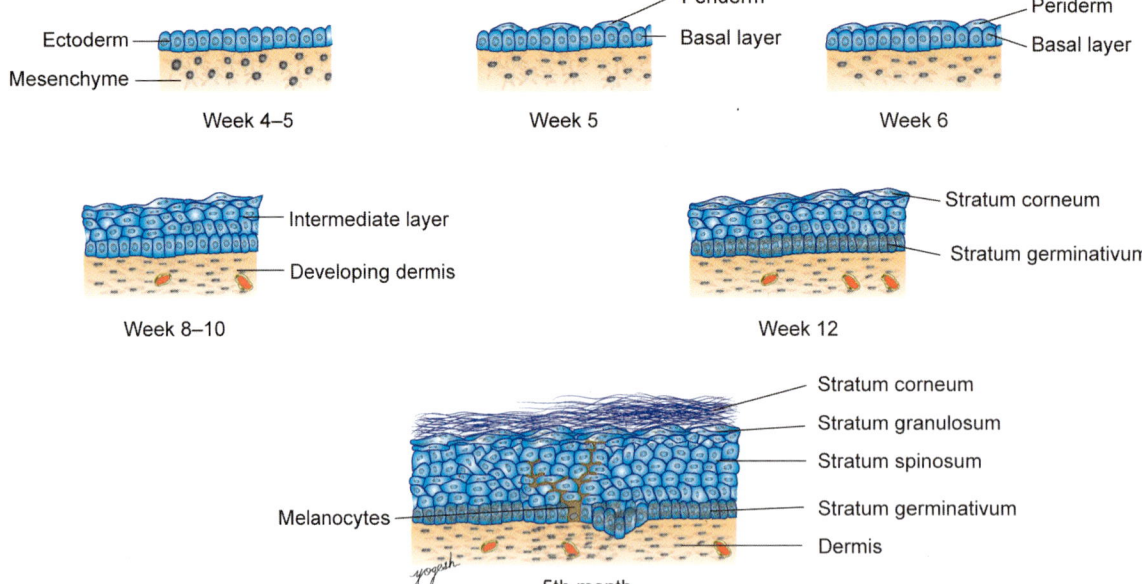

Fig. 10.1: Development of thin skin. Epidermis develops from surface ectoderm. Melanocytes are derived from neural crest cells. Dermis develops from somatopleuric mesoderm. Stratum lucidum is seen only in thick skin

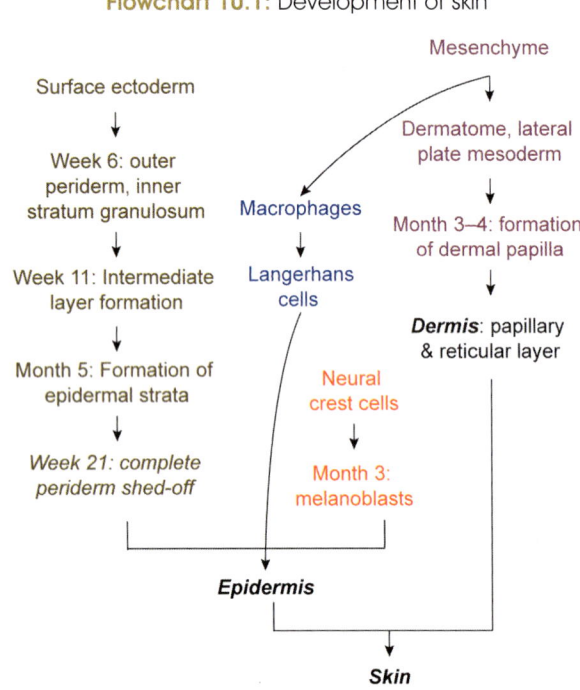

Flowchart 10.1: Development of skin

Stages of Development

Epidermis

- Epidermis develops from the surface ectoderm (Fig. 10.1, Flowchart 10.1).
- Initially, surface ectoderm is a single cell-layer thick.
- In the second month (6th week), ectoderm differentiates into two layers.
  – Outer flattened cell layer as *periderm* or *epitrichium*.
  – Inner cuboidal cell layer as *stratum germinativum* or *basal cell layer*.
- In 11th week, cells of the basal layer proliferate to form an intermediate layer.
- Cells of the intermediate layer produce keratin proteins.
- In 5th month, proliferating cells of stratum basale generate stratum spinosum, stratum granulosum and stratum corneum.
- Periderm layer gradually sloughed into the amniotic fluid. The **periderm shed off completely** by the 21st week.[MCQ]
- *Collodion babies* are the babies born with persistent periderm. This periderm usually shed during the first week of life spontaneously.[MCQ]
- *Vernix caseosa*: Cell of superficial layer of epidermis shed off slowly. These cells get mixed with secretions of sebaceous glands and hairs to form whitish sticky substance called *vernix caseosa*. It covers skin of the fetus and protects from maceration in amniotic fluid.[MCQ] Vernix caseosa is a whitish sticky coat on the skin of newborn.
- Formation of *epidermal ridges*: By 11th week, cells of the stratum basale proliferate and extend into the dermis to form epidermal ridges (become permanent by 18th week).[MCQ]
- Epidermal ridges form a specific pattern of fingerprints (also in palm and sole) that is genetically determined.
- At birth, all the layers of the adult epidermis are present.
- *Melanoblasts* (dendritic cells): Neural crest cells invade the epidermis during **3rd month** and become melanoblasts. These cells start producing melanin.[NEXT]
- Merkel cells are pressure-detecting mechanoreceptors in the skin (palms and soles). Their origin is not clear. They appear in 4th–6th months.

- *Langerhans cells* are the tissue macrophages. They arise in bone marrow and migrate into the skin from 7th week onward.^MCQ

Dermis

- Dermis is derived from the mesenchymal connective tissue underlying the epidermis (surface ectoderm) (Fig. 10.1, Flowchart 10.1).
- Sources of mesenchymal cells forming dermis:
  1. Dermatomes
  2. Lateral plate mesoderm
  3. Neural crest cells
- Dermatomes form dermis over the dorsal aspect of head and trunk.
- Lateral plate mesoderm forms dermis over lateral and ventral aspects of trunk.
- Neural crest cells form dermis over most of the part of head and anterior aspect of neck.
- *Dermal papillae:* During 3rd–4th month, the dermis shows regularly spaced thickenings that project into the overlying epidermis and form the dermal papillae.
- Later, the dermis differentiates into a superficial papillary layer and a deep reticular layer.

Anomalies of Skin and Appendages

1. *Aplasia of skin*: It is a failure of development of skin in some regions of body.
2. *Albinism*: Reduced or absent synthesis of melanin pigment produces depigmented zones in skin, hair and eyes. This condition is albinism. It is an autosomal recessive disorder.^MCQ
3. *Vitiligo*: It is an autoimmune disorder with patchy loss of pigmentation in skin, hair and oral mucosa due to loss of melanocytes.^MCQ
4. *Piebaldism* is a rare autosomal dominant disorder. In this condition, melanocytes are absent in patchy areas of hairs and skin, mostly affects forehead.^MCQ
5. *Ichthyosis* (Gr. *Icthyos* means fish): It is an autosomal recessive or X-linked disease characterized by fish-like scaling of skin due to hyperkeratinization.^MCQ
6. *Harlequin fetuses* have rigid, deeply cracked skin. Harlequin babies die shortly after birth. Harlequin fetus occurs due to failure of
   - maturation of keratinocytes
   - desquamation of keratinocytes (shed off property).^MCQ
7. *Gorlin syndrome:* It is also called *nevoid basal cell carcinoma syndrome* (NBCCS). It is an autosomal dominant disorder due to chromosome 9q22.3 gene defect. It is characterized by basal cell carcinoma, pathogenic dyskeratotic pitting of hands and feet.^MCQ

Some Interesting Facts
- Skin of the neonate contains 20 times more blood vessels than required for thermoregulation.

Box 10.1: Dermatoglyphics
- It is a study of specific pattern of *epidermal ridges*.
- In 11th week, epidermal ridges start appearing and they become permanent by 18th week.^MCQ
- The pattern of epidermal ridges is genetically determined and remains fixed throughout life.
- As epidermal ridge patterns are individual specific, they are commonly used for identification of genetic disorders.
- For details, read book *Principles of Clinical Genetics* by Dr Yogesh Sontakke.

DEVELOPMENT OF HAIR

Q. Write a short note on development of hair.

Summary (Examination Guide)
- Shaft of hair follicle develops from the surface ectoderm (Fig. 10.2, Flowchart 10.2).
- Dermal papilla develops from the mesenchyme of dermis.
- *Arrector pili* muscles develop from the *mesodermal* sheath.^NEXT

Stages of Development
- Hair follicles first appear at the end of the second month on eyebrows, eyelids, upper lip and chin.
- Hair follicles do not appear in other regions until the fourth month.

Phases of Development

1. *Formation of hair germ (hair bulb)*: It is a small concentration of ectodermal cells in the stratum basale of epidermis (Fig. 10.2, Flowchart 10.2).
2. *Formation of hair peg*: The hair bulb proliferates in the dermis to form a solid rod-like structure called *hair peg*. Later hair peg expands to form a bulbous peg.
3. *Formation of dermal papilla*: Underlying dermal cells of hair peg proliferate to form a small hillock called *dermal papilla*. Invagination of dermal papilla makes the hair bulb cup-shaped.
4. *Formation of germinal matrix*: Ectodermal cells covering dermal papilla become *germinal matrix* that produce root of hair.
5. *Formation of hair shaft*: Cells of hair root proliferate and get keratinized. These cells form hair shaft.
6. *Formation of follicular canal*: Growing hair shaft is pushed outwards by growth of hair root. Passage of hair shaft through the epidermis forms a *follicular canal*.

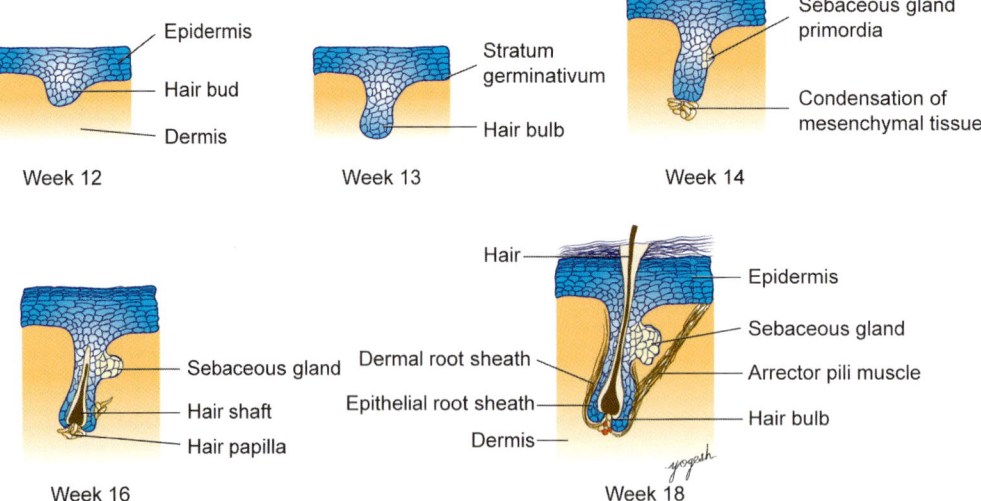

Fig. 10.2: Development of hair. Shaft of hair follicle develops from surface ectoderm. Dermal papilla develops from mesoderm of dermis. Arrector pili muscles develop from mesodermal sheath

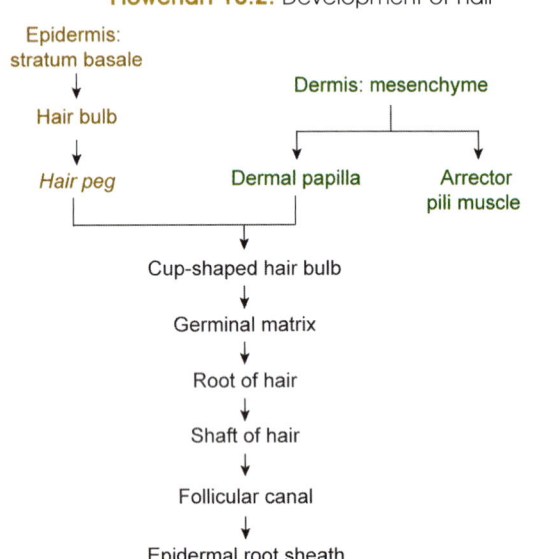

7. *Formation of epidermal root sheaths*: Cells lining follicular canal form inner and outer epidermal root sheaths.
8. *Development of arrector pili muscles*: Surrounding mesenchymal cells condense to form arrector pili muscles except for eyebrows and eyelashes.^MCQ

Some Interesting Facts

- Melanocytes migrate into hair bulbs and transfer melanin to proliferating cells of germinal matrix. This is responsible for the color of hair.
- *Lanugo*: These are fine, soft hairs that cover body and limbs of human fetus.
- Lanugo is replaced by coarser hairs during perinatal period.
- Terminal hair is more coarse and present in axilla and groin (moustache and beard only in males).
- *Definitive hair* once reaches to certain length, they cease to grow. Examples: Hairs of eyelashes and eyebrows, pubic hairs, axillary hairs.
- *Angora* is hairs that grow continuously. Examples: Hairs of scalp (hairs of moustache and beard only in males).

Anomalies Related to Hair (Clinical Facts)

1. *Hypertrichosis* is an excessive hair growth due to development of unusual abundance of hair follicles. It may be all over the body or may be patchy. It may be persistence of lanugo hairs that normally disappear after birth.^MCQ, Viva
2. *Congenital alopecia* is a lack or loss of hairs due to the absence of hair follicles.
3. *Trichorrhexis nodosa* is a defect of the hair shaft due to metabolic disorder (arginosuccinic aciduria and citrullinemia). In this disease, the hair shaft shows breaks.^MCQ
4. *Menkes syndrome* is an X-linked recessive disorder of copper metabolism (ATPTA gene defect) having depigmented brittle hairs, neurological abnormalities and low serum calcium levels.^MCQ
5. Curly hair is a result of asymmetrical hair follicles. It is an example of incomplete dominance.^MCQ

SWEAT GLANDS

Q. Write a short note on development of sweat glands.

- Sweat glands are also known as sudoriferous glands (*sudor* is sweat in Latin)
- Sweat glands are simple tubular exocrine glands that produce sweat on the surface of skin.

- There are two types of sweat glands: Eccrine and apocrine (Fig. 10.3).

Summary (Examination Guide)

- There are two types of sweat glands (Figs 10.3, 10.4)
  – Eccrine sweat glands – open directly on skin surface and develop from invagination of surface ectoderm.
  – Apocrine sweat glands – open into hair follicles and develop from outgrowth of hair follicle.
  – Myoepithelial cells are derived from mesoderm (dermis).

Eccrine Sweat Glands

- They are distributed almost all over the human body (more in number in palms and soles) (Fig. 10.4).
- These glands open directly on surface of skin and pour secretions directly on the skin surface.
- These are *merocrine* in nature (secrete by exocytosis).
- Their secretions are watery and help in maintenance of body temperature.
- Eccrine sweat glands develop from surface epithelium before birth as follows:
  1. At 20th week, epidermis develops down growth in the dermis.
  2. Cells of stratum germinativum proliferate to form enlarging solid mass (bud) of epithelial cells in dermis.
  3. Deeper end of bud continues to grow and becomes coiled.

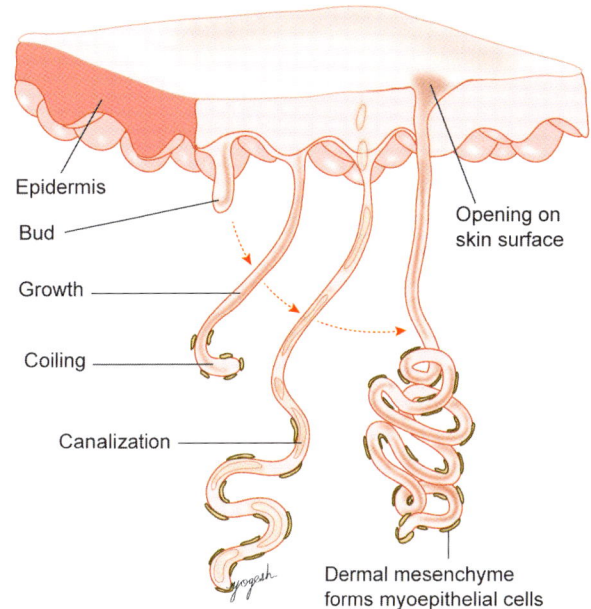

Fig. 10.4: Development of eccrine sweat gland. At 20th week, cells of stratum germinativum proliferate to form enlarging solid mass (bud) of epithelial cells in the dermis. Deeper end of bud continues to grow and becomes coiled and later, solid bud gets canalized to form lumen. Straight part of gland forms duct, whereas deeper coiled part forms secretory segment. Surrounding mesenchymal cells form myoepithelial cells. Arrow indicates advancing stages of gland development

  4. Later, solid buds get canalized to form lumen.
  5. Straight part of gland forms duct, whereas deeper coiled part forms secretory segment.
  6. Surrounding mesenchymal cells modify to form myoepithelial cells.

Apocrine Sweat Glands

- They are confined to axilla, pubic and perianal regions, areola of the nipple, ear and eyelids.
- These glands open into hair follicles.
- These are *apocrine* in nature (shed off a portion of cell in the form of secretion).
- Their secretion is thick and produces odor.
- These glands develop at puberty as epidermal outgrowths from hair follicles.

SEBACEOUS GLANDS

- Sebaceous glands are exocrine glands that secrete an oily substance called *sebum*.
- Sebaceous glands are distributed in the skin of all parts of the body except palms and soles.
- Meibomian glands of eyelid (tarsal glands), Montgomery's areolar tubercles surrounding female nipples, preputial (Tyson's) glands in genitalia are modified sebaceous glands. *MCQ*

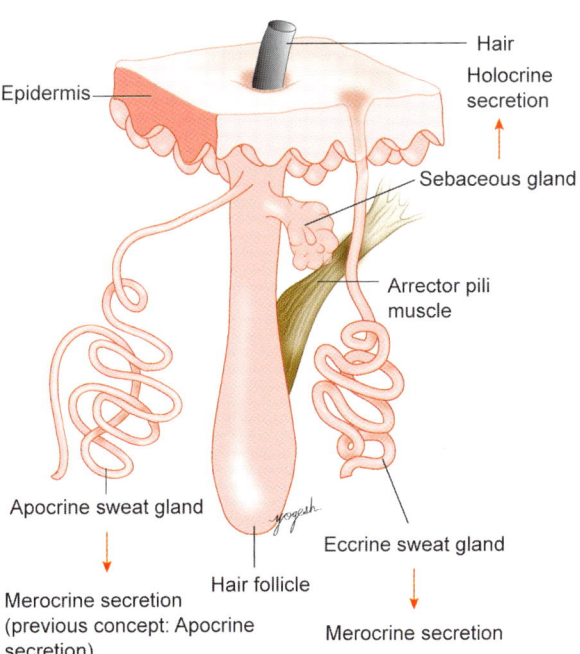

Fig. 10.3: Apocrine and eccrine sweat glands

Development (Fig. 10.2)

- Sebaceous gland develops as a bud that arises from epithelial root sheath of hair follicle in 13th–16th week of IUL.
- The bud grows and divides into number of branches to form acini and their ducts.

Mode of Secretion

- Sebaceous gland is *holocrine* in nature (whole cell rupture to become secretion).
- Note: *Merocrine* by exocytosis and *apocrine* by membrane budding or loss of cytoplasm.

NAILS

Q. Write a short note on development of nail.

- Nail is a horn-like covering at the tips of fingers and toes.
- Nails consist of a tough protein called *alpha-keratin*.

Structure of Nail

The nail shows the following parts (Fig. 10.5):

1. **Nail plate** (body) consists of keratinized cells. Nail plate grows over underlying nail bed.
2. **Nail bed** is a highly vascular connective tissue layer that lies deep to the nail plate.
3. **Hyponychium** is a part of epidermis that lies under free edge of the nail plate (Greek, *onyx* is nail).
4. **Germinal matrix** (nail root) is a growing area of nail.
5. **Lunula** is a proximal soft, half-moon shaped part of nail plate that overlies nail bed.
6. **Cuticle** is an overlapping epidermis around the base of nail (overlies matrix).
7. **Nail walls** are folds of skin that overlap sides of nail.
8. **Perionychium** includes nail wall and cuticle area.
9. **Eponychium** is an extension of base of nail plate under that nail plate emerges from the matrix.

Stages of Development

- *Nail field* appears by the end of 10th week as a thickened area at the tip and adjacent sides of fingers and toes (Fig. 10.6).
- At the base of nail field, U-shaped *epidermal nail folds* appear.
- Development of fingernails is followed by toenails.
- The underlayer of nailfold modifies to form a *germinal matrix*.
- In 5th month, a few cells of matrix get keratinized to form *nail plate*.
- Nail plate differentiates to form proximal lunula and remaining hard nail body.
- Adjacent epidermis forms *nailwall* and *cuticle*.
- Beneath the nail plate, surface epidermis pileup to form a mass called *hyponychium*.
- Nail plate reaches up to the tip of finger about 1 month before birth.^MCQ
- The fingernails reach the fingertips by 32 weeks and toenails reach toe tips by 36 weeks. After birth, nails grow about 0.5 mm a week.^MCQ

Clinical Aspects

1. *Anonychia* is partial or complete absence of nails due to failure of germinal matrix to form nails.

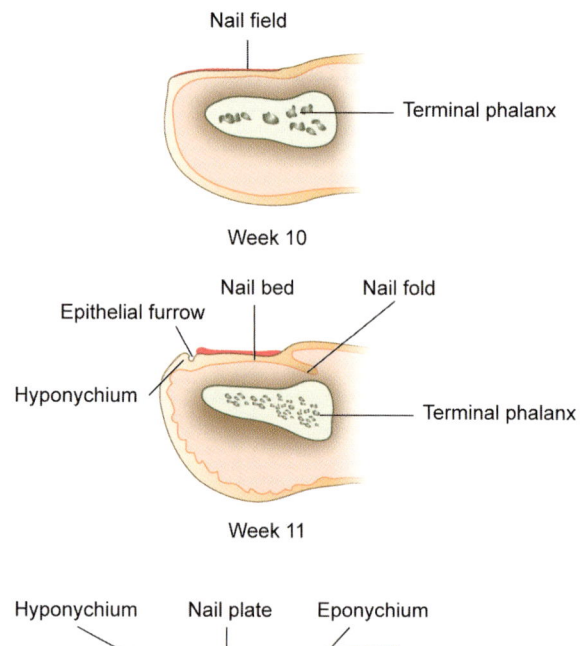

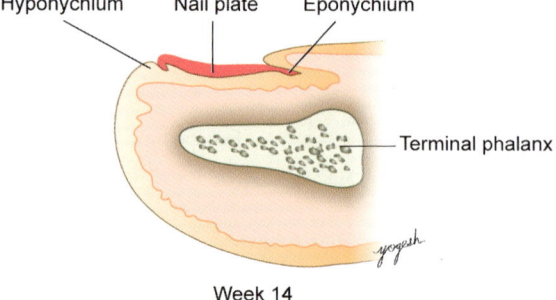

Fig. 10.6: Development of nail

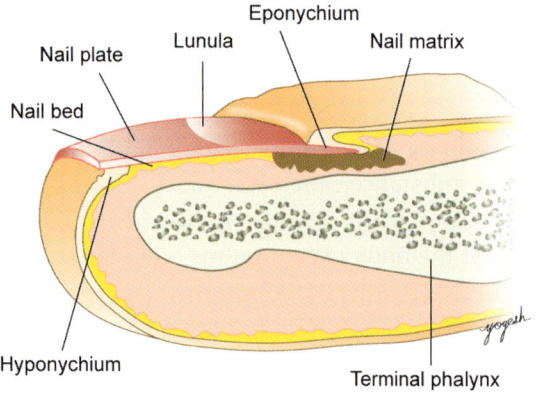

Fig. 10.5: Parts of nail

2. ***Dyskeratosis congenita*** (DKC) (*Zinsser-Cole-Engman syndrome*) is a rare progressive congenital disorder due to short telomeres. It shows triad of abnormal skin pigmentation, nail dystrophy, and leukoplakia of the oral mucosa. *MCQ*

MAMMARY GLANDS

Q. Write a short note on development of mammary gland.

Summary (Examination Guide)

- Mammary gland is a modified sweat gland (Table 10.2, Figs 10.7, 10.8, Practice Fig. 10.1, Flowchart 10.3).
- **Development of parenchyma:** Parenchyma of mammary gland develops from ectodermal bud raising from the mammary ridge. Mammary bud forms solid cords that grow into surrounding mesoderm. Later, these cords get canalized to form lactiferous ducts, whereas their terminal parts form secretory acini.
- **Fibrous stroma, fat and myoepithelial cells:** Surrounding mesoderm forms fibrous stroma, suspensory ligaments and myoepithelial cells.

Table 10.2	Development of mammary gland
Structure	Embryonic source
Parenchyma (secretory part)	Mammary buds arising from ectodermal mammary ridge (extend from axillae to groins)
Myoepithelial cells	Surrounding mesenchyme
Fibrous stroma, suspensory ligaments and fat	Surrounding mesenchyme

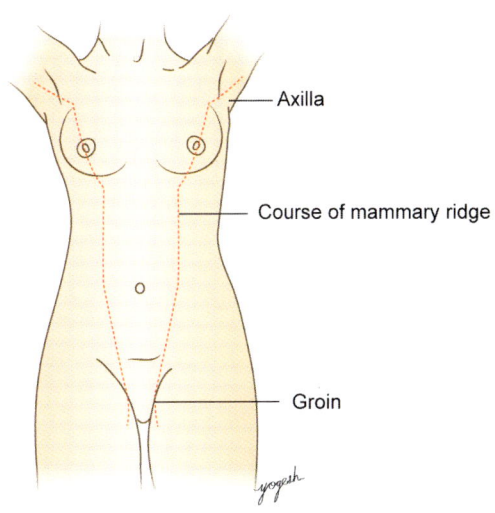

Fig. 10.7: Mammary ridge. In 6th week, surface ectoderm shows two thickened strips called primitive mammary ridges or milk lines. The ridges extend from axillae to inguinal regions. These ridges rapidly regress except in the thoracic region

Stages of Development

Formation of Mammary Ridge (Fig. 10.7)

- In 6th week, surface ectoderm shows two thickened strips called *primitive mammary ridges* or *milk lines*.
- The ridges extend from axillae to inguinal regions. In humans, these ridges rapidly regress except in the thoracic region.

Formation of mammary buds (Fig. 10.8, Practice Fig. 10.1, Flowchart 10.3)

- Mammary buds arise from the persistent thoracic part of the mammary ridges.

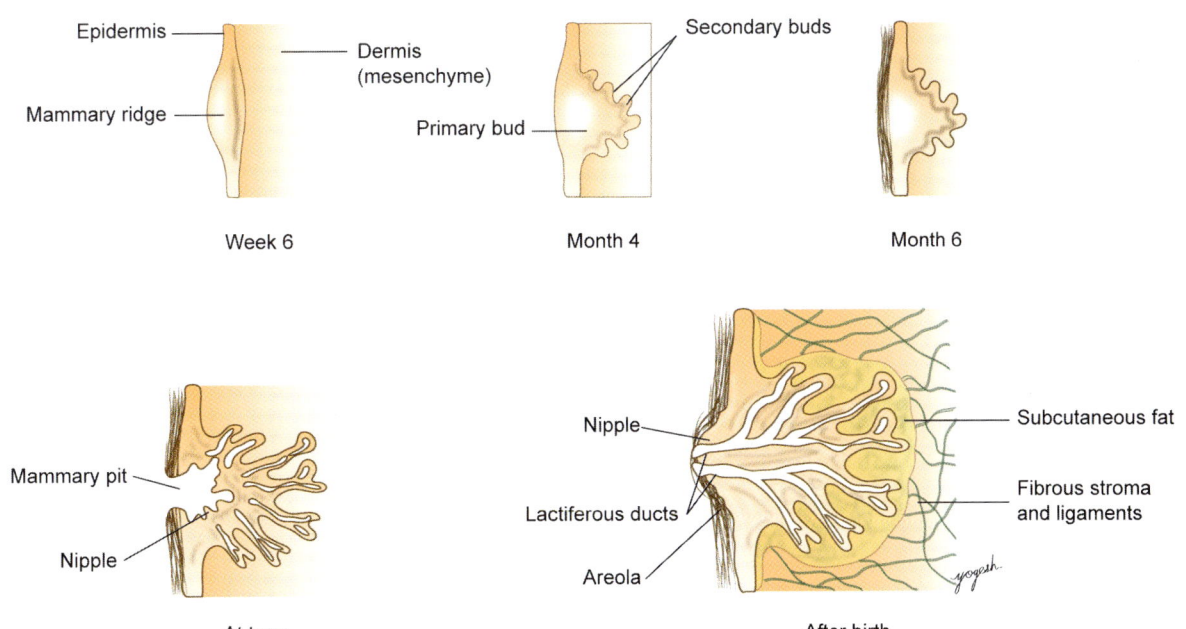

Fig. 10.8: Development of mammary gland

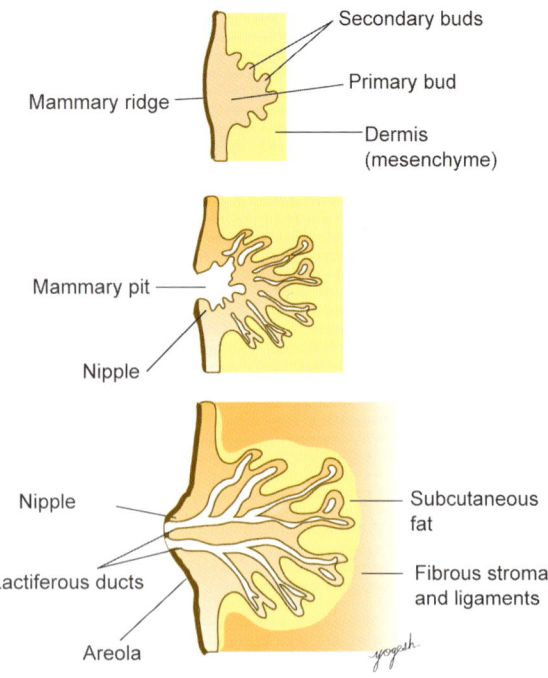

Practice Fig. 10.1: Development of mammary gland

- Mammary buds penetrate underlying mesenchyme and give rise to several secondary buds that later form lactiferous ducts and their branches.
- Lactiferous ducts canalize by the end of prenatal period.
- Only the main ducts are found at birth, and the gland remains undeveloped until puberty.

Formation of fibrous stroma

- The fibrous connective tissue, suspensory ligaments and fat of mammary gland develop from surrounding mesenchyme.

Formation of mammary pit

- During the late fetal period, the epidermis becomes depressed to form a shallow mammary pit (epithelial pit).
- Lactiferous ducts open onto this epithelial pit.

Formation of nipple

- Nipple develops during the perinatal period due to proliferation of the mesenchyme under areola (circular area of skin around nipple).

Development at puberty

- At puberty, owing to the deposition of fat and connective tissue, female mammary glands enlarge rapidly.
- Under the influence of estrogen and progesterone, duct system grows.

Development during pregnancy

- During pregnancy, the glandular tissue rapidly develops and form buds and alveoli.

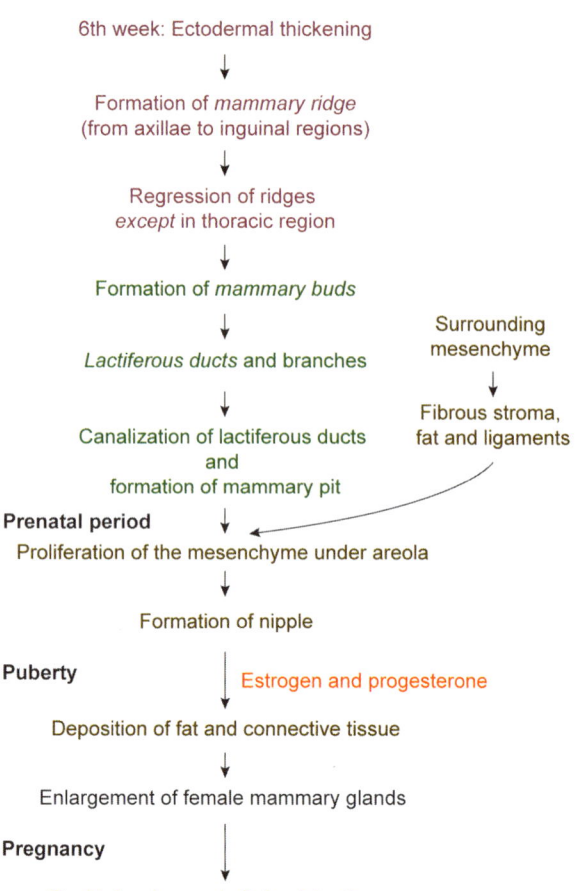

Flowchart 10.3: Development of mammary gland

Some Interesting Facts

- The male mammary glands undergo a little postnatal development.
- *Witch's milk*: The mammary glands of both newborn males and females are often enlarged and may secrete a small quantity of milk called *witch's milk* or *neonatal milk*. It occurs due to the influence of maternal hormones passing into fetal circulation.

Malformations of Mammary Gland

- Athelia is an absence of nipple.[NEXT]
- Amastia is an absence of mammary gland.[NEXT]
- Polythelia is presence of supernumerary nipples (Fig. 10.9).[NEXT]
- Polymastia is presence of supernumerary mammary glands. Polymastia is seen in about 1% of the female population.[NEXT]
- Inverted or *crater* nipple: Due to a failure of the underlying mesenchyme to proliferate and push nipple out, the nipple fails to develop and evert after birth.
- *Gynecomastia* is unusual enlargement of male mammary glands.

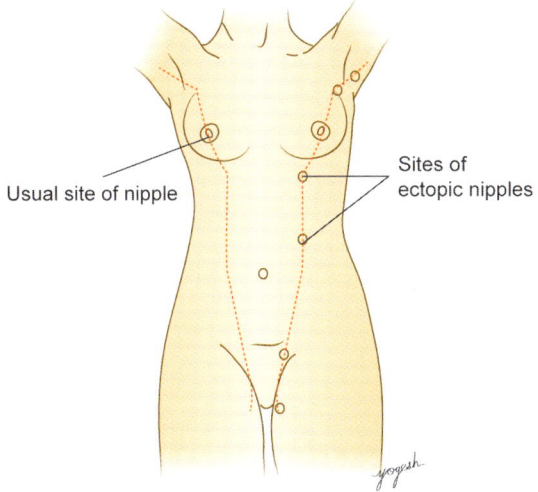

Fig. 10.9: Supernumerary nipples (polythelia)

Clinical Embryology

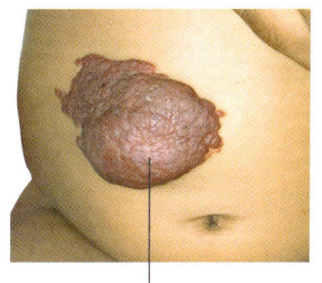 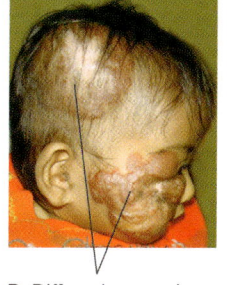

A. Focal hemangioma   *B.* Diffuse hemangioma

Clinical image 10.2: Infantile hemangioma: (A) Focal hemangioma; (B) Diffuse hemangioma. A hemangioma (infantile hemangioma) is a benign vascular tumor composed of collection of small blood vessels that form a lump under the skin (**strawberry mark**). It is one of the common benign tumors of infancy (occurs in 5–10% of infants). It appears during the first week of life and grows most rapidly during the first three to six months of life. Its involution commences by twelve months of age. Majority of infantile hemangioma regresses by five years of age. The cause of hemangiomas is not fully known. Probably it arises from placental tissue embolized to fetus. (Image courtesy: *Dr Kumaravel S*)

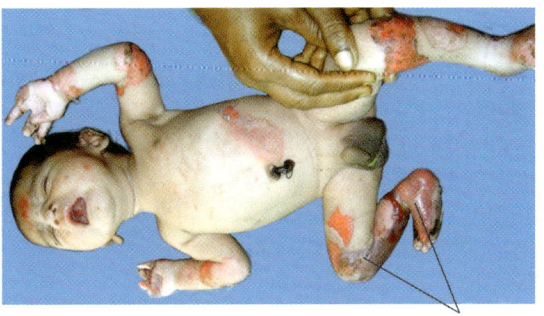

Clinical image 10.1: Epidermolysis bullosa (EB). It is a rare inherited connective tissue disorder that causes blisters on the skin and mucosal membranes. Its incidence is 20 per million newborns. It is a result of a defect in anchoring between the epidermis and dermis specifically type VII collagen. It results in skin fragility (even mild friction causes separation of epidermis from dermis). Hence, EB affected child is also called *butterfly children* (having fragile skin like butterfly) or *cotton wool babies*^MCQ (Image courtesy: *Dr Kumaravel S*)

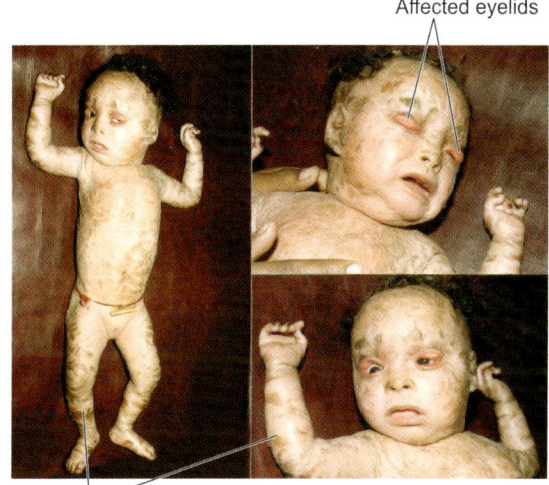

Clinical image 10.3: Harlequin ichthyosis. An infant with Harlequin ichthyosis has hard, thick skin with large diamond-shaped plates separated by deep cracks (fissures). It affects the shape of the eyelids, nose, mouth and ears. Restricted movement of the chest can lead to breathing difficulties. It occurs due to mutations of the ABCA12 genes that is inherited as an autosomal recessive disorder. ABCA12 gene product (protein) is essential for the normal development of skin cells and transport of lipids in the skin. This protein plays a major role in the transport of fats (lipids) in the outermost layer of skin. Its incidence is 1 in 300,000 births. (Image courtesy: *Dr Kumaravel S*)

Chapter 11

Pharyngeal Apparatus

eSmartQuiz

Chapter Outline

- Pharyngeal apparatus
- Pharyngeal arches
  - Skeletal elements
  - Muscular derivatives
  - Nerves of the pharyngeal arches
  - Arteries of arches
- Pharyngeal clefts
- Branchial cyst
- Branchial fistula
- DiGeorge's syndrome
- First arch syndromes
- Pharyngeal pouches
- Caudal pharyngeal complex
- Development of palatine tonsil, thymus, parathyroid and thyroid glands
  - Development of palatine tonsil
  - Development of thymus
    ➤ Involution
  - Development of parathyroid gland
  - Development of thyroid gland
    ➤ Anomalies of thyroid gland
- Thyroglossal cyst and fistula
- Goldenhar syndrome

Competency:
- **AN43.4:** Describe the development and developmental basis of congenital anomalies of face, palate, tongue, branchial apparatus, pituitary gland, thyroid gland, eye.
  This chapter includes branchial apparatus and thyroid gland development and their anomalies.

INTRODUCTION

- Pharynx is a part of the throat behind the mouth and nose. It is a funnel-shaped tubular structure that develops from the foregut.
- On the formation of embryonic folds, foregut develops from the part of yolk sac that lies within the head fold.
- Overgrowing forebrain vesicle brings the buccopharyngeal membrane in the depression called *stomodeum* that lies cranial to the pericardial bulge.
- Primitive pharynx lies dorsal and caudal to the stomodeum.
- The primitive pharyngeal part has floor, roof and two lateral walls.
- *Relations of the primitive pharynx*
  - Cranial: Forebrain
  - Ventral (floor): Stomodeum, pericardial bulge, and septum transversum
  - Dorsal (roof): Notochord and hindbrain vesicle
  - Lateral: Splanchnopleuric layer of the mesoderm, surface ectoderm
- In early developmental stages, the neck is not present. The neck is formed in between stomodeum and pericardial bulge due to mesodermal growth.
- In the neck zone, between stomodeum and pericardial bulge, mesoderm shows intermittent thickening. The thickened mesoderm forms bars (bulging) on the surface ectoderm. These bars extend ventrally and push and separate pericardial bulge from stomodeum (Fig. 11.1).
- Each mesodermal bar fuses with opposite bar in the midline to form arch-like, shoe-shaped structure called *pharyngeal arch or branchial arch* (Fig. 11.2).
- Subsequently, six arches appear, out of these, the fifth arch is small and rudimentary.*MCQ, Viva*
- When seen from the cavity of the foregut (primitive pharynx), endoderm of the foregut shows depressions between the adjacent pharyngeal arches. These six

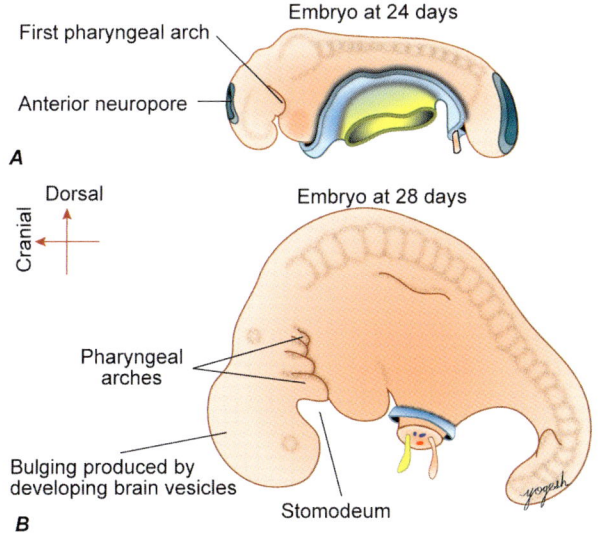
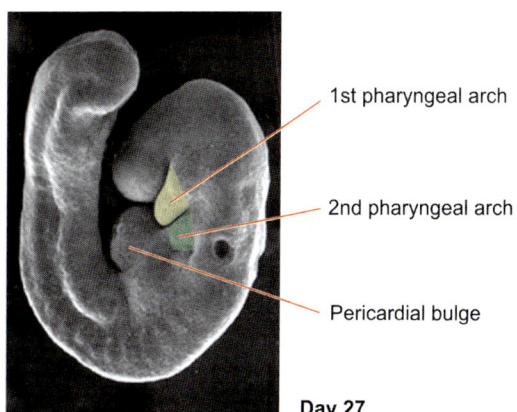

Scanning electron micrograph 11.1: SEM showing pharyngeal arches. On 27th day (by the time that anterior neuropore closes), the first and second pharyngeal arches are evident [Species: Mouse, approximate human age: 27 days, lateral view]

Fig. 11.1: Side view of the developing embryo with formation of pharyngeal arches. By 24th day, embryo shows the first pharyngeal arch. The number of arches increases to four by 28th day

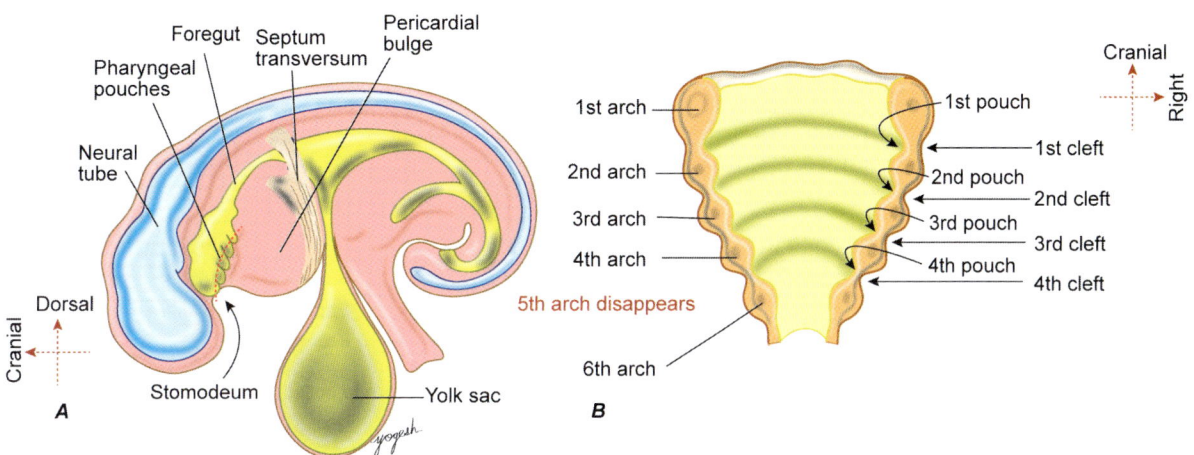

Fig. 11.2: (A) Section of the embryo showing the foregut and pharyngeal pouches; (B) Section of the embryo passing through the dotted red line shown in Fig. A. The mesodermal thickening forms six pharyngeal arches. Inner side of the foregut shows depressions in between adjacent pharyngeal arches. These depressions are called pharyngeal pouches. The surface ectoderm also shows depressions in between adjacent arches. These depressions are called pharyngeal clefts

endodermal depressions in the floor and the lateral wall of the pharynx are called *pharyngeal pouches*.
- Surface ectoderm also shows depressions or groove in between adjacent arches. These four grooves are called *pharyngeal clefts*.
- Pharyngeal arches appear in the fourth and fifth week of the development.^{MCQ}

PHARYNGEAL APPARATUS

Q. Define pharyngeal apparatus, pharyngeal arch, pharyngeal pouch and pharyngeal cleft.^{Viva}

- The pharyngeal apparatus consists of pharyngeal arches, pharyngeal pouches and pharyngeal clefts (Fig. 11.2, Flowchart 11.1).

Pharyngeal arches
- Thickened **mesodermal** bars present in the floor and lateral wall of the primitive pharynx are called pharyngeal arches.^{Viva}

Pharyngeal clefts
- Depressions (grooves) on the surface **ectoderm** in between adjacent arches are called pharyngeal clefts.^{Viva}

Pharyngeal pouches
- **Endodermal** depressions between adjacent pharyngeal arches in the floor and lateral wall of the primitive pharynx are called pharyngeal pouches.^{Viva}
- For study purpose, the derivatives of the pharyngeal apparatus are grouped into derivatives of pharyngeal arches, pharyngeal pouches and pharyngeal clefts.

Flowchart 11.1: Pharyngeal apparatus

```
                    Pharyngeal apparatus
    ┌───────────────┬───────────────┬───────────────┐
Pharyngeal      Pharyngeal      Pharyngeal      Pharyngeal
arches          clefts          pouches         membranes
Thick           Grooves on      Endodermal      Area of contact
mesodermal bars surface         depression in   of pharyngeal
in the floor of ectoderm in     between         pouches
lateral wall of between         adjacent        and pharyngeal
pharynx         adjacent        pharyngeal      clefts
                pharyngeal      arches
                arches
```

Some Interesting Facts

- **Pharyngeal membranes** are the area of contact between pharyngeal pouches (endoderm) and pharyngeal clefts (ectoderm). **Tympanic membrane** is derived from 1st pharyngeal membrane (separates 1st pouch from 1st cleft) and represents all three derms.^{NEXT}

- In fishes and other aquatic vertebrates, the pharyngeal membranes rupture to form gill slits. Gill slits work as respiratory organ and help to take dissolved oxygen from water that flows from mouth and exits from gill slits.

- In the human embryo, a thin layer of mesenchyme appears between pharyngeal membranes and form fibroareolar tissue of the neck. In human, pharyngeal membranes do not rupture.^{MCQ}

- By the fourth week, buccopharyngeal membrane ruptures and foregut communicates with the amniotic cavity.^{MCQ}

- By 4th week (22nd day) first and second pharyngeal arch appears.^{MCQ} By 29th day (5th week), four pharyngeal arches appear.

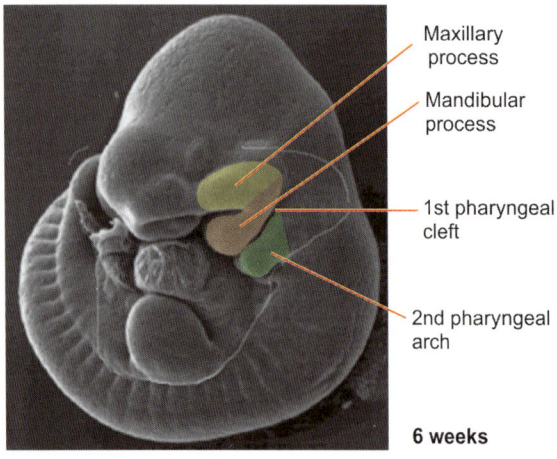

Scanning electron micrograph 11.2: SEM showing 6-week embryo with first and second pharyngeal arch. Maxillary and mandibular processes of first pharyngeal arch are also evident [Species: Mouse, approximate human age: 6 weeks, lateral view]

PHARYNGEAL ARCHES $^{High\ yielding\ facts}$

Q. List the derivatives of first pharyngeal arch.

Definition
- *Horseshoe-shaped* thickened mesodermal bars in lateral wall and the floor of the primitive pharynx are called *pharyngeal arches*.

Number
- There are *six* pharyngeal arches, but the fifth pharyngeal arch is rudimentary (small and disappears).

Components
- Each arch consists of splanchnopleuric mesoderm with invaded neural crest cells.
- These invading neural crest cells form skeletal elements and connective tissue of the head and neck region.$^{MCQ,\ Viva}$ Hence, facial skeleton or viscerocranium is derived from neural crest cells.^{NEXT}
- Each pharyngeal arch mesoderm differentiates to form muscle mass, pharyngeal arch artery and nerve (Fig. 11.3, Flowchart 11.2, Table 11.1).

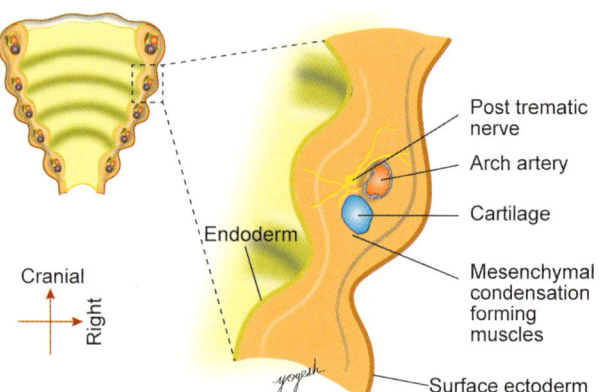

Fig. 11.3: Components of the pharyngeal arch. Each pharyngeal arch has one arch artery, cartilage, post-trematic nerve and muscles

Flowchart 11.2: Components of pharyngeal arch

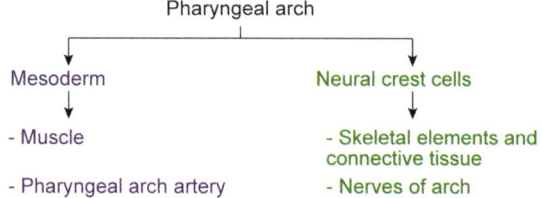

Skeletal Elements

Q. List the muscular and skeletal derivatives of first pharyngeal arch.

Q. Write a short note on Meckel's cartilage.

- Neural crest cells form the cartilaginous rod in the substance of the pharyngeal arch (Fig. 11.4, Flowchart 11.3, Practice Fig. 11.1).

Table 11.1: Derivatives of pharyngeal arches^{High yielding facts, NEXT}

Pharyngeal arch	Muscles NEXT	Nerve NEXT	Skeletal elements NEXT	Ligament NEXT
First arch (Meckel's cartilage)^{NEXT}	Muscles of mastication (temporalis, masseter, medial and lateral pterygoid) Tensor veli palatini Tensor tympani Anterior belly of digastric Mylohyoid	Pretrematic: Chorda tympani Post-trematic: Mandibular nerve^{NEXT}	Premaxilla Maxilla Zygomatic bone Temporal bone Incus Malleus	Anterior ligament of malleus Sphenomandibular ligament
Second arch (Reichert's cartilage)^{NEXT}	Muscles of facial expression Posterior belly of digastric Stylohyoid Stapedius	Facial nerve^{NEXT}	Stapes Styloid process Short (lesser) cornua of hyoid bone Superior part of body of hyoid bone	Stylohyoid ligament
Third arch	Stylopharyngeus ^{NEXT}	Glossopharyngeal nerve ^{NEXT}	Greater cornua of hyoid bone. Lower part of body of hyoid bone	—
Fourth arch	Cricothyroid, constrictors of pharynx, muscles of palate except tensor veli palatini ^{NEXT}	Superior laryngeal nerve ^{NEXT}	Laryngeal cartilages except epiglottis	—
Sixth arch	Intrinsic muscles of larynx except cricothyroid	Recurrent laryngeal nerve ^{NEXT}		—

Flowchart 11.3: Fate of neural crest cells in pharyngeal arches

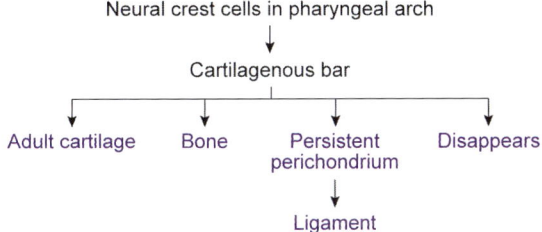

- The fate of cartilages of the pharyngeal arches:
  - Some part of the cartilage persists
  - Some part disappears
  - Some part is converted into bone
  - Some part of perichondrium persists as ligament

First Arch^{High yielding facts}

- The first arch is differentiated into smaller cranial maxillary process and larger caudal mandibular process (Fig. 11.4, Practice Fig. 11.1, Flowchart 11.4).
- Maxillary process form part of the upper lip, upper jaw and palate.
- Cartilage of mandibular part, the first arch, is called **Meckel's cartilage**.
- Meckel's cartilage forms –
  1. Malleus (ear ossicle) from dorsal part^{MCQ}
  2. Incus (ear ossicle) from dorsal part^{MCQ}
  3. Anterior ligament of malleus from perichondrium
  4. Sphenomandibular ligament

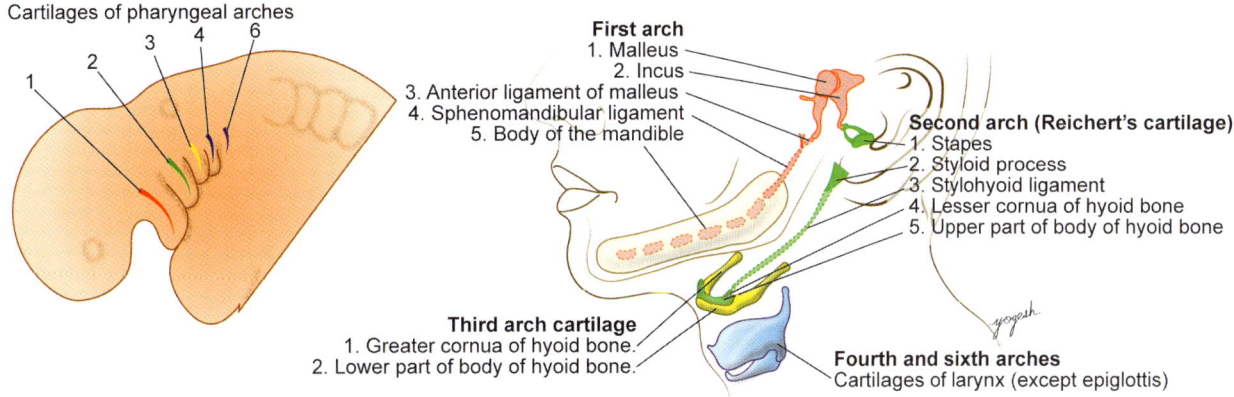

Fig. 11.4: Structures derived from cartilages of the pharyngeal arches. The first arch cartilage is Meckel's cartilage and the second one is Reichert's cartilage

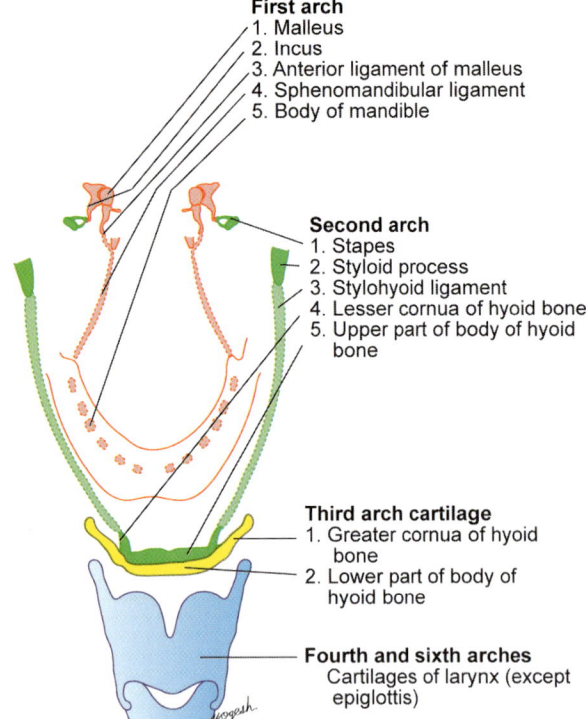

First arch
1. Malleus
2. Incus
3. Anterior ligament of malleus
4. Sphenomandibular ligament
5. Body of mandible

Second arch
1. Stapes
2. Styloid process
3. Stylohyoid ligament
4. Lesser cornua of hyoid bone
5. Upper part of body of hyoid bone

Third arch cartilage
1. Greater cornua of hyoid bone
2. Lower part of body of hyoid bone

Fourth and sixth arches
Cartilages of larynx (except epiglottis)

Practice Fig. 11.1: Structures derived from cartilages of the pharyngeal arches

5. Body of the mandible develops from fibrous surrounding of the Meckel's cartilage^MCQ

Note: Meckel's cartilage does not form mandible. Maxillary part of the first arch forms premaxilla, maxilla, zygomatic bone, part of the temporal bone.

Flowchart 11.4: Derivatives of 1st arch

Derivatives of 1st arch

Muscular derivatives	Skeletal elements	Ligaments

Muscles of mastication
  Temporalis
  Masseter
  Medial pterygoid
  Lateral pterygoid
Tensor veli palatini
Tensor tympani
Anterior belly of digastric
Mylohyoid
	Incus
	Malleus
	Premailla
	Zygomatic bone
	Temporal bone
		Anterior ligaments of malleus
		Sphenomandibular ligament

Nerves of first arch
Pretrematic: Chorda tympani
Posttrematic: Mandibular

Second Arch Cartilage^High yielding facts

Q. List the skeletal derivatives of second pharyngeal arch.

- Cartilage of second (hyoid) arch is called **Reichert's cartilage** (Fig. 11.4, Practice Fig. 11.1, Flowchart 11.5).

Reichert's cartilage forms:
1. Stapes (ear ossicle) from dorsal part^MCQ
2. Styloid process of temporal bone from dorsal part^MCQ
3. Short (lesser) cornua of hyoid bone from ventral part
4. Superior (upper) part of body of hyoid bone from ventral part

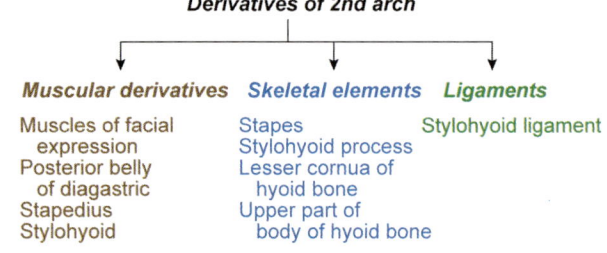

Flowchart 11.5: Second pharyngeal arch

Derivatives of 2nd arch

Muscular derivatives	Skeletal elements	Ligaments
Muscles of facial expression Posterior belly of diagastric Stapedius Stylohyoid	Stapes Stylohyoid process Lesser cornua of hyoid bone Upper part of body of hyoid bone	Stylohyoid ligament

Nerves of second arch: Facial nerve

5. Stylohyoid ligament from perichondrium of disappearing cartilage between styloid process and hyoid bone^NEXT

(Mnemonic: Note second arch derivatives starting from alphabet S.)

Third Arch Cartilage

- Dorsal part of the third arch cartilage disappears (Flowchart 11.6).
- Ventral part of the third arch cartilage forms –
  1. Greater cornua of hyoid bone
  2. Lower part of body of hyoid bone

Flowchart 11.6: Third pharyngeal arch

Derivatives of 3rd arch

Muscular derivatives	Skeletal elements	Nerve
Stylopharyngeus	Greater cornua of hyoid bone Lower part of body of hyoid bone	Glossopharyngeal nerve

Fourth and Sixth Arches

- Dorsal part of the fourth and sixth arch cartilage disappears (Flowchart 11.7).
- Ventral part of the fourth and sixth arches form cartilages of larynx (except epiglottis) such as
  - Thyroid cartilage
  - Cricoid cartilage
  - Arytenoid cartilage
  - Corniculate cartilage
  - Cuneiform cartilage

Note: Epiglottic cartilage develops from hypobranchial eminence.^MCQ

Flowchart 11.7: Fourth and sixth arches

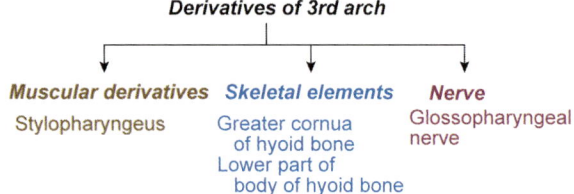

	Fourth arch	Sixth arch
Muscles	Cricothyroid Constrictors of pharynx Muscles of palate except tensor veli palatini	Intrinsic muscles of larynx except cricothyroid
Nerve	Superior laryngeal nerve	Recurrent laryngeal nerve
Skeletal elements	——— Laryngeal cartilages except epiglottis ———	

Note: Epiglottis is derived from hypobranchial eminence.

Muscular Derivatives

- Mesodermal cells of arches differentiate to form striated muscles.
- These striated muscles migrate from their site of development. During migration, they carry their nerves.

First Arch

- Muscles derived from the first arch are as follows:^{MCQ}
    1–4. Muscles of mastication: Temporalis, masseter, lateral pterygoid and medial pterygoid
    5. Tensor tympani
    6. Tensor veli palatini
    7. Anterior belly of digastric
    8. Mylohyoid muscle
- Nerve supply: Mandibular nerve

Second Arch

- Muscles derived from second arch are as follows:
    1. Muscles of facial expression
    2. Posterior belly of digastric
    3. Stapedius
    4. Stylohyoid
- Nerve supply: Facial nerve

Third Arch

- The *stylopharyngeus* muscle develops from third arch.
- Nerve supply: Glossopharyngeal nerve

Fourth Arch

- Muscles derived from fourth arch are:
    1. Cricothyroid
    2. Constrictor muscles of pharynx
    3. Muscles of palate except tensor veli palatini
- Nerve supply: Superior laryngeal branch of vagus nerve

Sixth Arch

- Muscles derived from the sixth arch are: All the intrinsic muscles of the larynx except cricothyroid muscle.^{MCQ}
- Nerve supply: Recurrent laryngeal branch of vagus nerve

> **Some Interesting Facts**
>
> - Carotid body is derived from the third arch, whereas aortic body is derived from the fourth arch.^{MCQ}

Nerves of Pharyngeal Arches

Q. Name the nerves of pharyngeal arches.

- Pharyngeal arches receive nerve supply from hindbrain vesicle.
- Each nerve appears at the dorsal end of the cleft and divides into pretrematic and post-trematic branches (Fig. 11.5).
- Pretrematic branch supplies the arch cranial to the cleft, whereas posttrematic branch supplies caudal to the cleft.
- Pretrematic nerve of all arches degenerate except the first arch. The pretrematic nerve of the first arch is chorda tympani nerve.^{MCQ}
- The nerve to the arch is mixed nerve as it supplies muscles and carry sensations from derivatives of pouches and clefts.

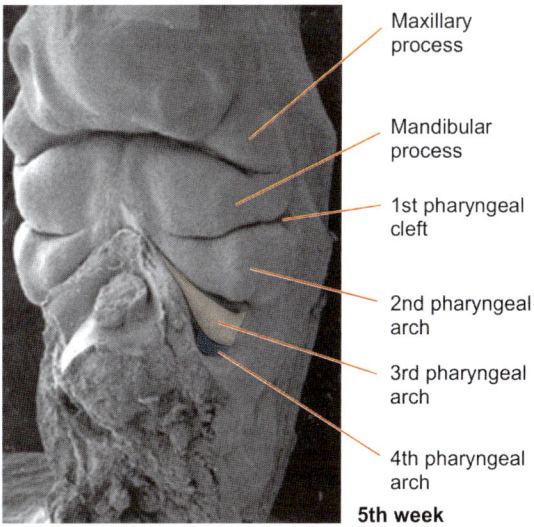

Scanning electron micrograph 11.3: SEM showing pharyngeal arches. The first, second, third and fourth arches are visible externally. The sixth arch does not form an external elevation. The heart has been removed in this specimen [Species: human, approximate age: fifth week]

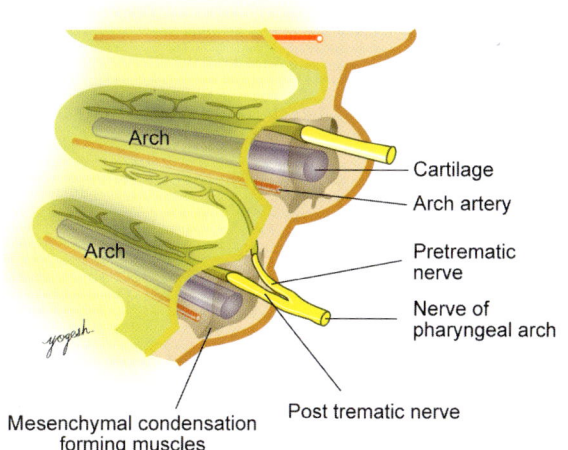

Fig. 11.5: Arrangement of nerves in the pharyngeal arch. The pretrematic branch supplies the structures of the preceding arch, whereas nerve of the pharyngeal arch continues as posttrematic nerve and supplies the structures of the same arch

- Nerves of arches are as follows (Fig. 11.6):
  1. First arch: Mandibular nerve (post-trematic) and chorda tympani branch of facial nerve (pretrematic)
  2. Second arch: Facial nerve
  3. Third arch: Glossopharyngeal nerve
  4. Fourth arch: Superior laryngeal nerve
  5. Sixth arch: Recurrent laryngeal nerve

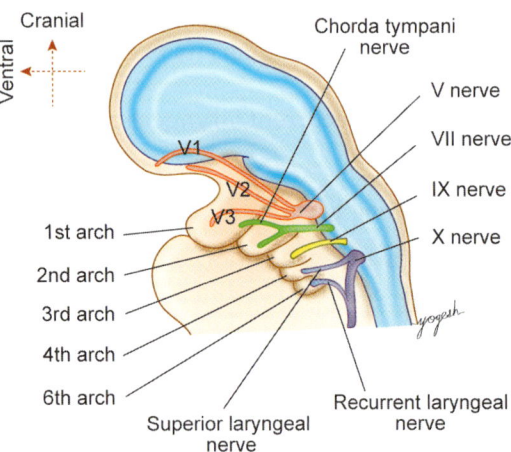

Fig. 11.6: Nerve supply of the pharyngeal arches. First arch is supplied by mandibular nerve (V3) and chorda tympani nerve. Second arch is supplied by facial nerve, third arch by glossopharyngeal nerve and fourth arch by superior laryngeal nerve, whereas sixth arch by recurrent laryngeal nerve. Sixth arch is not prominently visible on the surface. V1, ophthalmic nerve; V2, maxillary nerve; V3, mandibular nerve

Arteries of Arches

- Each arch contains one arch artery.
- These arch arteries connect dorsal aorta with aortic sac (that lies ventrally).
- Aortic arches modify and forms following structures:
  1. First aortic arch artery: A part of maxillary artery
  2. Second aortic arch artery: Stapedial artery, hyoid artery^{NEXT}
  3. Third aortic arch artery:
     a. *Common carotid artery* from ventral part of third aortic arch and
     b. stem of internal carotid artery from dorsal part of third aortic arch^{NEXT}
  4. Fourth aortic arch artery:
     a. On the right side – proximal part of right subclavian artery.
     b. On the left side – arch of aorta.
  5. Fifth aortic arch artery: Disappears completely
  6. Sixth aortic arch artery:
     a. On the right side – right pulmonary artery.
     b. On the left side – left pulmonary artery and ductus arteriosus (after birth, ligamentum arteriosum).

PHARYNGEAL CLEFTS

Definition

- The groove of the surface ectoderm between adjacent pharyngeal arches is called *ectodermal cleft*.
- There are *four* pharyngeal clefts.
- Only dorsal part of the *first* pharyngeal cleft **persists** and forms the epithelial lining of the external acoustic meatus and a cuticular layer of the tympanic membrane (Fig. 11.7).^{MCQ}

Cervical Sinus

Q. Write a short note on cervical sinus.

- The mesenchymal tissue of second pharyngeal arch grows rapidly and covers second, third and fourth clefts. This growing tissue fuses with epicardial ridge. Thus, second to fourth clefts bury under the bulging second arch and form a slit-like cavity called *cervical sinus* (Fig. 11.7).
- Cervical sinus is lined with ectoderm.
- Gradually cervical sinus disappears and neck becomes smooth (devoid of grooves).

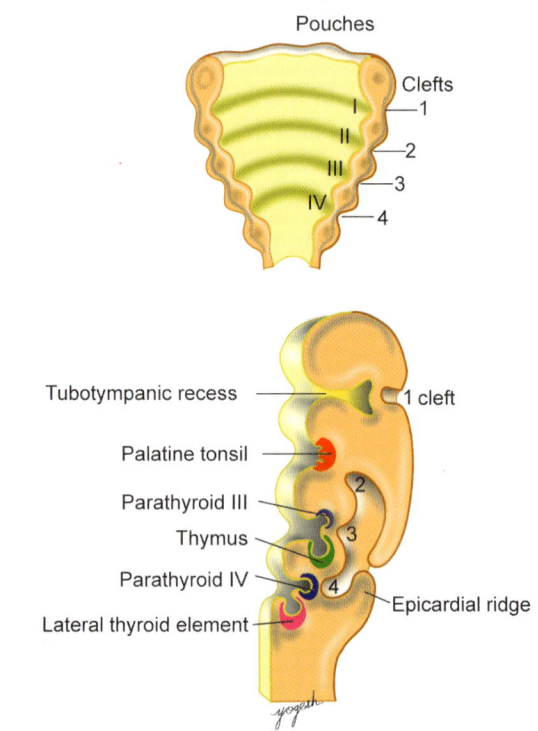

Fig. 11.7: Development of pharyngeal clefts and pouches. The second arch grows to cover the second, third and fourth clefts. Finally, fuses with the epicardial ridge. The trapped part of the second, third and fourth clefts forms the cervical sinus that later gets obliterated

Some Interesting Facts

- Ectodermal cells proliferate at the dorsal ends of the first, second and fourth pharyngeal clefts before their regression and form epibranchial placodes.
- Later epibranchial placodes contribute to sensory ganglia of 5th, 7th, 9th and 10th cranial nerves.

Box 11.1: Branchial cyst or cervical cyst

Q. Write a short note on branchial cyst.

Branchial Cyst (*Branchia* = gills, in Greek)

- Branchial cyst is a congenital cyst in the skin of the lateral part of the neck (Fig. 11.8, Flowchart 11.8).
- **Location**: Located along the *anterior border of the sternocleidomastoid muscle*, mostly close to the angle of the mandible.
- **Cause:** Branchial cyst is a result of *failure of obliteration of the branchial cleft*, mostly second cleft.
- **Symptoms**
  - Cyst presents as a smooth, slowly enlarging lateral neck mass.
  - Cyst is usually not present at birth. Its size increases with advancing age.
  - Cyst usually increases in size with upper respiratory tract infection.
- **Pathology**
  - Cyst wall may be lined by
    A. Stratified squamous cells or
    B. Simple columnar cells
- **Treatment**
  - Branchial cysts can be *removed surgically*, but mostly incomplete surgical removal leads to recurrence of the cyst.

Branchial Fistula

- If the branchial cyst opens both in the pharynx and externally on the skin of the neck, it is called **complete branchial** or **cervical fistula**.
- If the cyst shows only internal communication with pharynx, it is called **internal branchial fistula** or **sinus,** whereas if the cyst shows only external communication on the skin of the neck, it is called **external branchial sinus** or **fistula**.

Flowchart 11.8: Branchial cyst

Branchial cyst
Congenital cyst in the lateral part of neck

Location	Cause	Symptoms	Treatment
Anterior border of sternocleidomastoid muscle	Failure of obliteration of 2nd branchial cleft	Smooth, slowly enlarging cystic mass in neck Size increases with age	Surgical removal

Branchial fistula: Cyst opened internally in the pharynx and externally on the skin

PHARYNGEAL POUCHES

Q. Draw a well-labelled diagram showing derivatives of pharyngeal pouches.

- There are *five* pairs of pharyngeal pouches (Fig. 11.9, Practice Fig. 11.2, Flowchart 11.9).
- Pharyngeal pouches are numbered craniocaudally.
- The fifth pharyngeal pouch is rudimentary.
- Ventrally right and left pouches fuse to form floor of the pharynx where tongue develops.
- The derivatives of pharyngeal pouches are listed in Table 11.2.

Q. List the derivatives of pharyngeal pouches.

Table 11.2 Derivatives of pharyngeal pouches[MCQ, Viva]

Pouch	Derivatives
First pouch	Auditory tube Tympanic cavity Inner surface of tympanic membrane
Second pouch	Palatine tonsil Tonsillar fossa, intratonsillar cleft
Third pouch	Inferior parathyroid gland Thymus
Fourth pouch	Superior parathyroid gland
Caudal pharyngeal complex	Thymic element – part of thymus Lateral thyroid element – part of thyroid gland Ultimobranchial body – parafollicular cells of thyroid gland (neural crest cells)

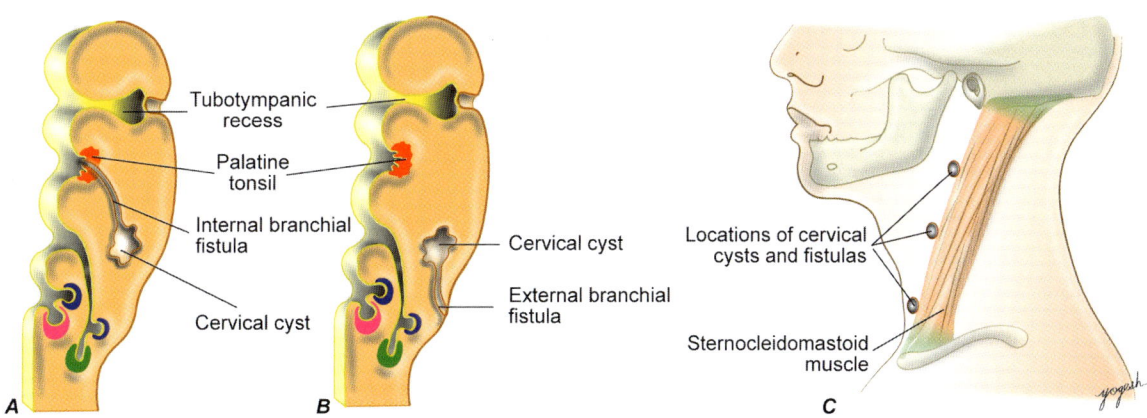

Fig. 11.8: (A and B) Cervical cysts and fistulas; (C) Locations of the openings of the cervical cysts in the neck

Some Interesting Facts

DiGeorge's Syndrome (22q11.2 deletion syndrome)
- Also known as a *velocardiofacial syndrome* or *Shprintzen syndrome*.
- Cause: Microdeletion of chromosome 22.[MCQ]
- Symptoms: It presents with congenital heart disease with fish mouth deformity (short philtrum), low sets of malformed ears, long face, small lower jaw bone.
- Incidence: 1 in 2000–4000 live births

Box 11.2: First arch syndromes

- First arch syndromes occur due to failure of migration of neural crest cells into the first arch.
- These neural crest cells form skeletal elements and connective tissue in the first arch.
- The first arch syndrome includes Treacher Collins syndrome and Pierre Robin syndrome.

A. Treacher Collins syndrome
- It is also called **mandibulofacial dystosis**.[MCQ]
- Described first by Edward Treacher Collin in 1900.
- It is *autosomal dominant* disorder due to mutation in TCOF1 gene located on chromosome 5.[MCQ]
- Incidence: 1:50,000 births
- Clinical presentation:
  - Underdeveloped lower jaw (mandibular hypoplasia)
  - Underdeveloped zygomatic bone (malar hypoplasia)
  - Down-slanting palpebral fissure
  - External ear malformations (malformed pinna and meatal atresia)[NEXT]

B. Pierre Robin Syndrome
- It has three main features:[MCQ]
  - Cleft palate
  - Retrognathia (small mandible) and
  - Glossoptosis (backward displacement of the tongue)
- Cause: Anomalies of chromosome 2, 11 and 17; mostly mutation in SOXG gene of chromosome 17.
- Incidence: 1 in 10,000 births

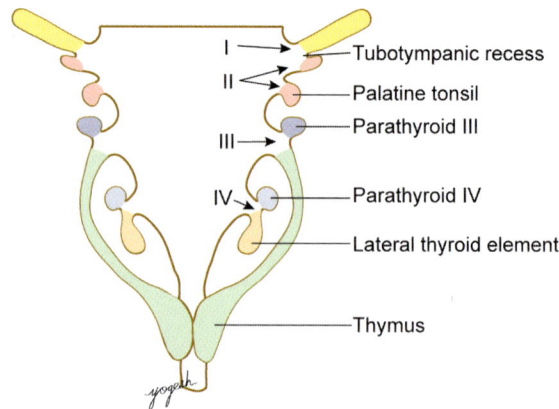

Practice Fig. 11.2: Derivatives of the pharyngeal pouches

First Pouch
- Ventral part of the first pouch is obliterated by the developing tongue.
- Dorsal part of the first pouch along with dorsal part of the second pouch form a diverticulum called **tubotympanic recess**.
- The proximal part of tubotympanic recess forms an *auditory (Eustachian) tube*.[NEXT]
- Distal part of the recess forms middle ear cavity, mastoid antrum, mastoid air cells and inner lining epithelium of the tympanic membrane.

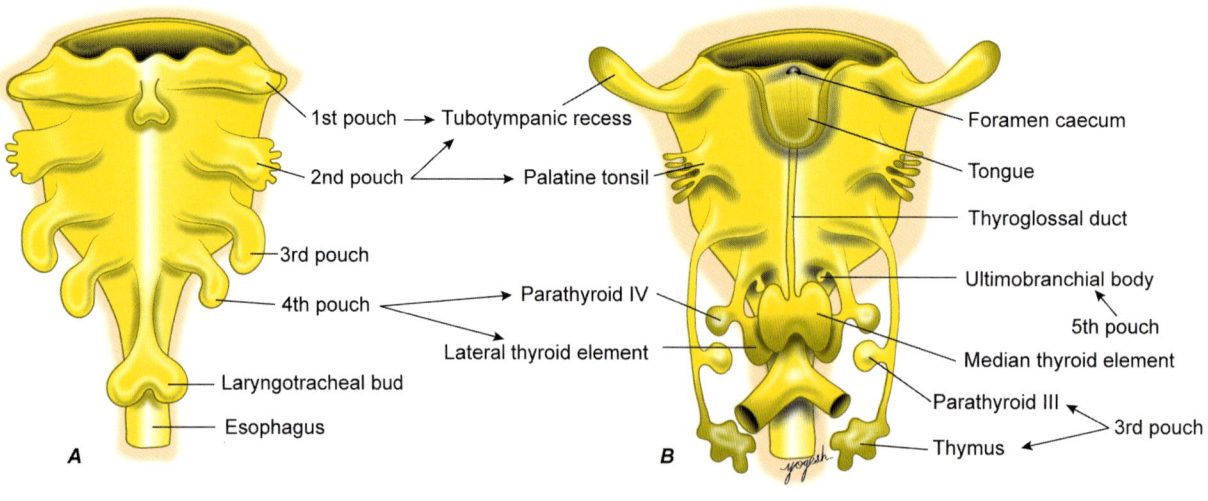

Fig. 11.9: Derivatives of the pharyngeal pouches: (A) In the fourth week, endoderm of the primitive pharynx outpouches to form pharyngeal pouches that later give rise to various structures as shown in this figure. (B) Inferior parathyroid develops from the third pharyngeal pouch, whereas superior parathyroid develops from the fourth pharyngeal pouch

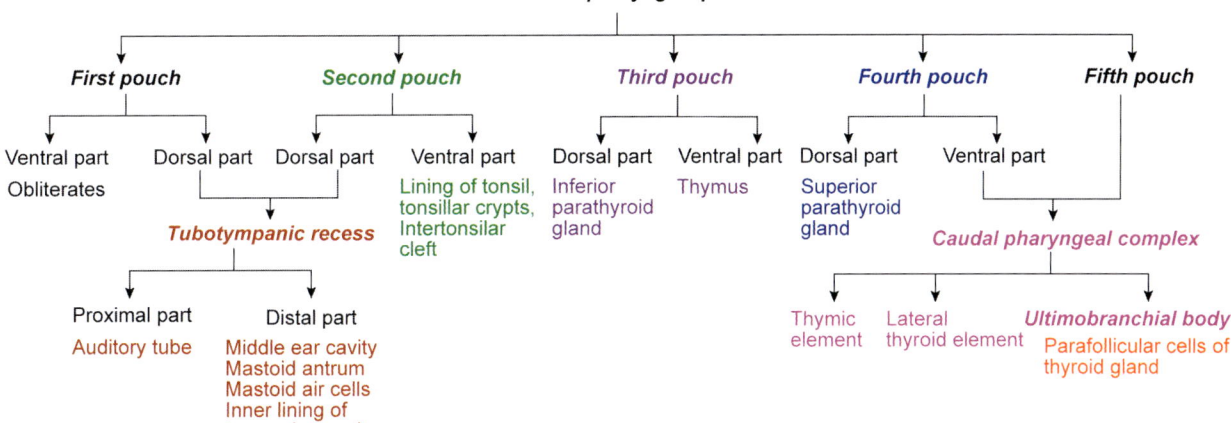

Flowchart 11.9: Derivatives of pharyngeal pouches

Second Pouch

- Dorsal part of second pouch fuses with dorsal part of the first pouch to form tubotympanic recess.
- Ventral part of the second pouch forms epithelial lining of *tonsil* and tonsillar crypts. Note: Lymphatic follicles of tonsil develop from mesoderm.
- *Intratonsillar cleft* (crypta magna) represents non-obliterated part of the second pouch.^{MCQ}

Third Pouch

- Dorsal part (wing) of third pouch forms *inferior parathyroid gland* (parathyroid III).^{MCQ}
- Ventral wing of the third pouch forms *thymus*.
- Both right and left wings lose their contact with pharynx and migrate caudally towards the developing heart.
- Finally, inferior parathyroid also lose its connection with thymus and gain permanent attachment with lower pole of the thyroid gland.
- Thymus further continues caudal migration and come to lie within developing anterior mediastinum.

Note: Thymocytes develop in bone narrow (mesoderm) and migrate to the thymus, whereas **Hassall's corpuscles** are derived from the third pouch (endoderm).^{MCQ}

Fourth Pouch

- Dorsal wing (part) of fourth pouch forms *superior parathyroid gland* (parathyroid IV).
- Dorsal wing loses contact with pharynx, migrate caudally and finally gain permanent attachment with posterior border of lateral lobe of the thyroid gland.

Fifth Pouch

- In some species, it forms the *ultimobranchial body*.
- In human, the fifth pouch is seen for a brief period.

Box 11.3: Caudal pharyngeal complex

- Ventral part of the fourth pouch fuses with a rudimentary fifth pouch to form caudal pharyngeal complex.
- Caudal pharyngeal complex shows three components:
  1. Thymic element: It gets incorporated in developing thymus.
  2. Lateral thyroid element: It fuses with median thyroid element (that derives from thyroglossal duct) and arrests caudal migration of median thyroid element.
  3. Ultimobranchial body: It forms parafollicular or C-cells of the thyroid gland.

Note: Neural crest cells migrate to thyroid gland via ultimobranchial body and forms parafollicular cells.^{MCQ}

DEVELOPMENT OF PALATINE TONSIL, THYMUS, PARATHYROID, AND THYROID GLANDS

Development of Palatine Tonsil *High yielding facts*

Q. Write a short note on development of palatine tonsil.

- Palatine tonsil develops from two sources
  - Endoderm of second pharyngeal pouch
  - Mesoderm (lymphocytes) (Flowchart 11.10)

Stages of Development

- During the third month of development, ventral part of the second pouch proliferates outwards in surrounding mesoderm as several solid cords called *tonsillar buds*.
- On degeneration of central cells, tonsillar buds cannulate to form hollow *tonsillar crypts*.
- During 3rd to 5th month, lymphocytes aggregate on the mesoderm that surrounds crypts and form lymphatic follicles.

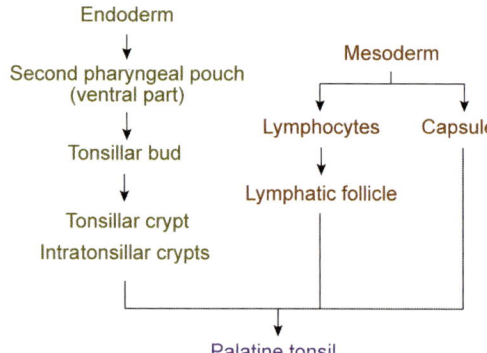

Flowchart 11.10: Development of the palatine tonsil

- Mesodermal cells condense to form a *capsule* of the tonsil.
- Lymphocyte proliferates and forms pharyngeal tonsillar bulging.
- The remnant of the pouch is represented by an intratonsillar cleft and tonsillar fossa.^{MCQ}

Development of Thymus^{High yielding facts}

Q. Write a short note on development of thymus.

- Thymus develops from the following two sources:
  A. Endoderm of the third pharyngeal pouch
  B. Mesoderm forms thymocytes and other connective tissue.

Stages of Development

- Ventral part of the third pharyngeal pouch descends caudally and forms thymic rudiment.
- The thymic rudiment and inferior parathyroid gland (that develops from the dorsal part of the third pharyngeal pouch) descend caudally and lose contact with pharynx.
- Finally, thymic rudiment loses contact with inferior parathyroid and continues to descent caudally.
- Endodermal third pouch forms cytoreticulum and Hassall's corpuscles of thymus.^{MCQ}
- Thymocytes (lymphocytes) migrate from bone marrow and infiltrate the thymic rudiment.^{MCQ}

Involution

- Thymus continues to grow from birth till puberty and then undergo gradual atrophy called *thymic involution*.

Development of Parathyroid Gland

Q. Write a short note on development of parathyroid gland.

- There are four parathyroid glands.
- *Two superior parathyroid glands are derived from fourth pharyngeal pouch, whereas two inferior parathyroid glands are derived from third pharyngeal pouch.*^{MCQ}

Stages of Development

- Dorsal part of the *third* pouch grows and loses contact with pharynx and then descends caudally along with thymus. Finally, it loses contact with thymus and forms *inferior parathyroid gland* (*parathyroid* III).
- Dorsal part of *fourth* pharyngeal pouch grows and loses contact with the pharynx. Later it descends caudally to form *superior parathyroid gland* (*parathyroid* III).

Development of Thyroid Gland

Q. Write a short note on development of thyroid gland.

Q. Write a short note on thyroglossal duct.

Summary (Examination Guide)^{High yielding facts}

Thyroid gland develops from the following two sources (Fig. 11.10, Practice Fig. 11.3, Flowchart 11.11):

A. *Follicles* from thyroglossal duct.

B. *Parafollicular cells* from ultimobranchial body (a part of caudal pharyngeal complex).

- By the end of the third month (12th week) follicular cells start producing thyroid hormones.^{MCQ}
- The thyroid gland is the first gland that develops after fertilization.^{MCQ}

Stages of Development

- In the floor of the primitive pharynx, over the first arch in the midline, there is a swelling called *tuberculum impar*.
- By the 24th day, just behind tuberculum impar, pharyngeal epithelium forms a depression (diverticulum) called *thyroglossal duct*.

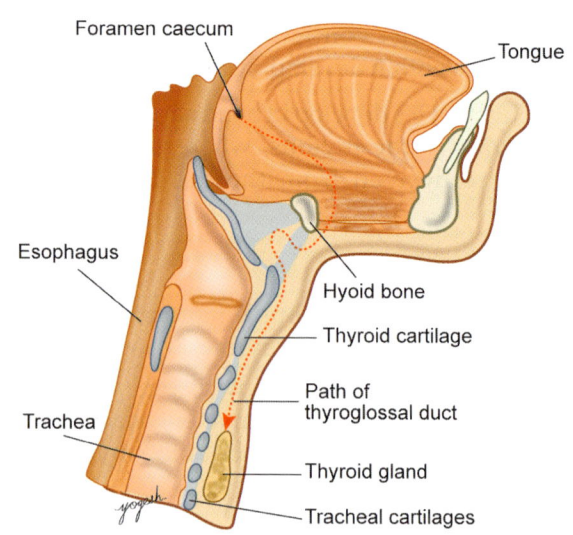

Fig. 11.10: Pathway of the thyroglossal duct. It extends from the foramen caecum to the neck

Practice Fig. 11.3: Development of thyroid gland

Flowchart 11.11: Development of thyroid gland

```
          Development of thyroid gland
          Starts functioning by 12th week
         ┌──────────────────┴──────────────────┐
   Thyroid follicles                    Parafollicular cells
   Pharyngeal endothelium               Ventral part of 4th pouch
            ↓                           + 5th pouch
   Foramen caecum and                         ↓
   thyroglossal duct                   Caudopharyngeal complex
            ↓                                 ↓
   Duct grows toward                   Ultimobranchial body
   pericardial bulge                         ↓
            ↓                           Parafollicular cell
   Duct bifurcates
      ┌─────┴─────┐
  Proximal     Distal part
  part         bifurcates
  Regresses        ↓
               Follicles of
               thyroid gland
```

Anomalies: Pyramidal lobe, abnormal position: lingual, intralingual, suprahyoid, infrahyoid, intrathoracic

- The opening of thyroglossal duct in the pharynx is represented by the *foramen caecum*.
- Thyroglossal duct grows caudally (towards pericardial bulge) in the midline.
- Tip of the thyroglossal duct bifurcates to give rise to two lobes of the thyroid gland (by 7th week).
- Ultimobranchial body (a part of caudal pharyngeal complex meets thyroid gland and contribute as *parafollicular cells*).

Anomalies of the Thyroid Gland

1. *Pyramidal lobe*: It may arise from the isthmus or any one of the lobes. It is variable in the length. It is derived from thyroglossal duct.
2. Sometimes isthmus or one lobe of the thyroid gland may be absent or small.
3. Anomalies of location
   - The thyroid gland may lie at any position at the passage of thyroglossal duct.
   - Anomalies of the locations are listed in Table 11.3.
4. Ectopic thyroid tissue: Ectopic thyroid is the presence of thyroid tissue in locations other than usual (normal) thyroid gland locations. It is mostly found in larynx, trachea, esophagus, pericardium and ovaries.

Table 11.3 Anomalies of position of thyroid gland

Anomaly	Location
1. Lingual thyroid	Under mucosa of the dorsum of tongue
2. Intralingual thyroid	Embedded in substance of tongue
3. Suprahyoid thyroid	Lie in the midline of neck above the hyoid bone
4. Infrahyoid thyroid	Lie in the midline of neck below the hyoid bone but superior to its usual position
5. Intrathoracic thyroid	Lie in thorax

Box 11.4: Thyroglossal cyst and fistula

- Thyroid gland develops from thyroglossal duct (parafollicular cells from ultimobranchial body).
- Usually, thyroglossal duct regresses. Remnant of the thyroglossal duct may form thyroglossal cyst or fistula anywhere along the course of thyroglossal duct (Fig. 11.11, Practice Fig. 11.4).
- Thyroglossal cyst is an irregular mass or lump in the midline of the neck.
- Occasionally thyroglossal cyst ruptures externally, resulting in a draining sinus called a *thyroglossal fistula*.
- Rarely it forms *thyroglossal cyst carcinoma*.

Box 11.5: Goldenhar syndrome

- Also called *oculo-auriculo-vertebral (OAV) syndrome*.
- It is a congenital anomaly characterized by hemifacial microsomia.
- Incidence: 1 in 5600 births
- Clinical presentation
  - Anotia or microtia (absent or small deformed ear)
  - Eye deformity
  - Fused hemivertebrae
  - Spina bifida
  - Heart defects

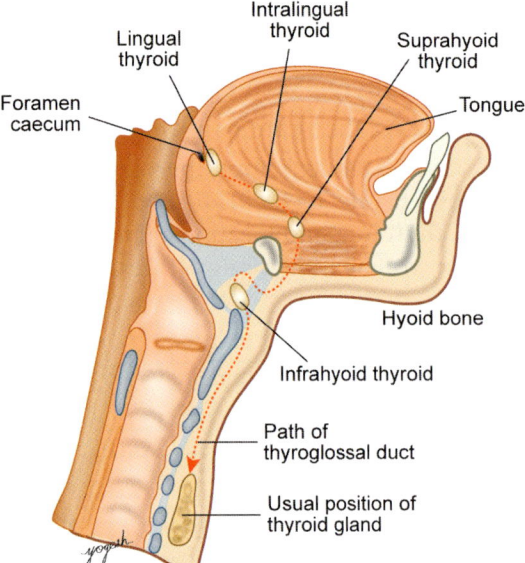

Fig. 11.11: Anomalies of the position of the thyroid gland and locations of the thyroglossal cyst. Thyroid gland may lie anywhere along the pathway of the thyroglossal duct. Thyroglossal cyst also may be present as the persistent pathway for the thyroglossal duct

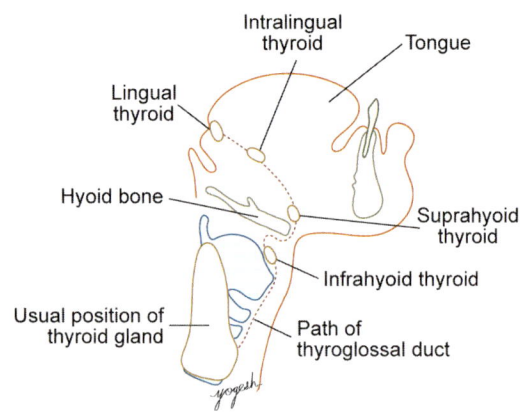

Practice Fig. 11.4: Anomalies of the position of the thyroid gland and locations of the thyroglossal cyst

Clinical Embryology

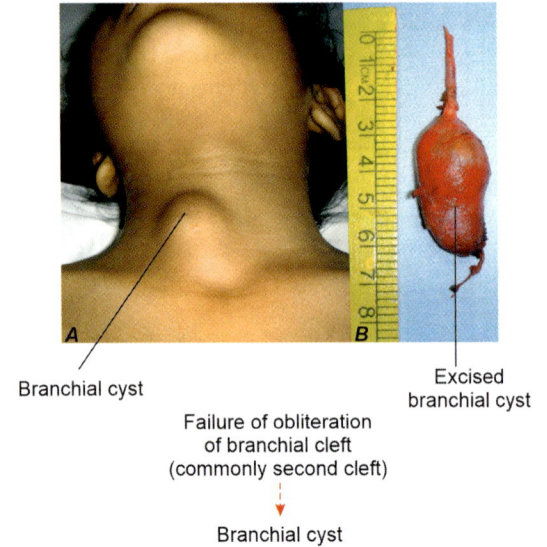

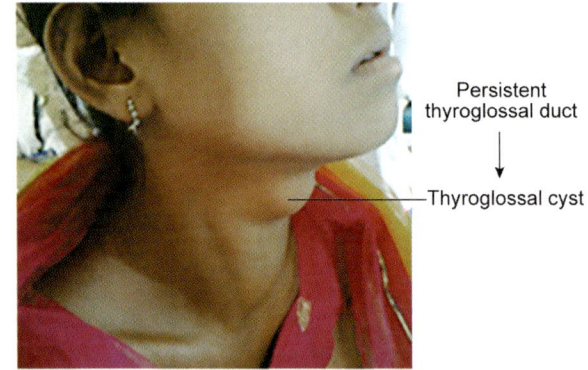

Clinical image 11.2: Thyroglossal cyst: adult presentation (Image courtesy: *Dr Uday Kumbhar*)

Clinical image 11.1: (A) Unilateral branchial cleft cyst (right); (B) Excised branchial cyst from the same case. It is a cyst in the skin of the lateral part of the neck without any opening to the skin surface (In case of branchial fistula, there is opening on the surface of the skin) (Image courtesy: *Dr Kumaravel S*)

Chapter 12

Alimentary Tract I: Development of Face, Nose and Palate

eSmartQuiz

Chapter Outline

- Development of face
- Development of nasolacrimal duct
- Development of nose
- Development of paranasal air sinuses
- Intermaxillary segment
- Development of Palate
- Cleft lip
- Developmental anomalies of face
- Cleft palate

Competency:

- **AN43.4:** Describe the development and developmental basis of congenital anomalies of face, palate (included in this chapter), tongue, branchial apparatus, pituitary gland, thyroid gland, eye.

INTRODUCTION

- At the end of fourth week, embryo shows *stomodeum* as a depression in between bulging brain vesicle and pericardial bulge.
- *Buccopharyngeal membrane* lies in floor of the stomodeum.
- Mesoderm surrounding the stomodeum proliferates and forms elevations (processes) that later form face, palate and nose.

DEVELOPMENT OF FACE

- Face develops from *five mesodermal processes* that appears in 4th week surrounding the stomodeum^{NEXT} (Fig. 12.1, Practice Fig. 12.1). These processes are:
  1. Frontonasal process (unpaired)
  2. Maxillary process (paired)
  3. Mandibular process (paired).
- The mesoderm surrounding the stomodeum thickens and produces abovementioned processes (elevations) on the surface ectoderm.
- Facial development takes place between 4 and 8 weeks.^{NEXT} The embryo has human-like appearance by the end of 8th week of IUL. The final facial appearance results from gradual changes in the proportion and relative positions of the facial features occurring during the fetal period.^{NEXT}

Steps in Development of Face

- In the 4th week of IUL, the stomodeum is bounded cranially by the bulging *forebrain vesicle* and caudally by first pharyngeal (mandibular) arch (Fig. 12.1A).
- In the fifth week of IUL, mesoderm covering the bulging forebrain vesicle proliferates to form *frontonasal process* (Fig. 12.1A).
- On the frontonasal process, bilateral localized oval thickening appears as *nasal placodes* or *olfactory placode* on either side of the median plane (Fig. 12.1B).
- On the olfactory placodes, depression called *nasal pit* or *olfactory pit* develops. Nasal pit later becomes continuous with roof of the stomodeum (Fig. 12.1C).
- Margins of the nasal pit form horseshoe-shaped elevated ridges. Medial margin of the nasal pit forms *medial nasal prominence* (process), whereas lateral margin forms *lateral nasal prominence* (process).
- During the development of the nasal pit and nasal processes, the *maxillary process* develops from cranial side of dorsal part of the first pharyngeal arch (Fig. 12.1B, C, D).
- The maxillary process grows medially and finally fuses with the medial nasal process and later with lateral nasal process.

- *Note:* Lateral and cranial to the nasal placodes, a pair of lens placodes appears (Fig. 12.1E).
- Between 7th and 10th weeks, a fusion of the maxillary process with medial and lateral nasal processes separates the *nasal pit* from the stomodeum and thus, convert it into the *primitive anterior nares* (Fig. 12.1F).
- Continuous growth of the nasal process produces elevated bridge of the nose (Fig. 12.1G).
- Fusion of medial nasal processes form the *intermaxillary segment*. This segment forms philtrum (middle part) of the upper lip, premaxillary part of the maxilla and primitive palate.
- The entire upper lip is being formed by the maxillary processes. The middle part (philtrum) of the upper lip formed by the fusion of the medial nasal processes is covered by the medially growing extensions of the maxillary processes. Lateral nasal processes form the alae of the nose (Figs 12.1F, G, 12.2).^{MCQ}
- Stomodeum gets separated from pericardial bulge by first (mandibular) arch and later by the other arches (Fig. 12.1A).

Box 12.1: Development of nasolacrimal duct

- The maxillary process grows medially and fuses with lateral nasal process along *naso-optic furrow* (nasolacrimal groove) (Fig. 12.1E).
- During fusion of maxillary process with the lateral nasal process, some ectodermal cells along naso-optic furrow get buried into mesenchyme and form a solid cellular cord. Later this cord forms the *nasolacrimal duct*.
- Upper part of the nasolacrimal duct dilates and forms the *lacrimal sac*.
- Failure of canalization of nasolacrimal duct results into an atresia of the nasolacrimal duct.

- Mandibular processes form the lower lip, chin and also contribute in the formation of the cheeks (Fig. 12.1F).
- *Note:* Both the maxillary process and mandibular process arise from the first pharyngeal arch and fusion of these processes forms lateral angles of mouth.

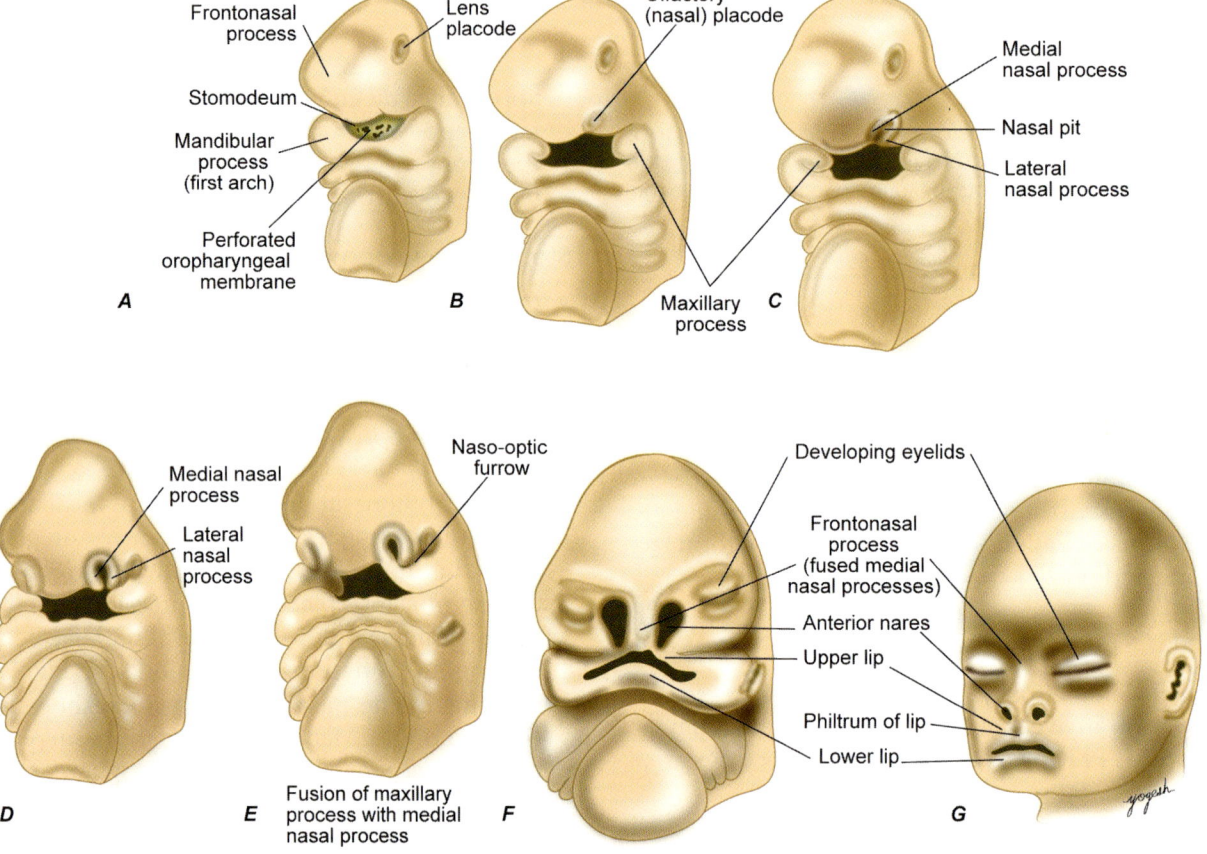

Fig. 12.1: Development of the face. Five facial primordia that appear as prominences around the stomodeum are: Single frontonasal process, paired maxillary process and paired mandibular processes. On appearance of the nasal placode and later nasal pit, the frontonasal process gives rise to medial and lateral nasal processes. The frontal nasal process forms the forehead and dorsum and apex of the nose. The lateral nasal processes form the alae of the nose. The medial nasal processes form the nasal septum. The maxillary processes form the upper cheek regions and the upper lip. The mandibular processes form chin, lower lip and lower cheek regions

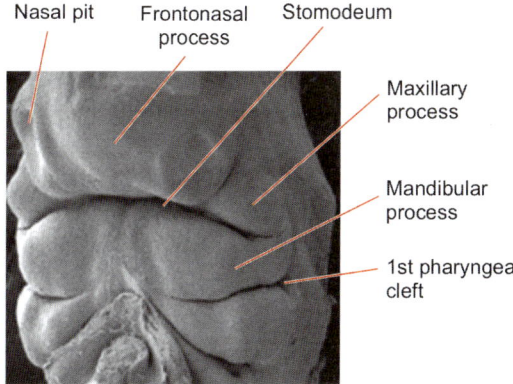

Scanning electron micrograph 12.1: SEM showing developing face. Frontonasal, maxillary and mandibular processes and nasal pits are visible. [Species: Human, approximate age: Fifth week]

- Fusion of the maxillary process and the mandibular process continues on the lateral side, and reduces oral fissure (earlier stomodeum) and forms cheeks (Fig. 12.1F).
- Nerve supply: Derivatives of the frontonasal process are supplied by ophthalmic nerve, the maxillary process by maxillary nerve and the mandibular process by mandibular nerve.

Summary of Development of Face (Examination Guide) (Flowchart 12.1)

Q. Write a short note on development of face.

- Lower lip: Bilateral mandibular processes fuse in the midline to form a lower lip and jaw bone.
- Upper lip:
  - Central part (philtrum) of upper lip is derived from medial nasal process.
  - Lateral parts of upper lip are derived from bilateral maxillary processes.

Note:
- The ectoderm (skin) of maxillary process overgrows and covers central part (philtrum) of the upper lip;

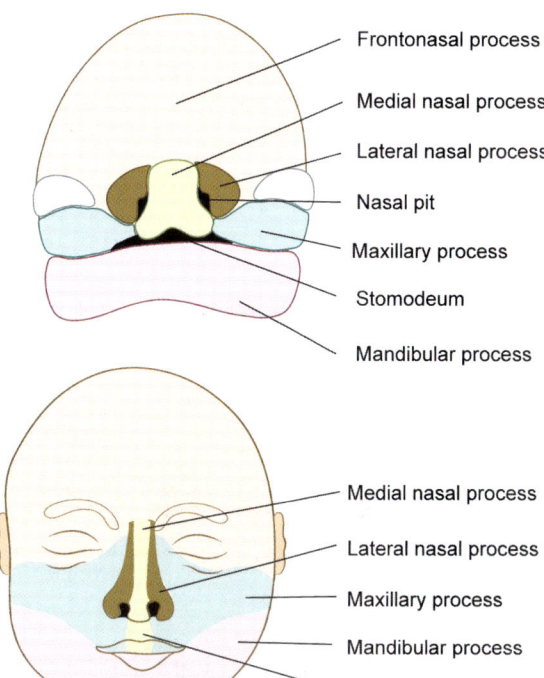

Practice Fig. 12.1: Development of the face

hence, skin of the upper lip is supplied by maxillary nerve (Fig. 12.2). *MCQ, Viva*

- Muscles of face are derived from second arch; hence supplied by facial nerve. *MCQ*

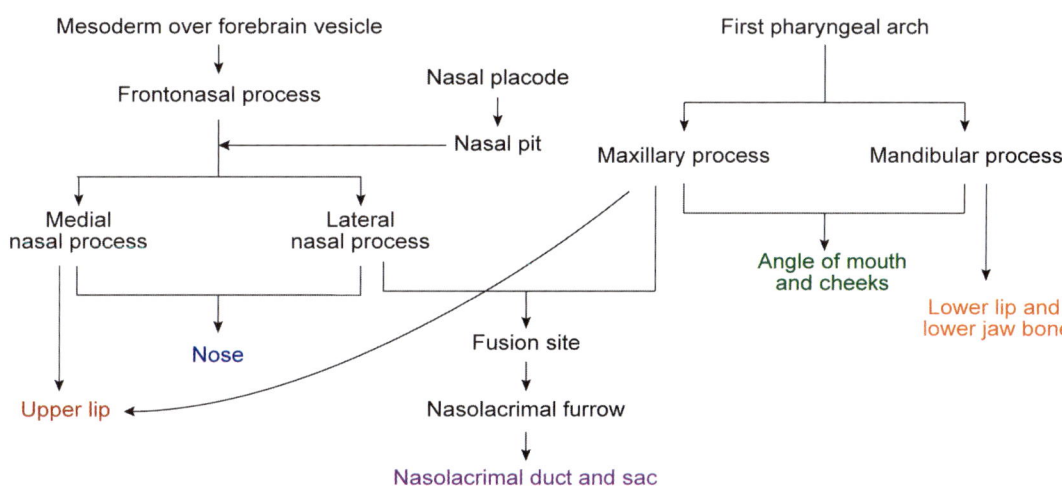

Flowchart 12.1: Development of face

- Cheeks:
    - Stomodeum is bounded by the maxillary, frontonasal and mandibular processes.
    - The maxillary and mandibular processes undergo fusion from the lateral side and form smaller stomodeum or normal oral fissure, whereas fused part forms cheek.
- For details of the development of eye and ear, read Chapters 23 and 24.

DEVELOPMENT OF NOSE

Summary (Examination Guide)

- External nose is derived as follows:
  1. Bridge of nose from frontonasal process.
  2. Dorsum and tip of the nose from fused medial nasal processes.

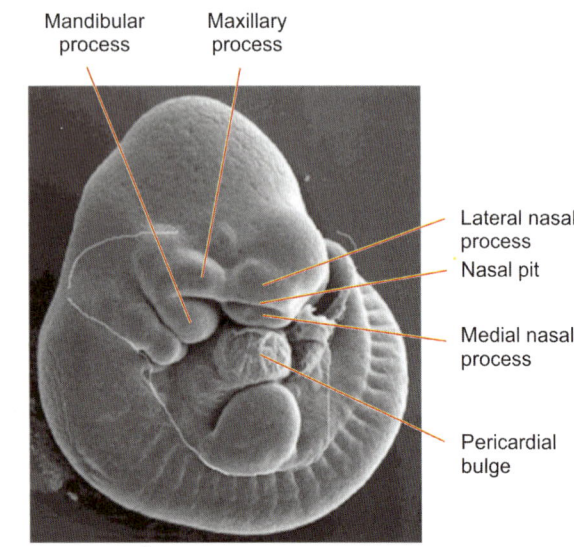

Scanning electron micrograph 12.2: SEM showing 6-week embryo with medial nasal, lateral nasal, maxillary and mandibular processes. [Species: Mouse, approximate human age: 6 weeks, lateral view]

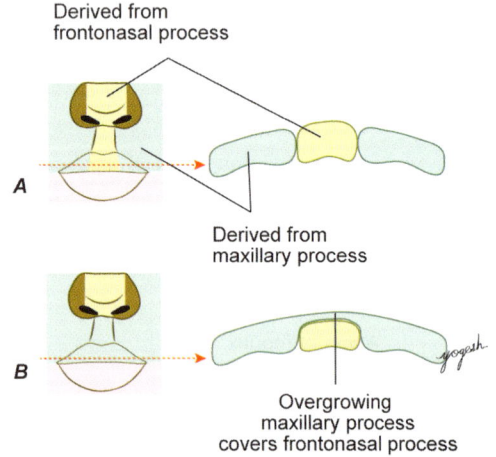

Fig. 12.2: Formation of the upper lip. The ectoderm of the maxillary process overgrows the frontonasal process. Hence, skin of the upper lip is supplied by the maxillary nerve

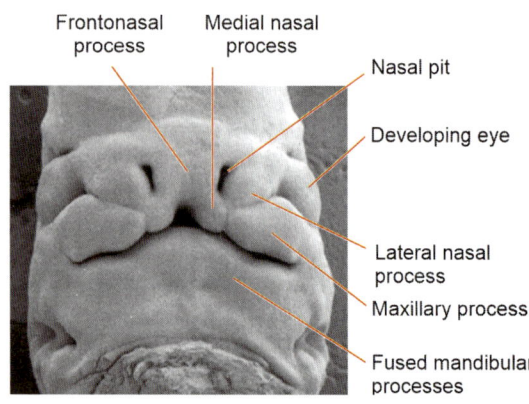

Scanning electron micrograph 12.3: SEM showing development of face, nose and upper lip. The medial nasal prominences merge in the midline to smooth the median furrow. [Species: Human, approximate age: Sixth week, frontal view]

  3. Ala of nose from lateral nasal processes.
  4. Anterior nares (nostrils) from nasal pit.
  5. Nasal cavity from nasal sacs.
  6. Posterior nares (choanae) from rupture of bucconasal membrane.

Stages of Development of Nose and Cavities

- During development of face, the *nasal pits* appear on the frontonasal process (Fig. 12.1C).
- Nasal pits sink deep and form communication with stomodeum (Fig. 12.1D).
- Elevated margins of nasal pits form *medial* and *lateral nasal processes* (Fig. 12.1D).
- Maxillary process first fuses with the lateral nasal process and later with medial nasal process (Fig. 12.1E).
- Lateral and medial nasal processes also fuse with each other and thus, nasal pits get separated from stomodeum by *developing palate* (Fig. 12.1F).
- Nasal pit forms *anterior nares* (Fig. 12.3A).
- Nasal pit sinks deep to develop *nasal sac* (Fig. 12.3A).
- Nasal sac enlarges dorsally and caudally. Dorsal to the primitive palate, the nasal sac is separated from stomodeum by a thin membrane called *bucconasal membrane* or *nasal fin* (Fig. 12.3B).
- Later bucconasal membrane ruptures and develops communication between nasal sac and stomodeum that ultimately forms a *posterior nasal aperture* (Fig. 12.3C).
- Continuous narrowing of frontonasal process brings nasal sac close to each other and frontonasal process forms *nasal septum* and bridge of the nose.
- Medial nasal process forms dorsum and tip of the nose (Fig. 12.1F, G).
- Expanding lateral nasal process forms *lateral wall* of the nose (Fig. 12.1F, G).
- Inner elevated masses of lateral nasal process form *nasal conchae* (Fig. 12.3D).

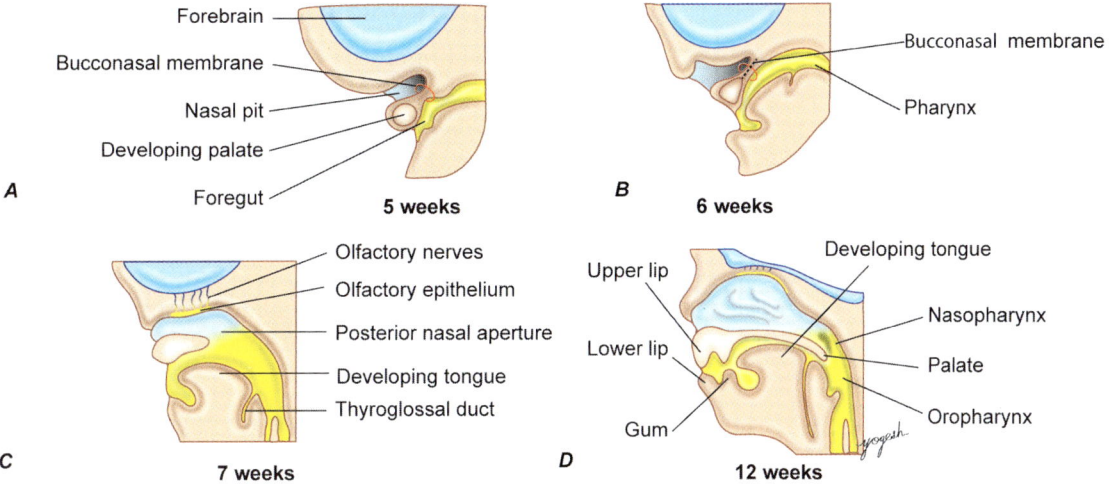

Fig. 12.3: Development of the nasal cavity. Nasal pits appear on the frontonasal process and it gets separated from stomodeum by the developing palate. Nasal pit forms anterior nares. Dorsal to the palate, the nasal sac is separated from stomodeum by bucconasal membrane. Later, the bucconasal membrane ruptures and forms posterior nasal aperture. Inner elevated masses of the lateral nasal process form nasal conchae. Olfactory epithelium develops from the thickened ectodermal lining of roof of the nasal cavity. The olfactory nerves develop from extension of neural processes of the olfactory bulb of the brain

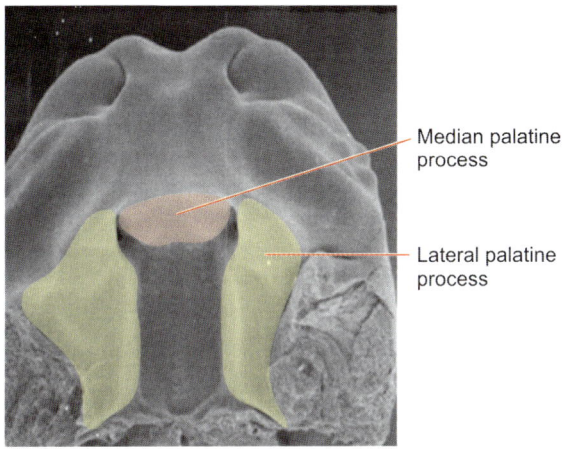

Scanning electron micrograph 12.4: Development of palate. The secondary palatal shelves are considered to be part of the maxillary prominences. The medial nasal prominences contribute the tissues that will form the anterior part of palate, primary palate. [Species: Mouse, approximate human age: Seventh week]

- *Olfactory epithelium* (receptor cells) develops from the thickened ectodermal lining of the roof of the nasal cavity (Fig. 12.3C, D).
- The olfactory nerves develop from extension of neural processes of olfactory bulb of brain.

DEVELOPMENT OF PALATE

Q. Explain development of soft and hard palate.

Summary (Examination Guide) (Flowchart 12.2)*High yielding facts*

- During the development, the palate develops from two components: Primary palate and secondary palate (Practice Fig. 12.2, Fig. 12.4).

Box 12.2: Development of paranasal air sinuses

- Paranasal sinuses are ectodermal in origin.
- Diverticulae (outpouching) develop from the nasal cavity. These diverticulae invade bones adjacent to the nasal cavity (frontal, sphenoid, ethmoid and maxilla) and enlarge to form paranasal air sinuses.
- Nasal opening of these diverticulae persists as orifices of the paranasal air sinuses in the nasal cavity.
- All paranasal air sinuses start developing before birth *except* frontal air sinus that develops after birth during 5th or 6th year of life.*MCQ*
- The maxillary sinus is the first sinus to develop (in the third month of intrauterine life).*MCQ, Viva*
- Paranasal air sinuses continue their growth till puberty.

Box 12.3: Intermaxillary segment

- In between maxillary processes, fused part of medial nasal processes forms the *intermaxillary segment* (Fig. 12.4A).
- The intermaxillary segment has the following parts:
  1. *Labial component*: Forms philtrum of upper lip.
  2. *Upper jaw component* is related to upper four incisor teeth.
  3. *Palatal component*: Forms triangular primary palate.

- Frontonasal process forms *primary palate*, whereas maxillary process forms *secondary palate*.
- Primary palate fuse with secondary palate to form definitive palate.

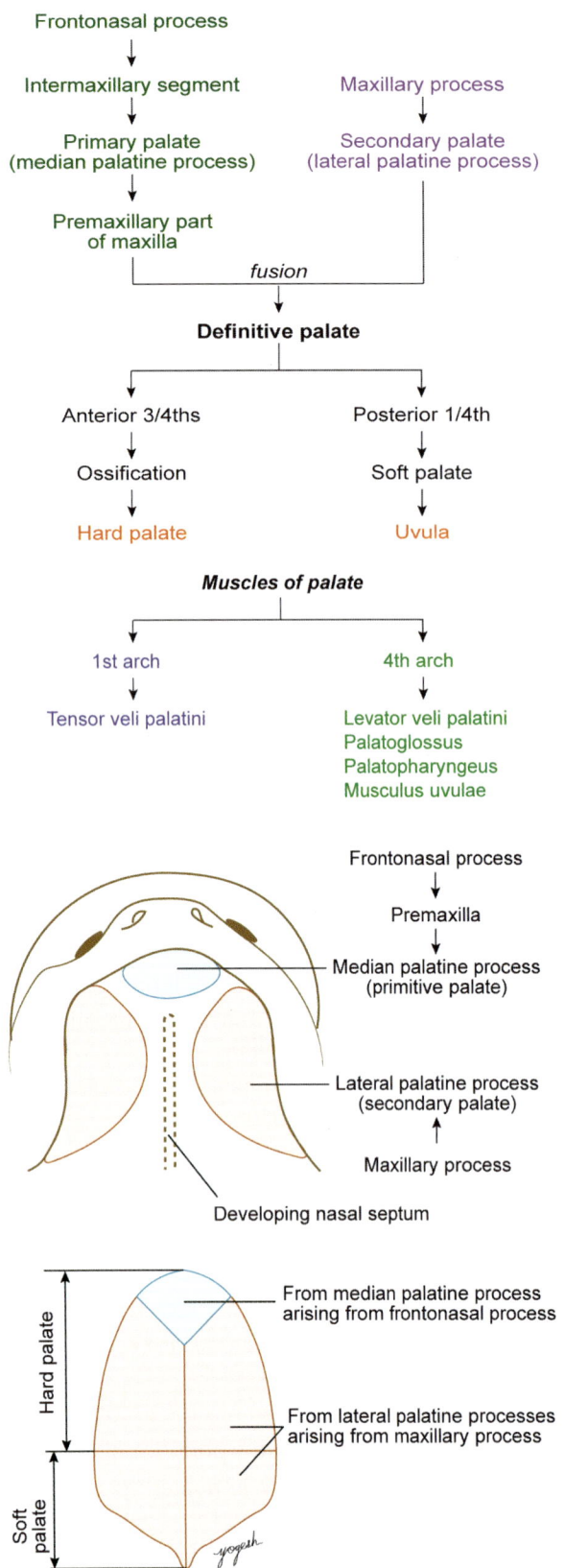

Flowchart 12.2: Development of palate

Practice Fig. 12.2: Development of palate

- Anterior 3/4ths of definitive palate ossifies to form hard palate, whereas posterior 1/4th forms soft palate and uvula.

Stages of Palate Development

- Palatogenesis takes place between 5th week and 12th week of IUL.
- *Primary palate*
  - In sixth week, the *intermaxillary segment* forms a shelf-like projection (that later bear upper four incisor teeth) called *primary palate* or *median palatine process* (Fig. 12.4A).
  - Later primary palate forms *premaxillary part* of the maxilla (Fig. 12.4B to D).
- Secondary palate
  - In sixth week, two mesenchymal projections extend from the inner aspects of maxillary processes. These projections are called *secondary palate* or *lateral palatine processes* (Fig. 12.4A).
- During 7th–8th weeks, the lateral palatine processes elongate and fuse (Fig. 12.4C):
  1. With each other in the midline.
  2. With nasal septum.
  3. With posterior part of the primary palate.

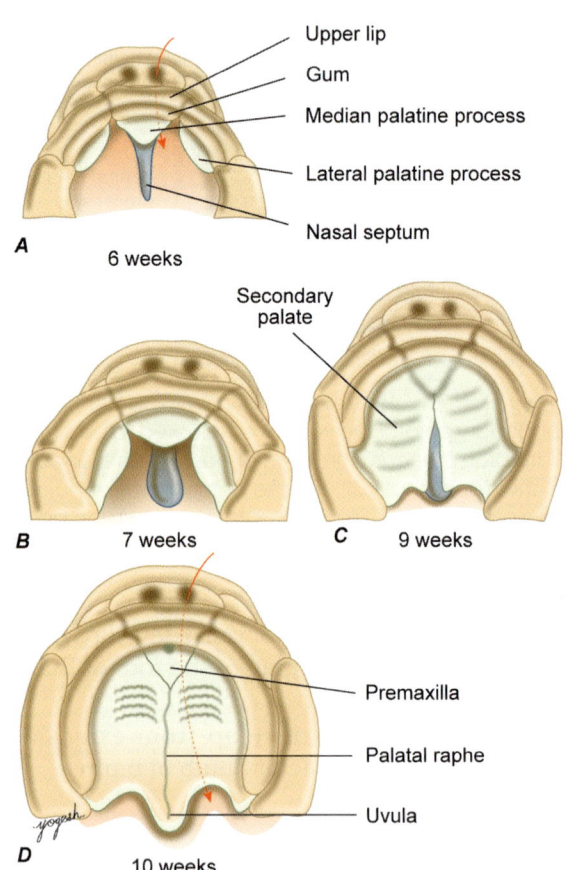

Fig. 12.4: Development of the palate. The intermaxillary segment forms median palatine process and later it forms premaxillary part of the maxilla. Two mesenchymal projections of the maxillary processes form lateral palatine processes. The lateral palatine processes elongate and fuse with each other in the midline, with the nasal septum and with posterior part of the primary palate

- Formation of definitive palate:
  Primary palate fuses with secondary palate to form *definitive palate*. Incisive foramen divides primary and secondary palates.^{NEXT}
  - Anterior three-fourths of the definitive palate ossifies and forms *hard palate*.
  - Posterior one-fourth of the definitive palate remains unossified and forms *soft palate* with *uvula*.
  - Small persistent *nasopalatine canal* in the median plane of premaxilla forms the *incisive fossa*. In the incisive fossa, right and left incisive canals open.
- Muscles of palate:
  - Mesoderm of branchial arches invade soft palate to form muscles.
  - Tensor veli palatini – from 1st arch
  - Levator veli palatini, palatoglossus, palatopharyngeus, musculus uvulae – from 4th arch.

Box 12.4: Cleft lip (harelip)

Q. Write a short note on cleft lip.

- **Definition:** Cleft lip is a congenital split in the upper lip of one or both sides of its center (Fig. 12.5).
- Usually, upper lip of hare has cleft; hence, cleft lip is commonly called *harelip*.
- **Embryological basis:** Failure of fusion of the maxillary processes with the medial nasal process (part of frontonasal process) results in cleft lip. Midline cleft lip is due to failure of fusion of two medial nasal processes.^{NEXT}
- Harelip may be unilateral, bilateral or midline harelip.
- Cleft lip occurs more frequently (80%) in males than in females.
- Incidence of cleft lip is 1 in 1000 births.
- Incidence of cleft lip increases with increasing maternal age.
- If a couple has a cleft lip child, there are 4% chances that the next baby will have a cleft lip.^{MCQ}
- If two babies of a couple are affected, then the chances of cleft lip increase up to 9%.^{MCQ}
- **Treatment:** Cleft lip can be corrected surgically.

Developmental Anomalies of Face

Q. Name the developmental anomalies of the face.

- *Oblique facial cleft* may result due to nonfusion of maxillary and lateral nasal process. It results in a cleft from medial angle of the eye to the mouth and nonformation of nasolacrimal duct.
- *Macrostomia* is a wide mouth due to incomplete fusion of mandibular and maxillary processes.
- *Microstomia* is a small mouth due to excessive fusion of mandibular and maxillary processes.
- *Proboscis* is an elongated cylindrical projecting nose. In some cases of proboscis, cyclops (fusion of both the eyes) is present.
- *Retrognathia* is a small mandible in that chin does not reach the rest of the face.
- *Agnathia* is the absence of jaw, may be due to failure of mandible development.
- *Hypertelorism* is widely placed eyes due to broad nasal bridge. It is caused by wide frontonasal process.
- Harelip or cleft lip. Refer to Box 12.4.

Box 12.5: Cleft palate

Q. Write a short note on cleft palate. *High yielding facts*

- **Definition:** Cleft palate is a congenital split defect of palate that causes communication between oral and nasal cavities (Fig. 12.5, Practice Fig. 12.3, Flowchart 12.3).
- Patient with cleft palate usually has eating, speech, and dental problems.
- The commonest cause of cleft lip with or without cleft palate is multifactorial inheritance.
- **Incidence**
  - 1 in 2500 births.
  - Cleft palate is more common in females (67%).
  - Incidence of cleft palate is not related to the maternal age.
  - If a couple has a child with cleft palate, there are 2% chances that another baby will have cleft palate.^{MCQ}
  - Unilateral cleft of upper lip is the commonest congenital anomaly of face.^{MCQ}

Embryological basis
  - Nonfusion of median and lateral palatine processes, and the nasal septum results in cleft palate.

Classification
- Cleft palate may be complete or incomplete (partial).
- *Complete cleft palate* may be unilateral or bilateral.
  - *Unilateral complete cleft palate:* It results due to nonfusion of one lateral palatine process of the maxilla with the median palatine process of premaxilla and also the nonfusion of the two lateral palatine processes.
  - It is always associated with harelip on the same side of the defect.
  - *Bilateral complete cleft palate*: It results due to nonfusion of both the lateral palatine process of maxilla with the median palatine process of premaxilla.
- *Incomplete cleft palate* may be cleft of hard and soft palate or only the cleft of soft palate or uvula.

Treatment
- Cleft palate can be corrected surgically.

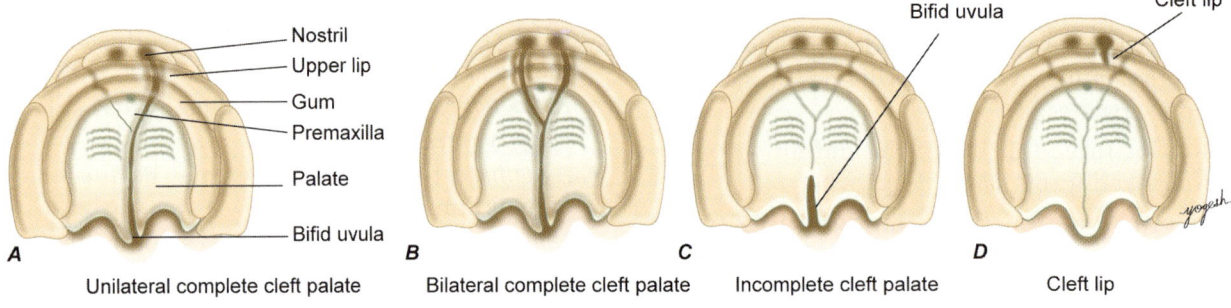

Fig. 12.5: Cleft lip and cleft palate. Nonfusion of the median and later palatine processes results in the cleft palate. It may be unilateral or bilateral complete cleft palate or incomplete cleft palate. Failure of fusion of the maxillary processes with medial nasal process results in the cleft lip

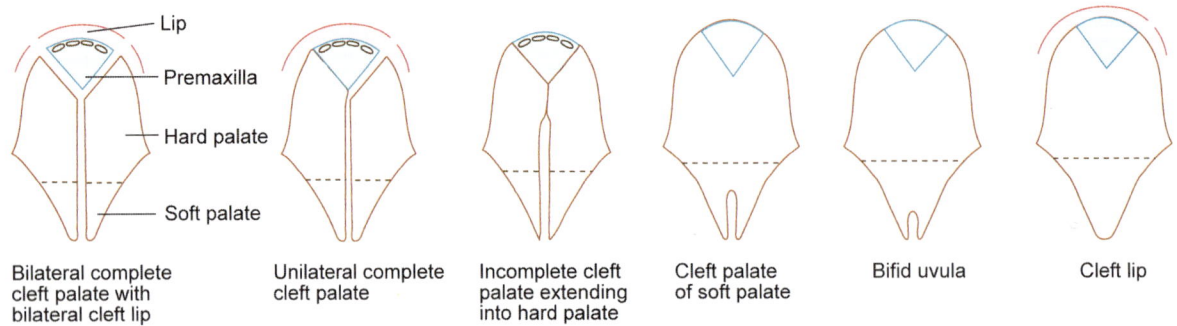

Practice Fig. 12.3: Cleft lip and cleft palate

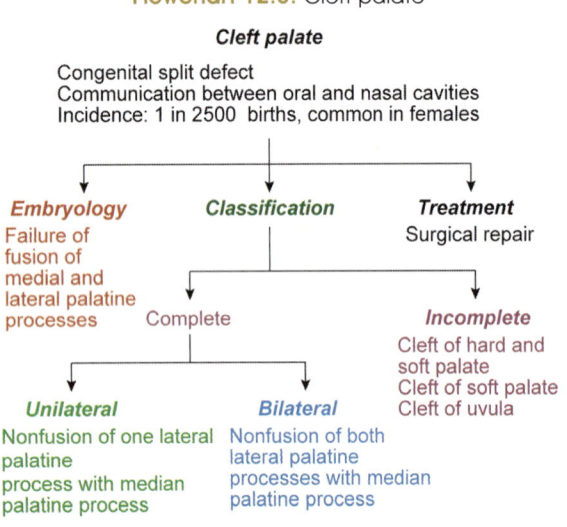

Flowchart 12.3: Cleft palate

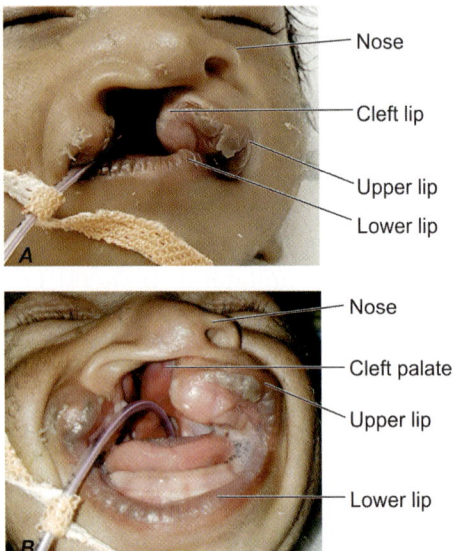

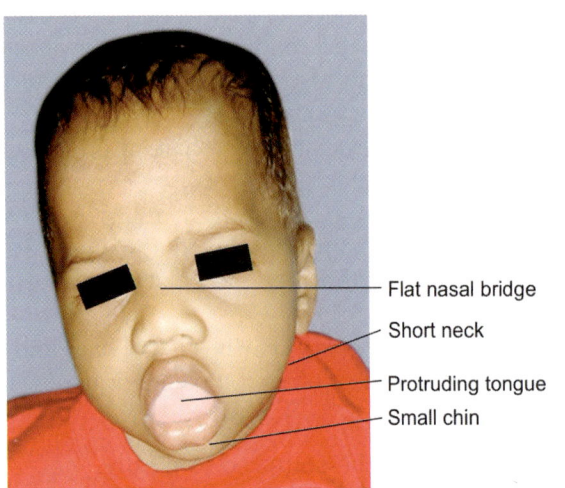

Clinical image 12.1: A 5-day-old baby with unilateral cleft lip and cleft palate (on the right side). Cleft lip is a congenital split in the upper lip that occurs due to failure of fusion of the maxillary processes with the medial nasal process (part of frontonasal process). Cleft palate is a congenital split defect of the palate that causes communication between oral and nasal cavities. Cleft palate occurs due to the nonfusion of the median and lateral palatine processes (Image courtesy: *Dr Prakhar Mohniya*)

Clinical image 12.2: Facial features in a baby of Down syndrome showing flat and wide face, small chin, flat nasal bridge, protruding tongue due to small oral cavity and short neck (Image courtesy: *Dr Adhisivam B*)

Chapter 13

Alimentary Tract II: Development of Teeth, Pharynx, Tongue and Salivary Glands

eSmartQuiz

Chapter Outline

- Development of mouth cavity
  - Primitive oral cavity
  - Definitive oral cavity
- Development of teeth
  - Structure of tooth
  - Stages of teeth development
  - Development of permanent teeth
  - Anomalies of teeth
- Development of pharynx
- Development of tongue
  - Mucous membrane
  - Muscles of tongue
  - Nerve supply
  - Developmental anomalies
- Development of salivary glands
  - Parotid gland
  - Submandibular gland
  - Sublingual gland

Competencies:
- **AN43.4:** Describe the development and developmental basis of congenital anomalies of face, palate, tongue (included in this chapter), branchial apparatus, pituitary gland, thyroid gland, eye.
- **AN39.1:** Describe the embryological basis of nerve supply of tongue.

DEVELOPMENT OF MOUTH CAVITY

- Mouth cavity develops from contribution of two derms:
  1. Ectoderm (stomodeum) forms the *primitive mouth cavity*.
  2. Endoderm (cephalic part of foregut) forms *definitive mouth cavity*.
- In the fourth week, *buccopharyngeal membrane* ruptures and endoderm becomes continuous with ectoderm (Fig. 13.1).

Primitive Oral Cavity

- *Primitive oral cavity* develops from stomodeum (ectoderm).
- *Stomodeum* is divided into nasal and oral part by the developing *palate*.
- Nasal part forms the mucous membrane of nasal cavity, nasal septum and palate.

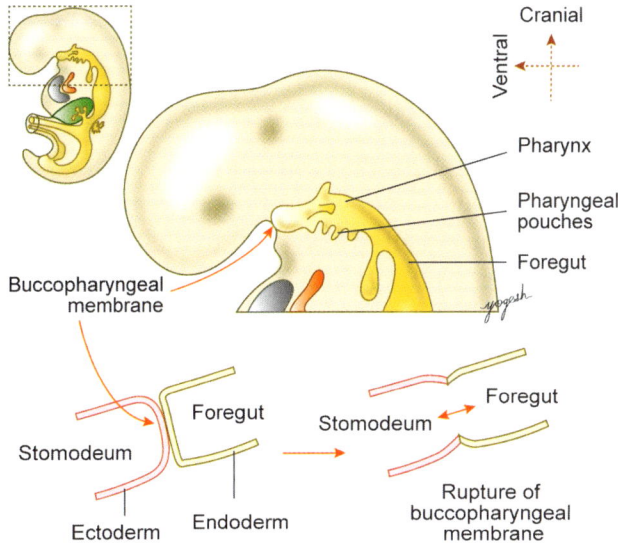

Fig. 13.1: Buccopharyngeal membrane

- Oral part forms the mucous membrane of cheek, lips, gums and enamel of the teeth.

Definitive Oral Cavity

- The cephalic part of foregut (endoderm) forms definitive oral cavity.

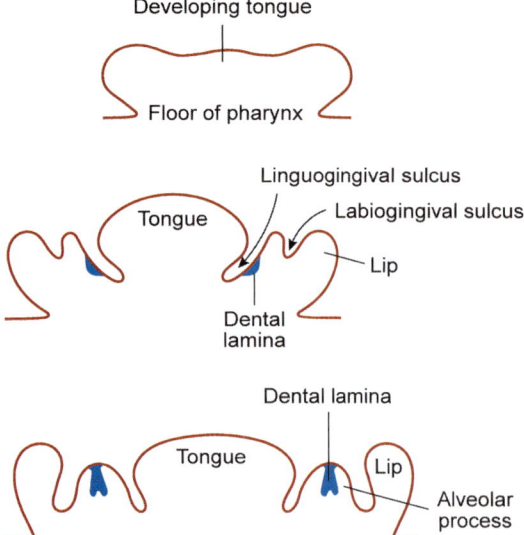

Practice Fig. 13.1: Developing floor of pharynx

- In the floor of oral cavity, the developing tongue gets separated from mandibular process by *linguogingival sulcus* (endodermal zone) (Fig. 13.2, Practice Fig. 13.1).
- Lateral to the linguogingival sulcus, in the ectodermal zone, a *labiogingival sulcus* appears.
- Labiogingival sulcus deepens. Expanding mandibular arch forms the lower lips, lower part of cheeks and lower jaw.
- The area between linguogingival sulcus and labiogingival sulcus elevates and develops an alveolar process that later forms jaw and teeth.
- Upper lip also gets separated from developing alveolar process by the labiogingival furrow (Practice Fig. 13.2).

DEVELOPMENT OF TEETH

- Human have two sets of teeth:
  A. Deciduous or milk teeth: Twenty in number.
  B. Permanent teeth: Thirty-two in number.
- *Successional teeth* are permanent incisors, canine and premolars as these teeth preceded by milk teeth.
- *Superadded teeth* are permanent molars as these do not precede by milk teeth.

Source of Development

Each tooth develops from:
- Surface ectoderm – that forms the enamel.
- Mesoderm that forms dentine, tooth pulp, cementum and periodontal ligament.

Structure of Tooth

Each tooth has the following parts:
- Enamel
- Dentine
- Cementum
- Pulp and periodontal ligament.

Stages of Teeth Development

Q. Describe the stages of development of tooth.

Tooth develops in the following stages (Figs 13.3, 13.4, Flowchart 13.1, Practice Fig. 13.3):

1. *Stages of dental lamina:* During the 6th week of development, epithelium (ectoderm) in the region of developing an alveolar process (U-shaped zone) thickens to form *dental lamina* (Fig. 13.3).

2. *Bud stage:* In each alveolar process, the dental lamina thickens at ten places and form *tooth buds* (*enamel organ*) that grow towards underlying mesoderm (Fig. 13.3).

3. *Cap stage:* Mass of mesenchyme (mostly neural crest cells) occupies the core of enamel organ and makes enamel organ cap-shaped. In 8th week: Enamel organs appear (Fig. 13.3).

   This mass of the mesenchyme forms the *dental papilla*. In 10th week: Enamel organs become cap-shaped.

4. *Bell stage:* Cells of the enamel organ facing dental papilla become columnar and form *ameloblasts* (Fig. 13.3).

   Cells of the dental papilla facing ameloblasts, later form an epithelium-like layer called *odontoblasts*. Enamel organ soon forms:
   - outer cell layer as *outer dental epithelium,*
   - inner cell layer as *inner dental epithelium* (*ameloblasts*) and

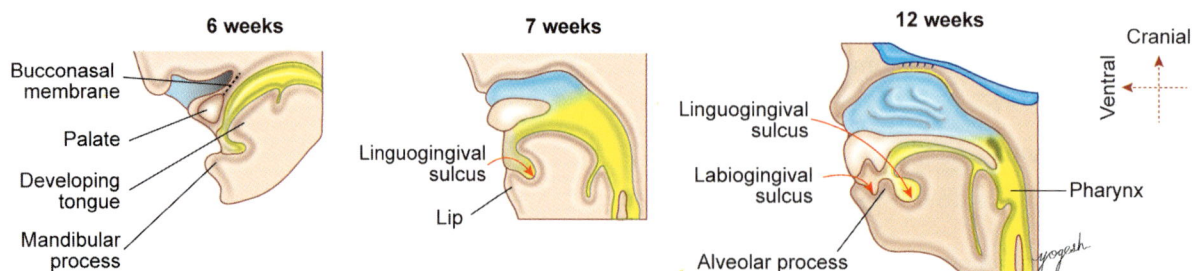

Fig. 13.2: Formation of oral cavity. The cephalic part of foregut forms definitive oral cavity. In the floor of oral cavity, the developing tongue gets separated from mandibular process by the linguogingival sulcus. Lateral to the linguogingival sulcus, in ectodermal zone, labiogingival sulcus appears. Area between linguogingival sulcus and labiogingival sulcus forms alveolar process

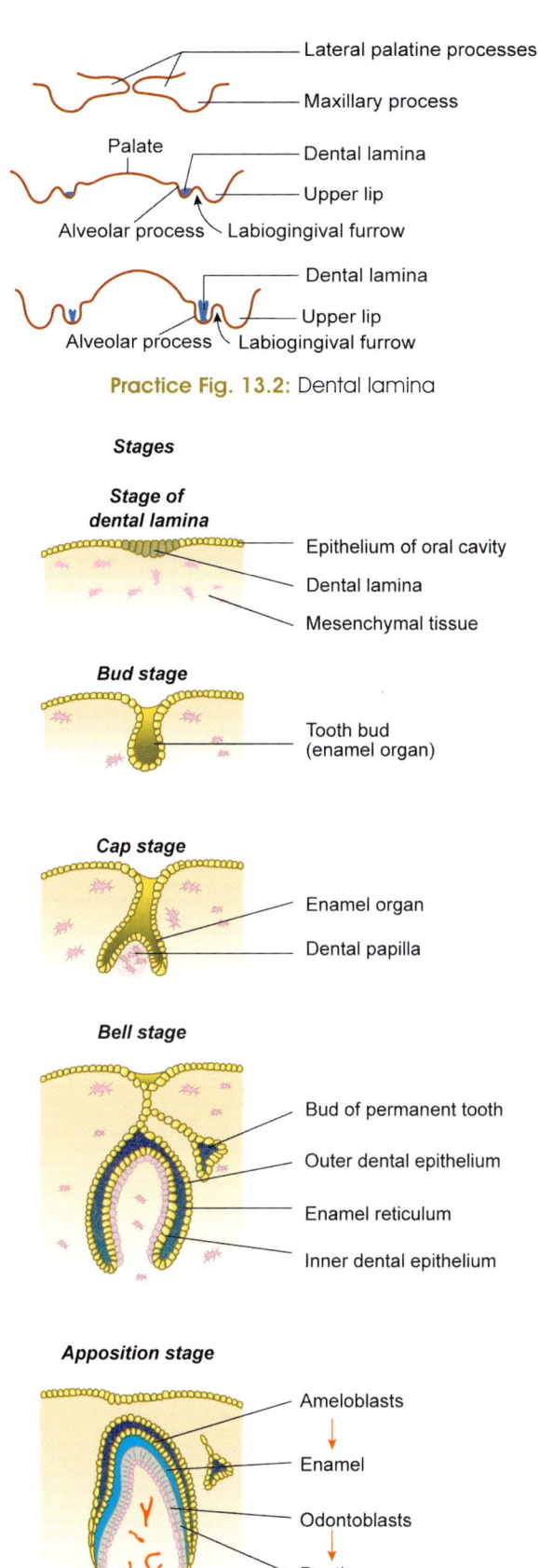

Practice Fig. 13.2: Dental lamina

Fig. 13.3: Development of tooth: Stages of the dental lamina, bud stage, cap stage, bell stage and apposition stage

- central core loose mesenchymal cells as *stellate reticulum* or enamel reticulum.

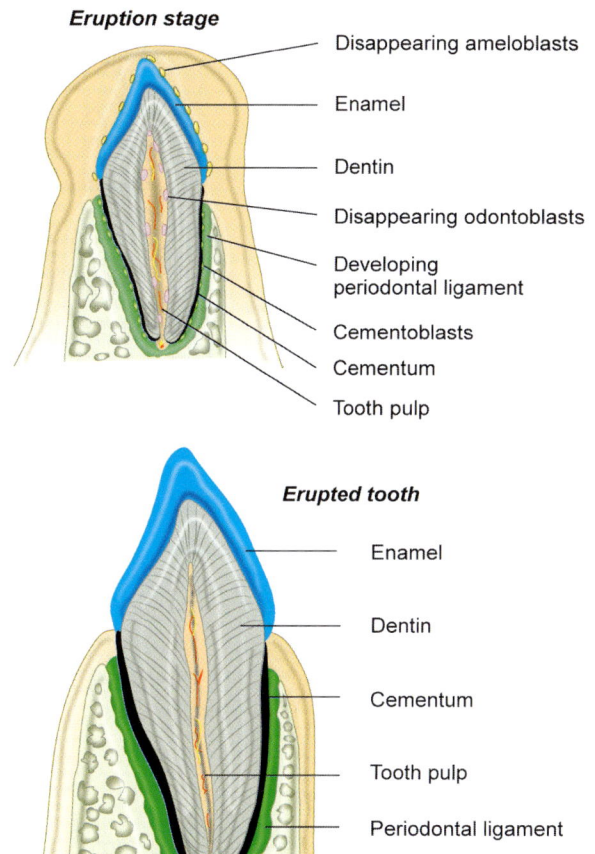

Fig. 13.4: Development of tooth: Stage of the eruption and structure of the erupted tooth

Flowchart 13.1: Formation of tooth

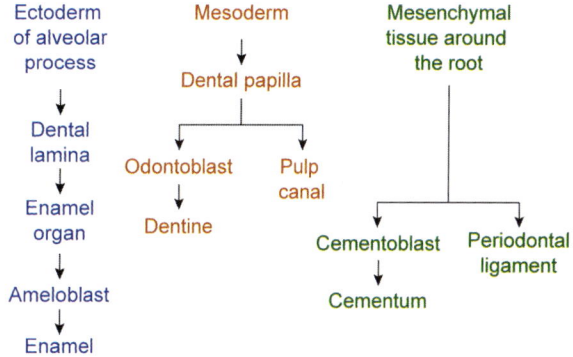

Growing dental cap forms a bell-shaped structure over underlying dental papilla; hence called *bell stage*.

5. *Apposition stage:* Ameloblasts lay down *enamel* on the outer surface of basement membrane separating ameloblasts and odontoblasts, whereas odontoblast laydown *dentine* on deeper surface of basement membrane (Fig. 13.3).

The ameloblasts move towards outer dental epithelium through satellite reticulum. Finally, outer epithelium, reticulum and ameloblasts disappear, leaving behind *dental cuticle of Nasmyth* (a thin layer) over enamel.

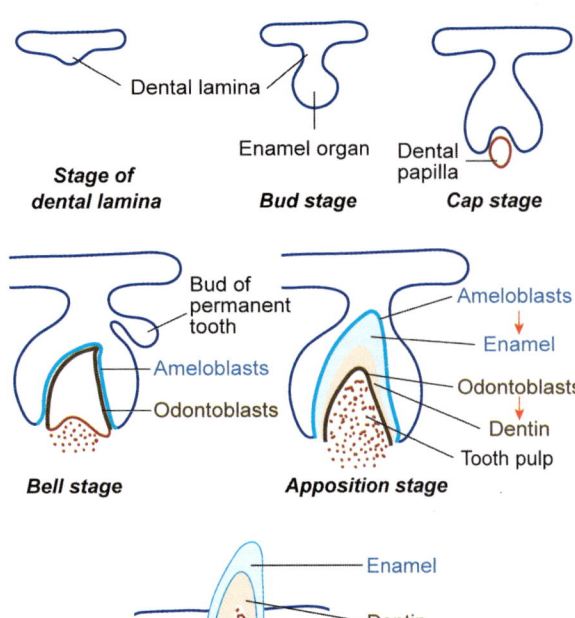

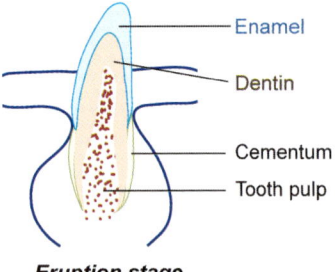

Practice Fig. 13.3: Development of tooth

On the formation of dentine, regressing odontoblast leaves behind their cytoplasmic processes (called odontoblastic processes or Tomes processes) that remains trapped in dentine.

Q. Enlist the timings of eruption of temporary and permanent teeth.

Table 13.1	Time of eruption of teeth
Teeth	Time of eruption
Deciduous	
Lower central incisors	6–9 months
Upper incisors	8–10 months
Lower lateral incisors	12–20 months
First molar	12–20 months
Canines	16–20 months
Second molars	20–39 months
Permanent	
Central incisor	7–8 years
Lateral incisor	8–9 years
Canine	10–12 years
First premolar	10–11 years
Second premolar	11–12 years
First molar	6–7 years^NEXT
Second molar	12 years
Third molar	18–25 years

Continuous deposition of dentine reduces pulp cavity to a narrow *pulp canal*. Blood vessels and nerves reach tooth through the pulp canal.

Mesenchymal cells covering the root of the tooth modifies to form *cementoblasts*.

The cementoblasts lay down a layer of dense bone called *cementum*. Cementum is produced just before the birth.

Mesenchymal cells covering cementum form periodontal ligament that connects root of the tooth with jaw bone. After birth, before eruption of tooth, periodontal ligament appears.

6. Eruption stage: Growth of the root produces eruption of tooth. Eruption age of various teeth is listed in Table 13.1 (Fig. 13.4).

Development of Permanent Teeth

- There are thirty-two permanent teeth.
- During the 3rd month of intrauterine life, a series of *tooth buds* arise from dental lamina from lingual side of milk tooth (Fig. 13.3).
- These buds remain dormant till six to seven years after birth and then form permanent incisors, canines and premolars (Table 13.1).
- Developing permanent tooth pushes deciduous tooth outward and finally, deciduous tooth shed off.
- For permanent molars, tooth buds arise from dental lamina and remain dormant till the age of eruption of permanent molars.
- Enamel is the hardest tissue of body, whereas dentin is the second hardest.

Anomalies of Teeth

1. *Anodontia*: Anodontia is a complete absence of teeth.
2. Supernumerary tooth (extra tooth) may be present that cause malocclusion (improper alignment of teeth).
3. *Natal teeth*: Occasionally, teeth may be present at birth. These teeth are called natal teeth.
4. Germination is fusion of two or more teeth.
5. *Impaction of tooth:* It is the failure of a tooth to erupt. The third molar is most commonly impacted tooth.^MCQ
6. *Amelogenesis imperfecta* is a condition due to hypocalcification of enamel in vitamin D deficiency (rickets). The enamel becomes soft, friable and yellowish–brown in color.^MCQ
7. *Dentinogenesis imperfecta* is an autosomal dominant disorder that involves long arm of chromosome 4 (4q). Enamel lose easily and dentine gets exposed.
8. *Dentigerous cyst* develops from unerupted permanent tooth.

Some Interesting Facts

- Development of tooth is a classic example of an epithelio-mesenchymal interaction.^MCQ
- Ameloblasts and thus, enamel is derived from ectoderm, whereas mesenchyme of dental papilla from neural crest cells.^NEXT
- Teeth have *enamel knot* as a circumscribed region of the dental epithelium at the tooth buds. Enamel knot acts as a signalling center (organiser).^MCQ
- Humans are *diphyodont* (having only two successive sets of teeth). Many vertebrates (fishes, crocodiles) are *polyphyodont* (having continuously replacing teeth).
- Tooth regeneration from stem cell is new possibility developed in the field of tissue engineering and stem cell biology by Young et al. (2002).
- *Hertwig epithelial root sheath* (HERS) is a proliferation of epithelial cells of enamel organ. HERS stimulates differentiation of odontoblast in dental papilla and thus help in the formation of dentine. HERS cells completely disappear.
- *Epithelial cell rests of Malassez* (ERM) are residual cells of the HERS in the periodontal ligament. These residual cells may form odontogenic cysts.

DEVELOPMENT OF PHARYNX

- Pharynx develops from the cranial part of the foregut.
- In the lateral wall and floor of pharynx, the pharyngeal pouches form various structures (for details, refer to Chapter 11).
- Laryngotracheal groove (furcula of His) develops in the floor of the pharynx caudal to the hypobranchial eminence. This groove deepens to form a diverticulum that gives rise to the respiratory system (for details, refer to Chapter 16).
- Formation of the nose, palate and respiratory diverticulum divides the pharynx into nasopharynx, oropharynx and laryngopharynx.
- *Pharyngeal bursa* or *pouch of Luschka* is a cystic notochordal remnant in the posterior wall of nasopharynx at the lower end of the pharyngeal tonsil.^MCQ

Box 13.1: Luschka

- Hubert von Luschka (1820–75) was a German anatomist.
- *Luschka's crypts* are mucous membrane indentation of the inner wall of the gallbladder.
- *Luschka's joint* (uncovertebral joint or neurocentral joint) is formed between uncinate process and uncus. These joints are present in the cervical region of vertebral column between C3 and C7 vertebrae.
- *Duct of Luschka* is an accessory bile duct.
- *Foramina of Luschka* are two lateral opening of the fourth ventricle of the brain.
- Pharyngeal bursa or *pouch of Luschka* is a cystic notochordal remnant in the posterior wall of nasopharynx at the lower end of pharyngeal tonsil.

DEVELOPMENT OF TONGUE

Q. Write a short note on development of tongue.

- Tongue develops in the floor of primitive pharynx and developing mouth.

Summary (Examination Guide) High yielding facts

- The tongue is derived from three different sources as follows (refer to Table 13.2, Fig. 13.5, Practice Figs 13.4, 13.5, Flowchart 13.2):
  1. Endoderm covering the pharyngeal arches forms mucous membrane covering the tongue.
  2. Mesenchyme of arches forms fibroareolar stroma of the tongue.
  3. Occipital myotomes form muscles of the tongue.

Mucous Membrane

- Mandibular arches show three swellings: Single midline swelling as *tuberculum impar* and two lateral *lingual swellings*. In 4th week, two lingual swellings and tuberculum impar become visible (Fig. 13.5A).
- Caudal to tuberculum impar, proliferating epithelium forms thyroglossal duct and its pharyngeal site is marked by a depression called *foramen caecum* (Fig. 13.5A to C).

Table 13.2	Development and nerve supply of tongue^MCQ, Viva	
Structure	Embryonic source	Nerve supply
Mucosa of tongue Anterior two-thirds of tongue	Endodermal lining of first arch Two lingual swellings Tuberculum impar	**General sensory:** Lingual nerve (branch of mandibular nerve) **Special sensory:** Chorda tympani branch of facial nerve
Posterior one-third of tongue and circumvallate papillae	Endodermal lining of third arch	**General and special sensory:** Glossopharyngeal nerve
Posterior most part	Endodermal lining of fourth arch	**General and special sensory:** Superior laryngeal branch of vagus nerve
Muscles All extrinsic and intrinsic muscles except palatoglossus	Occipital myotomes	Hypoglossal nerve (palatoglossus by vagus nerve)

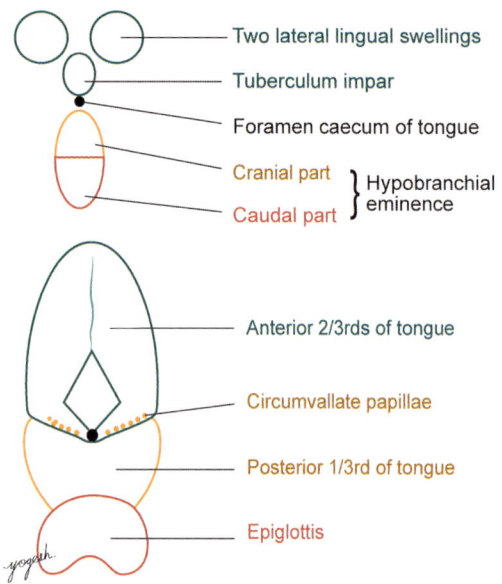

Practice Fig. 13.4: Development of tongue

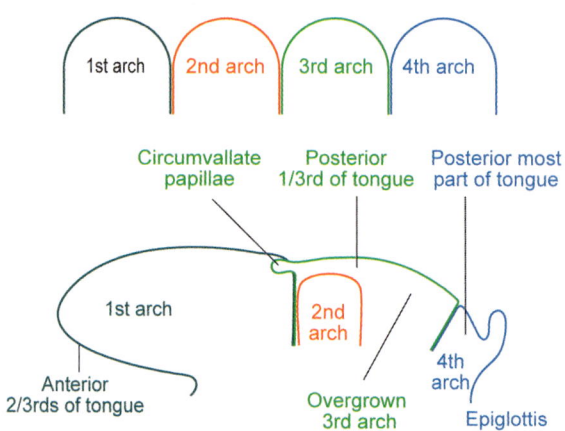

Practice Fig 13.5: Development of tongue: Overgrowing third arch burries the second arch

- The lingual swellings grow and fuse with each other and with tuberculum impar. These combined swellings form anterior two-thirds of the tongue (Fig. 13.5C, Practice Fig. 13.4).
- Developing alveololingual sulcus gradually separates tongue from floor of mouth.
- In relation to third and fourth arch, pharyngeal surface shows a midline swelling called *hypobranchial eminence* or *copula of His*. In 5th week, hypobranchial eminence becomes visible (Fig. 13.5A, B).
- The hypobranchial eminence is divided into ventral and dorsal parts. Ventral part expands to form posterior one-third of the tongue. Fusion of anterior and posterior part is represented by *sulcus terminalis* (Fig. 13.5C).
- Caudal part of the hypobranchial eminence forms *epiglottis*. Some cells migrate from posterior one-third of tongue and cross sulcus terminalis to form *circumvallate papillae* (Fig. 13.5C, Practice Fig. 13.4).

Flowchart 13.2: Development of tongue

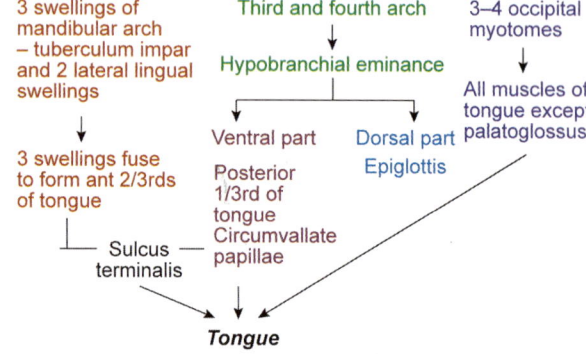

- The third arch overgrows over the second arch and fuses with the first arch, thus the second arch mesoderm gets burried in the substance of the tongue (Practice Fig. 13.5).

Muscles of Tongue

- 3–4 *occipital myotomes* migrate ventrally to the mesenchyme of the tongue and forms all extrinsic and intrinsic muscles of tongue.

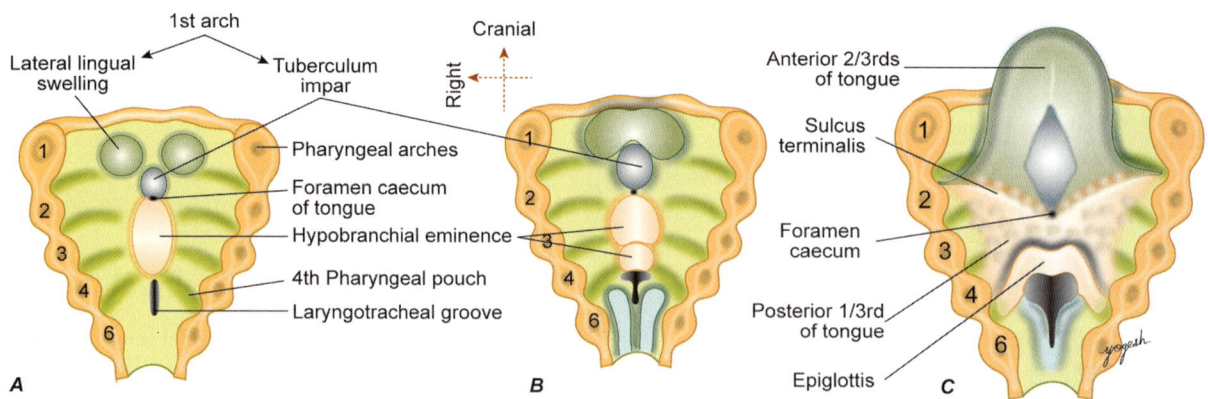

Fig. 13.5: Development of the tongue: (A) A section of pharynx of the embryo at 4th week. In the floor of pharynx two lateral lingual swellings, one median lingual swelling and more caudally hypobranchial eminence appear; (B) 6 weeks and; (C) 10 weeks: One medial and two lateral lingual swellings fuse to form anterior two-thirds of the tongue, whereas cranial part of the hypobranchial eminence forms posterior one-third of the tongue and circumvallate papillae

- The occipital myotomes pull their nerve (hypoglossal nerve) during migration; hence hypoglossal nerve crosses both external and internal carotid arteries superficially.

Nerve Supply

Q. Correlate the nerve supply of tongue with its development.

- Mucosa of anterior two-thirds of tongue develops from mandibular (1st) pharyngeal arch. Hence, supplied by the mandibular branch of trigeminal nerve (post-trematic nerve of 1st arch) and for a taste sensation, supplied by chorda tympani branch of facial nerve (pretrematic nerve of 1st arch).
- Mucosa of posterior one-third of tongue and circumvallate papillae develop from mucosa of the third arch by hypobranchial eminence; hence supplied by glossopharyngeal nerve (nerve of 3rd arch).
- Mucosa of posterior part of the tongue (near vallecula) develops from mucosa of fourth arch by hypobranchial eminence; hence, supplied by vagus nerve (nerve of the fourth arch).
- Muscles of tongue *except* palatoglossus are derived from occipital myotomes; hence, supplied by hypoglossal nerve (Fig. 13.6).

Developmental Anomalies of Tongue

1. *Aglossia* is complete agenesis of tongue.
2. *Hemiglossia* is produced due to failure of one lingual swelling to form half part of the tongue.
3. *Bifid tongue* is split tongue in anterior two-thirds due to nonfusion of two lingual swellings.
4. *Tongue tie* or *ankyloglossia* occurs due to incomplete formation of alveololingual sulcus. The tongue is connected with a floor of mouth by short frenulum.

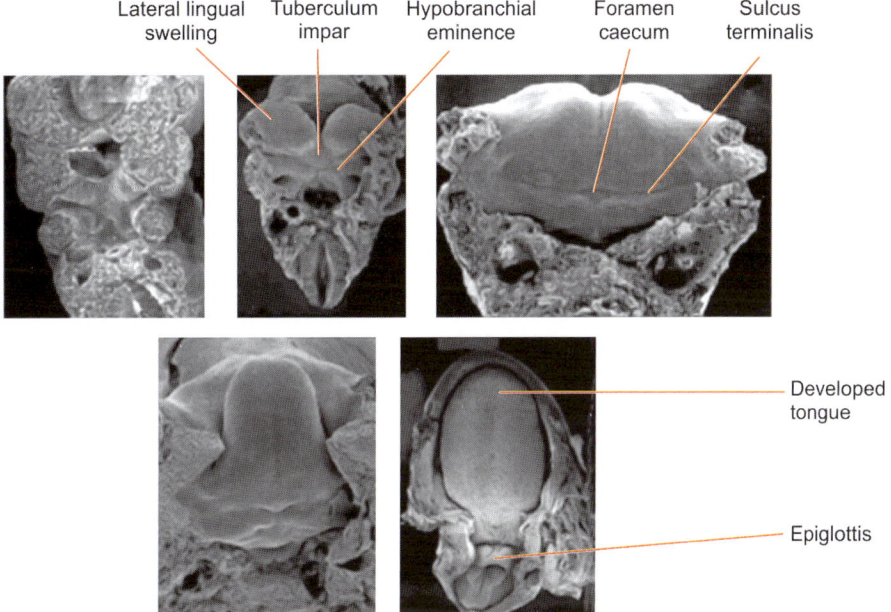

Scanning electron micrograph 13.1: SEM showing contribution of the pharyngeal arches to the developing tongue and epiglottis. A series of micrographs of sequentially older embryos also illustrate the contribution of arches to tongue. [Species: Mouse, approximate human age: Early 5th week, dorsal view]

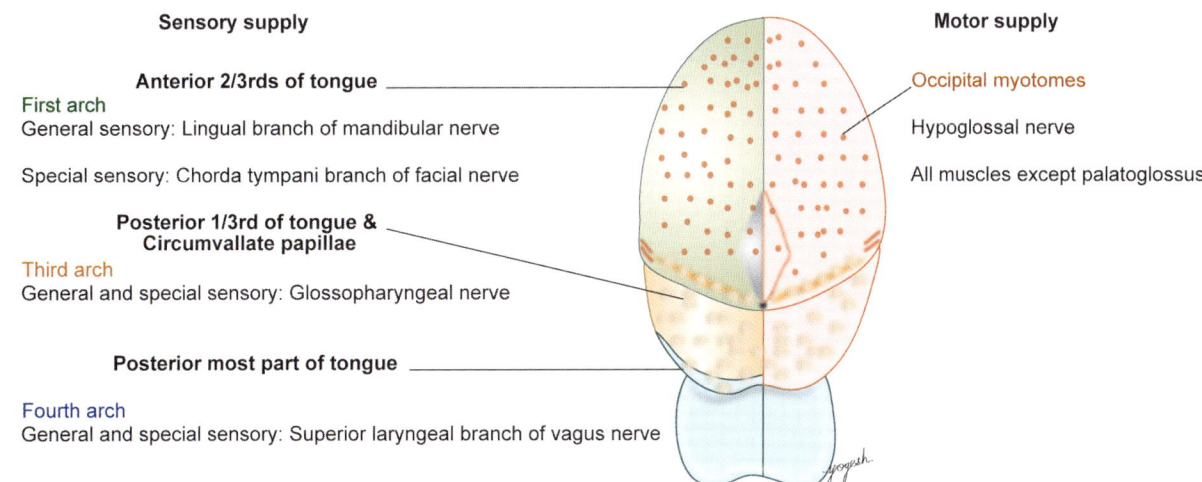

Fig. 13.6: Nerve supply of the tongue

5. *Microglossia* is a small tongue and *macroglossia* is a large tongue.
6. *Ankyloglossia superior* is a condition of adherent tongue with palate.
7. *Lingual thyroid* occurs due to failure of migration of the thyroid gland.

DEVELOPMENT OF SALIVARY GLANDS

Q. Write a short note on development of parotid and submandibular salivary glands.

- There are three pairs of salivary glands, namely parotid, submandibular and sublingual.
- The parotid gland develops from ectoderm, whereas sublingual and submandibular salivary glands develop from endoderm.
- Each salivary gland develops as epithelial outgrowth that forms solid cords.
- Solid cords later get canalized and then they divide and redivide. Each cord at the end gets converted into acini.
- Main canalized cord form duct of salivary gland and its oral opening forms papilla of ductal opening of salivary gland (Fig. 13.7).

Parotid Gland

- The parotid gland develops during *fifth week* from an ectodermal outgrowth or furrow from cheek at the angle of stomodeum (between mandibular arch and maxillary process).
- Later the furrow gets canalized and forms parotid duct.
- Lateral end of duct proliferates and divides to form ductules and acini of parotid gland.
- Maxillary and mandibular processes fuse and reduce size of oral fissure. This fusion increases the length of parotid duct.
- Finally, the duct of parotid gland opens into vestibule of mouth (in adult opposite to upper second molar teeth).^MCQ
- Presence of myoepithelial cells surrounding parotid acini confirms its ectodermal origin.^MCQ

Submandibular Gland

- During *sixth week*, a solid endodermal outgrowth arises from floor of stomodeum, from floor of alveololingual groove.
- Later furrow gets canalized and forms submandibular duct.
- Lateral end of the duct proliferates and divides to form ductules and acini of submandibular gland.

Sublingual Gland

- During *seventh week*, multiple endodermal outgrowths arise from linguogingival sulcus and submandibular duct and finally these outgrowths form sublingual glands.
- Developmentally salivary gland shows prebud stage, initial bud stage, pseudoglandular stage, canalicular stage, and finally terminal bud stage (Fig. 13.7).

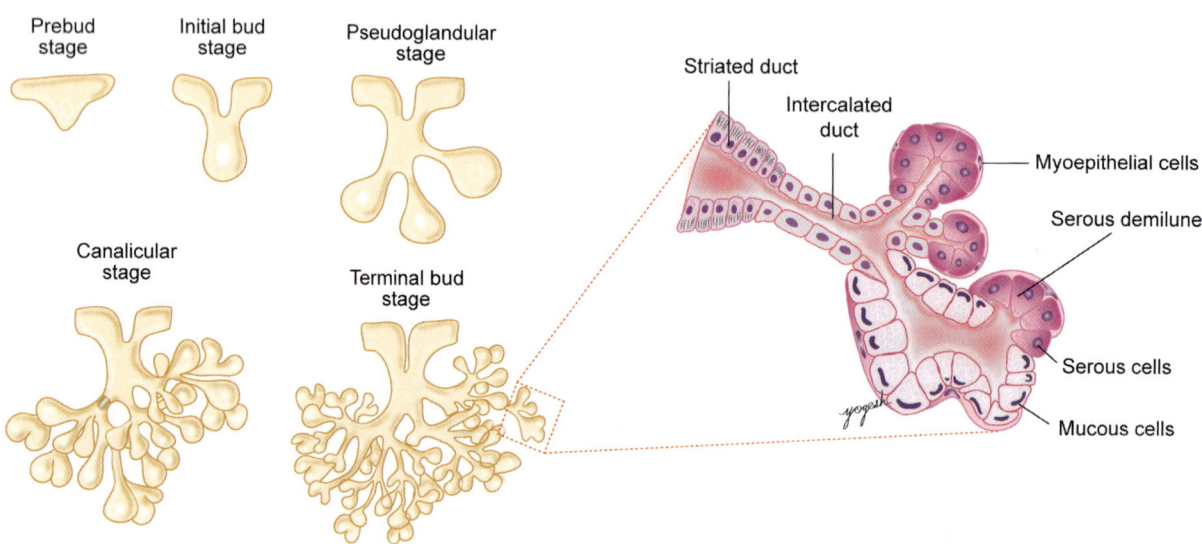

Fig. 13.7: Development of salivary gland

Clinical Embryology

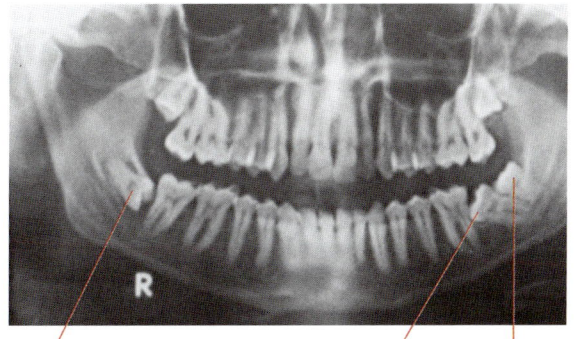

Clinical image 13.1: Orthopantomogram (OPG) showing impacted teeth. Right lower third molar (48) tooth is horizontal impacted, whereas left lower second and third molar teeth (37, 38) are mesioangular impacted. Note OPG is a panoramic dental X-ray that produces a two-dimensional view of maxilla and mandible. While recording OPG, the machine rotates around patient's head. For reference purpose, dentition is divided into four quadrants: (1) upper right, (2) upper left, (3) lower left and (4) lower right. Hence, right lower third molar is referred to as tooth 48 (Image courtesy: *Dr Saikat Chakraborty*)

Chapter 14

Alimentary Tract III: Development of Intestine

eSmartQuiz

Chapter Outline

- Development of esophagus
  - Stages of development
  - Congenital anomalies
- Development of stomach
  - Stages of development
  - Rotation of stomach
  - Changes in mesenteries
  - Histogenesis of stomach
- Congenital hypertrophic pyloric stenosis
- Development of duodenum
  - Stages of development
  - Anomalies of duodenum
- Development of midgut
- Physiological umbilical hernia
- Rotation of gut
  - Stages of rotation
  - Congenital anomalies of midgut
- Malrotation
- Meckel's diverticulum
- Development of caecum and appendix
- Development of hindgut
  - Development of urorectal septum
- Development of anal canal
- Meconium

Competency:
- **AN52.6:** Describe the development and congenital anomalies of foregut, midgut and hindgut.

INTRODUCTION

- The alimentary tract develops from *primitive gut*.
- On formation of head and tail folds, the part of *definitive yolk sac* gets trapped within the embryo. This trapped part forms *primitive gut*^NEXT (Fig. 14.1, Practice Fig. 14.1, Flowchart 14.1).
- The primitive gut extends from *buccopharyngeal membrane* cranially to *cloacal membrane* caudally. Buccopharyngeal membrane and cloacal membrane are the regions where ectoderm and endoderm are opposed without intervening mesoderm.^NEXT
- Developing primitive gut communicates with
  1. Yolk sac through vitellointestinal duct.
  2. Allantoic diverticulum (Fig. 14.1C).
- Cranial part of the gut that lies in the head fold is *foregut*.
- Caudal part of gut that lies in the tail fold is *hindgut*.
- The part of gut that communicates with vitello-intestinal duct is *midgut*.
- Vitellointestinal duct disappears by 5th week.^MCQ
- *Anterior (cranial) intestinal portal* is the communication between foregut and midgut, whereas *posterior (caudal) intestinal portal* is the communication between midgut and hindgut.
- The *buccopharyngeal membrane* separates stomodeum from foregut, whereas *cloacal membrane* separates hindgut from proctodeum.
- Gut is attached to body wall by ventral and dorsal mesenteries.
- The primitive gut is supplied by coeliac artery for the foregut, superior mesenteric artery for the midgut and inferior mesenteric artery for the hindgut (Fig. 14.2, Practice Fig. 14.2).^NEXT
- During early development, *allantois* opens in caudal part of hindgut called *cloaca*.
- The *urorectal septum* divide cloaca in ventral *primitive urogenital sinus* and dorsal *primitive rectum* or *primitive anorectal canal*.^NEXT

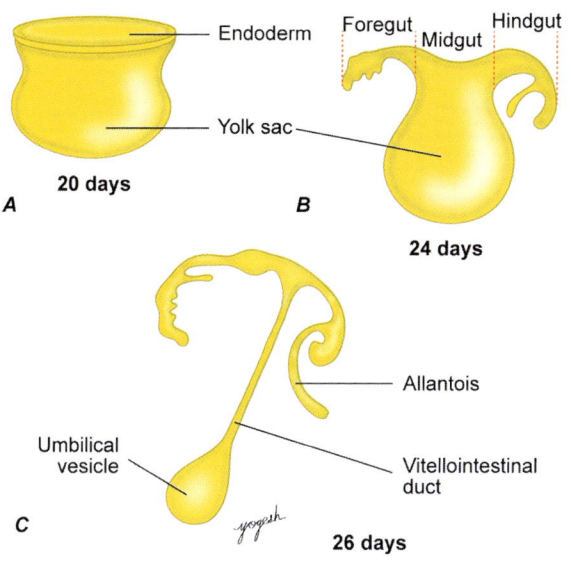

Fig. 14.1: Conversion of endoderm and yolk sac to gut

Flowchart 14.1: Gut tube

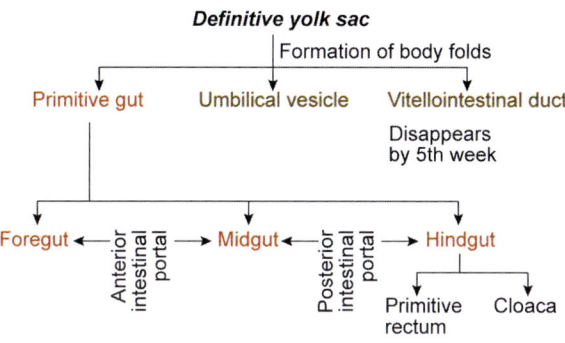

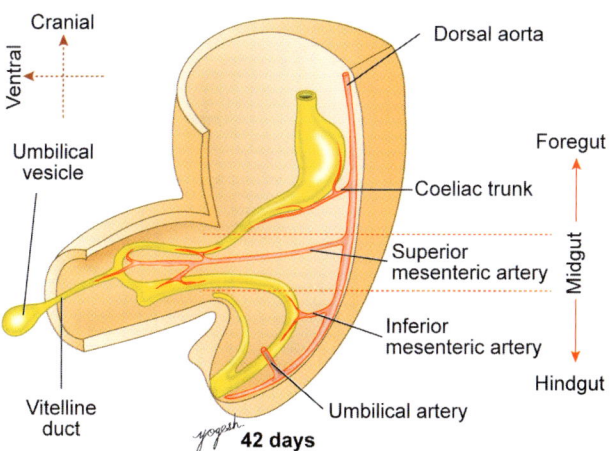

Fig. 14.2: Blood supply of developing gut. Foregut and its derivatives are supplied by the branches from coeliac trunk. Midgut is supplied by superior mesenteric artery, whereas hindgut by inferior mesenteric artery

- Attachment of urorectal septum also divides the cloacal membrane into ventral *urogenital membrane* and dorsal *anal membrane*.

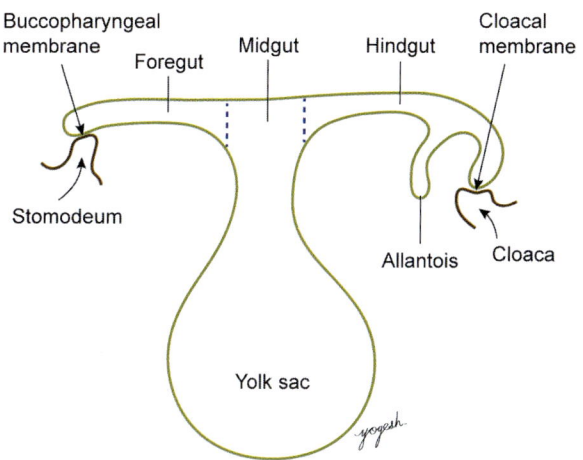

Practice Fig. 14.1: Parts of primitive gut

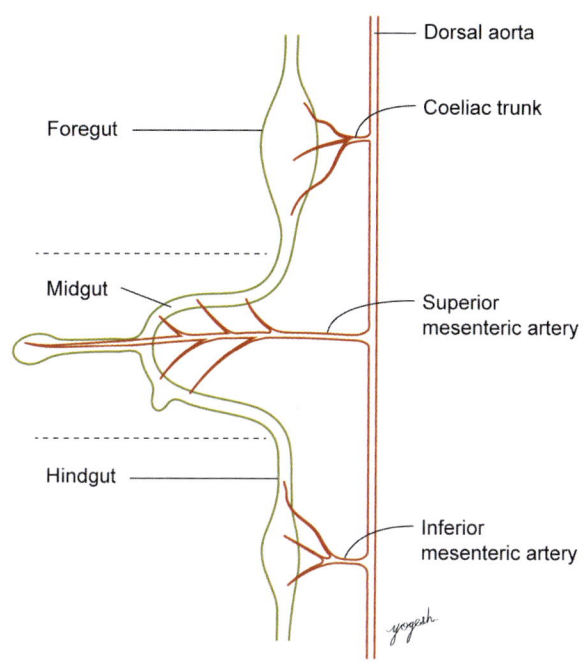

Practice Fig. 14.2: Blood supply of primitive gut

DEVELOPMENT OF ESOPHAGUS

Q. Write a short note on development of esophagus.

- Esophagus develops from the part of foregut between the pharynx and stomach.

Summary (Examination Guide)

- Derivation of the components of esophagus:
  – Epithelium – from endoderm of foregut.
  – Muscles and connective tissue – from the splanchnopleuric mesoderm surrounding the foregut.
- Refer to Flowchart 14.2.

Stages of Development

- In lower part of the pharynx, a *laryngotracheal groove* appears that later forms tracheobronchial (respiratory) diverticulum (Fig. 14.3A).

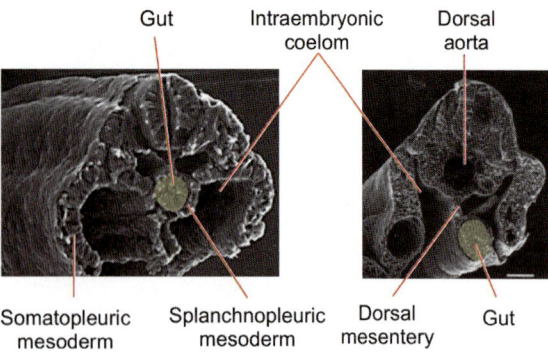

Scanning electron micrograph 14.1: Gut is suspended by dorsal mesentery. Intraembryonic coelom splits mesoderm into splanchnopleuric and somatopleuric mesoderm [Species: Mouse, approximate human age: 27–28 days. Transverse section]

- Tracheoesophageal septum divides the part of foregut caudal to tracheobronchial diverticulum as ventral trachea and dorsal esophagus (Fig. 14.3B and C).
- Small esophagus elongates due to formation of neck and descent of diaphragm, lungs and heart.

> **Some Interesting Facts**
>
> - Auerbach's and Meissner's plexus are derivatives of neural crest.*NEXT*
> - Esophagus has striated muscles in upper one-third, smooth muscles in lower one-third and mixed (both smooth and striated muscles) in middle one-third.*MCQ, Viva*

Congenital Anomalies of Esophagus

1. *Esophageal stenosis*: Failure of canalization of esophagus results in esophageal atresia (obliterated lumen). Esophageal atresia results in *polyhydramnios* (excessive amniotic fluid) due to inability of ingestion of amniotic fluid by fetus.

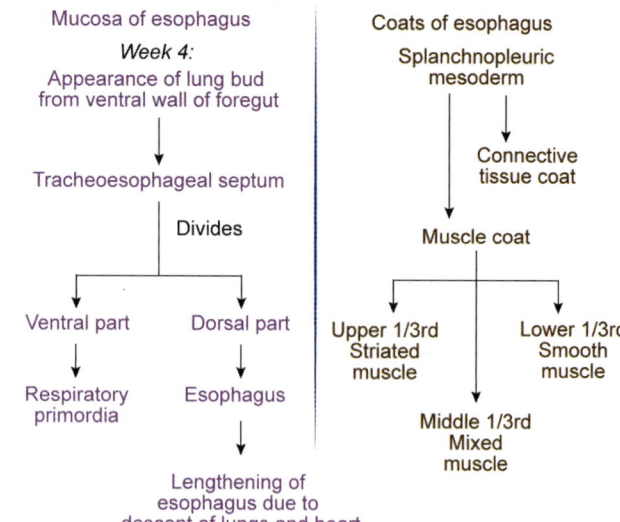

Flowchart 14.2: Development of esophagus

2. *Esophageal atresia*: It is a failure of development of part of the esophagus. Continuous pouring of saliva from the mouth is the most important confirmatory sign of esophageal atresia.*MCQ*

3. *Tracheoesophageal fistula*: It is a communication of trachea with esophagus due to the failure of proper development of tracheoesophageal septum. In this condition, proximal part of the esophagus ends as blind pouch; whereas distal part of the esophagus communicates with the trachea.

Q. Write a short note on tracheoesophageal fistula.

4. *Achalasia cardia* or *cardiospasm*: Loss of the ganglionic cells in Auerbach's plexus of the esophageal wall results in a failure of muscle relaxation in lower part of the esophagus. This deformity is *achalasia cardia*. Barium swallow shows *bird-beak deformity* (pencil-shaped narrowing of the esophagus).*MCQ*

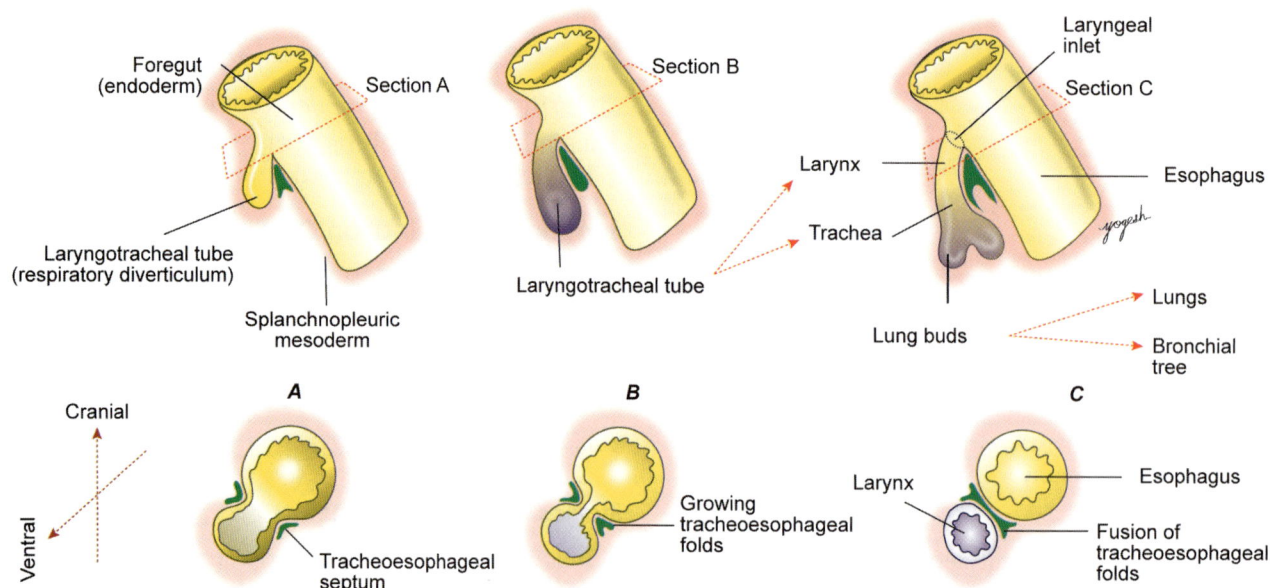

Fig. 14.3: Formation of tracheal bud and lung bud. Tracheoesophageal septum separates trachea from esophagus

DEVELOPMENT OF STOMACH

Q. Write a short note on development of stomach.

Summary (Examination Guide)

- Stomach develops during 4th–5th week as a fusiform dilatation of part of foregut distal to the esophagus.
- Refer to Flowcharts 14.3 and 14.4.

Stages of Development

- Adult stomach has anterior and posterior surfaces, lesser and greater curvature and fundus (Figs 14.4, 14.5, Practice Fig. 14.3, Flowchart 14.3, Practice Fig. 14.1).
- Tubular foregut segment dilates and forms fusiform sac with ventral and dorsal borders (Fig. 14.5A).
- Dorsal border overgrows to form *greater curvature* of stomach (Fig. 14.5B, C).
- Ventral border grows slowly and forms *lesser curvature* (Fig. 14.5C).
- Ventral border is attached with septum transversum by *ventral mesogastrium*, whereas dorsal border is attached with dorsal body wall by *dorsal mesogastrium* (mesentery). Spleen, coeliac trunk and dorsal pancreatic bud develop in dorsal mesogastrium, whereas ventral pancreatic bud, liver and gallbladder develop in ventral mesogastrium (Fig. 14.4).^{NEXT}

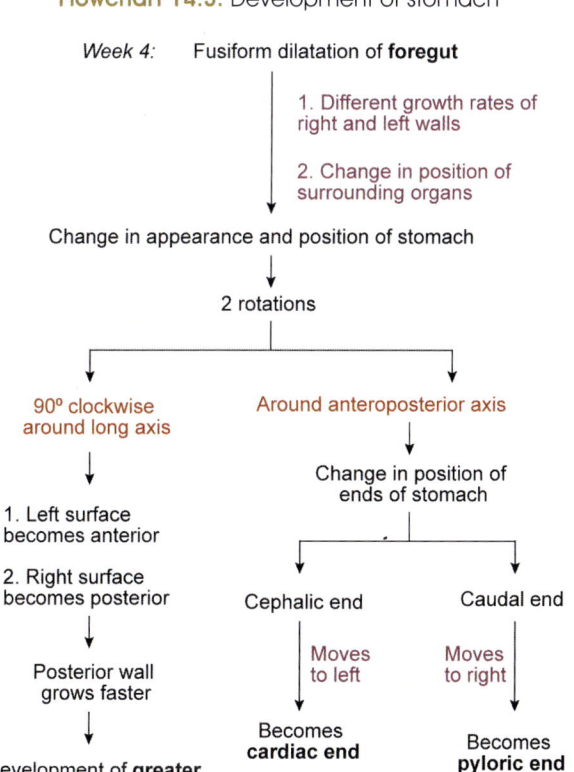

Flowchart 14.3: Development of stomach

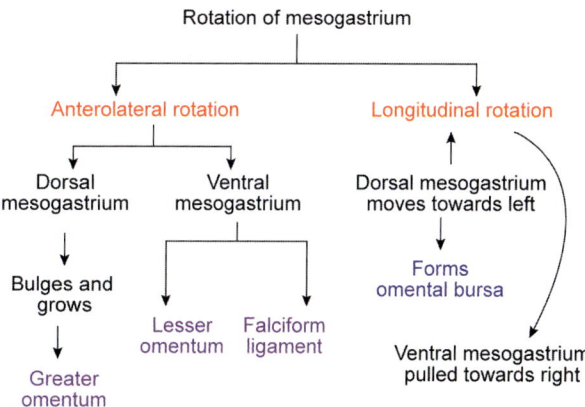

Flowchart 14.4: Development of mesogastrium

Rotation of Stomach

- Stomach rotates to the *right clockwise* (around 90°) along longitudinal axis and thus left surface of foregut forms anterior surface of adult stomach and right surface of foregut forms posterior surface of adult stomach (Fig. 14.5B).
- Hence, anterior surface of stomach is supplied by left vagus nerve, whereas posterior surface is by right vagus nerve.
- Stomach rotates *along transverse* (anteroposterior) *axis* and lower end rotates to the right. The right end forms pyloric end of stomach (Fig. 14.5C).

Changes in Mesenteries

- Liver develops in the ventral mesogastrium (Figs 14.4, 14.5, Flowchart 14.4).
- The developing liver divides ventral mesogastrium into two parts (Fig. 14.4):
  - Falciform ligament – lies between liver and anterior abdominal wall.^{NEXT}
  - lesser omentum – lies between liver and stomach (lesser curvature).^{NEXT}
- Ventral mesogastrium also forms coronary and triangular ligaments.^{NEXT}
- Spleen develops in dorsal mesogastrium.^{NEXT}
- Developing spleen divides dorsal mesogastrium into two parts:
  - Gastrosplenic ligament – lies between greater curvature of stomach (fundus) and spleen (contains short gastric arteries)^{NEXT}.
  - Lienorenal ligament – lies between the spleen and posterior body wall.
- Dorsal mesogastrium from rest of the greater curvature extends to form a *greater omentum*.
- Space behind lesser omentum, stomach and greater omentum form a *lesser sac* (lesser bursa).

Histogenesis of Stomach

- Epithelial lining and gastric gland – develop from endoderm of foregut.

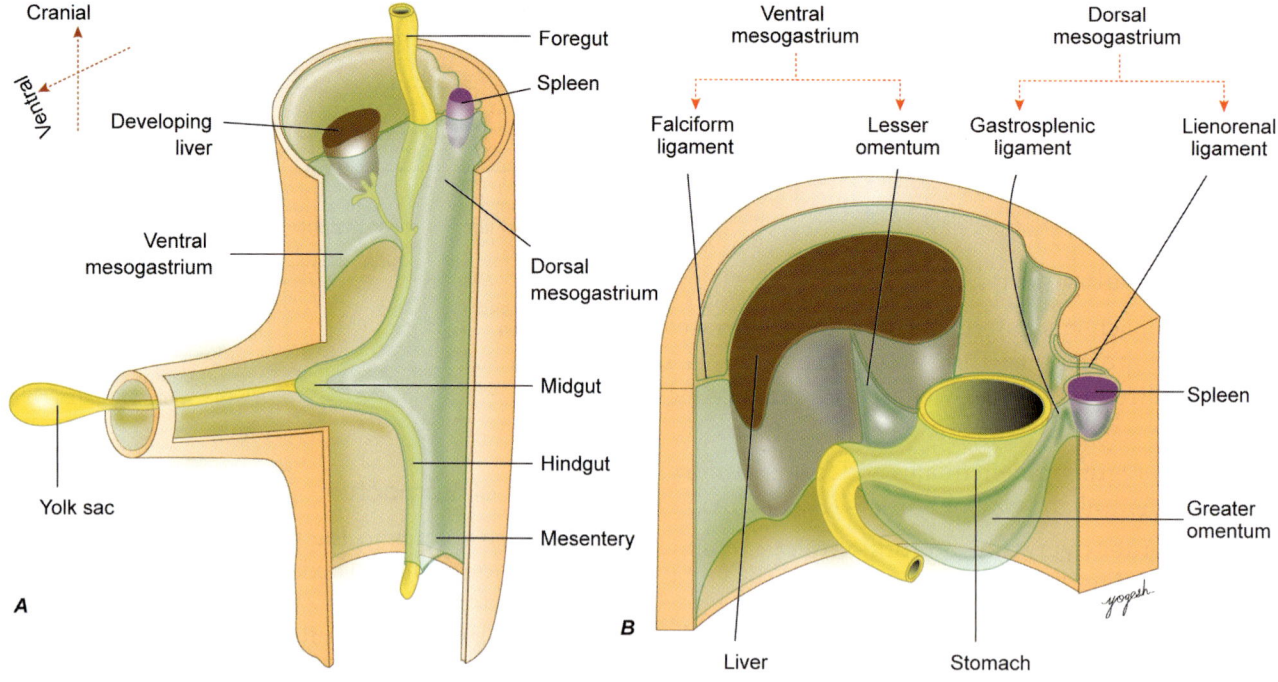

Fig.14.4: Transverse section through the region of stomach showing changes in the position of stomach, liver and spleen: (A) Positions at the end of 5th week; (B) Position at the end of 11th week. Ventral mesogastrium forms falciform ligament and lesser omentum, whereas dorsal mesogastrium forms gastrosplenic and lienorenal ligaments and greater omentum

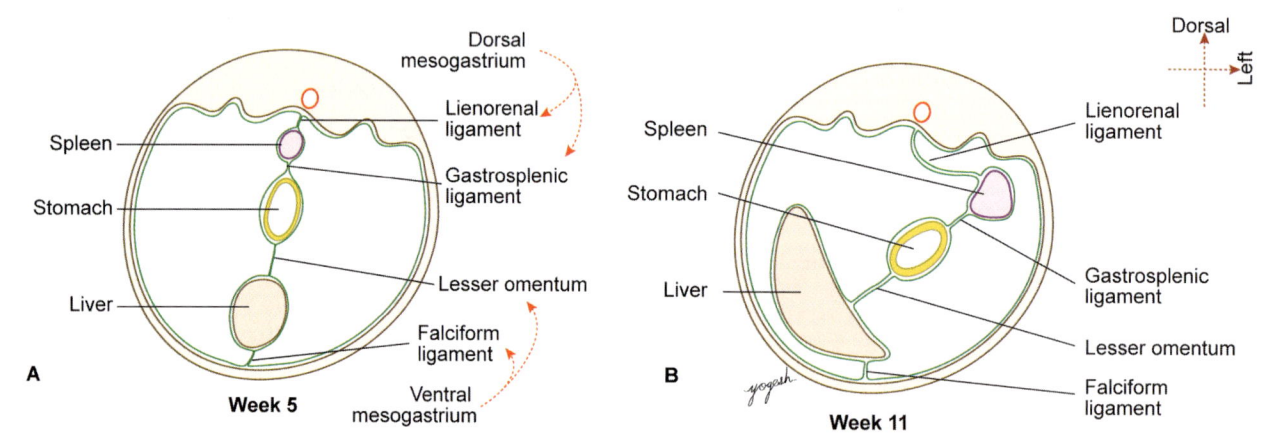

Practice Fig. 14.3: Development of transverse mesocolon and lesser sac (omental bursa, transverse section of abdomen)

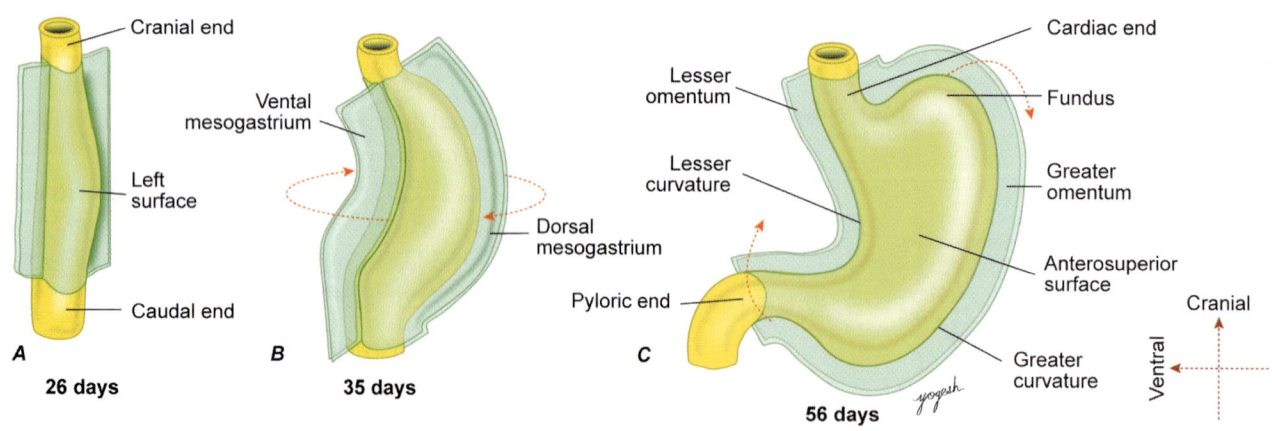

Fig. 14.5: Development of stomach

- Muscles and connective tissue – develop from the splanchnopleuric mesoderm.
- Gastric glands appear in the third month, whereas oxyntic and zymogenic cells are differentiated in the fourth month of intrauterine life.^{MCQ}

> **Box 14.1: Congenital hypertrophic pyloric stenosis**
>
> - It is a congenital defect due to the hypertrophy of circular muscle layer at the pylorus. *Pyloric stenosis is one of the most common abnormalities of the stomach in infants.*
> - **Incidence**: 1 in every 150 male infants and 1 in every 750 female infants *(common in males)*.
> - **Presentation**: Newborn is normal until first feed.
> - Newborn present projectile forceful vomiting after 2–3 hours after each feed. Vomitus does not contain bile.
> - **Treatment**: Surgical treatment of pyloric obstruction.

DEVELOPMENT OF DUODENUM

Q. Write a short note on development of duodenum.

Summary (Examination Guide)

- Duodenum develops from two sources:^{NEXT}
  a. Foregut forms the part of duodenum proximal to the opening of common bile duct.
  b. Midgut forms the part of duodenum distal to the opening of bile duct.

Stages of Development

1. Rotation of stomach brings midline duodenum to the right side (Flowchart 14.5).
2. Initially, duodenum is connected to posterior abdominal wall by dorsal mesentery (*mesoduodenum*).
   - Most of the part of mesoduodenum undergo *zygosis* and duodenum becomes retroperitoneal organ except small proximal part of the duodenum near pylorus of stomach (Figs 14.6, 14.7).

Flowchart 14.5: Development of duodenum

Stages of development
Rotation of stomach
↓
Shift duodenum to the right

Mesoduodenum
↓ Zygosis
Retroperitoneal duodenum

Blood supply
Foregut – proximal to opening of CBD – celiac trunk
Midgut – distal to opening of CBD – superior mesenteric art

Anomalies
Duodenal stenosis – partial occlusion
Duodenal atresia – complete occlusion
Duodenal diverticula

CBD = Common bile duct

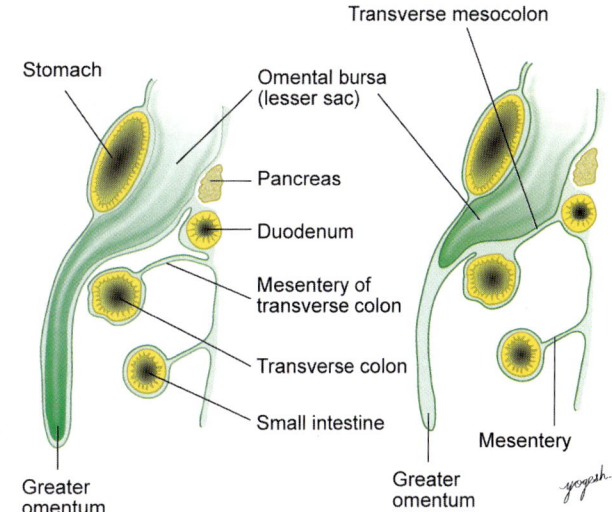

Fig. 14.6: Development of transverse mesocolon and lesser sac (omental bursa)

- Blood supply:
  - Part of the duodenum derived from foregut is supplied by branches of *coeliac trunk*.
  - Part of the duodenum derived from midgut is supplied by branches of *superior mesenteric artery*.
- Proliferation of the endodermal cells obliterates lumen by 8th week and it gets recanalized by 3rd month of intrauterine life (Fig. 14.8).^{MCQ}

Anomalies of Duodenum

1. *Duodenal stenosis*: Partial occlusion of duodenal lumen is *duodenal stenosis*. Incomplete recanalization produces the duodenal stenosis. Newborn baby with duodenal stenosis vomits the feed that contains bile.^{MCQ}
2. *Duodenal atresia*: Complete occlusion of the duodenal lumen is *duodenal atresia*. It occurs mostly distal to the opening of hepatopancreatic ampulla. A newborn baby with duodenal atresia vomits the feed that always contains bile. *Duodenal atresia is the most common intestinal atresia.* Duodenal atresia produces *polyhydramnios*. On ultrasonography, distended gas-filled stomach and duodenum produce *double-bubble sign*.^{MCQ}
3. *Duodenal diverticula*: Duodenal diverticulum usually arises from the second part of the duodenum.

DEVELOPMENT OF MIDGUT

Q. List the derivatives of midgut.

- Primitive midgut extends from *cranial intestinal portal* to *caudal intestinal portal*.
- Midgut is suspended with *dorsal mesentery* from posterior abdominal wall.
- Midgut communicates with a yolk sac through a *vitellointestinal duct* (vitelline duct or yolk stalk).

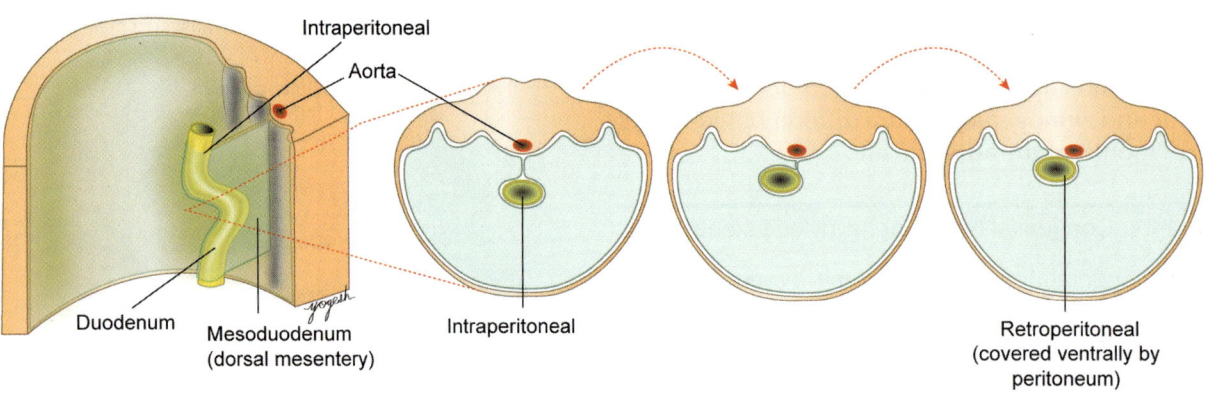

Fig. 14.7: Process of zygosis

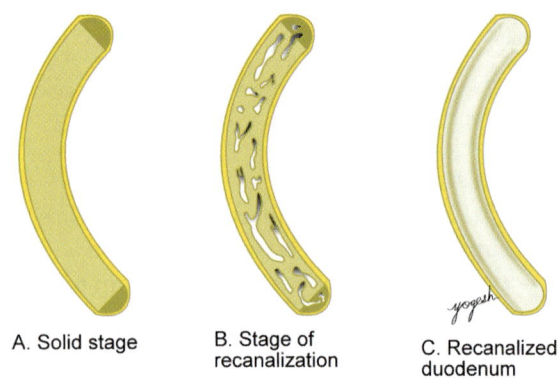

A. Solid stage   B. Stage of recanalization   C. Recanalized duodenum

Fig. 14.8: Development of duodenum: (A) Solid stage: Endodermal cells proliferate to obliterate the lumen of the duodenum; (B, C) Stage of recanalisation: Small lacunae appear, enlarge and fuse to form the lumen of the duodenum

- Midgut is supplied by superior mesenteric artery.^{MCQ}
- Superior mesenteric artery divides the midgut into
  - Prearterial (proximal) segment
  - Postarterial (distal) segment
- Prearterial segment forms^{NEXT}
  - Distal part of duodenum
  - Jejunum
  - Ileum
- Postarterial segment forms^{NEXT}
  - Terminal part of ileum
  - Caecum
  - Appendix
  - Ascending colon
  - Right two-thirds of transverse colon.

Rotation of Gut

Q. Write a short note on rotation of gut.

- Midgut undergoes 270° counterclockwise rotation (Flowchart 14.6, Fig. 14.9, Practice Fig. 14.2).^{MCQ}
- *Purpose of rotation*: To accommodate herniated midgut loop in the small abdominal cavity.

Flowchart 14.6: Rotation of gut

Midgut rotates 270° counterclockwise
Purpose: to accommodate gut in abdomen
Axis Around superior mesenteric artery (SMA)
Before rotation
  Prearterial segment – Cranial to SMA ⎤ in midline
  Post arterial segment – Caudal to SMA ⎦
First 90° rotation:
  Prearterial segment → on right SMA ⎤ in hoizontal plane
  Postarterial segment → on left SMA ⎦
Second 90° rotation:
  Prearterial segment elongates → forms jejunum and ileum
        ↓ Rotation
  Coils of jejunum and ileum pass behind SMA
Third 90° rotation:
  Postarterial segment come to lie on the right of SMA
        ↓ Growth
  Cecum and appendix reach right iliac fossa

Box 14.2: Physiological umbilical hernia

Q. Write a short note on physiological umbilical hernia.

- Physiological umbilical hernia is a natural, normal phenomenon.
- It is the protrusion of midgut loop (herniation) outside the abdominal cavity through umbilical opening.
- Duration: From 6th week to 12th week of intrauterine life. Reduction of physiological hernia occurs at ~10 weeks of embryonic period.^{NEXT}
- Physiology: Abdominal cavity is smaller to accommodate rapidly elongating gut. It results into the midgut loop herniation. The midgut rotation and increase in abdomen size accommodates midgut in the abdominal cavity.

Stages of Rotation

- Midgut is divided into prearterial and postarterial segment by centrally passing superior mesenteric artery.
- Midgut rotates 270° counterclockwise around the axis passing through the superior mesenteric artery.

- Before rotation, prearterial segment lies cranial to the superior mesenteric artery in the midline, whereas postarterial segment lies caudal (Fig. 14.9A).
- Rotation of midgut can be divided into two stages, first 90° rotation and remaining 180° rotation.
- First 90° rotation brings back the midgut loop in the abdominal cavity, whereas remaining 180° rotation occurs within the abdominal cavity.
  1. First 90° rotation: Midgut rotates 90° counterclockwise around the superior mesenteric artery. This rotation brings prearterial segment on the right side and postarterial segment on the left side in the horizontal plane (Fig. 14.9B).
  2. Remaining 180°: Prearterial segment elongates to form coils of the jejunum and ileum. The midgut again undergoes counterclockwise rotation. Thus, prearterial segment (coils of jejunum and ileum) come to lie behind the superior mesenteric artery. This brings the superior mesenteric artery ventral to duodenum (Fig. 14.9C).

Midgut rotates further counterclockwise around the superior mesenteric artery. It brings the postarterial segment (caecum, appendix) on the right side (Fig. 14.9D). Postarterial segment elongates and cecal bud come to lie in right iliac fossa (adult position). Due to the this rotation, transverse colon crosses the superior mesenteric artery (Fig. 14.9E).

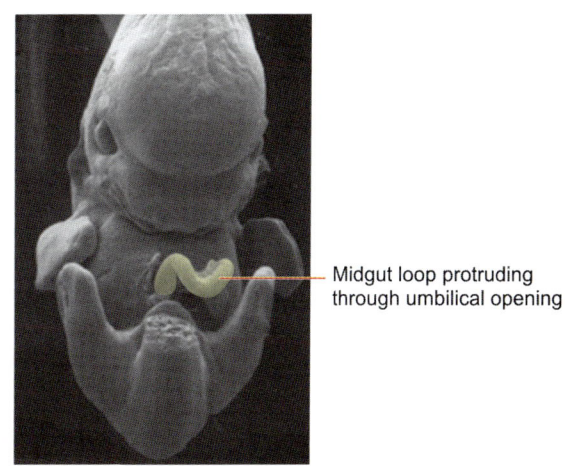

Scanning electron micrograph 14.2: Physiological hernia. Midgut elongates rapidly and during sixth week of development, it extends beyond body wall in umbilical cord (physiological umbilical herniation). [Species: Mouse, approximate human age: 40 days, ventral view]

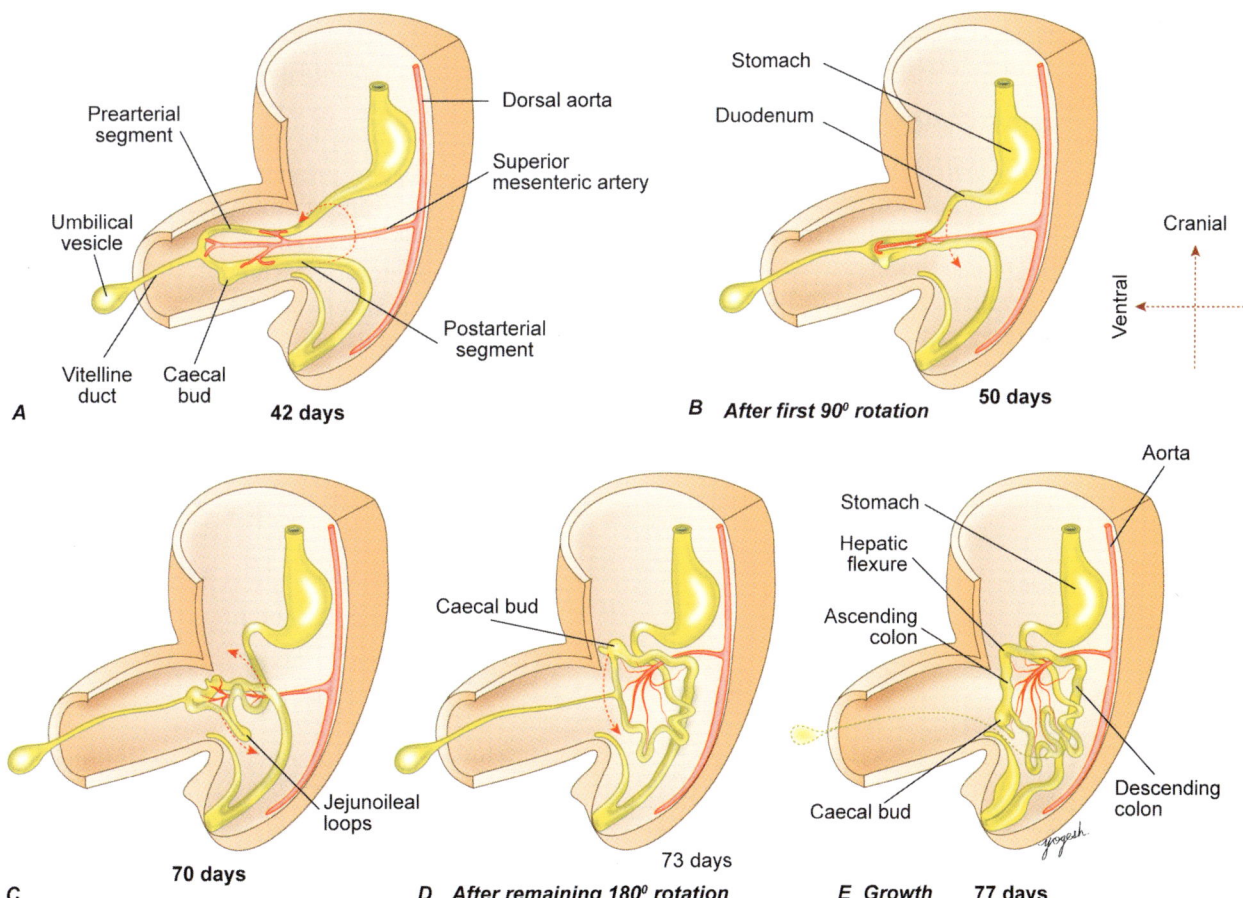

Fig. 14.9: Rotation of gut: (A) Position of the gut before rotation; (B) Position of the gut after first 90° counterclockwise rotation; (C) The position of the intestine during remaining 180° counterclockwise rotation of gut; (D) The position of the intestine after remaining 180° counterclockwise rotation of gut; (E) Cecal bud and appendix moves towards the right iliac fossa

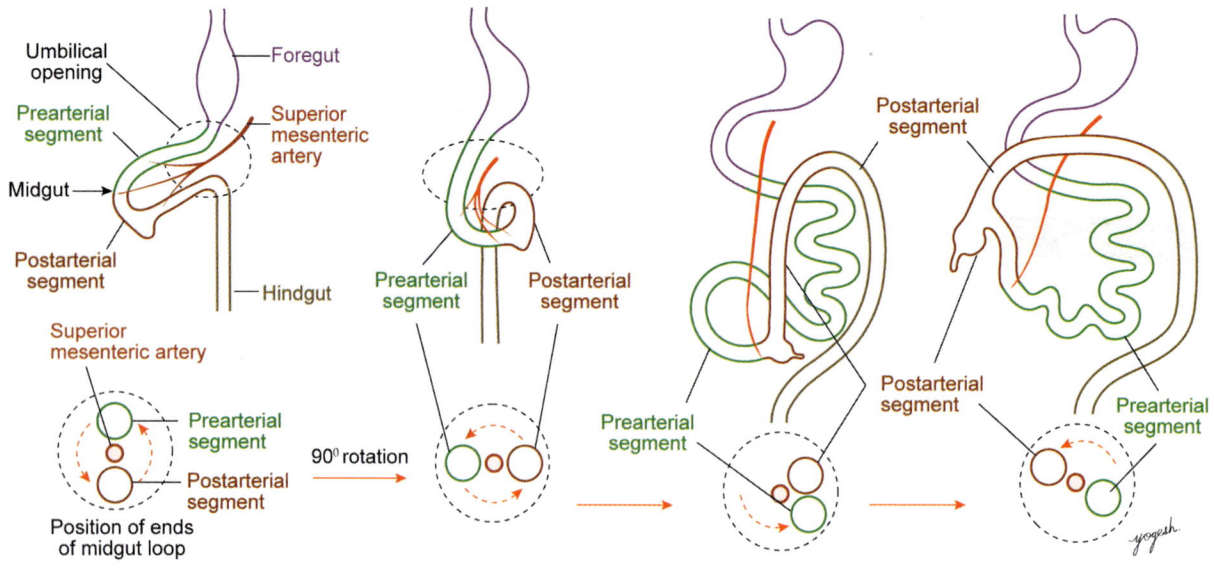

Practice Fig. 14.4: Rotation of gut

- Initially, all parts of midgut are connected with the dorsal wall by dorsal mesentery. After intestinal rotations, dorsal mesentery of duodenum, ascending colon, descending colon and rectum undergo zygosis and these organs become retroperitoneal (covered by peritoneum anteriorly).^{NEXT}
- A persistent part of mesentery forms the mesentery of small intestine and mesocolon of transverse and sigmoid colon and mesoappendix for appendix.

Congenital Anomalies of Midgut

1. *Umbilical fecal fistula (vitelline fistula)*: It is caused by patent vitellointestinal duct. It involves communication of the small intestine with exterior and results in discharge of fecal matter (Fig. 14.10).
2. *Meckel's diverticulum*: Box 14.3 (Fig. 14.10).
3. *Enterocystoma (Vitelline cyst)*: It is the cyst of the vitellointestinal duct that occurs due to small persistent middle part of the duct (Fig. 14.10). Persistent vitellointestinal duct → Meckel's diverticulum, vitelline cyst (enterocystoma), umbilical fistula and umbilical (vitelline) sinus.^{NEXT}

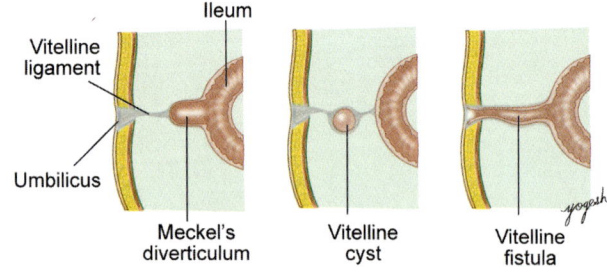

Fig. 14.10: Remnants of the vitellointestinal (vitelline) duct: (A) Meckel's diverticulum; (B) Vitelline cyst; (C) Vitelline fistula that connects the lumen of the ileum with the umbilicus. Persistent part of vitelline duct may be present as vitelline ligament (omphalomesenteric ligament)

Box 14.3: Meckel's diverticulum (diverticulum ilei)
High yielding facts, NEXT

Q. Write a short note on Meckel's diverticulum.

- Meckel's diverticulum was first explained by GF Hildanus in the sixteenth century and later named after Johann Friedrich Meckel in 1809.
- Meckel's diverticulum is *true* congenital diverticulum of the *small intestine* as it consists of *all layers* of GIT.^{NEXT} Meckel's diverticulum is the commonest congenital anomaly of intestine.^{MCQ}
- It is the persistent proximal part of *vitellointestinal duct* that is present in embryo (Fig. 14.10).
- Usually, vitellointestinal duct disappears during the 6th week of intrauterine life.
- Persistent part of vitelline duct may form vitelline cyst or vitelline fistula.

Features

- It occurs in 2% subjects.
- Male : Female ratio is 2:1.
- The most common age at clinical presentation is 2 years.
- Length of the diverticulum is 2 inches (5 cm).^{NEXT}
- Situation: About 2 feet or 60 cm proximal to ileocecal valve.
- It shows 2 types of common ectopic tissues (gastric and pancreatic).
- Attachment: It is attached to the antimesenteric border of ileum.
- Its caliber is equal to that of ileum.
- The apex of diverticulum: Apex may be free or may be attached to umbilicus, to mesentery, or to any other abdominal structure by a fibrous band.

Contd

Contd

Clinical Anatomy
- Meckel's diverticulum may cause intestinal obstruction.
- It may have small regions of gastric mucosa.
- Acute inflammation of diverticulum (diverticulitis) may produce symptoms that resemble those of appendicitis.

Treatment
- Cases with complications can be treated with *surgical resection*, preferably laparoscopic resection.

---

4. *Raspberry tumor* at umbilicus: Persistent distal part of the vitellointestinal duct (at the umbilicus) produces raspberry red tumor.
5. *Exomphalos* or *omphalocele*: Usually, physiological hernia reduces by 12th week of IUL. After birth, persistent gut loops at the closed umbilicus produces rounded mass called exomphalos.[NEXT]
6. *Congenital umbilical hernia*: It is the protrusion of the coils of intestine at umbilicus. The content is covered by skin, connective tissue and peritoneum. Congenital umbilical hernia can be reduced by pushing back coils of intestine through umbilical opening, whereas it reappears on coughing or crying. It gets reduced, within 2–3 years on its own and if not reduced then can be treated surgically.
7. *Gastroschisis*: It is a congenital defect of the **anterior abdominal wall** through which the abdominal content protrudes outside. It occurs due to the ***failure of complete lateral folding*** of the embryo. Gastroschisis occurs in 1 in 10,000 births.[NEXT]
8. *Errors of rotation*: Rotation of gut may fail partially or completely, even there may be reverse rotation. All these defects result in the change of usual positions of abdominal viscera. Suspensory ligament of duodenum (ligament of Treitz) is a key element for diagnosis of rotational anomalies of gut; usually it is on the left of body of first or second lumbar vertebrae.[NEXT] Left-sided colon occurs if the midgut loop has not rotated at all.[NEXT] Mixed rotation may result in the caecum lying inferior to the pylorus.[NEXT] Nonrotation results in left-sided large intestine, right-sided small intestine, reversed rotation of duodenum (it lies anterior to transverse colon), transverse colon lies posterior to superior mesenteric artery.[NEXT]
9. *Apple-peel atresia (Christmas tree intestinal atresia or type IIIb atresia)*: These are atresia of small intestine and account for 10% of all intestine atresias. In the apple-peel atresia, duodenum or proximal jejunum ends in a blind pouch and distal small intestine wraps around its vascular supply resembling an apple peel (spiral).[MCQ]

Box 14.4: Malrotation[NEXT]

- It is a congenital anomaly of rotation of the gut that commonly causes intestinal obstruction.
- Ladd's band is present in malrotation. It is a fibrous stalk of peritoneal tissue that attach caecum to retroperitoneum in right lower abdominal quadrant.

Classical presentation
- Sudden onset of bilious vomiting in newborn or
- Recurrent abdominal pain with bilious vomiting in child due to obstruction.

Diagnosis
- S-shaped duodenum on barium follow through
- Abnormal position of ligament of Treitz
- Management: Ladd's pressure: It includes dissection of Ladd's band, broadening of mesentery base to reduce incidence of volvulus and appendectomy.

DEVELOPMENT OF CAECUM AND APPENDIX

- Caecum and appendix develop from a *cecal bud* that arises as dilatation of postarterial segment of the midgut loop (Fig. 14.11, Practice Fig. 14.5).
- Caecal bud appears in the 6th week of intrauterine life (Fig. 14.11A).[MCQ]
- Proximal part of caecal bud dilates to form *caecum*, whereas distal part persists as narrow tube that forms a *vermiform appendix* (Fig. 14.11B, C).
- Caecal bud grows rapidly and forms two saccule one on either side. The right saccule grows faster than the left saccule, hence, attachment of appendix shift towards left (near ileocaecal junction) (Fig. 14.11D).

DEVELOPMENT OF HINDGUT

- Hindgut gives rise to the following structures:
  1. Left one-third of the transverse colon
  2. Descending colon
  3. Sigmoid colon
  4. Rectum
  5. Upper part of the anal canal

Development of Urorectal Septum
- Distal part of hindgut that communicates with allantois is *cloaca*.
- Cloaca is divided into ventral broad *primitive urogenital sinus* and dorsal narrow *primitive rectum* by growing *urorectal septum* (Fig. 14.12, Practice Fig. 14.6).[NEXT]
- Urorectal septum also divides the *cloacal membrane* into anterior *urogenital membrane* and posterior *anal membrane*. Cloacal membrane ruptures by seventh week.[NEXT] Anal membrane lies at the proximal part of proctodeum.[NEXT]

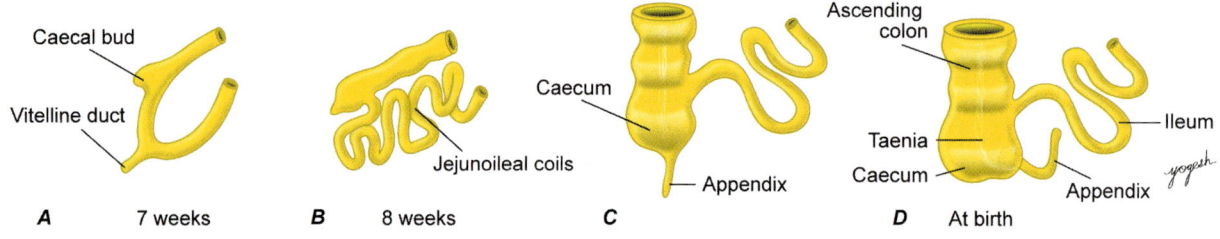

Fig. 14.11: Development of caecum and appendix

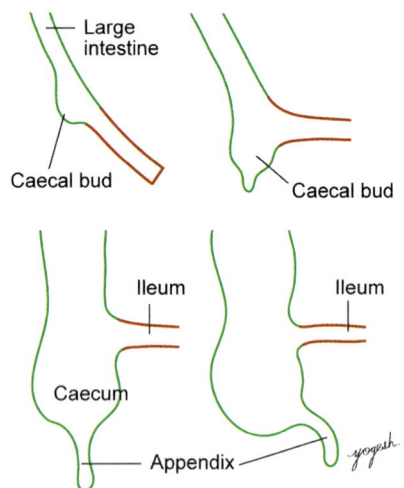

Practice Fig. 14.5: Development of caecum and appendix

- Urogenital sinus forms urinary bladder and urethra, whereas primitive rectum forms rectum and upper part of the anal canal.
- Urorectal septum shows
  - *Tourneux fold* as vertical element that grows caudally between rectum and urogenital sinus.
  - *Folds of Rathke* project inwards from the lateral wall of cloaca.

DEVELOPMENT OF ANAL CANAL

Q. Write a short note on development of anal canal. *High yielding facts*

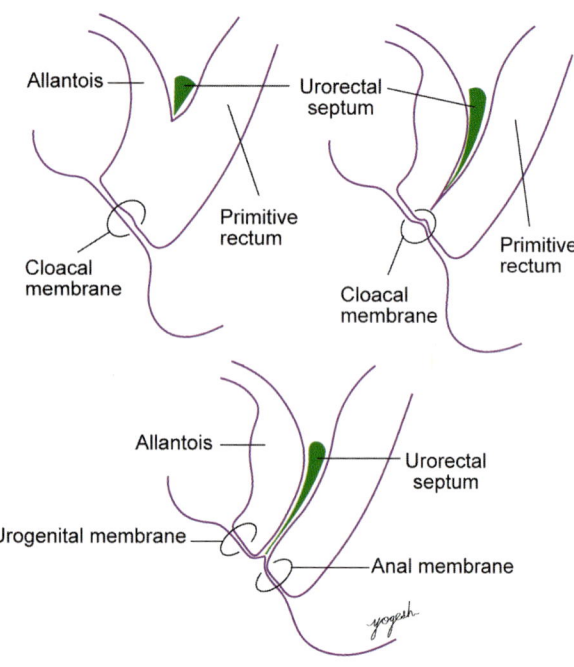

Practice Fig. 14.6: Formation of urorectal septum

Summary (Examination Guide)

- Anal canal is derived from two sources:
  1. *Endodermal cloaca* (distal part of primitive rectum) forms upper part of anal canal above the pectinate line.
  2. *Ectodermal anal pit* (proctodeum) forms lower part of anal canal below the pectinate line.
- Refer to Table 14.1, Fig. 14.12, Practice Fig. 14.7, Flowchart 14.7.

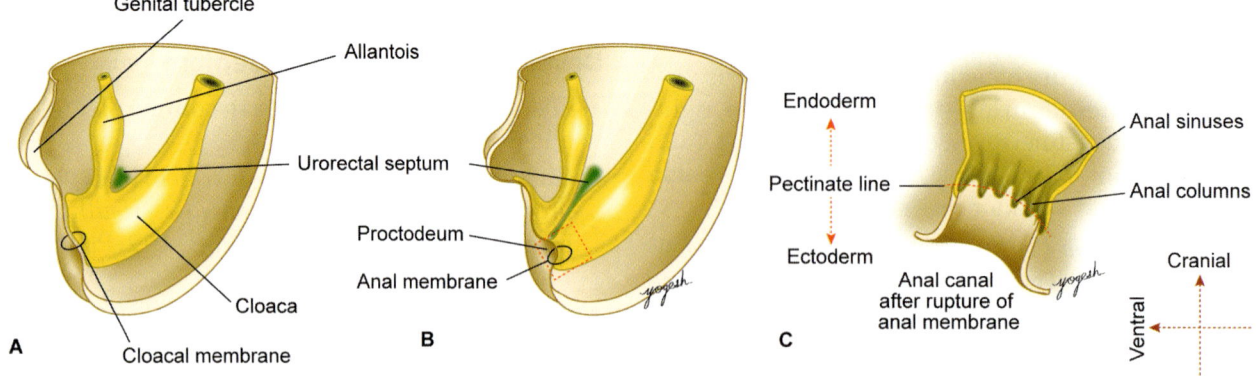

Fig. 14.12: Development of the anal canal. Urorectal septum divides cloaca into ventral primitive urogenital sinus and dorsal primitive rectum (A, B) and cloacal membrane into urogenital membrane and anal membrane. Surface ectoderm and lower part of primitive rectum (endoderm) forms the anal canal (C)

Table 14.1 Development of anal canal

	Above pectinate line (upper part of anal canal)	Below pectinate line (lower part of anal canal)
Origin	Endoderm	Ectoderm
Develops from	Endodermal cloaca (primitive rectum)	Proctodeum or anal pit
Arterial supply	Superior rectal artery	Inferior rectal artery
Venous drainage	Portal vein via superior rectal vein	Systemic vein (inferior vena cava) via inferior rectal vein
Nerve supply	Autonomic nerves	Somatic nerves

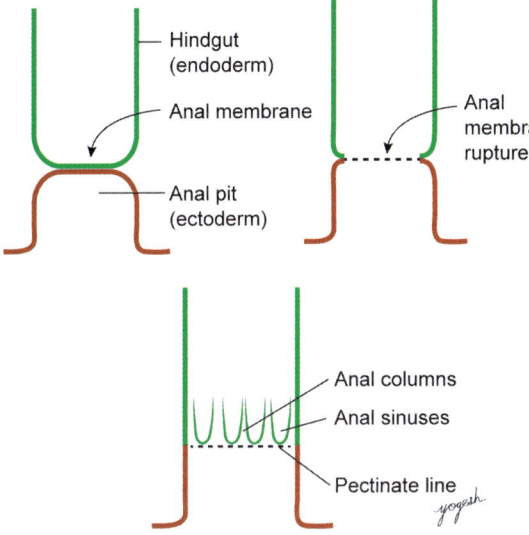

Practice Fig. 14.7: Development of anal canal

Flowchart 14.7: Development of anal canal

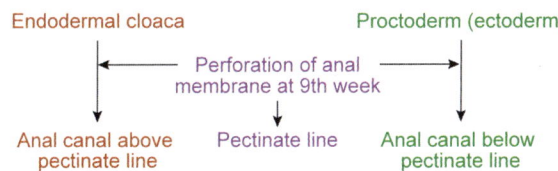

Stages of Development

- Proctodeum (anal pit) is a depression of the surface ectoderm. In the bottom of proctodeum, anal membrane and urogenital membranes are present (Fig. 14.12).

- The *anal membrane* perforates at 9 weeks and hindgut communicates with exterior (Fig. 14.12B). (In later life, anal membrane is represented by anal valves or pectinate line.)^NEXT

- Location of the anal membrane is represented by pectinate line of anal canal. Thus, part of anal canal above pectinate line is derived from endodermal cloaca, whereas part below pectinate line is derived from ectodermal proctodeum (Fig. 14.12C).^MCQ

- Hence, the blood supply, lymphatic drainage and nerve supply above and below pectinate line are different (Table 14.1).

Congenital Anomalies

Q. Write a short note on congenital anomalies of anal canal.

1. *Hirschsprung's disease* (congenital megacolon)^NEXT
   - It is a congenital anomaly of the large intestine.
   - It shows a dilated segment of a colon due to congenital absence of parasympathetic ganglia in the wall of gut (myenteric and submucous plexuses).
   - It occurs due to failure of migration of neural crest cells before reaching anus.^NEXT
   - A segment without parasympathetic supply (aganglionated) shows constriction due to unopposed activity of sympathetic nerves and proximal part of colon to such constricted segment shows dilatation due to accumulated food.
   - Incidence: 1 in 5,000 newborns.
   - Treatment: Surgical resection of constricted segment.

Q. Write a short note on imperforate anus.

2. Imperforate anus
   - The distal part of gut does not communicate with exterior.
   - Causes of imperforate anus
     a. Failure of rupture of anal membrane.
     b. Failure of development of ectodermal proctodeum.
     c. Failure of rectal development (rectal atresia).

3. Ectopic anus
   - Posterior growth of perineal body divides the cloacal membrane into ventral urogenital and dorsal anal membrane.
   - Failure or abnormality in this division may result into ectopic anal opening at the following sites:
     a. In female: Within vestibule.
     b. In male: At the base of scrotum, in intrabulbar fossa of spongy urethra.

4. Rectal fistula
   - A fistula is abnormal communicating tunnel between two organs.

– Rectal fistulas are of the following types:
   a. Rectovesical fistula (high fistula): Rectum communicates with urinary bladder.
   b. Rectourethral fistula (low fistula): Rectum communicates with urethra.
   c. Rectovaginal fistula (low fistula): Rectum communicates with vagina.

Box 14.5: Meconium

Q. Write a short note on meconium.

- Meconium is the earliest *stool* of newborn.
- Meconium consists of material that is ingested by fetus during intrauterine life such as lanugo (very thin, soft fetal hairs), mucus, amniotic fluid, bile, intestinal epithelial cells and water.
- Meconium is viscous, sticky, dark olive green and odorless. Meconium (in Greek) means poppy (due to its appearance).
- *Meconium stained liquor*: If the fetus defecates before birth, the meconium stains amniotic fluid. This condition is *meconium stained liquor*.
- Aspiration of meconium by fetus results in *meconium aspiration syndrome*.
- In Hirschsprung's disease and cystic fibrosis, the newborn does not pass meconium.^{MCQ}
- *Meconium ileus*: Thickened and congested meconium in intestine is *meconium ileus*. It is first sign of the cystic fibrosis.^{MCQ}

DERIVATIVES OF GUT

- Derivatives of the gut are listed in Table 14.2.

Q. List the derivatives of foregut, midgut and hindgut.

Table 14.2	Derivatives of the gut
Part of gut	Derivatives
Foregut	• Part of floor of mouth • Tongue • Pharynx • Esophagus • Stomach • Proximal part of the duodenum up to major duodenal papilla • Pharyngeal pouches and their derivatives • Liver with intrahepatic biliary apparatus • Pancreas • Gallbladder with extrahepatic biliary apparatus • Respiratory system
Midgut	• Part of the duodenum distal to major duodenal papilla • Jejunum • Ileum • Caecum • Appendix • Ascending colon • Right two-thirds of transverse colon
Hindgut	• Left one-third of the transverse colon • Descending colon • Sigmoid colon • Rectum • Upper part of anal canal • Mucosal lining of urinary bladder and urethra

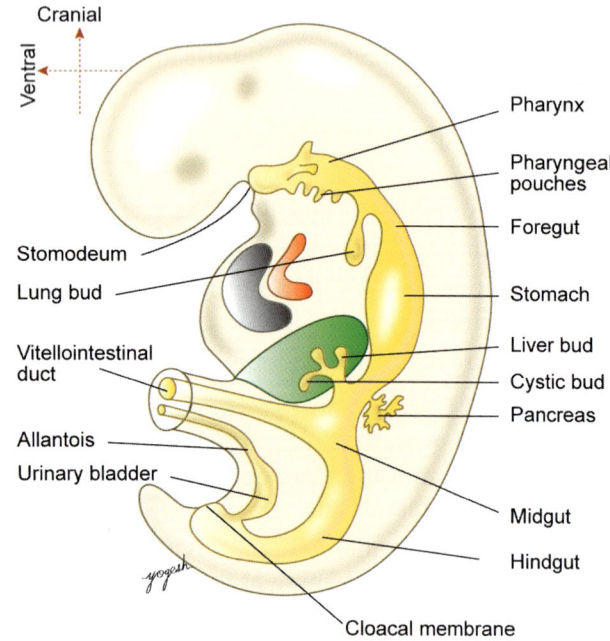

Fig. 14.13: Sagittal section of the embryo showing the derivatives of the endoderm. For understanding, other structures such as neural tube, dorsal aorta are not shown

Clinical Embryology

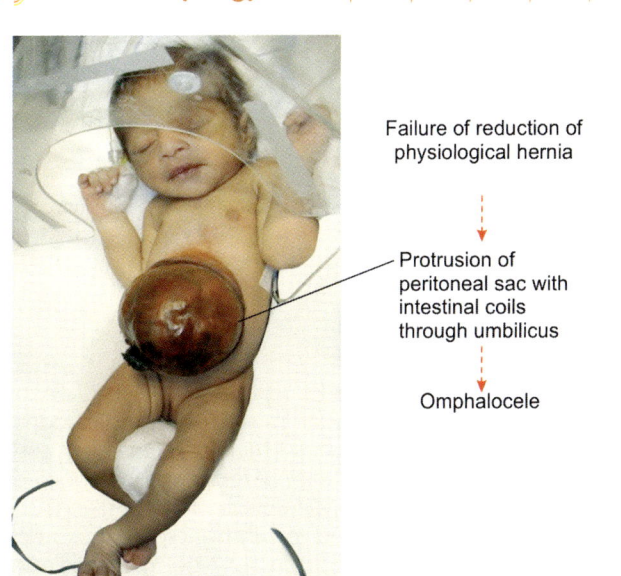

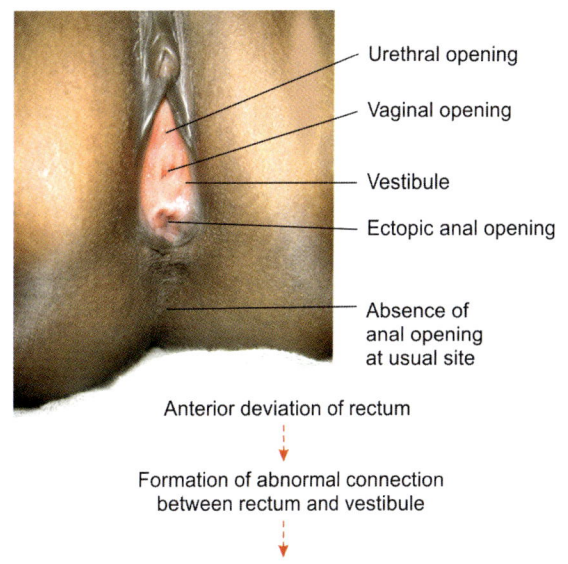

Clinical image 14.1: *Omphalocele*. It is a rare abdominal wall defect in that intestine (occasionally liver and other organs) remains outside of the abdomen in a sac because of failure of normal return of intestines and other contents back to abdominal cavity during around ninth week of intrauterine life. The sac is formed from an outpouching of peritoneum, protrudes in the midline, through the umbilicus (Image courtesy: *Dr Adhisivam B*)

Clinical image 14.2: *Rectovestibular fistula* is an abnormal connection (fistula) between the rectum and vestibule of the female genitalia. It is the most common anorectal malformation in female patients. In the present case, vestibule has urethral, vaginal and rectal opening. There is no separate anal opening (in other cases, small anal opening may be present) (Image courtesy: *Dr Kumaravel S*)

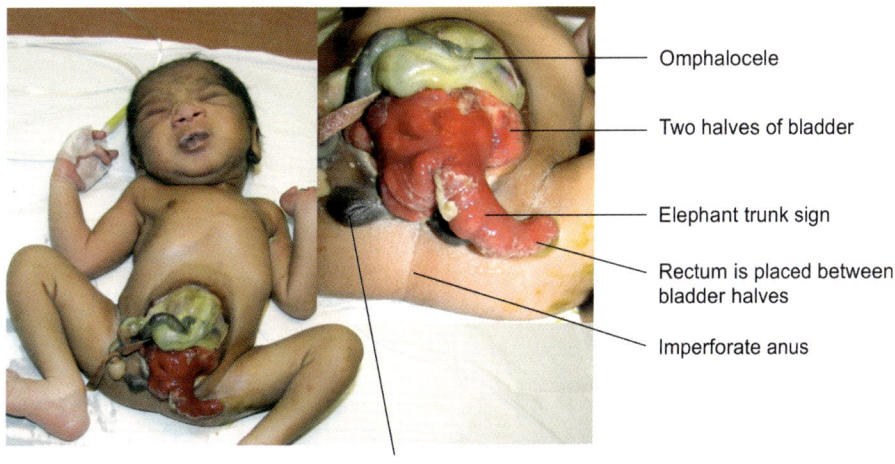

Clinical image 14.3: *Cloacal exstrophy*. The case shows 'elephant trunk sign' representing the intussuscepted ileum. It is a rare condition having incidence of 1 in 200,000 pregnancies and 1 in 400,000 live births. It shows omphalocele (large intestine lies outside of the body), exstrophy of the bladder (bladder is open and separated into two halves) and rectum is placed between the bladder halves on the surface of the abdomen, imperforate anus (anus has not been formed or perforated) (Image courtesy: *Dr Kumaravel S*)

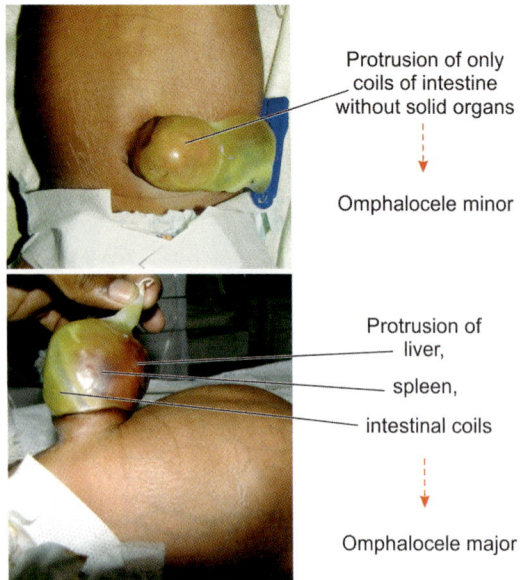

Clinical image 14.4: Omphalocele minor and major. Omphalocele is an abdominal wall defect in that abdominal contents are present in the cord outside the abdominal cavity. Omphalocele can be classified as *omphalocele minor* (only a few loops of gut in the sac) and *omphalocele major* (contain most of abdominal organs, including liver) (Image courtesy: *Dr Kumaravel S*)

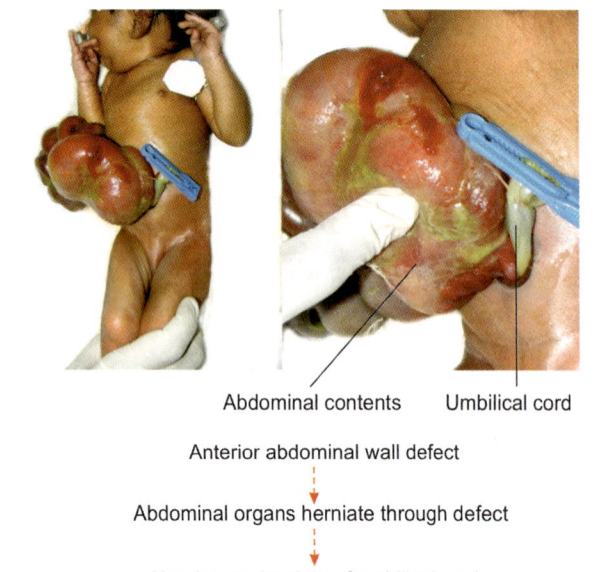

Clinical image 14.5: Gastroschisis. It is the condition of defective anterior abdominal wall. Through the defect coils of intestine and other abdominal viscera protrude outside. It differs from omphalocele in that there is the absence of parietal sac covering the contents and it lies on the right side of umbilical cord (in omphalocele, cord attaches to the herniated peritoneal sac) (Image courtesy: *Dr Kumaravel S*)

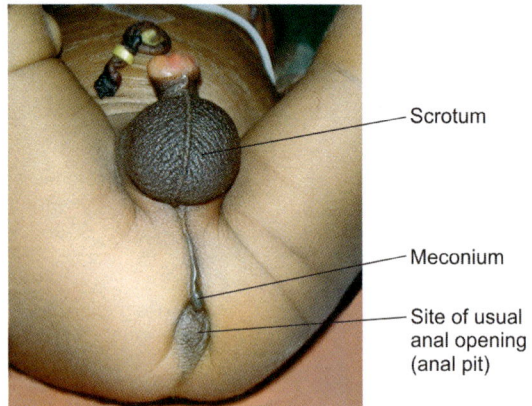

Clinical image 14.6: *Male anorectal malformation*. Anorectal malformation is a disorder in which anal canal does not open at its usual site. Anorectal malformations are classified based on location of the rectum in relation to the puborectalis sling into two types: High imperforate anus (rectum ends above the puborectalis sling) and low imperforate anus (rectum traverses the puborectalis sling). In high type, there is no external opening. In low type, there is a small opening covered by a layer of skin or other type of membrane through which meconium passes. The anorectal malformations also include *rectoperineal fistula* (slightly anterior, small anus), rectourethral fistula (rectum opening into urethra rather than its usual anal opening), rectovesical fistula (rectum opens into the urinary bladder), rectal/anal agenesis (no communication between genitourinary tract and rectum and no external anal opening), rectovaginal, rectouterine and rectovestibular fistula (rectum opens in vagina, uterus and vestibule respectively). Confirmation of anorectal fistula needs micturating cystourethrogram (radiograph) (Image courtesy: *Dr Kumaravel S*)

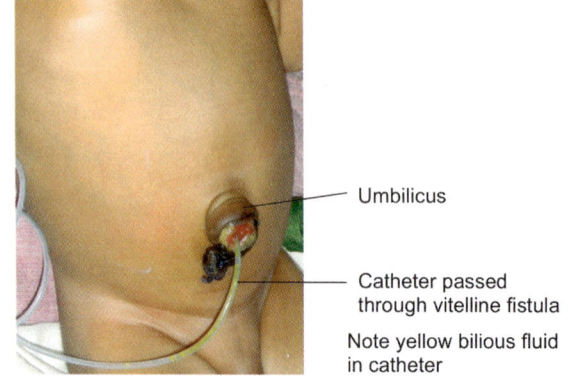

Clinical image 14.7: Patent vitellointestinal duct. The vitellointestinal duct connects midgut loop to the umbilical vesicle. Usually, vitellointestinal duct obliterates during 5th–6th weeks of IUL. Persistent vitellointestinal duct produces vitelline fistula causing discharge of yellow bilious fluid from the umbilicus (Image courtesy: *Dr Kumaravel S*)

Chapter 15

Alimentary Tract IV: Development of Liver, Gallbladder, Pancreas and Spleen

eSmartQuiz

Chapter Outline

- Development of liver
  - Stages of development
  - Molecular regulation of liver induction
  - Congenital anomalies of liver
- Histogenesis of liver
- Development of gallbladder and extrahepatic biliary apparatus
  - Stages of development
  - Anomalies of gallbladder
  - Anomalies of extrahepatic biliary ducts
- Development of pancreas
  - Stages of development of pancreas
  - Molecular regulation of pancreas development
  - Anomalies of pancreas
- Annular pancreas
- Development of spleen
  - Stages of development
  - Anomalies of spleen

Competency:

- **AN52.6:** Describe the development and congenital anomalies of foregut, midut and hindgut.
  Note: Liver, gallbladder, pancreas and spleen develop in relation to gut tube.

INTRODUCTION

- Gastrointestinal tract develops to form foregut, midgut and hindgut.
- The liver, gallbladder, pancreas and spleen develop in relation to the foregut and midgut.
- This chapter includes development of liver, gallbladder, pancreas, and spleen.

DEVELOPMENT OF LIVER

Q. Write a short note of development of liver.

Summary (Examination Guide) (Table 15.1)

- Liver develops from the following sources:
  1. Endodermal hepatic bud forms the hepatocytes and intrahepatic biliary apparatus.
  2. Septum transversum (mesoderm) forms connective tissue of liver including fibrous capsule, Kupffer's cells, and blood vessels.

Table 15.1 Development of liver

Part of liver	Embryonic source
Lobes of liver – Liver parenchyma – Bile canaliculi – Bile ductules	Endoderm: Hepatic bud arising from the second part of the duodenum (that develops from foregut)
Connective tissue – Glisson's capsule – Connective tissue stroma – Kupffer's cells – Blood vessels	Mesoderm: Septum transversum
Liver sinusoids	Vitelline and umbilical veins
Ligaments of liver – Falciform ligament – Lesser omentum – Coronary ligaments – Triangular ligaments	Ventral mesogastrium
Ligamentum teres hepatis	Left umbilical vein
Ligamentum venosum	Ductus venosus

  3. Vitelline and umbilical veins form sinusoids.
  4. Ventral mesentery forms lesser omentum, falciform, coronary and triangular ligaments. *NEXT*

Stages of Development (Figs 15.1 to 15.3, Practice Fig. 15.1, Flowchart 15.1)

1. *Formation of hepatic bud*: During the 3rd week of IUL, *hepatic bud* arises from ventral border of terminal part

of the foregut (developing second part of duodenum) (Fig. 15.1).

2. *Growth of hepatic bud*: The hepatic bud grows ventrally and cranially in the *ventral mesogastrium* and reaches the *septum transversum*.^{VIVA}

3. *Division of hepatic bud*: The hepatic bud divides into cranial *pars hepatica* and smaller caudal *pars cystica* (forms gallbladder). The pars hepatica divides into *right* and *left hepatic ducts*. Each hepatic duct forms solid cord of cells (interlacing columns) called *hepatic trabeculae*.

4. *Formation of hepatic sinusoids*: The hepatic trabeculae soon separate from each other to form *hepatic sinusoids*. The vitelline and umbilical veins that are passing through the septum transversum, breakup and establish a communication with the hepatic sinusoids.

5. *Formation of bile canaliculi*: The hepatic ducts branch to form intrahepatic biliary passages.

6. *Formation of peritoneal ligaments and liver capsule*: The mesenchyme of septum transversum form blood vessels, Kupffer's cells, hematopoietic cells, and capsule of the liver.

7. Developing liver divides the *mesogastrium* into a *falciform ligament* and *lesser omentum*. Reflections of peritoneal covering (part of ventral mesogastrium) from liver to diaphragm form *triangular* and *coronary ligaments*.

Some Interesting Facts

- During early development, both the lobes (right and left) are of equal size.
- In 10th week, weight of liver is approximately 10% of the total body weight, whereas at birth it is 5% of the total body weight. By third month of IUL, the liver contributes one-tenth of the total body weight. By seventh month, it contributes one-fifth of the body weight.
- From the sixth week of IUL till birth, the liver also functions for hematopoiesis.^{MCQ}
- Liver starts bile secretion by 12th week of IUL.^{MCQ}

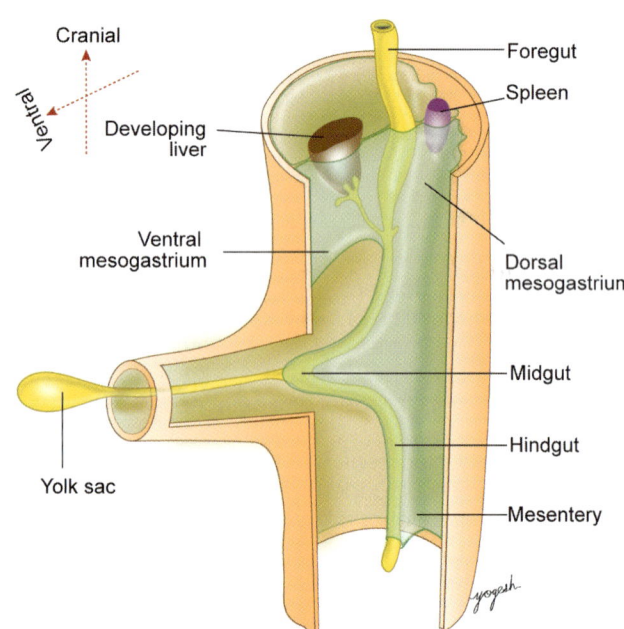

Fig. 15.1: Development of the liver and gallbladder. The liver develops in ventral mesogastrium with the contribution of the right and left hepatic buds (endoderm) and septum transversum (mesoderm). The gallbladder develops from cystic bud (endoderm)

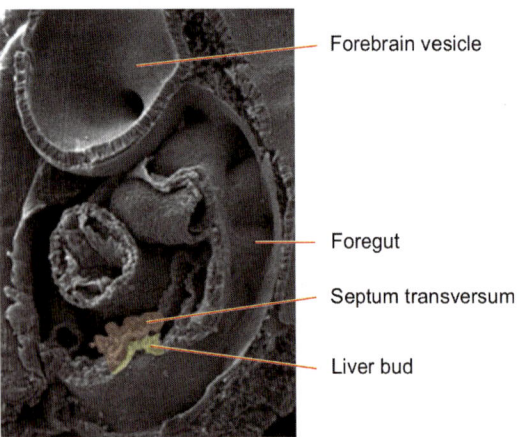

Scanning electron micrograph 15.1: SEM showing a midsagittal cut that illustrates endoderm-lined foregut and a diverticulum (hepatic bud) extending ventrally into tissue of the septum transversum. [Species: Mouse, approximate human age: 27 days, sagittal section]

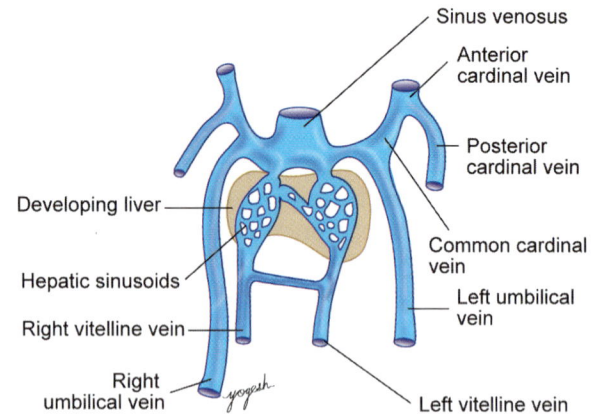

Fig. 15.2: Formation of hepatic sinusoids

Molecular Regulation of Liver Induction

- The cardiac mesoderm secretes fibroblast growth factor 2 (FGF2) that induces expression of the liver-specific genes in gut tissue and form hepatic bud.
- Bone morphogenic proteins (BMPs) enhances action of FGF2 on the gut.
- Hepatocyte nuclear transcription factors (HNF3 and 4) control differentiation of cells into hepatocytes and biliary cells.

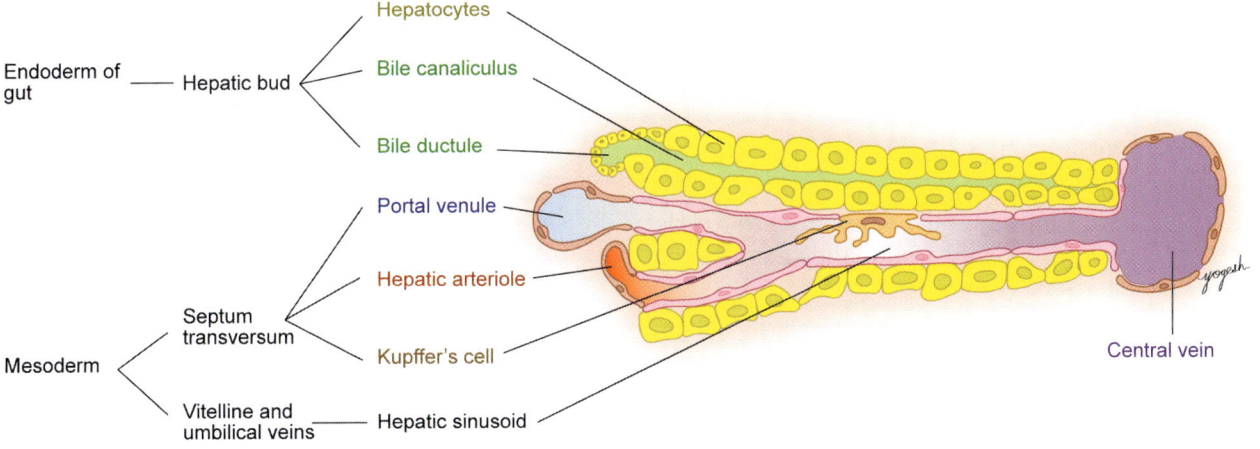

Fig. 15.3: Development of various components of liver

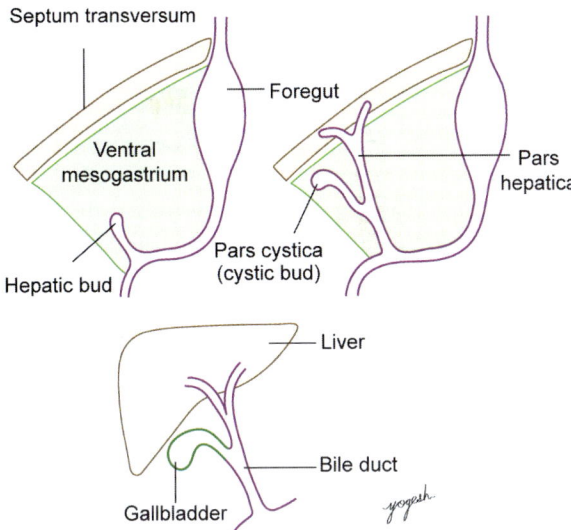

Practice Fig. 15.1: Development of liver and gallbladder

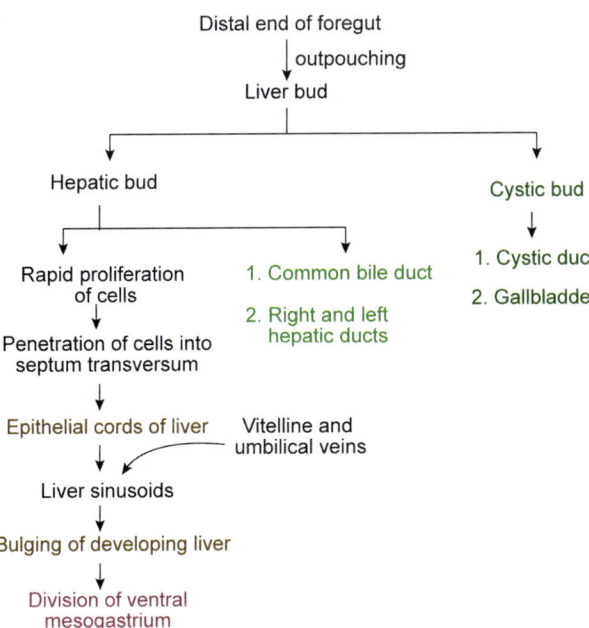

Flowchart 15.1: Development of liver

Congenital Anomalies of Liver

1. *Riedel's lobe*: It is a downward tongue-like extension of the right lobe of the liver. Often, it is mistaken for abnormal abdominal mass and lead to surgery.
2. *Polycystic liver disease* (PLD): It is a rare condition that results due to failure of union of intrahepatic biliary canaliculi and ductules with extrahepatic bile ducts. It results in formation of cysts within the liver. PLD is frequently associated with polycystic kidney disease and cystic pancreas.^MCQ These are transmitted as autosomal dominant disorder.
3. *Intrahepatic biliary atresia*: A failure of development of intrahepatic biliary system (atresia) is a serious condition that can be treated only with liver transplantation.
4. *Caroli's disease*: It involves congenital cystic dilatation (ectasia) of intrahepatic biliary tree.^MCQ
5. *Congenital hepatic fibrosis* is the inherited fibrocystic liver disease. Hepatic fibrosis produces portal hypertension.
6. One lobe or part of a lobe of liver may be absent. An extra lobe may be present. Complete liver may be rudimentary. Ectopic liver tissue may be present in the lesser omentum or falciform ligament.

Box 15.1: Histogenesis of liver

- Hepatic bud is derived from endoderm of the gut.
- From this bud, solid extensions grow into mesentery and form trabeculae that break up vitelline and umbilical veins into smaller channels.
- Trabeculae latter anastomose freely with one another. Lumen begin to appear in the trabeculae at about the fourth week.
- The hepatic trabeculae later form cords of liver cells. Lumen appears in the cord to form bile capillary.
- Trabeculae are broken up into hepatic cords by the ingrowth of branches from the sinusoids.

Contd.

Contd.

- Initially, in primary hepatic lobules, the trabeculae are not arranged radially and there are several central veins in each lobule.
- Branches of the portal vein invade the primary lobules and divide them into several secondary lobules and simultaneously hepatocyte cords become arranged radially around the central veins in a characteristic manner.
- Hepatic artery grows in the liver secondarily and its branches follow the course of branches of the portal vein.

DEVELOPMENT OF GALLBLADDER AND EXTRAHEPATIC BILIARY APPARATUS

Q. Write a short note on development of gallbladder.
Q. Write a short note on development of extrahepatic biliary apparatus.

Summary (Examination Guide)

- Refer to Table 15.2.

Table 15.2	Development of extrahepatic biliary apparatus
Part	Embryological source
Gallbladder	Cystic bud
Cystic duct	Cystic bud
Right and left hepatic ducts	Hepatic bud proper
Common bile duct	Proximal part of hepatic bud

Stages of Development (Figs 15.4, 15.5, Practice Fig. 15.2)

- Extrahepatic biliary apparatus is endodermal in origin.
- Gallbladder develops from *cystic bud* that arises from the *hepatic bud*. Originally hepatic bud arises from terminal part of the foregut (later it forms second part of duodenum).
- The hepatic bud grows ventrally and cranially in the ventral mesogastrium. The hepatic bud divides into pars cystica (cystic bud) and pars hepatica (hepatic bud proper). The pars hepatica divides into right and left hepatic ducts.
- Cystic bud enlarges to form gallbladder and cystic duct.
- Common hepatic ducts and cystic duct join to form common bile duct.
- Differential growth of duodenal wall turns opening of the common bile duct from ventral aspects to dorsomedial aspects of duodenum along with ventral pancreatic bud.

Anomalies of Gallbladder (Fig. 15.4)

1. *Agenesis of gallbladder:* It is absence of gallbladder.
2. *Sessile gallbladder:* It is an absence of cystic duct that results in direct fusion of gallbladder with common bile duct (Fig. 15.4D).

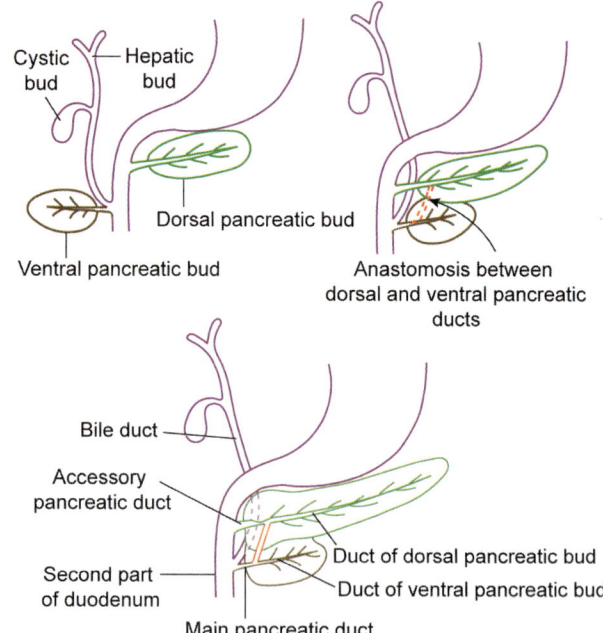

Practice Fig. 15.2: Development of pancreas

3. *Phrygian cap:* It is a gallbladder with fundus folded on itself to form cap-like structure (Fig. 15.4B).
4. *Hartmann's pouch:* It is an outpouching of neck of the gallbladder (Fig. 15.4C).
5. *Septate gallbladder:* Lumen of the gallbladder is divided into several segments with partial septae (Fig. 15.4E).
6. *Double gallbladder:* In double gallbladder, two gallbladders are present that are connected with the cystic duct.
7. *Intrahepatic gallbladder:* In this case, the gallbladder is embedded in the substance of liver.
8. *Floating gallbladder:* This gallbladder is lined by peritoneum on both surfaces and is free from liver.

Anomalies of Extrahepatic Biliary Ducts

1. *Atresia of ducts:* Ducts of extrahepatic biliary apparatus such as bile duct, common hepatic duct, hepatic ducts may be partially or completely absent.
2. *Accessory ducts:* Small accessory bile duct connecting liver with the gallbladder may be present.

DEVELOPMENT OF PANCREAS

Q. Write a short note on development of pancreas.[High yielding facts]

Summary (Examination Guide) (Table 15.3)

- Pancreas develops from endodermal ventral and dorsal pancreatic buds that arise from caudal part of the foregut (junctional zone of foregut and midgut).
- Proliferation of these endodermal buds form ducts, parenchyma (acini) and islets of Langerhans.

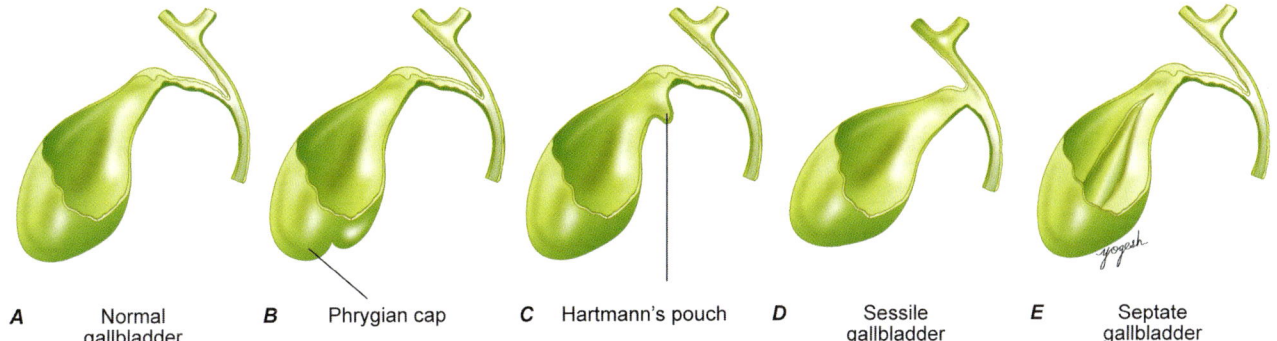

A	B	C	D	E
Normal gallbladder	Phrygian cap	Hartmann's pouch	Sessile gallbladder	Septate gallbladder

Fig. 15.4: Developmental anomalies of gallbladder

Table 15.3 Development of pancreas^{High yielding facts, NEXT}

Part	Embryological source
Lower part of head and uncinate process	Ventral pancreatic bud
Upper part of head and neck, body and tail	Dorsal pancreatic bud
Main pancreatic duct	Duct of ventral pancreatic bud Distal part of duct of dorsal pancreatic bud^{NEXT}
Accessory pancreatic duct	Proximal part of duct of dorsal pancreatic bud^{NEXT}
Connective tissue	Mesoderm

Note: The pancreatic acini and islets of Langerhans are derived from endodermal pancreatic buds. ^{MCQ}

By 7th week, α-cells start secreting glucagon and by 10th week, β-cells start secreting insulin. ^{MCQ} Glucagon can be detected in fetal plasma 15th week onward.

- Adjacent splanchnopleuric mesoderm condenses to form capsule, blood vessels and other connective tissue of pancreas.

Stages of Development of Pancreas (Figs 15.5 to 15.7, Flowchart 15.2, Practice Figs 15.2, 15.3)

1. *Formation of pancreatic bud*
   - By 3rd week, *ventral* and *dorsal pancreatic buds* arise from ventral and dorsal wall of terminal part of the foregut (Fig. 15.5B).^{MCQ} (Dorsal pancreatic bud appears earlier than ventral.)
   - Ventral pancreatic bud arises in combination of hepatic bud and they share a combined opening in the duodenum (Fig. 15.5B).
   - Ventral pancreatic bud is smaller and appears distal to dorsal pancreatic bud.
   - Ventral pancreatic bud grows in ventral duodenal mesentery, whereas dorsal pancreatic bud grows in dorsal duodenal mesentery (Fig. 15.5C).
2. *Rotation of buds*
   - Differential growth wall of duodenum, and rotation of duodenum brings ventral pancreatic bud with common bile duct (arise from hepatic bud) to the right of duodenum and dorsal bud to the left of duodenum (Fig. 15.5D).
   - Continuous differential growth of duodenal wall brings the ventral pancreatic bud closer and proximal to the dorsal bud (Fig. 15.5D, E).
   - Finally, both the buds fuse with each other in 7th week of IUL (Fig. 15.5E).
3. *Formation of pancreatic ducts*
   - Ducts of dorsal and ventral pancreatic bud anastomose and derive the following ducts:
     a. *Main pancreatic duct:* It is formed by duct of ventral pancreatic bud, distal part of duct of dorsal pancreatic bud and anastomosing channel between these ducts (Fig. 15.6).
     b. *Accessory pancreatic duct:* It is formed by proximal part of duct of the dorsal pancreatic bud (Fig. 15.6).
4. *Formation of acini and islet of Langerhans:*
   - Both ventral and dorsal pancreatic buds branch enormously.
   - At the end of each branch, pancreatic acini appear.
   - Some cells of pancreatic duct get separated and form islet of Langerhans by third week and start secretion of insulin by 10th week. ^{MCQ}
5. Surrounding mesoderm forms capsule, connective tissue, septae and blood vessels of the pancreas.
6. Along with duodenum, pancreas also becomes retroperitoneal except at its tail that lies in lienorenal ligament.

Molecular Regulation of Pancreas Development

- FGF2 and activin are produced by notochord and dorsal aorta upregulate pancreatic and duodenal homeobox1 (PDX) genes.
- PDX6 expressing cells form *alpha cells* that secrete glucagon.
- PDX4 and PDX6 expressing cells form *beta cells* that secrete insulin, *delta cells* that secrete somatostatin and *gamma cells* that secret pancreatic polypeptides.

Anomalies of Pancreas

Q. Write a short note on developmental anomalies of pancreas.

1. Annular pancreas (Box 15.2).
2. *Divided pancreas* **(pancreatic divisum):** It occurs due to failure of fusion of dorsal and ventral pancreatic

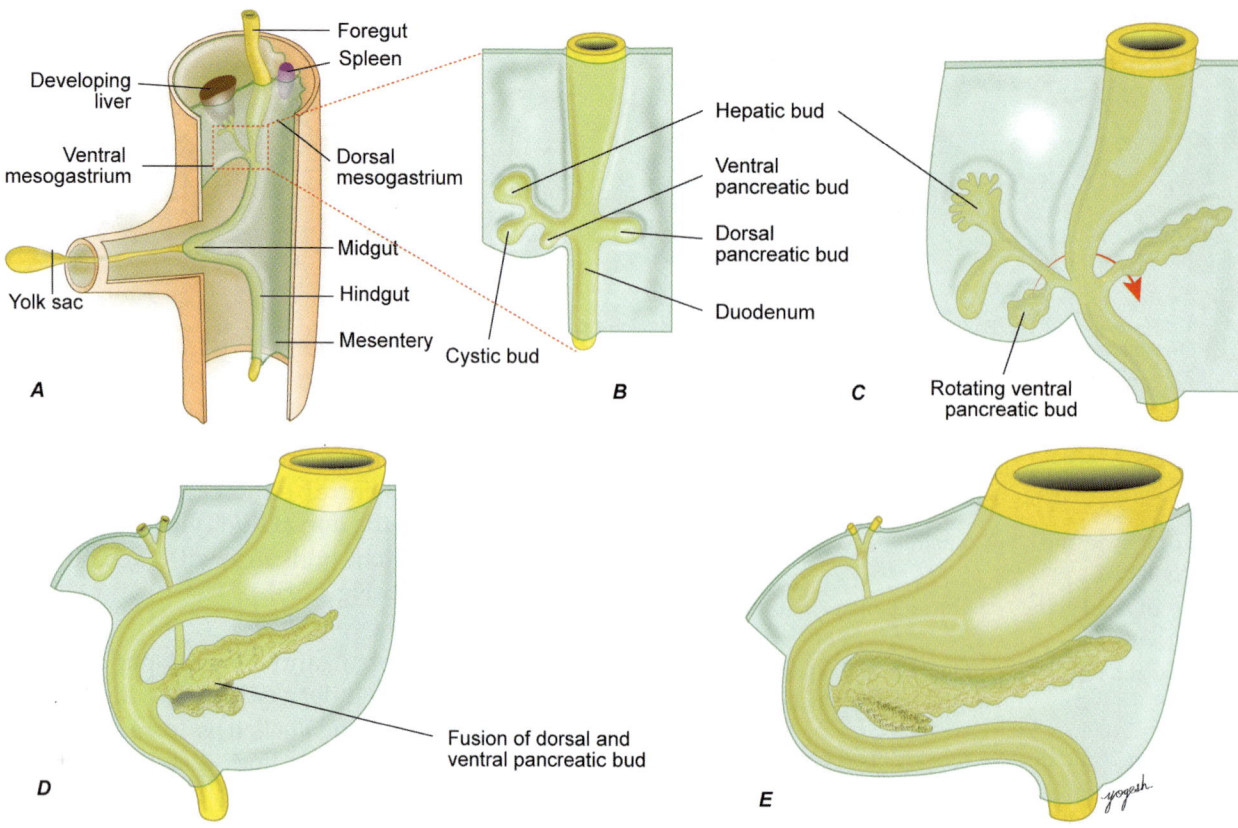

Fig. 15.5: Successive stages of development of pancreas. Pancreas develops by fusion of ventral and dorsal pancreatic bud

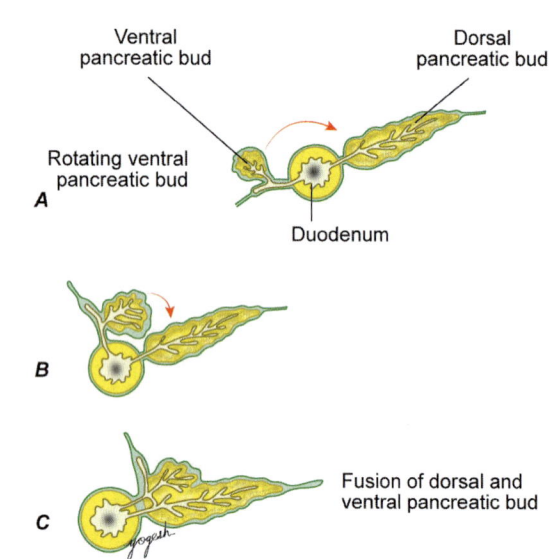

Fig. 15.6: Rotation of the ventral pancreatic bud during the development of the pancreas

buds. It is most common congenital anomaly of pancreas.^{NEXT}

3. *Accessory pancreatic tissue*: This ectopic pancreatic tissue that lies in the wall of stomach, duodenum, gallbladder, and Meckel's diverticulum.^{NEXT} Most common site of ectopic pancreatic tissue is stomach.^{NEXT}
4. *Inversion of pancreatic duct*: In this condition, the main pancreatic duct is formed by duct of dorsal pancreatic

---

Box 15.2: Annular pancreas (Fig. 15.8)

Q. Write a short note on annular pancreas.

- It is a congenital anomaly where second part of duodenum is surrounded by a ring of pancreatic tissue.
- Incidence: 1 in 12,000–15,000 newborns, males are affected more than females.
- Cause: Usually pancreas develops from ventral and dorsal pancreatic buds. Differential growth of duodenal wall and rotation of duodenum brings ventral and dorsal pancreatic bud together and they fuse. Bifid ventral pancreatic bud (main reason) or failure of rotation of the ventral pancreatic bud may result in annular pancreas.
- Effect: Annular pancreas may cause pancreatitis, peptic ulcers, duodenal obstruction. In intraembryonic life, it may result in polyhydramnios.
- Radiograph of abdomen shows *double bubble* appearance due to gas in stomach and proximal part of duodenum.
- Treatment: Surgical treatment to bypass the obstructed segment of duodenum by duodenojejunostomy is required.

bud and opens at minor duodenal papilla, whereas duct of ventral pancreatic bud joins common bile duct and opens at the major duodenal papilla.

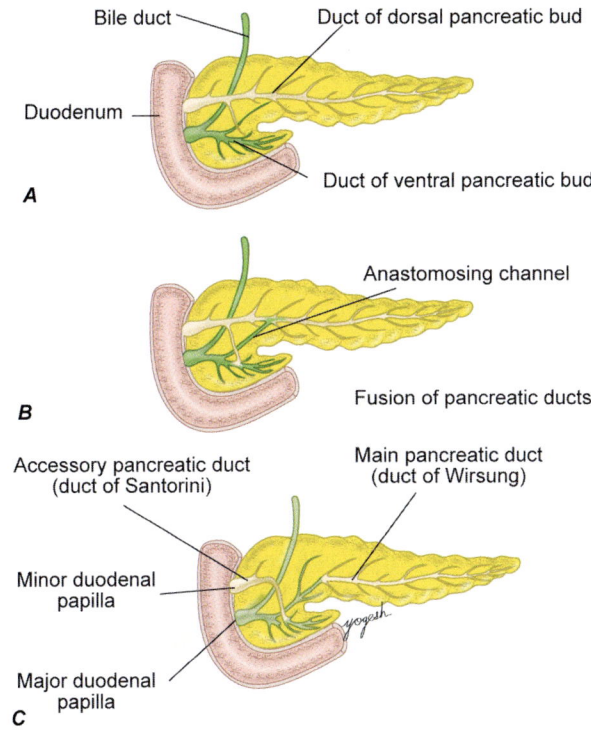

Fig. 15.7: Development of pancreatic duct system

Flowchart 15.2: Development of pancreas

A. Parenchyma

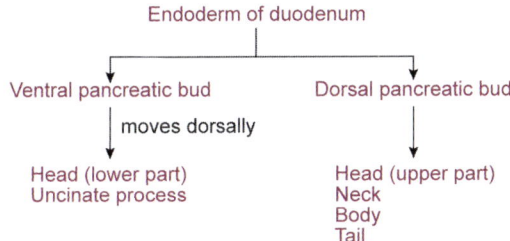

B. Islets of Langerhans

3rd week: Formation of Islets
Seventh week: Alpha-cells start secreting glucagon
Tenth week: Beta-cells start secreting insulin

C. Pancreatic ducts

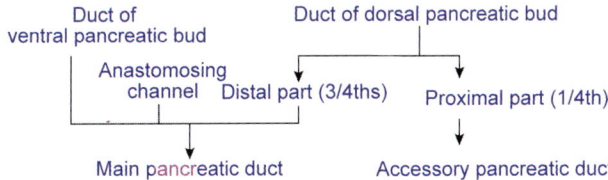

DEVELOPMENT OF SPLEEN

Q. Write a short note on development of spleen.

- Spleen develops in the dorsal mesogastrium from mesoderm.^{NEXT}
- The dorsal mesogastrium is divided by developing spleen into ventral gastrosplenic ligament and dorsal lienorenal ligament (Fig. 15.8).
- Mesoderm gives rise to capsule, septa, connective tissue network, reticular fibres, lymphocytes, and hematopoietic cells.

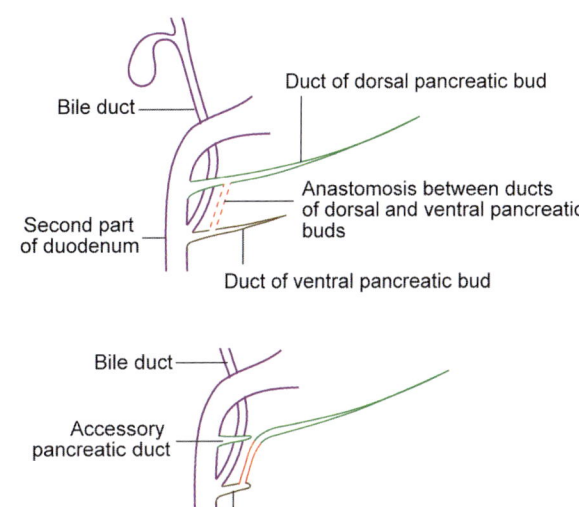

Practice Fig. 15.3: Formation of duct system of pancreas

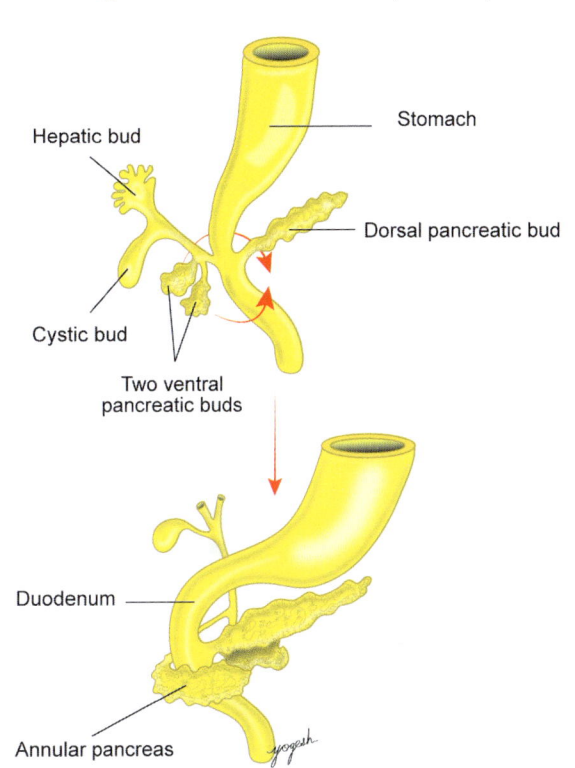

Fig. 15.8: Formation of annular pancreas. There may be two ventral pancreatic buds that fuse with dorsal pancreatic bud surrounding duodenum to form annular pancreas

Stages of Development (Fig. 15.9, Flowchart 15.3)

1. *Formation of spleniculi*: During the 5th week of IUL, mesenchymal cells in dorsal mesogastrium form small mesenchymal masses called *spleniculi* or *splenic lobules*.
2. *Fusion of spleniculi*: Spleniculi fuses to form a single splenic mass.
3. Lobulated development of spleen in an adult is indicated by splenic notches (usually lies along the superior border of spleen).^{NEXT}
4. *Formation of ligaments*: Developing spleen divides dorsal mesogastrium into *gastrosplenic* and *lienorenal*

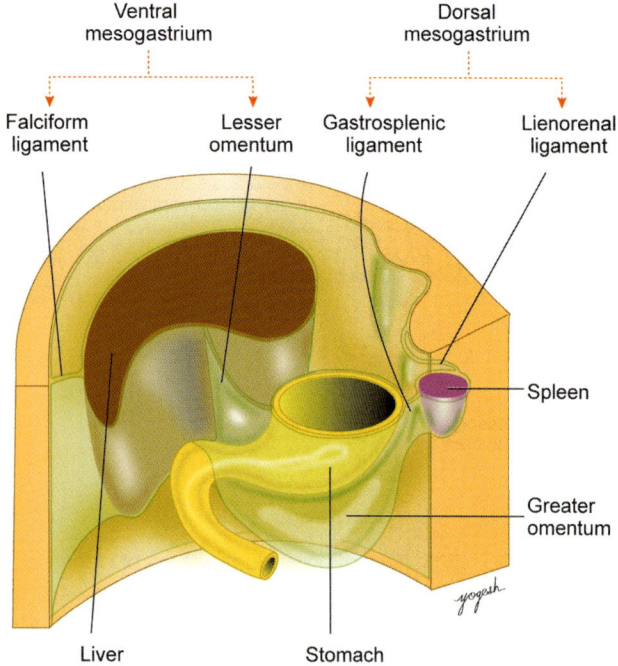

Fig. 15.9: Developing spleen in dorsal mesogastrium

ligaments. Lienorenal (splenorenal) ligament contains splenic artery.^{NEXT}

5. *Change in splenic position*: The following factors bring the spleen to its usual position:
   – Rotation of stomach
   – Fusion of posterior layer of dorsal mesogastrium with posterior abdominal wall.
6. *Hematopoiesis:* Spleen acts as hematopoietic organ in fetal life until birth.

Flowchart 15.3: Development of spleen

5th week of IUL: Formation of speniculi in dorsal mesogastrium
↓
Fusion of spelniculi
↓
Formation of single spleen with splenic notches
↓
Division of dorsal mesogastrium → Gastrosplenic ligament
                                 → Linorenal ligament
↓
Hematopoiesis

Anomalies Accessory spleen, lobulated spleen, polysplenia, asplenia

7. *Molecular regulation:* Spleen development is mainly regulated by Hox11, Bapx 1, and capsulin genes.

Anomalies of Spleen

1. *Accessory spleen*: Failure of fusion of spleniculi with the main splenic tissue give rise to accessory spleen at the following sites:
   – Hilus of spleen
   – Gastrosplenic ligament
   – Lienorenal ligament
   – Tail of pancreas
   – Along the splenic artery
   – Left spermatic cord
2. *Lobulated spleen*: Incomplete fusion of spleniculi (persistent fetal spleen) produces lobulated spleen.
3. *Right-sided bilaterality or isomerism* is characterized by *asplenia* or *hypoplastic spleen*, whereas *left-sided bilaterality* is characterized by *polysplenia*.^{NEXT}

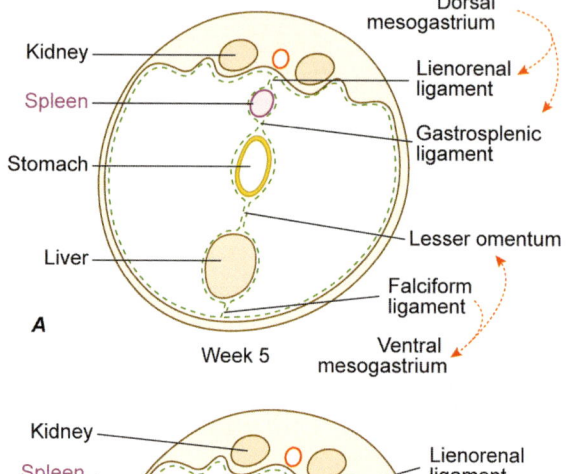
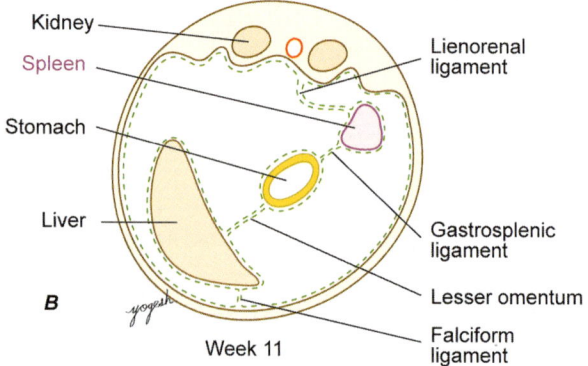

Practice Fig. 15.4: Development of spleen

Chapter 16

Respiratory System

eSmartQuiz

Chapter Outline

- Introduction
  - Formation of lung bud
- Development of larynx
  - Stages of development
  - Anomalies of larynx
- Development of trachea
  - Anomalies of trachea
- Tracheoesophageal fistula
- Development of bronchi and lungs
  - Formation of pleural cavity and pleura
  - Formation of intrapulmonary bronchi
  - Parenchyma of lung
  - Maturation of lungs
  - Anomalies of lungs
- Hyaline membrane disease

Competencies:
- **AN25.2:** Describe development of pleura, lung and heart. (Lung development is included in this chapter.)
- **AN25.4:** Describe embryological basis of atrial septal defect, ventricular septal defect, Fallot's tetralogy, tracheoesophageal fistula. (Tracheoesophageal fistula is included in this chapter.)

INTRODUCTION

Formation of Lung Bud

- Respiratory system develops from
  - *Lung bud* that arises from foregut and
  - Connective tissue from *splanchnic mesoderm*.
- During 4th week, *laryngotracheal groove* appears caudal to the hypobranchial eminence in the floor of pharynx (Fig. 16.1 and Flowchart 16.1).
- The laryngotracheal groove deepens to form a *laryngotracheal tube (respiratory diverticulum)* that grows caudally (Fig. 16.2A, B, Practice Fig. 16.1).
- Laryngotracheal tube bifurcates to form *two (right and left) lung buds* (Fig. 16.2C).
- Pharyngeal cells expressing **TBX4** factor form lung buds.
- Fate of laryngotracheal tube and lung bud:
  - Proximal part of laryngotracheal tube forms *larynx*, whereas its distal part forms *trachea*.

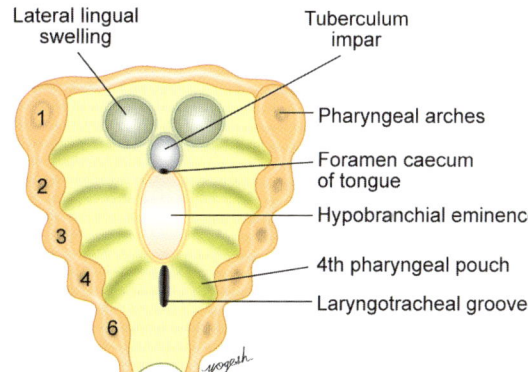

Fig. 16.1: A section of the pharynx of the embryo at 4th week. Laryngotracheal groove appears in the floor of the pharynx just caudal to the hypobranchial eminence

- Lung buds form primordium of *bronchial tree* and *lungs*.
- Splanchnic mesoderm forms surrounding connective tissue.
- On either side of laryngotracheal tube (diverticulum), two *tracheoesophageal folds* arise.
- These folds fuse to form *tracheoesophageal septum* that separates laryngotracheal tube from the esophagus (Fig. 16.2A to C).

Flowchart 16.1: Development of respiratory system

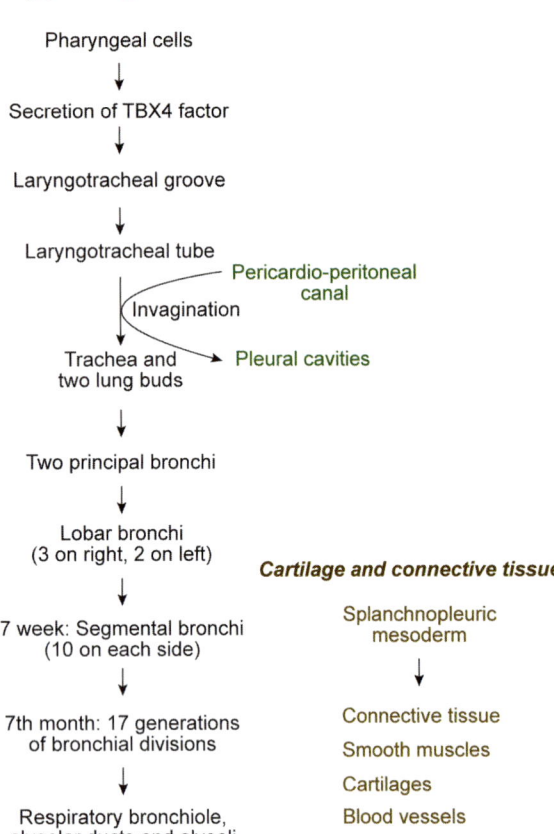

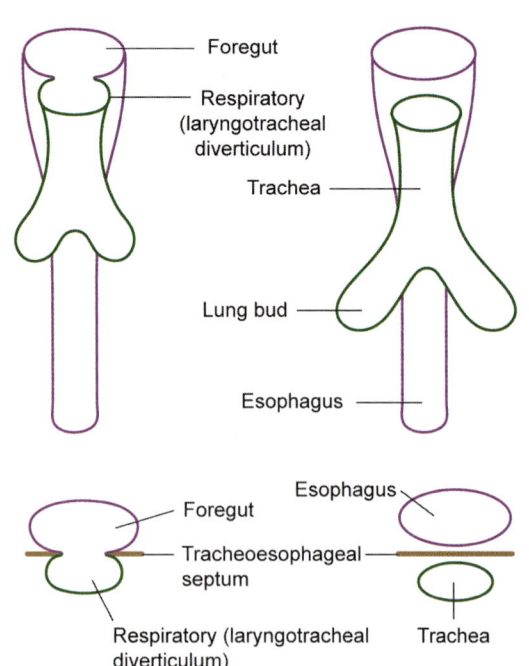

Practice Fig. 16.1: Formation of respiratory diverticulum

Table 16.1	Development of larynx
Part	*Embryological source*
Mucosa	Proximal part of laryngotracheal tube
Vestibular and vocal folds	Endodermal folds of laryngotracheal tube
Cartilages	All cartilages – fourth and sixth arches *except* epiglottis – hypobranchial eminence
Intrinsic muscles	All from sixth arch except cricothyroid from fourth arch.
Nerve supply	Motor All muscles by recurrent laryngeal nerve except cricothyroid by external laryngeal branch of superior laryngeal nerve Sensory Above vocal folds – internal laryngeal branch of superior laryngeal nerve Below vocal folds – recurrent laryngeal nerve

- Cranial extension of tracheoesophageal septum is arrested by the inlet of larynx (*furcula of His*) through which the larynx communicates with pharynx.^MCQ
- Lung buds invaginate into *pericardio-peritoneal canals* that later form *pleural cavities*.

DEVELOPMENT OF LARYNX

Q. Write a short note on development of larynx.

- The larynx is a voice box, a part of respiratory system that has a laryngeal inlet, vestibular and vocal folds, cartilages and muscles in the wall (Flowchart 16.2).

Summary (Examination Guide)

- Components of larynx are derived as follows (Table 16.1):
  1. *Lining epithelium* develops from endoderm of *laryngotracheal diverticulum*.
  2. *Vestibular and vocal folds* develop from endodermal folds arising from a laryngotracheal diverticulum.
  3. *Cartilages of larynx*: All the cartilages (thyroid, cricoid, cuneiform, corniculate, arytenoids) of larynx develop from the fourth and sixth arches, except epiglottis that develops from hypobranchial eminence.^MCQ
  4. *Muscles of larynx*: All muscles of larynx develop from sixth pharyngeal arches except cricothyroid that develops from fourth pharyngeal arch.
  5. Nerve supply is derived from superior laryngeal nerve (fourth arch) and recurrent laryngeal nerve (sixth arch).

Stages of Development

- Larynx develops from cranial part of *laryngotracheal diverticulum* that arises from the floor of the pharynx.
- Communication between laryngotracheal diverticulum and pharynx forms the *inlet of larynx* (Fig. 16.3A).
- Due to differential growth of fourth and sixth arches, mesenchyme surrounding the larynx converts the laryngeal opening into a T-shaped orifice (Fig. 16.3B).
- Endoderm of larynx proliferates to block the lumen. Later, the lumen gets recanalized.

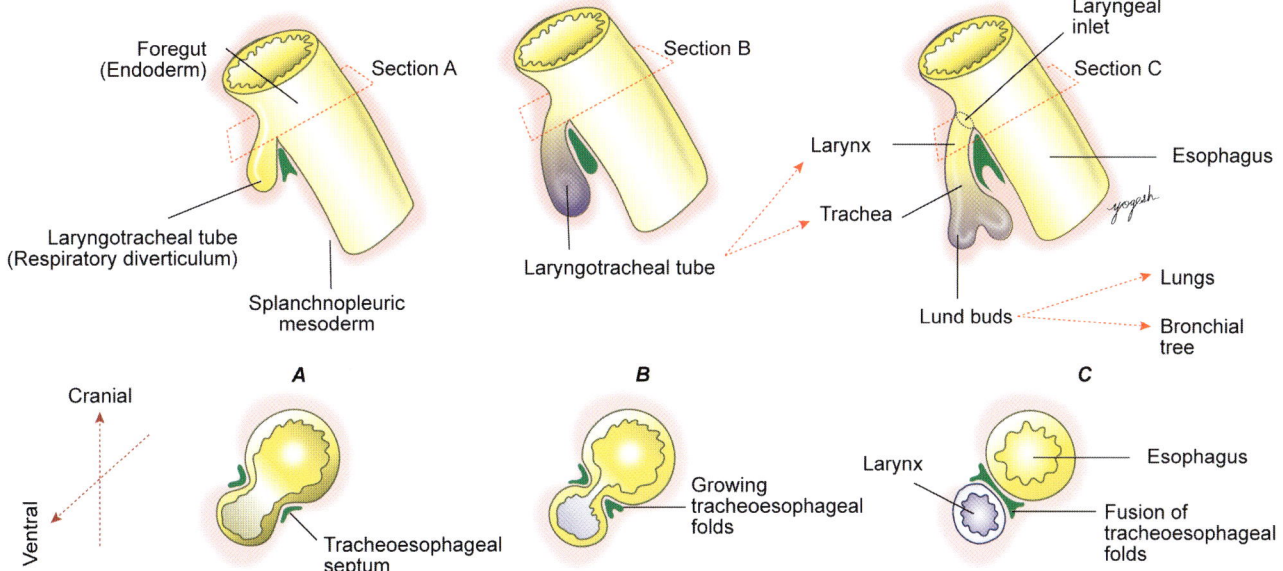

Fig. 16.2: Formation of tracheal bud and lung bud. Tracheoesophageal septum separates trachea from esophagus

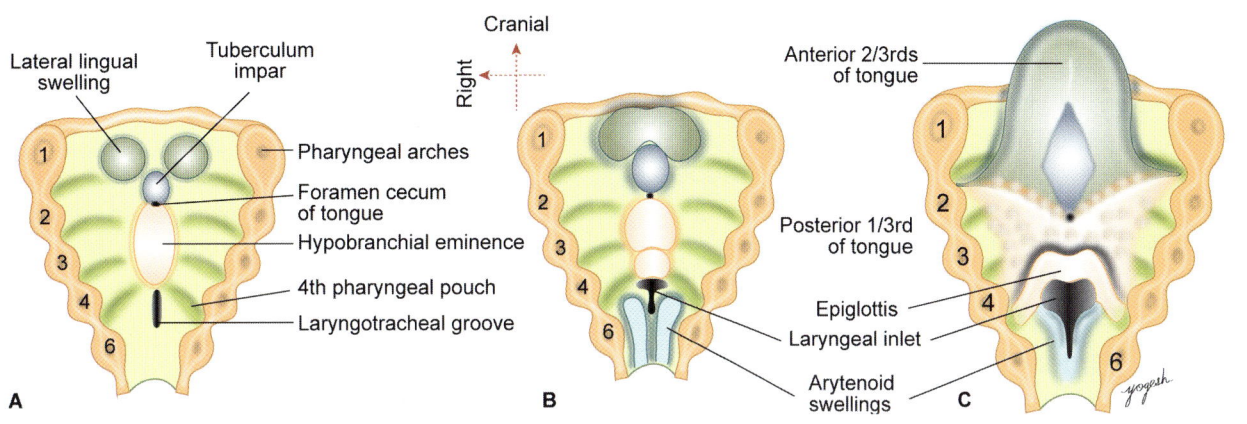

Fig. 16.3: (A) A section of pharynx of the embryo at 4th week. Slit-shaped laryngotracheal groove appears in the floor of pharynx just caudal to hypobranchial eminence; (B) 6 weeks; and (C) 10 weeks: On development of arytenoid swellings and epiglottis, laryngotracheal groove (later that forms inlet of the larynx) becomes T-shaped

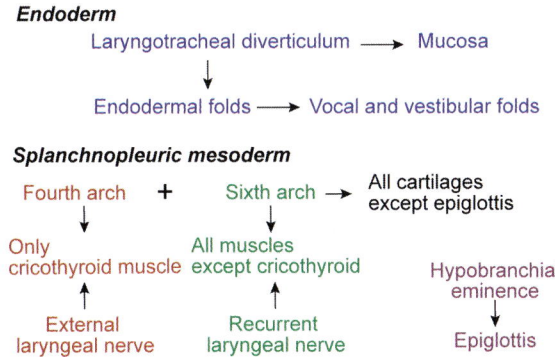

Flowchart 16.2: Development of larynx

- During luminal recanalization, the endoderm forms two pairs of folding, proximal vestibular and distal vocal pair of folds.
- *Vestibular fold* gives rise to false vocal cord and *vocal fold* to true vocal cord.
- The recess between vestibular fold and vocal fold forms *ventricle of larynx*.
- Mesenchyme of fourth and sixth arches forms all *cartilages of larynx* (thyroid, cricoid, arytenoids, corniculate and cuneiform) except epiglottis that derives from hypobranchial eminence.^{MCQ}
- All intrinsic muscles are derived from sixth arch except cricothyroid. Hence, all muscles of the larynx are supplied by recurrent laryngeal nerve except cricothyroid that is supplied by an external laryngeal branch of superior laryngeal nerve.^{MCQ}
- Vocal folds lie at the junction of fourth and sixth arches, hence mucosa above the vocal fold is innervated from an internal laryngeal branch of the vagus nerve (4th arch) and below the vocal fold is innervated by recurrent laryngeal nerve (6th arch).

Anomalies of Larynx

1. *Laryngocele*: It is congenital anomalous air sac in the neck communicating with the cavity of larynx.
2. *Congenital laryngeal atresia and stenosis*: It results from failure of the laryngeal recanalization (atresia is blockage and stenosis means narrowing).
3. *Larygoptosis*: Larynx is localized in a lower position than its usual position, may be due to absence of some of laryngeal cartilages.
4. *Laryngeal web*: Lumen of larynx has membrane-like structure. It may result due to incomplete recanalization of laryngeal lumen. It produces partial airway obstruction.

DEVELOPMENT OF TRACHEA

- Trachea develops from a part of *laryngotracheal tube* that lies between developing larynx and point of bifurcation of the tube (lung buds).

Summary (Examination Guide)

- Components of trachea develop as follows:
  1. Lining epithelium and glands develop from endoderm of *laryngotracheal tube*.
  2. Cartilages, connective tissue and trachealis muscle develop from *splanchnopleuric mesoderm* surrounding laryngotracheal tube.
- Trachea is separated from esophagus by a *tracheoesophageal septum* that is derived from tracheoesophageal folds.

Anomalies of Trachea

1. *Agenesis of trachea*: Failure of formation of laryngotracheal tube results in agenesis of trachea.
2. *Tracheoesophageal fistula*: Box 16.1.
3. *Tracheal stenosis*: It occurs due to ventral deviation of the tracheoesophageal septum.

Box 16.1: Tracheoesophageal fistula (TEF)

Q. Write a short note on tracheoesophageal fistula.

- Definition: Tracheoesophageal fistula is an abnormal congenital communication between the trachea and esophagus.
- Incidence: 1:3000–4500 births.
- Causes:
  Right and left tracheoesophageal folds on fusion form tracheoesophageal septum that separates the trachea from the esophagus. Failure of fusion of tracheoesophageal septum results in TEF.
- Types (Fig. 16.4):
  TEF can be classified according to morphology and anatomical locations as follows:
  – *Type A*: It is not true TEF. Both proximal and distal esophageal segments do not communicate with each other or with the trachea (Fig. 16.4A).
  – *Type B*: Proximal esophageal segment communicates with lower tracheal segment and distal esophageal segment forms blind pouch (Fig. 16.4B).
  – *Type C*: Proximal esophageal atresia (blind pouch) and distal esophagus arise from the trachea (Fig. 16.4C).
  – *Type D*: Proximal and distal esophageal segments communicate with the trachea (Fig. 16.4D).
  – *Type E*: Esophagus communicates with the trachea without any atresia (Fig. 16.4E).
- Clinical presentation:
  Esophageal atresia and subsequent inability to swallow amniotic fluid results in *polyhydramnios* (excess accumulation of amniotic fluid).
  TEF presents with coughing, vomiting, *cyanosis* in newborn with the onset of feeding (entry of milk in the lungs).
- Treatment: *Emergency surgical repair* is required to save the newborn. It involves surgical resection of fistula and anastomosis of proximal and distal esophageal segments.

---

4. *Tracheal bronchus*: There may be a blind diverticulum (*tracheal bronchus*) arising from trachea.
5. *Tracheal lobe*: A separate bronchus may rise from trachea and supply an isolated lobe of lung called tracheal lobe.

DEVELOPMENT OF BRONCHI AND LUNGS

- During the 5th week of IUL, *laryngotracheal diverticulum* divides into right and left principal bronchus (initially *lung buds*) (Practice Fig. 16.2).

Formation of Pleural Cavity and Pleura

- Lung buds grow in caudal and lateral direction and bulge into *pleuroperitoneal canals*.

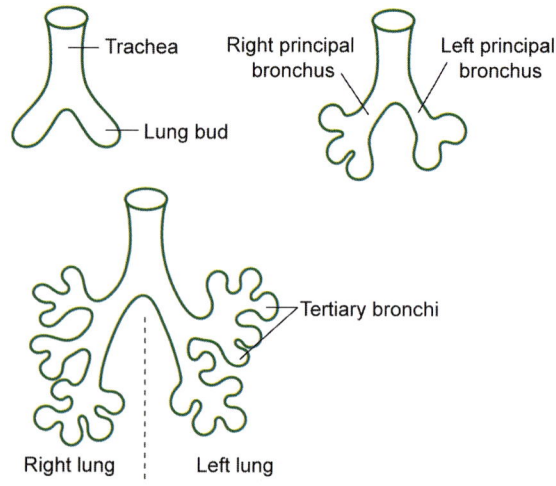

Practice Fig. 16.2: Development of lungs

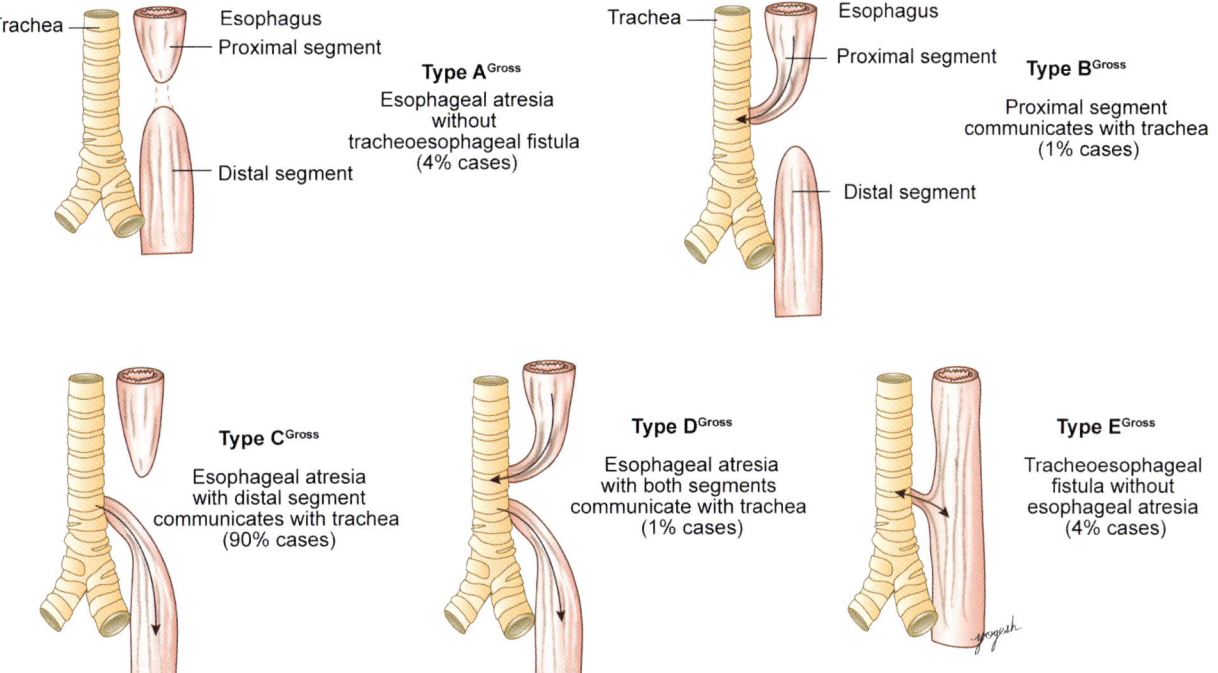

Fig. 16.4: Types of tracheoesophageal fistula: Types A to E according to Gross classification

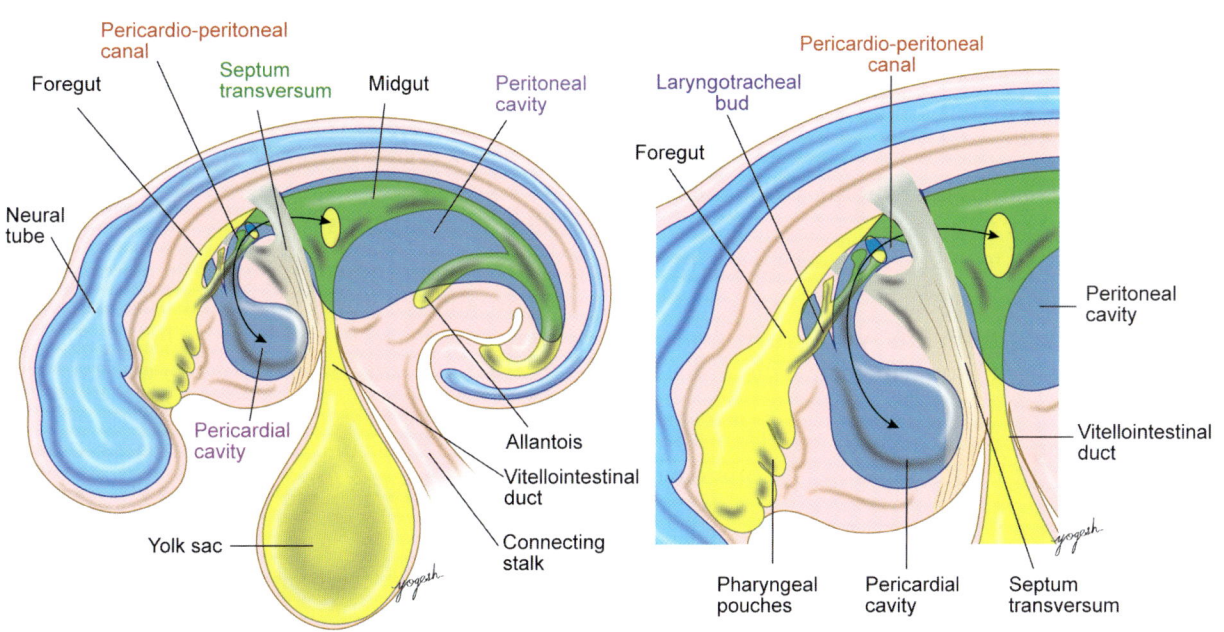

Fig. 16.5: Section of the embryo at 4th week. The laryngotracheal bud raises from the foregut and grows caudally. The laryngotracheal bud divides into two lung buds. Each one of the lung buds enters in the pericardio-peritoneal canal (shown by arrow) and enlarges to form lung. The pericardio-peritoneal canal communicates between the pericardial cavity cranially and peritoneal cavity caudally. Two pericardio-peritoneal canals run on either side of the foregut, behind the septum transversum

- Soon small pleuroperitoneal canals get filled with the growing lungs. Later, the canals start enlarging to accommodate the growing lungs (Figs 16.5 to 16.7).
- Pleuropericardial and pleuroperitoneal folds separate the pleuroperitoneal canals from pericardial and peritoneal cavities respectively. Thus, isolated pleuroperitoneal canal forms pleural cavities (for details, refer Chapter 17).
- A layer of *splanchnopleuric mesoderm* in contact with lung bud forms *visceral pleura* and *somatopleuric layer* forms *parietal pleura*.

Formation of Intrapulmonary Bronchi

Q. Write a short note on development of lung.

- *Left principal bronchus* divides into upper and lower secondary or lobar bronchi, whereas *right principal bronchus* divides into superior, middle and lower lobar bronchi (Figs 16.6, 16.7, 16.9).

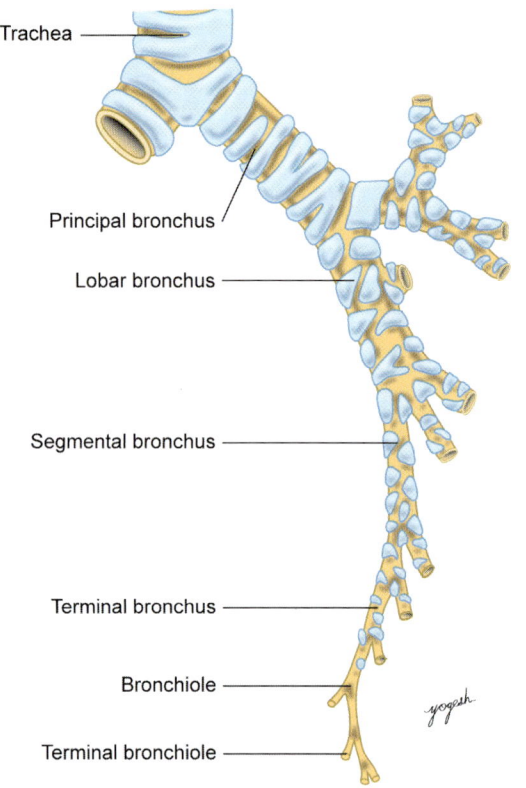

Fig. 16.6: Structures in conducting part of respiratory tract (no gaseous excahge)

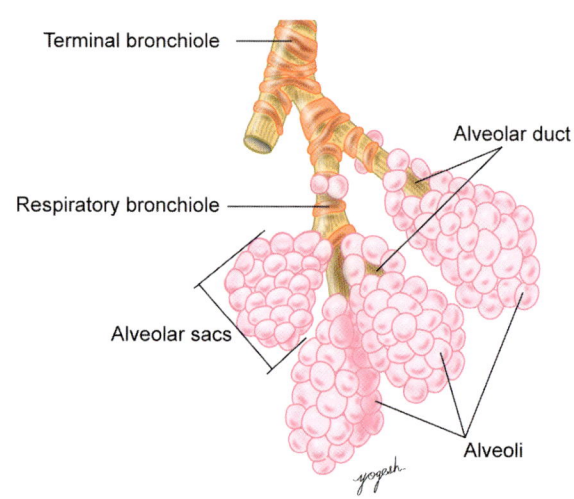

Fig. 16.7: Structures in respiratory part (zone of gaseous exchange)

- Each *secondary bronchus* later supplies a lobe of lung that is separated by fissures.
- In the 7th week of IUL, the secondary bronchi divide to form *10 segmental bronchi*.
- Each segmental bronchus with surrounding splanchnopleuric mesoderm forms the *bronchopulmonary segments*.
- Up to the end of 7th month of IUL, about 17 generations of bronchial subdivisions occur.

- About 6–7 divisions take place after birth before formation of adult lung.^{MCQ}
- Distal bronchial subdivisions form bronchioles, respiratory bronchioles, alveolar ducts and alveoli.

Parenchyma of Lung

- Lining epithelium of bronchial tree and alveoli develop from *endoderm of respiratory diverticulum*.
- Cartilages, blood vessels and other connective tissue elements develop from *splanchnopleuric mesoderm*.

Maturation of Lungs

Q. Write a short note on stages of maturation of lung.

- Maturation of lungs is divided into four phases or periods (Fig. 16.10 and Practice Fig. 16.3)
  1. Pseudoglandular period (6–16 weeks)
  2. Canalicular period (16–26 weeks)
  3. Terminal saccular period (26 weeks to birth) and
  4. Alveolar period (32 weeks to 8 years)

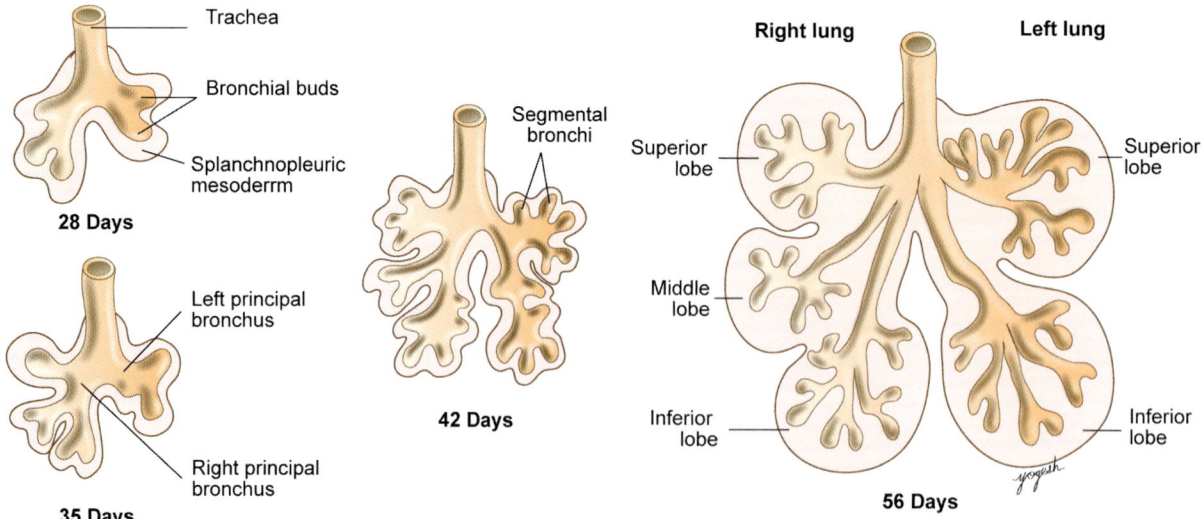

Fig. 16.8: Development of the lungs

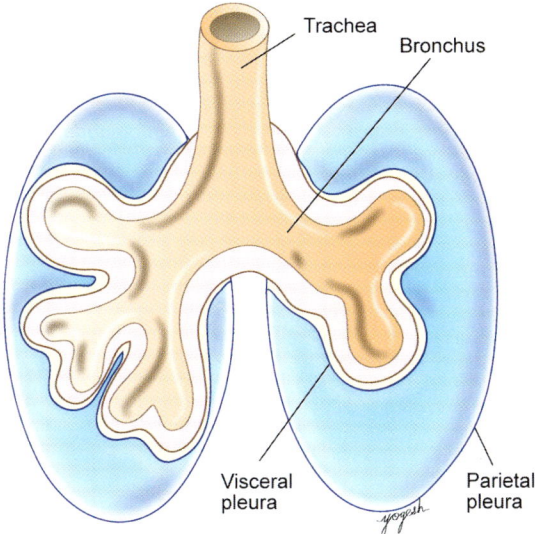

Fig. 16.9: Expanding lungs in pericardio-peritoneal canal. Splanchnopleuric mesoderm forms visceral pleura, whereas somatopleuric mesoderm forms parietal pleura. The cavity of pleuroperitoneal canal forms pleural cavity

Some Interesting Facts

1. Fetal kidneys maintain amniotic fluid volume that helps in fetal lung development. Hence, renal agenesis is associated with pulmonary hypoplasia (failure of lung development).
2. By the 7th month, pulmonary circulation becomes enough to provide adequate oxygen for sustaining the life. Hence, a newborn becomes viable at this age. *MCQ, Clinical fact*
3. TBX4 factor (T-box transcription factor) is a transcription factor that belongs to a T-box gene family and involved in the regulation of embryonic developmental processes. This transcription factor is encoded by TBX4 gene located on human chromosome 17.

1. Pseudoglandular period
– Developing lung resembles an exocrine gland, hence called *pseudoglandular period*. At the end of this period, all the major elements of lung up to terminal bronchiole are formed.
– As respiratory bronchioles and alveoli are not yet developed, the fetus is not viable.

2. Canalicular period
– During this stage, respiratory bronchiole, alveolar ducts and primary alveoli are formed.
– Fetus born at the end of canalicular period can survive with intensive care. *Clinical Fact*

3. Terminal sac period
– During this stage, a substantial number of primary alveoli are formed.
– Blood–air barrier (endothelio-epithelial barrier) thin out.

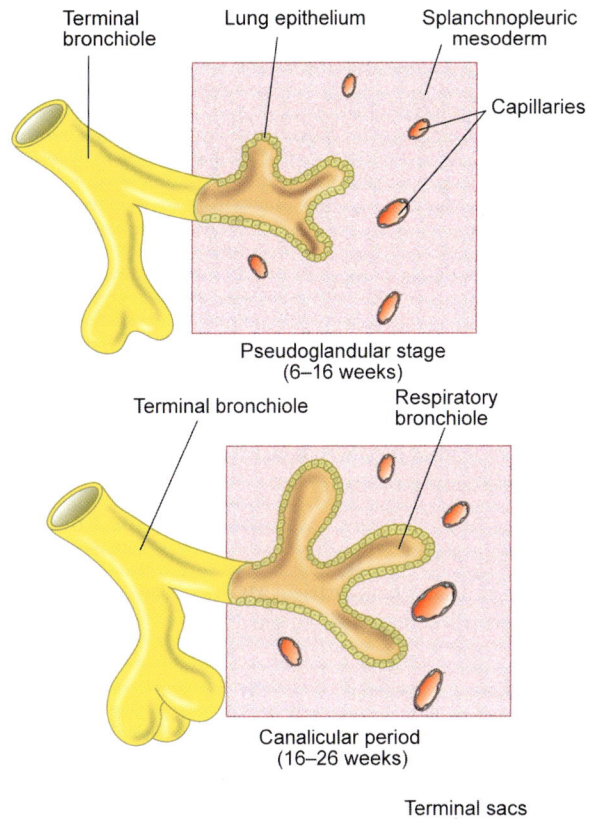

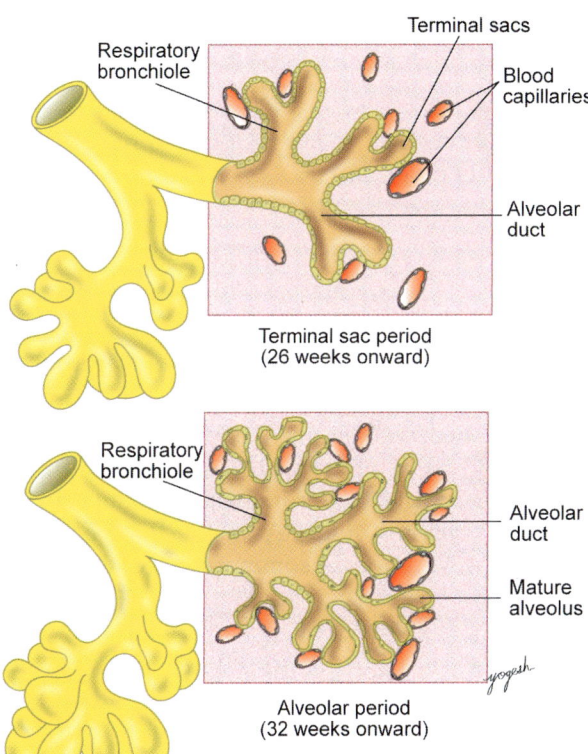

Fig. 16.10: Maturation of the lung. Alveoli are lined by simple squamous epithelium (type I pneumocytes) and some type II pneumocytes (Flowchart 16.3)

– Alveoli are lined with type I and a few type II pneumocytes. Type II pneumocytes produce surfactant.
– The quantity of surfactant increases gradually toward the full-term.

Flowchart 16.3: Maturation of lung

6–16 weeks	Pseudoglandular stage	Lungs resemble exocrine glands
16–26 weeks	Canalicular period	Formation of respiratory bronchioles, alveolar ducts, primary alveoli
26–32 weeks	Terminal sac period	Thinning of blood–air barrier Increase in quantity of surfactant
32 weeks onward	Alveolar period	Formation of definitive alveoli Increasing quantity of surfactant

4. **Alveolar period**
   – During this period, definitive alveoli develop and increases in number.
   – Type II pneumocytes continue production of more surfactant.
   – Formation of definitive alveoli continues after the birth up to the age of 8th years.

Anomalies of Lungs

Q. Write a short note on azygos lobe.

1. *Hyaline membrane disease* (Box 16.2).
2. *Agenesis and hypoplasia*: Part or complete lung on one side may be absent or underdeveloped.
3. *Abnormal lobulation*:
   - The absence of fissure results in a reduction of a number of lobes.
   - Extra fissure: It includes following cases:
     – A transverse fissure in left lung
     – A separate medial basal segment called *cardiac lobe*
     – A separate superior segment of lower lobe
4. *Azygos lobe (lobe of Wrisberg)*: Part of upper lobe of the right lung that lies medial to arch of azygos vein is called *azygos lobe* (Fig. 16.11). A vertical fissure separates azygos lobe from rest of the superior lobe of lung. Azygos vein lies on the floor of vertical fissure. Azygos lobe is commonest accessory lobe of the lung.^{MCQ}

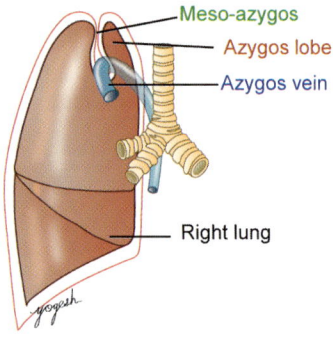

Fig. 16.11: Azygos lobe. Azygos lobe is separated from the apex of the right lung by meso-azygos. In the floor of the vertical fissure, the azygos vein is present

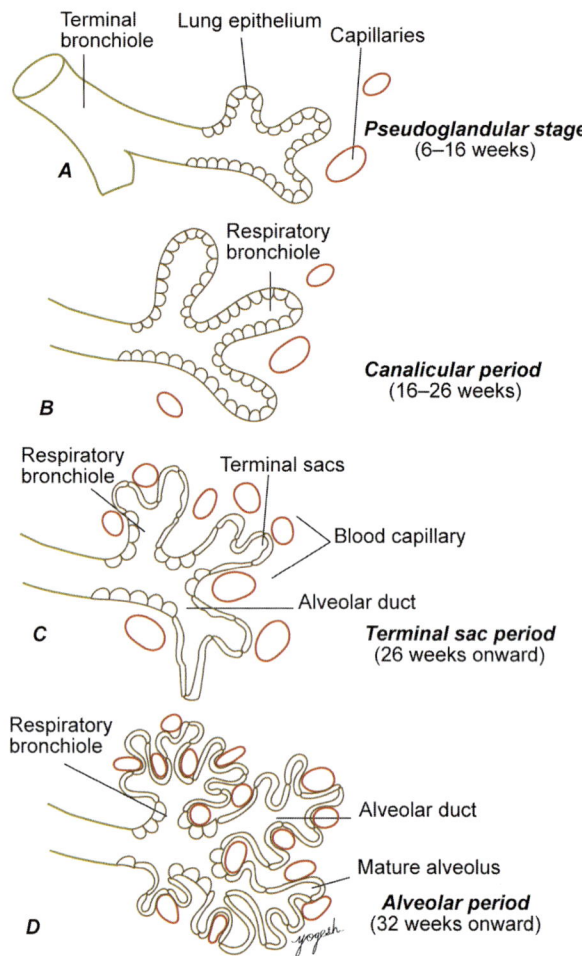

Practice Fig.16.3: Maturation of the lung

Box 16.2: Hyaline membrane disease or infant respiratory distress syndrome (IRDS)

Q. Write a short note on hyaline membrane disease.

- It is also called *surfactant deficiency disorder or infant respiratory distress syndrome.*
- It is produced in premature infants due to deficiency of *surfactant*.
- Production of surfactant begins by the 20th week of IUL.^{MCQ} The quantity of surfactant increases during last two weeks before birth.
- Incidence:
  – It affects about 1% of newborn infants and it is one of the leading causes of death in preterm infants.
  – Hyaline membrane disease accounts for 20% of deaths among newborns.^{MCQ}

Signs and symptoms
  – rapid breathing (tachypnoea)
  – faster heart rate (tachycardia)
  – bluish discoloration of the skin (cyanosis).

Contd.

Contd.

Pathological finding
- Waxy appearing layers of hyaline membrane that line collapsed alveoli of lung.

Prevention
- To speed up production of surfactant, injectable *glucocorticoids* are given to the mother during last trimester (after the 7th month of pregnancy).

Diagnostic amniocentesis
- Lecithin sphingomyelin (L/S) ratio in amniotic fluid: L/S ratio less than 2:1 indicates insufficient surfactant.^{MCQ}
- Surfactant/albumin (S/A) ratio in amniotic fluid: The S/A ratio <35 indicates immature lungs, 35–55 indicates intermediate maturity and >55 indicates sufficient maturity of lungs.

Treatment
- A newborn can be supported with oxygen therapy, continuous positive airway pressure (CPAP). Exogenous surfactant can also be useful.

5. *Sequestration* of the lung tissue: A separation of area of embryonic lung tissue from tracheobronchial tree is called sequestration (means separation).
6. *Ectopic lung*: It occurs due to development of additional lung bud from esophagus.
7. *Congenital polycystic lung*: The terminal bronchioles dilate to form multiple cysts and thus, produces honeycomb appearance on radiographs.
8. *Medicolegal aspect*: Lungs of newborn (live-born) contain air and hence float in water, whereas lungs of stillborn babies (dead born) do not contain air and hence their lungs sink in the water. This fact can be used to differentiate between stillborn and killed live-born baby.
9. **Vacteral association** have the following components: ^{MCQ}
    - Vertebral anomalies
    - Anal atresia
    - Cardiac defects
    - Tracheoesophageal fistula
    - Esophageal atresia
    - Renal anomalies
    - Limb defect

Chapter 17

Development of Body Cavities and Diaphragm

eSmartQuiz

Chapter Outline

- Development of pericardial cavity
  - Stages of development
- Development of pleural cavity
  - Stages of development
- Development of peritoneal cavity
- Development of diaphragm
  - Stages of development
- Descent of septum transversum
- Factors producing descent of diaphragm
- Congenital anomalies
- Congenital diaphragmatic hernia
- Formation of mesenteries
- Development of lesser sac
  - Stages of development

Competencies:

- **AN25.2:** Describe development of pleura, lung and heart. (Development of pleura is included in this chapter).
- **AN52.5:** Describe the development and congenital anomalies of diaphragm.

INTRODUCTION

- In the 3rd week, the small intercellular spaces appear in lateral plate mesoderm and pericardial bar. Later these spaces fuse to form U-shaped *primitive intraembryonic coelom* (Fig. 17.1, Practice Figs 17.1, 17.2, Flowchart 17.1).
- Central part of intraembryonic coelom forms the *pericardial sac*.
- Limbs of intraembryonic coelom are called *coelomic ducts*.
- Coelomic ducts communicate with extraembryonic coelom and thus, help in better nutrition.
- Pericardial, pleural and peritoneal cavities (serous sacs) are derived from the intraembryonic coelom.
- Intraembryonic coelom splits intraembryonic mesoderm into somatopleuric (parietal) layer and splanchnopleuric (visceral) layer.

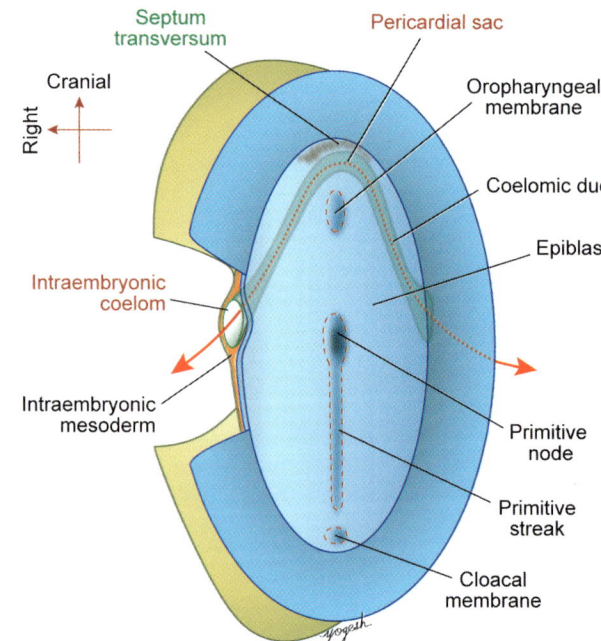

Fig. 17.1: Intraembryonic coelom. It lies in the lateral plate mesoderm and pericardial bar. In the figure red arrow is shown to be passing through the coelomic cavity. Pericardial bar lies between septum transversum and oropharyngeal membrane (not shown in this figure to maintain clarity)

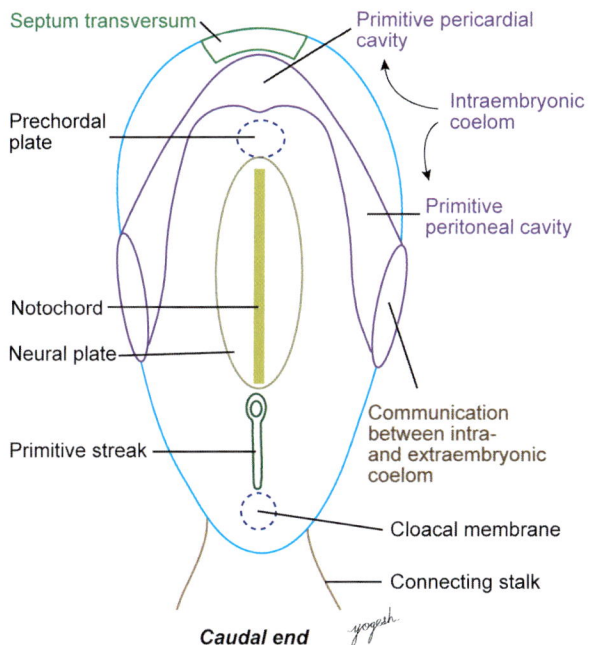

Practice Fig. 17.1: Divisions of intraembryonic coelom

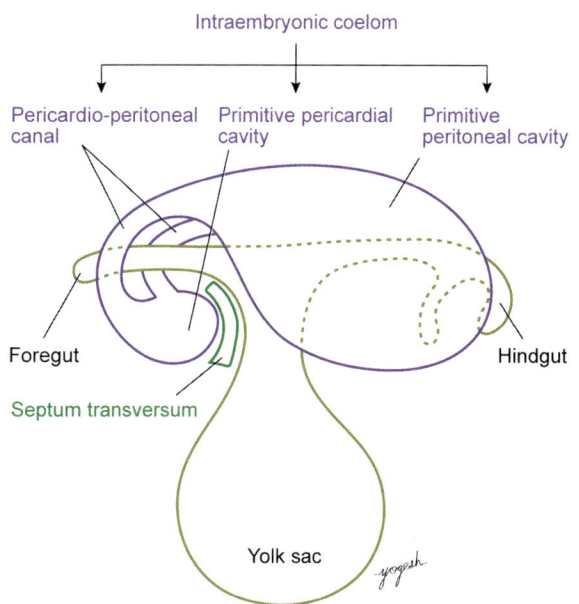

Practice Fig. 17.2: Relationship of intraembryonic coelom and gut tube

Flowchart 17.1: Formation and divisions of intraembryonic coelom

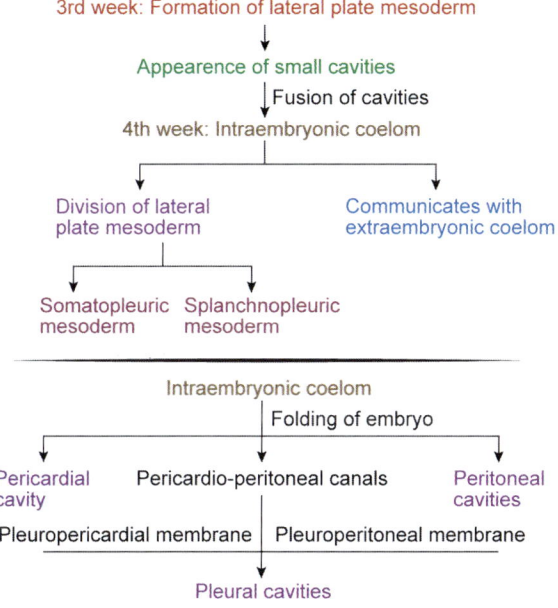

- Somatopleuric intraembryonic layer lies in contact with ectoderm and laterally it is continuous with somatopleuric extraembryonic mesoderm layer.
- Splanchnopleuric intraembryonic mesoderm lies in contact with endoderm and laterally it is continuous with extraembryonic splanchnopleuric mesoderm.

Changes due to Formation of Embryonic Folds

- Formation of embryonic folds changes the orientation of coelomic cavity.
- On the formation of the head fold, the pericardial sac becomes ventral to foregut and it lies between stomodeum cranially and septum transversum caudally (*see* Figs 8.7, 8.8, Chapter 8).
- On formation of lateral folds, ventrally coelomic ducts fuse with each other to form a peritoneal cavity.
- Part of coelomic ducts that communicates pericardial cavity with peritoneal cavity is called *pericardio-peritoneal canals*. These canals lie on the lateral sides of developing foregut.
- Lung buds arising from foregut invaginate pericardio-peritoneal canals and convert (by expansion) these canals into *pleural cavities*.
- Later, pleuropericardial membranes, pleuroperitoneal membranes and diaphragm divide the coelomic cavity into peritoneal, pleural and pericardial cavities.

DEVELOPMENT OF PERICARDIAL CAVITY

A pericardial cavity develops from midline part of intraembryonic coelom that lies in pericardial bar.

Stages of Development

1. Before formation of headfold: Pericardial cavity lies between septum transversum cranially and prechordal plate caudally.
2. After formation of headfold: Pericardial cavity lies between stomodeum (cranially) and septum transversum (caudally). Dorsally pericardial cavity is related to cardiogenic area and foregut.
3. Formation of layers of pericardium:
   - Fibrous pericardium and parietal layer of serous pericardium develop from *somatopleuric layer* of intraembryonic mesoderm.
   - Visceral layer of serous pericardium develops from *splanchnopleuric layer* of intraembryonic mesoderm.

Further details of development pericardial cavity are included in Chapter 18.

DEVELOPMENT OF PLEURAL CAVITY

Pleural cavities develop from the right and left pericardio-peritoneal canals that connect pericardial cavity with peritoneal cavities (Flowchart 17.2).

Stages of Development (Fig. 17.4)

1. *Invagination stage*: Lung buds invaginate pericardio-peritoneal canals.
2. *Enlargement*: Pericardio-peritoneal canals enlarge to accommodate enlarging lung buds.
3. *Separation*: Two folds of somatopleuric mesoderm appear in relation to invaginated lung buds as follows (Figs 17.2 to 17.4, Practice Figs 17.3 to 17.5):
   - Cranial pleuropericardial fold (membrane) separates pericardial cavity from pleural cavity.
   - Caudal pleuroperitoneal fold (membrane) separates pleural cavity from the peritoneal cavity.
   - Both membranes become continuous with posterior border of septum transversum.
4. *Closure of pleuropericardial opening*:
   - During the sixth week, pleuropericardial opening closes due to fusion of pleuropericardial membrane (pulmonary ridge of Mall) with the mesodermal tissue surrounding esophagus.
   - Overgrowing lung bud turns pleuropericardial membrane and makes it vertical (initially oblique).
5. *Closure of pleuroperitoneal opening*:
   - Boundaries of pleuroperitoneal opening are as follows (Fig. 17.2):
     Ventral: Dorsal border of septum transversum
     Medial: Esophagus, dorsal mesentery of esophagus and dorsal aorta
     Dorsal: Mesonephric ridge with gonads
     Lateral: Pleuroperitoneal membrane
   - Pleuroperitoneal membranes grow ventrally and fuse with dorsal border of septum transversum and other structures forming boundaries of pleuro-peritoneal openings. These membranes overgrow to cover the septum transversum completely.
6. *Expansion of pleural cavities in the body wall*: Expanding lung buds cause expansion of pleural cavities and descent of septum transversum (Fig. 17.4D).
7. *Splitting of mesoderm of body wall*: Expanding pleural cavity splits mesoderm into two layers (Fig. 17.4):
   a. Outer layer forms wall of thorax
   b. Inner layer lines pericardial cavity. This layer is called pleuropericardial membrane and it later forms fibrous pericardium.

DEVELOPMENT OF PERITONEAL CAVITY

- Peritoneal cavity develops from horseshoe-shaped limbs of intraembryonic coelom.
- Formation of lateral folds bring right and left intraembryonic coelomic ducts (limbs) closer and they fuse to form a peritoneal cavity.
- Peritoneal cavity initially communicates with pericardial cavity through pericardio-peritoneal canals. On formation of pleural cavity from pericardio-peritoneal canal, later peritoneal cavity separated from pleural cavity by septum transversum and pleuroperitoneal membranes.
- Up to 10th week, peritoneal cavity communicates with extraembryonic coelom at umbilicus (site for a physiological hernia).
- Layers of peritoneum: Parietal peritoneum develops from somatopleuric layer of mesoderm, whereas visceral peritoneum develops from splanchnopleuric layer of mesoderm.

DEVELOPMENT OF DIAPHRAGM

Q. *Write a short note on development of diaphragm.*[High yielding facts]

Summary (Examination Guide) (Table 17.1, Fig. 17.5, Practice Fig. 17.6, Flowchart 17.3)

- Diaphragm is a musculotendinous partition between thoracic and abdominal cavities.
- Diaphragm consists of central tendon and two crura.
- Various parts of diaphragm develop as follows:
  1. Central tendon from pleuro-peritoneal membranes
  2. Crura of diaphragm from dorsal mesentery of esophagus
  3. Muscular components form cervical somites (level C3–C5)
  4. Ventrolateral peripheral part from mesoderm of lateral body wall.
- Previous concept: Central tendon develops from septum transversum.

Table 17.1 Development of diaphragm[MCQ]

Part of diaphragm	Embryonic source
1. Central tendon	Pleuroperitoneal membranes
2. Right and left crura	Dorsal mesentery of esophagus
3. Muscular components	Cervical somites (level C3–C5)
4. Peripheral part (venterolateral)	Mesoderm of lateral body wall

Flowchart 17.2: Development of pleural cavity

Invagination Lung bud invaginates pleuroperitoneal canals
↓
Enlargement To accommodate enlarging lungs → Future pleural cavity
↓
Separation Pleuropericardial and pleuroperitoneal folds separate pleural cavity from peritoneal and pericardial cavities
↓
Closure of pleuropericardial and pleuroperitoneal openings
↓
Expansion of pleural cavities

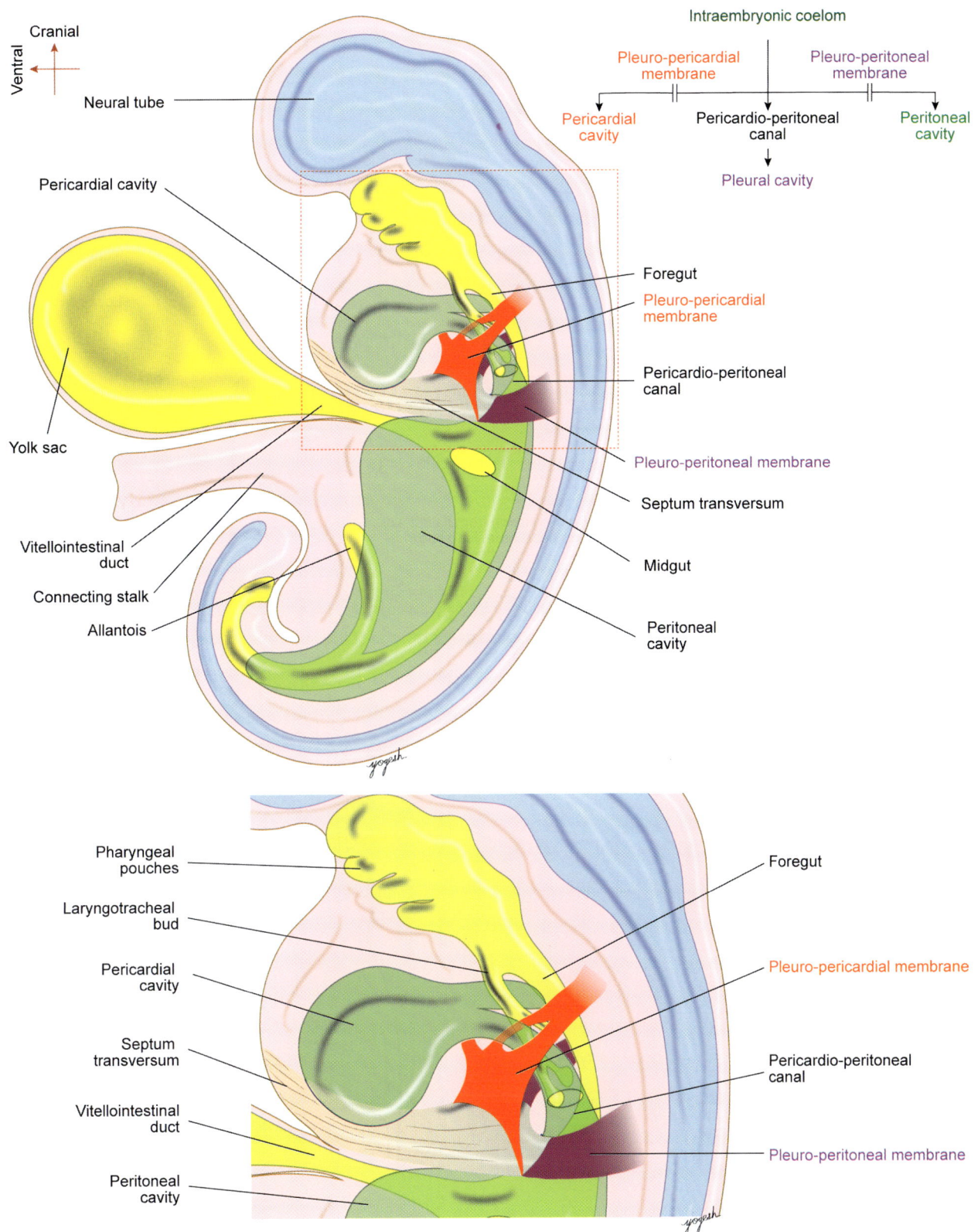

Fig. 17.2: Formation of coelomic cavities of body. Two folds of somatopleuric mesoderm, namely cranial pleuropericardial membrane (separates pericardial cavity from pleural cavity) and caudal pleuroperitoneal membrane (separates pleural cavity from peritoneal cavity) become continuous with the posterior border of the septum transversum

Stages of Development (Fig. 17.5)

1. **Septum transversum:** Septum transversum lies between thoracic and peritoneal cavities.
   Relations of septum transversum:
   Cranial: Pleural and pericardial cavities
   Caudal: Peritoneal cavity
   Dorsal: Esophagus and dorsal mesentery of esophagus

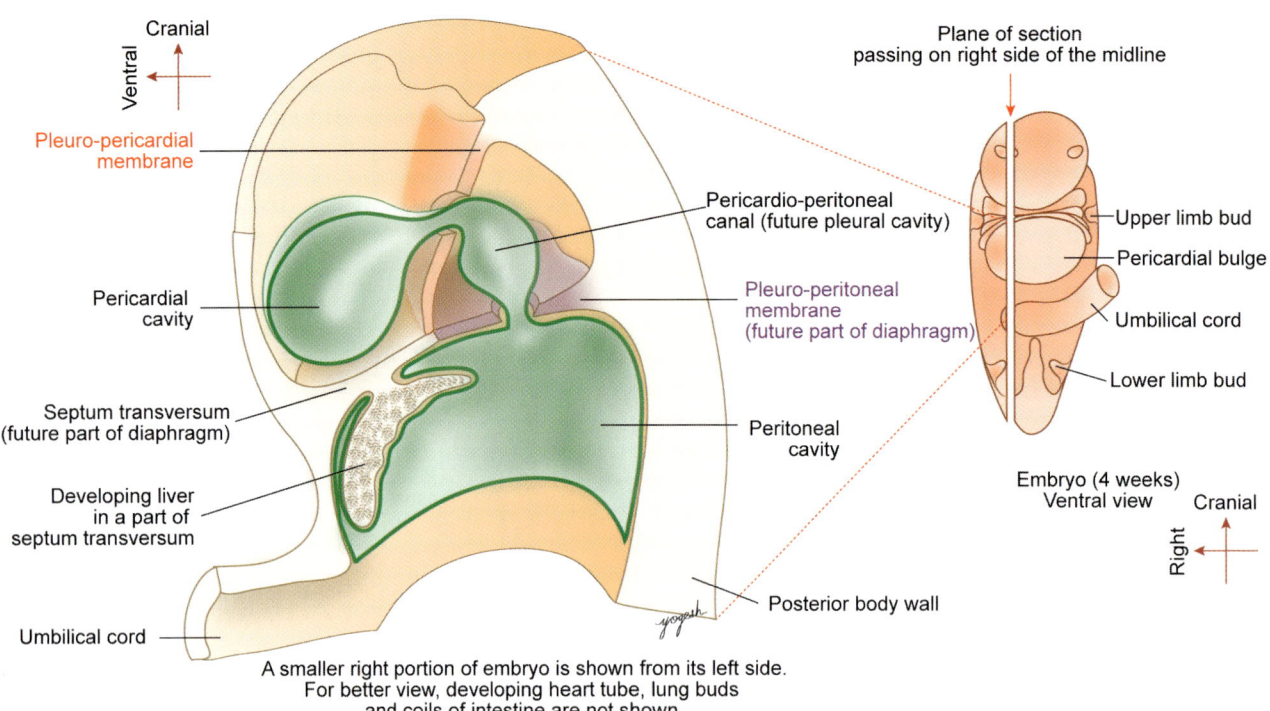

Fig. 17.3: Separations of pericardial, pleural and peritoneal cavities from each other. Cranial pericardiopleural membrane separates pericardial cavity from pleural cavity. Caudal pleuroperitoneal membrane separates pleural cavity from the peritoneal cavity. Both of these membranes become continuous with the posterior border of the septum transversum

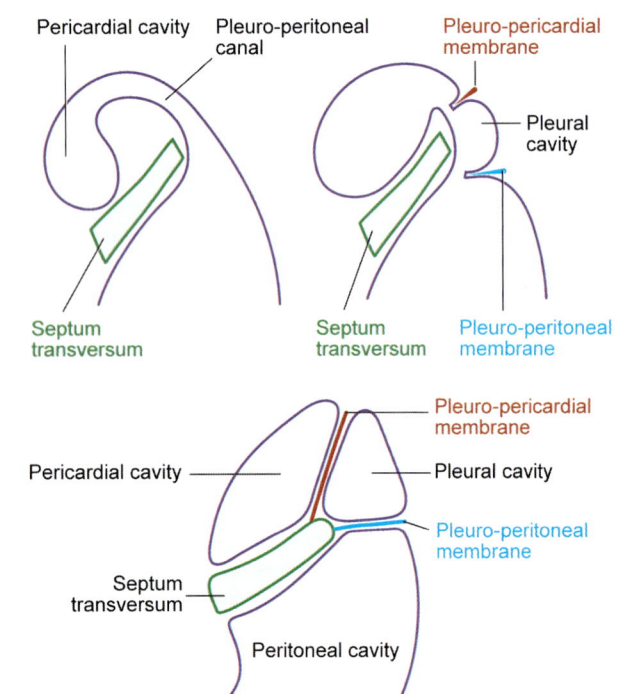

Practice Fig. 17.3: Separation of pericardial, pleural and peritoneal cavities

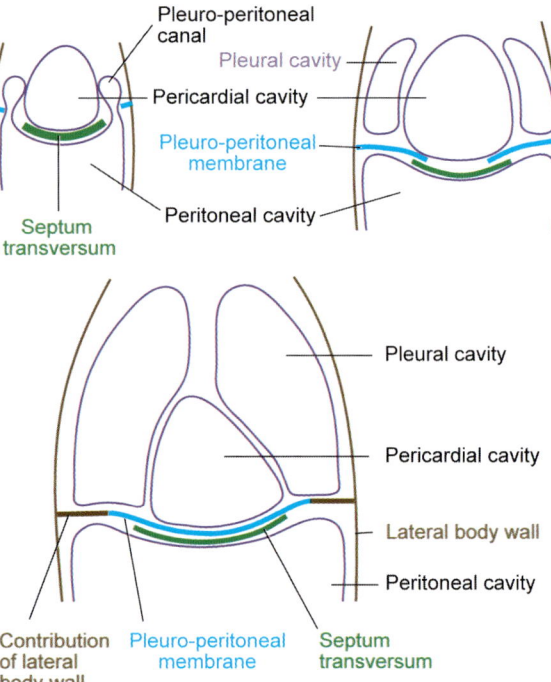

Note: Dorsal mesentery of esophagus also contributes to diaphragm.

Practice Fig. 17.4: Development of diaphragm and pleural cavity

Dorsolateral: Pleuroperitoneal canals
Note: Liver develops in caudal part of septum transversum, whereas central tendon of diaphragm develops from the cranial part.
2. Derivative of pleuroperitoneal membranes: Right and left pleuroperitoneal membranes separate pleural cavities from peritoneal cavity and form a central tendon of the diaphragm (Figs 17.3, 17.5). [*Previous concept:* Central tendon from septum transversum.]

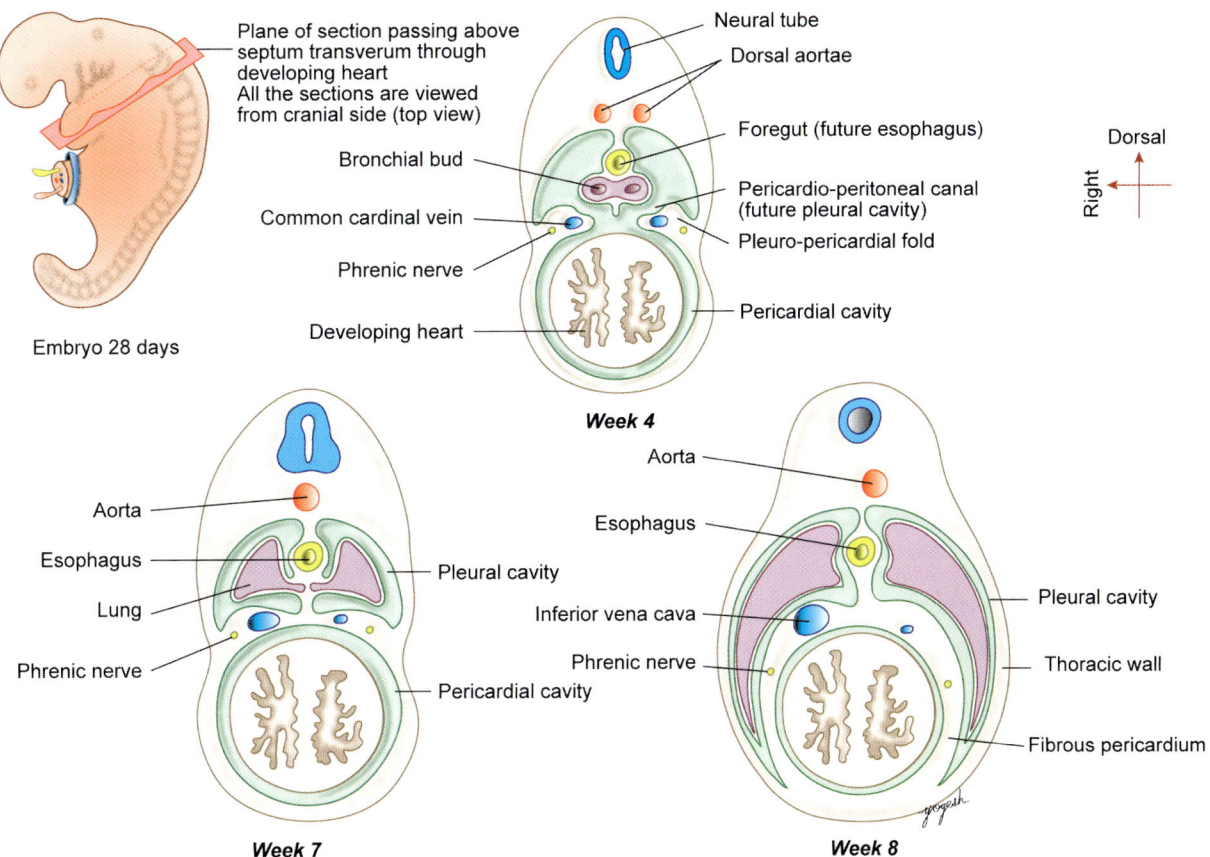

Fig. 17.4: Development of pleural cavities. Pleural cavities develop from right and left pericardio-peritoneal canals that connect pericardial cavity with peritoneal cavities. Lung buds invaginates into pericardio-peritoneal canals. These pericardio-peritoneal canals enlarge to accommodate enlarging lung buds. Pericardiopleural folds (membrane) separate pericardial cavity from pleural cavity. Pleuroperitoneal fold (membrane) (not shown in this figure) separates pleural cavity from the peritoneal cavity. During the sixth week of IUL, pleuropericardial opening closes due to fusion of membrane with mesodermal tissue surrounding esophagus. Expanding lung buds cause expansion of pleural cavities anteroposteriorly and craniocaudally. Expanding pleural cavity splits mesoderm into two layers, outer layer forms wall of thorax and inner layer forms fibrous pericardium

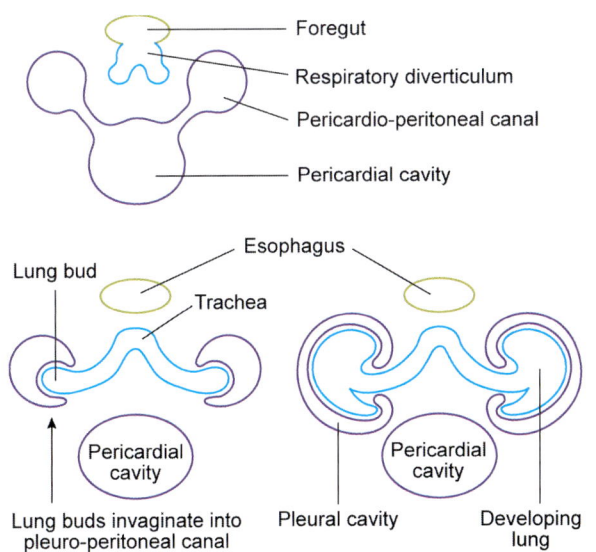

Practice Fig. 17.5: Conversion of pericardio-peritoneal canals into pleural cavities

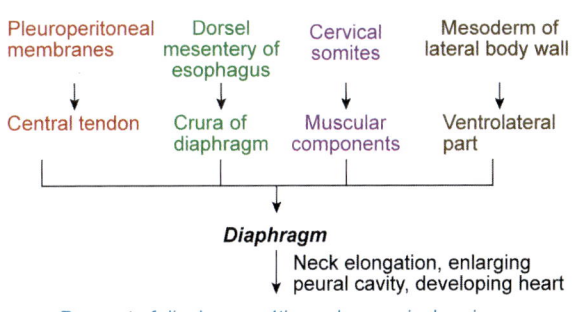

Flowchart 17.3: Development of diaphragm

Descent of diaphragm: 4th week – cervical region
6th week – definitive position

Congenital anomalies: Congenital diaphragmatic hernia, congenital hiatal hernia, retrosternal hernia, eventration
Note: Previous concept: Septum transversum forms central tendon of diaphragm.

3. Derivative of dorsal mesentery of esophagus: It forms crura of the diaphragm.
4. Derivative of lateral thoracic wall: Developing pleural cavity divides lateral body wall into external and internal layers. External layer forms definitive body wall, whereas internal layer forms ingrowth to develop ventrolateral part of the diaphragm, peripheral to pleuroperitoneal membrane derivative.

Descent of Septum Transversum

- In 4th week, septum transversum lies in cervical region at the level of third, fourth and fifth cervical

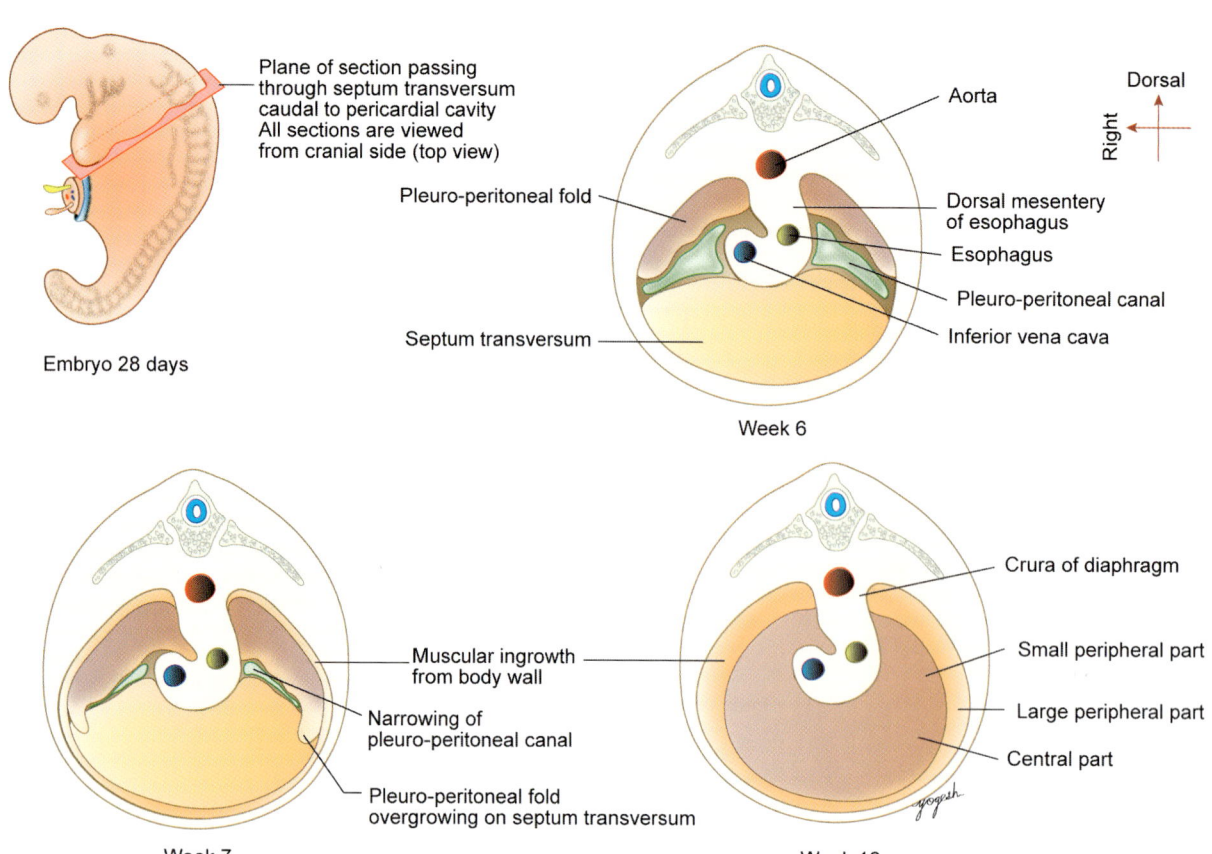

Fig. 17.5: Development of abdominothoracic diaphragm. Central tendon of diaphragm develops from septum transversum, crus of diaphragm from dorsal mesentery of esophagus, small dorsal peripheral part from pleuro-peritoneal membranes, ventro-lateral (large) peripheral part from mesoderm of the lateral body wall

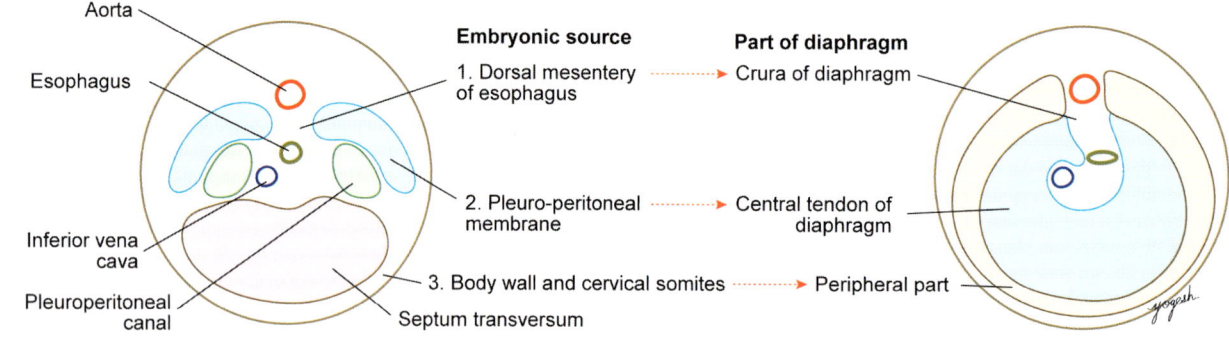

Practice Fig. 17.6: Development of diaphragm

somatic nerves (later, it develops phrenic nerve, C3–5 root value).
- Due to growth of lung buds in pericardio-peritoneal canals and heart development, diaphragm reaches to its definitive position by sixth week (opposite to T7 to T12 spinal segments).^{MCQ}
- Descending diaphragm pulls its original nerve supply (phrenic nerve) with it.

Factors Producing Descent of Diaphragm
The following factors causes descent of diaphragm:
1. Elongation of neck (developing pharyngeal arches)
2. Enlarging pleural cavities
3. Development of heart

Congenital Anomalies
1. Congenital diaphragmatic hernia (CDH): Box 17.1, Fig. 17.6
2. Congenital hiatal hernia
   - It is herniation of abdominal contents (mostly stomach) through esophageal opening of the diaphragm.
3. Retrosternal (parasternal) hernia: It is herniation of abdominal contents through enlarged foramen of Morgagni (gap between sternal and costal slips of diaphragm).
4. Eventration of diaphragm: It is an abnormal contour of diaphragmatic dome due to underdeveloped musculature of anyone dome of the diaphragm. Thin

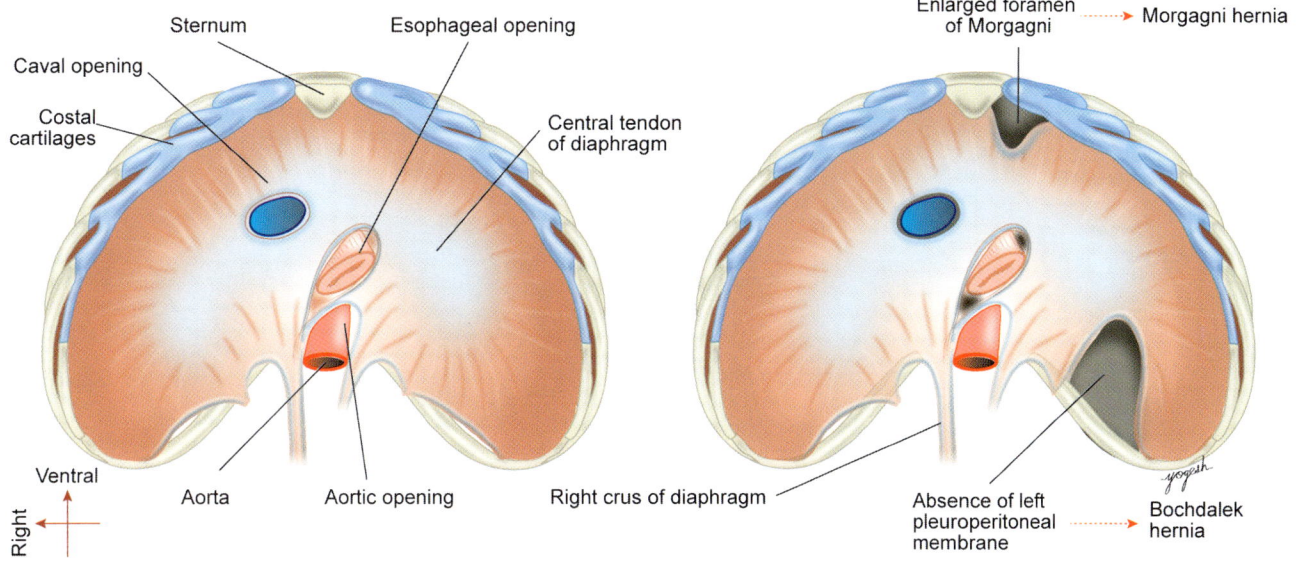

Fig. 17.6: Congenital diaphragmatic hernia. It is herniation of abdominal content into thoracic cavity due to failure of proper formation of the diaphragm. Bochdalek hernia occurs due to failure of pleuroperitoneal membrane contribution to the diaphragm, whereas Morgagni hernia involves protrusion of abdominal contents through enlarged foramen of Morgagni

diaphragmatic zone outpouches with abdominal contents in thoracic cavity.

Box 17.1: Congenital diaphragmatic hernia (CDH)

Q. Write a short note on congenital diaphragmatic hernia.

- It is herniation of abdominal content into thoracic cavity due to failure of proper formation of the diaphragm (Fig. 17.6B).
- CDH is a life-threatening condition in infants as it may result in pulmonary hypoplasia.
- Incidence: 1:2000 births
- Most common cause of pulmonary hypoplasia is CDH. Respiratory distress is the commonest cause of death in CDH.^{MCQ}
- There are *three cardinal signs* of CDH: Breathlessness, cyanosis, unusual flat abdomen.^{MCQ}
- Genetic cause: Microdeletion of chromosome 15 in the region 15q26.^{MCQ}
- Classification (Fig. 17.6B):
  The congenital diaphragmatic hernia has three types as follows:
  A. Bochdalek hernia: It is also called posterolateral hernia. About 95% case of CDH are Bochdalek hernia.^{MCQ} It occurs due to the failure of pleuroperitoneal membrane contribution to the diaphragm. It is more common on left side (85–90% cases).
  B. Morgagni hernia (retrosternal or parasternal hernia, right anterior part of diaphragm): It is CDH that involves protrusion of abdominal contents through foramen of Morgagni.
  C. Diaphragmatic eventration: It refers to abnormal contour of diaphragmatic dome because of paralysis, aplasia, or atrophy to varying degrees of muscle fibres.

FORMATION OF MESENTERIES

- Mesentery is a connective tissue fold formed by two layers of peritoneum that connects abdominal viscera (intestine) with abdominal walls.
- There are two mesenteries (Fig. 17.7)
  – Ventral mesentery – connects gut with anterior body wall.
  – Dorsal mesentery – connects gut with posterior body wall.
- Ventral mesentery disappears except for the following parts:
  a. Caudal part of esophagus
  b. Stomach
  c. Proximal part of duodenum
- Ventral mesentery of stomach is called *ventral mesogastrium.*
- On formation of lateral folds, owing to fusion of splanchnopleuric layers of mesoderm, the midgut and hindgut have only dorsal mesentery.
- Rotation of gut and zygosis converts the dorsal mesentery into mesentery of jejunum and ileum, mesoappendix, transverse and sigmoid mesocolons (Fig. 17.8).

DEVELOPMENT OF LESSER SAC

Q. Write a short note on development of lesser sac.

- Lesser sac is also called *omental bursa*. It is a part of peritoneal cavity.
- Lesser sac lies behind stomach and lesser omentum.

Stages of Development

1. Formation of pneumoenteric recess in dorsal mesogastrium (Figs 17.9, 17.10, Table 17.2).

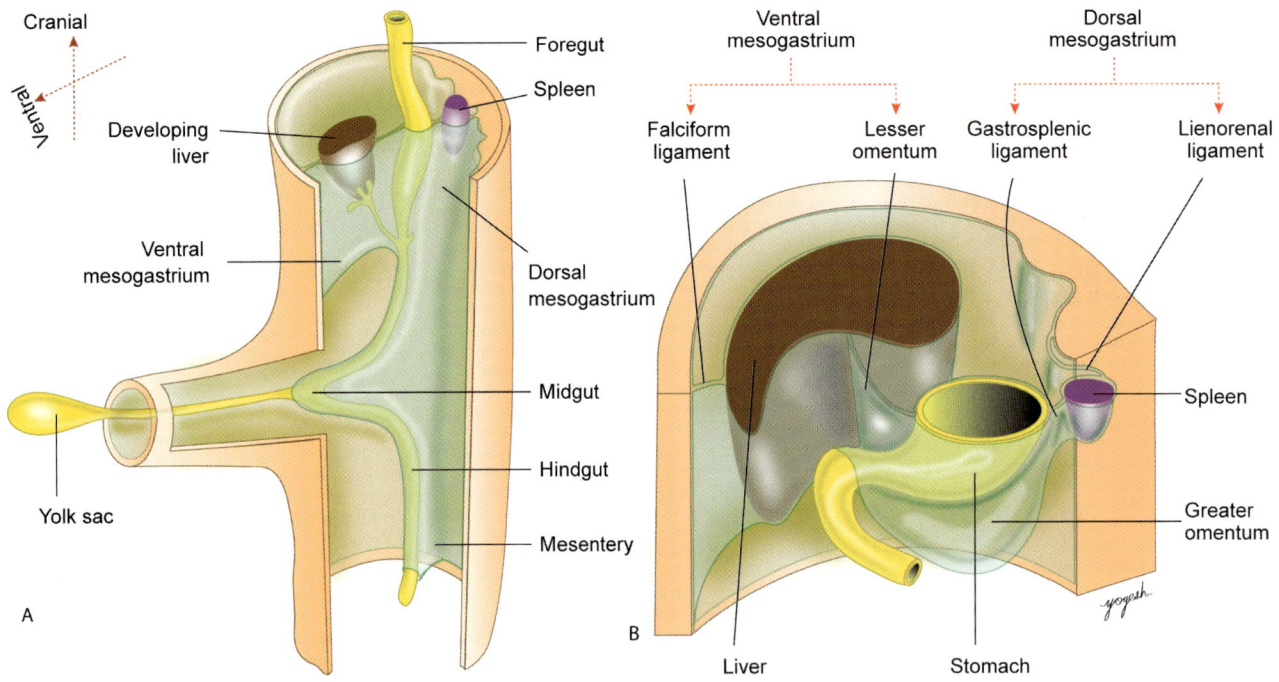

Fig. 17.7: Dorsal and ventral mesenteries of the gut. Transverse section through the region of the stomach showing the changes in the position of stomach, liver, spleen, and mesogastrium: (A) Positions at the end of the fifth week; (B) Positions at the end of the 11th week. Ventral mesogastrium forms falciform ligament and lesser omentum, whereas dorsal mesogastrium forms gastrosplenic and lienorenal ligaments and greater omentum

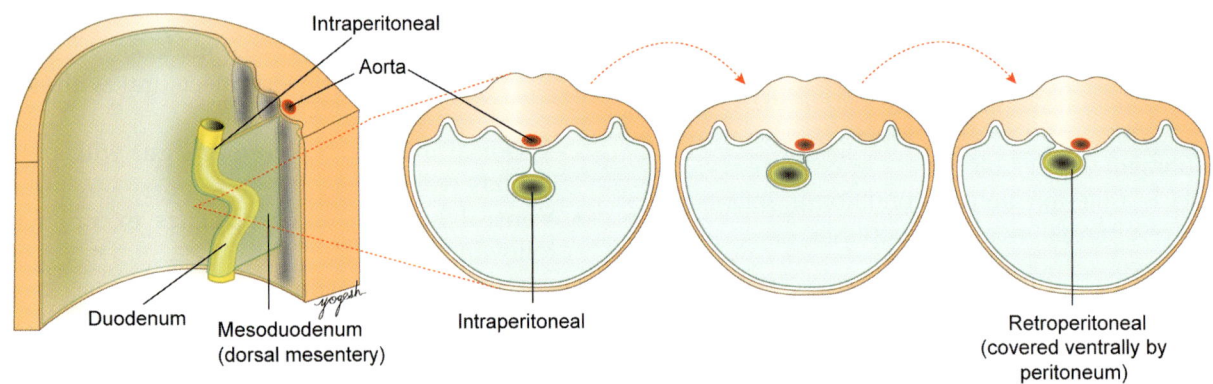

Fig. 17.8: Process of zygosis

Table 17.2	Development of lesser sac
Part	*Source*
Vestibule	On rotation of stomach, a part of peritoneal cavity that lies behind ventral mesogastrium
Superior recess	Cranial extension of right pneumoenteric recess below diaphragm
Inferior recess	Caudal extension of cavity in elongating greater omentum
Splenic recess	Part of lesser sac extending between gastrosplenic and lienorenal ligaments

- Right and left pneumoenteric recess (small cavities) appear in dorsal mesogastrium.
- Left one disappears soon.
- Right recess fuse with peritoneal cavity and later expands on left side to form a major part of lesser sac behind the stomach.
- Cavity of right recess expands cranially behind liver and forms superior recess of lesser sac.
- Cranial extension of right pneumoenteric bursa above the diaphragm forms *infracardiac bursa*.

2. Formation of part of lesser sac behind lesser omentum:
   - Due to rotation of stomach and development of liver, the part of peritoneal cavity (forms vestibule of lesser sac) comes to lie behind the lesser omentum (derived from ventral mesogastrium).

3. Formation of lower part of lesser sac:
   - Developing spleen and stomach rotation (counter-clockwise) divide dorsal mesogastrium into gastrosplenic and lienorenal ligaments (that lies on left side of lesser sac).
   - Part of lesser sac extending between gastrosplenic and lienorenal ligaments is *splenic recess*.

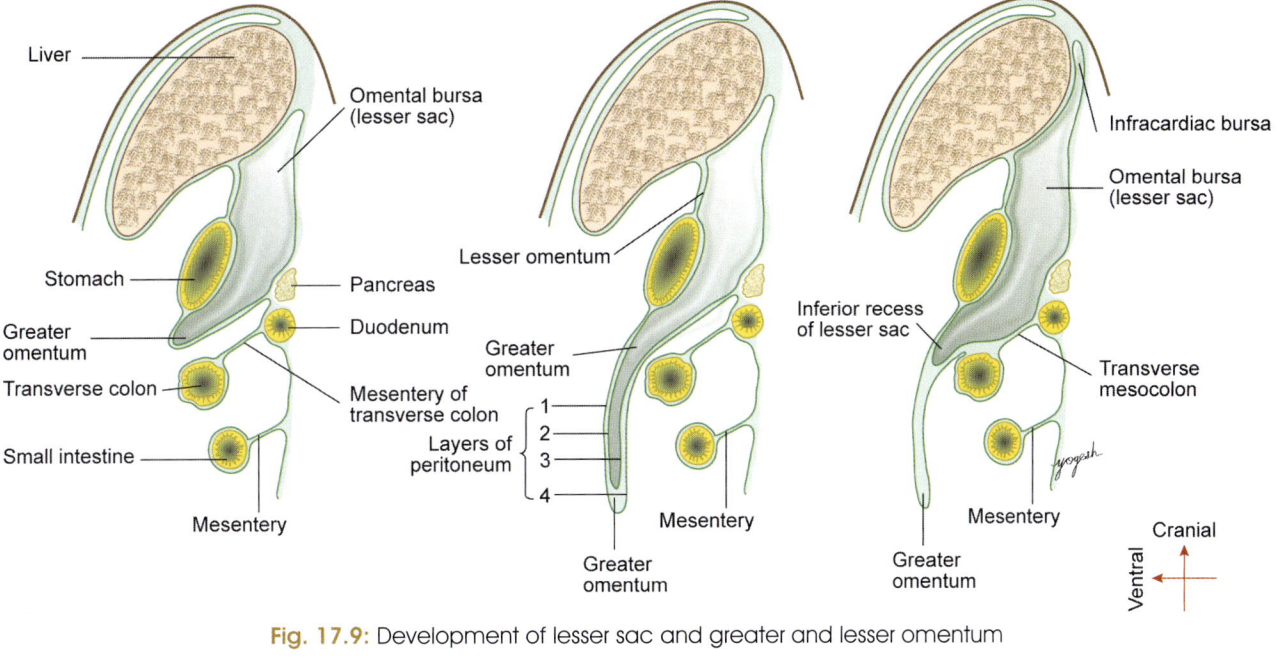

Fig. 17.9: Development of lesser sac and greater and lesser omentum

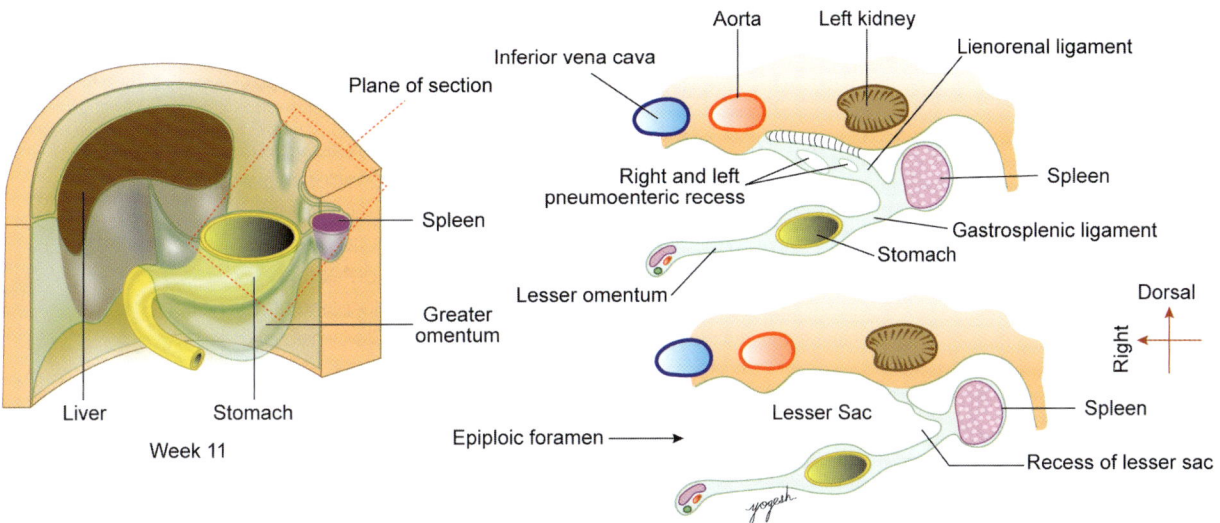

Fig. 17.10: Development of lesser sac

- The part of dorsal mesogastrium attached to greater curvature of stomach extends and forms greater omentum. Part of the lesser sac that lies within greater omentum is *inferior recess of lesser*

- Cavity of the lesser sac communicates with rest of the peritoneal cavity through epiploic foramen of Winslow, that lies behind right free margin of the lesser omentum.

Clinical Embryology

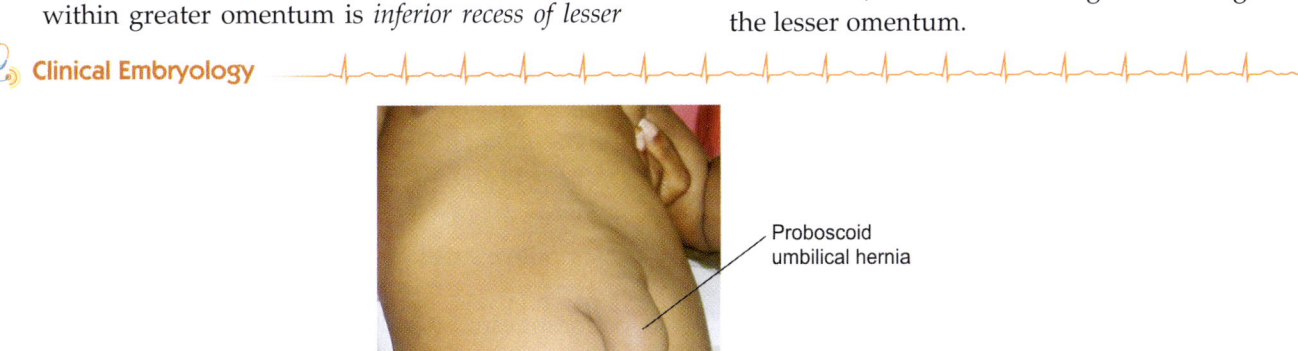

Clinical image 17.1: Proboscoid umbilical hernia. Umbilical hernia is the protrusion of abdominal contents through a defective anterior abdominal wall at the umbilicus. If the umbilical hernia is elongated, it is called proboscoid umbilical hernia (like elephant trunk). Usually, umbilical hernia regresses spontaneously by 2–3 years of age, but proboscoid umbilical hernia often requires surgical correction (Image courtesy: *Dr Kumaravel S*)

Chapter 18

Cardiovascular System I: Development of Heart

eSmartQuiz

Chapter Outline

- Fate of heart tube
- Acquisition of external features of the adult heart
- Development of atria
  - Right atrium
  - Left atrium
  - Sinus venosus
  - Atrioventricular canal
  - Interatrial septum
- Dextrocardia
- Atrial septal defects
- Development of ventricles
  - Bulbus cordis
  - Interventricular septum
  - Aorticopulmonary septum
- Development of valves of heart
  - Atrioventricular valves
  - Pulmonary and aortic valves
- Development of conducting system of heart
- Development of pericardium
- Tetralogy of Fallot
- Ventricular septal defects
- Timing of embryologic heart formation
- Probe patency of foramen ovale

Competencies:
- AN25.2: Describe development of pleura, lungs, and heart.
- AN25.4: Describe embryological basis of (1) atrial septal defect, (2) ventricular septal defect, (3) Fallot's tetralogy, (4) tracheoesophageal fistula.

INTRODUCTION

Nutrition of the Embryo at Various Stages of Development

- The nutritional supply of embryo changes according to development as follows:
  - During the first week, before implantation, deutoplasm (accumulated cytoplasmic nutrients) of oocyte supplies nutrition.
  - During the second week, breakdown products of endometrium (due to implantation) nourish the embryo by simple diffusion.
  - After the third week, maternal blood nourishes embryo through uteroplacental circulation.
- Increasing nutritional demand of growing embryo initiates development of cardiovascular system in the third week of intrauterine life.

- All components of cardiovascular system develop from mesoderm.
- The components of cardiovascular system can be studied as
  1. Development of heart
  2. Development of blood vessels
- This chapter deals with development of the heart.

Establishment of Cardiogenic Area (Field)

- *Progenitor heart cells:* During the third week, *cardiac progenitor cells* develop in the epiblast just lateral to the primitive streak.
- *Primary heart field/area:* These cells migrate through primitive streak cranially and form horseshoe-shaped *primitive/primary heart field* in the splanchnopleuric mesoderm by end of the third week (Fig. 18.1).
- On formation of head fold, primary heart field comes to lie on dorsal side of pericardial sac. *Secondary heart field:* On day 20–21, ventral to the pharynx, the cells of splanchnopleuric mesoderm form secondary heart field. Most of the heart develops from primary heart

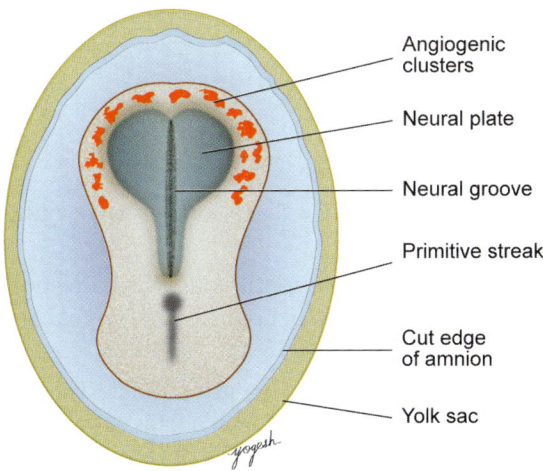

Fig. 18.1: Cardiogenic area is derived from intraembryonic mesoderm in the third week

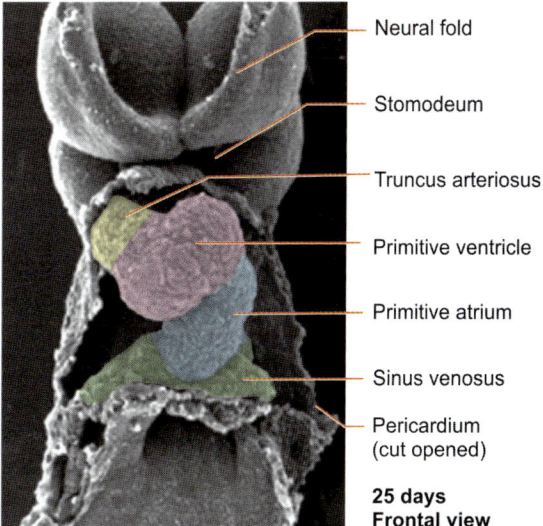

Scanning electron micrograph 18.2: Developing heart tube at week 4 development [Species: Mouse, approximate human age: 25 days, frontal view]

field. Secondary heart field forms part of the right ventricle and outflow tracts of both the ventricles. Circulatory system in the first system to start working.^MCQ

- *Formation of heart tube:* Endoderm of primitive pharynx induces vasculogenesis (formation of blood cells and vessels) in the primary heart field.
  Small vessels join to form two (right and left) *endothelial heart tubes* that give rise to the endocardium.
- *Splanchnopleuric mesoderm* that lies between heart tube and pericardial cavity forms a *myoepicardial mantle*.
- The myoepicardial mantle condenses to form
  – Myocardium (cardiac muscles) [cardiac muscles develop from splanchnopleuric mesoderm.^NEXT]
  – Epicardium (visceral layer of pericardium)
- Somatopleuric mesoderm that surrounds pericardial cavity forms parietal layer of pericardium.
- Primitive heart starts beating on the 22nd day.^MCQ
- Blood begins to circulate within the embryo by 24th day.^MCQ

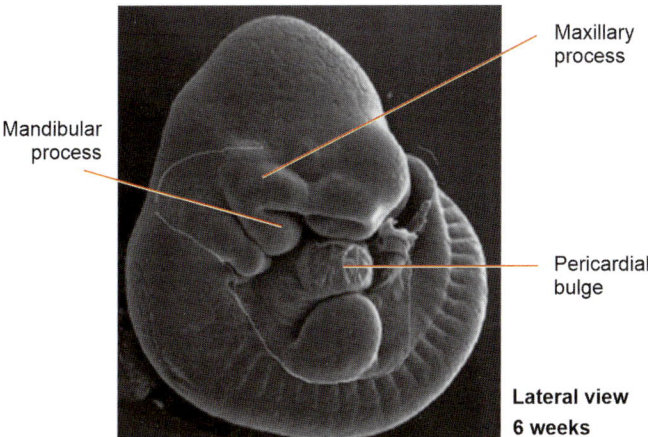

Scanning electron micrograph 18.1: SEM showing 6-week embryo showing pericardial bulge [Species: Mouse, approximate human age: 6 weeks, lateral view]

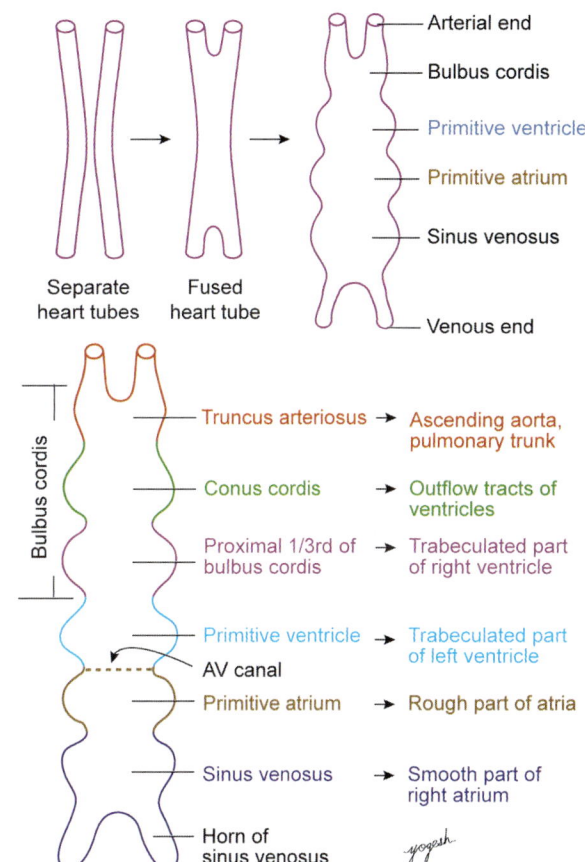

Practice Fig. 18.1: Parts of heart tube

Heart Tubes

- *Formation of single heart tube:* In the third week, two heart tubes fuse and form a single heart tube. Ends of the heart tube remain bifurcated. Its cranial end is called *arterial end*, whereas caudal end is called *venous end* (Fig. 18.2, Flowchart 18.1).

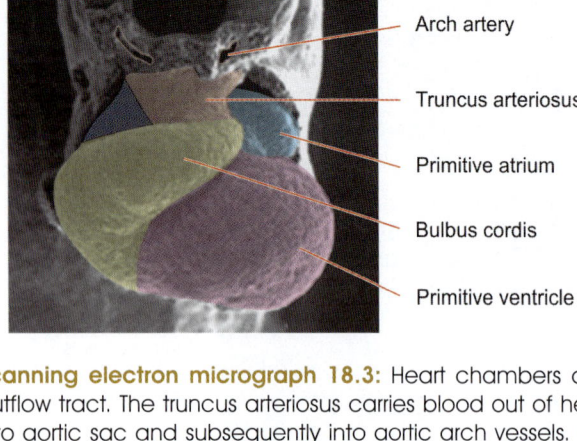

Scanning electron micrograph 18.3: Heart chambers and outflow tract. The truncus arteriosus carries blood out of heart into aortic sac and subsequently into aortic arch vessels. The conus cordis is a major contributor to the right ventricle [Species: Mouse, approx. human age: 27 days]

- *Dilatations of heart tube:* Heart tube soon forms dilatations from cranial to caudal end as follows (Fig. 18.3, Practice Fig. 18.1, Flowchart 18.1):*Viva*
  1. Bulbus cordis
     - Truncus arteriosus
     - Conus cordis
     - Bulbar part
  2. Primitive ventricle
  3. Primitive atrium
  4. Sinus venosus

Ends of Heart Tube

- Arterial end or truncus arteriosus shows right and left limbs.
- These limbs (horns) are continuous with corresponding dorsal aorta through first pair of pharyngeal arteries (Fig. 18.2, Practice Fig. 18.2).
- Soon six pairs of pharyngeal arch arteries connect truncus arteriosus with dorsal aorta. All pharyngeal arch arteries run on either side of foregut (primitive pharynx).

Venous End of Heart Tube

- Unfused part of sinus venosus (venous end of heart tube) forms two horns (right and left).
- Each horn receives three veins (from lateral to medial)*NEXT* (Figs 18.2, 18.3, Practice Fig. 18.2):
  1. Common cardinal vein from the body wall
  2. Umbilical vein from the placenta
  3. Vitelline vein from the yolk sac.*MCQ*

Flowchart 18.1: Heart tube

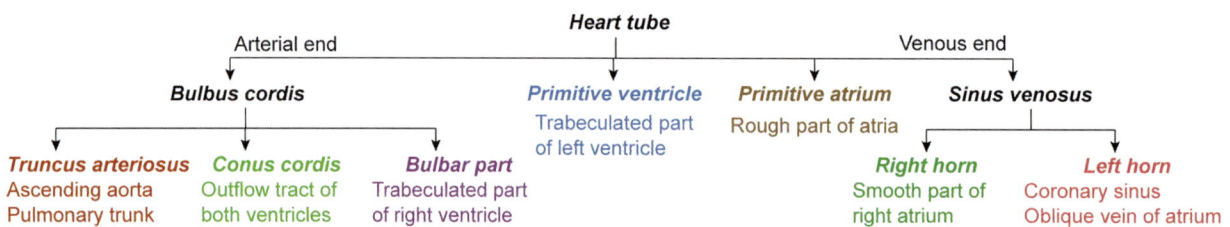

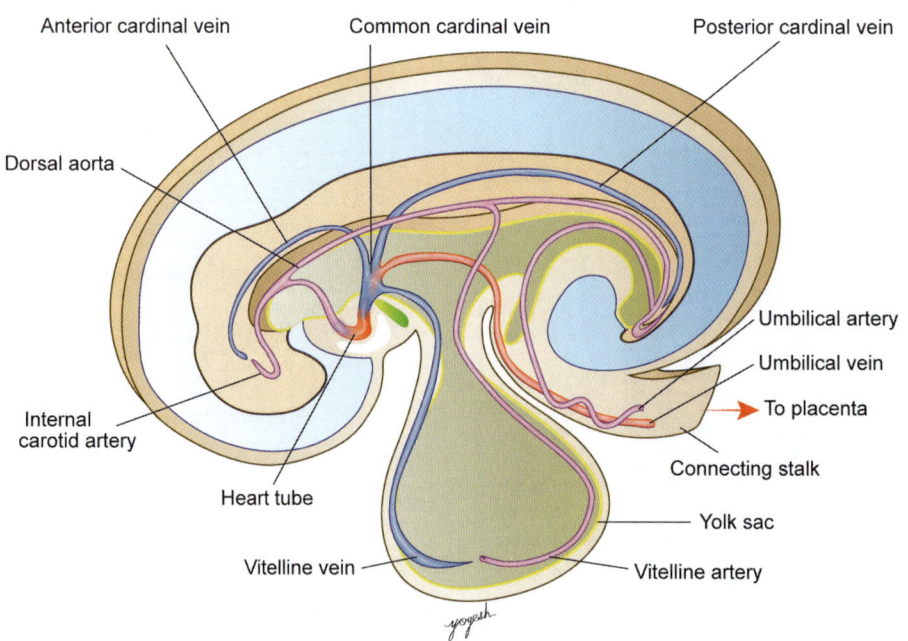

Fig. 18.2: Major vessels of embryo

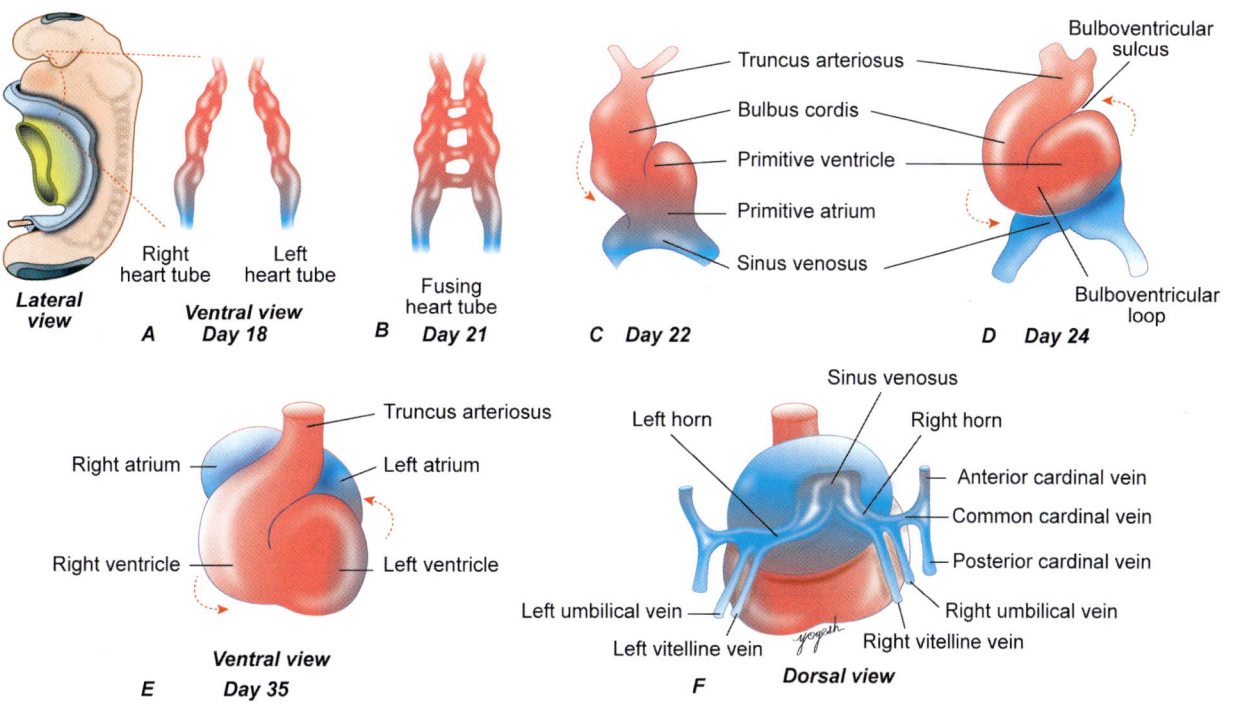

Fig. 18.3: Development of heart (external views)

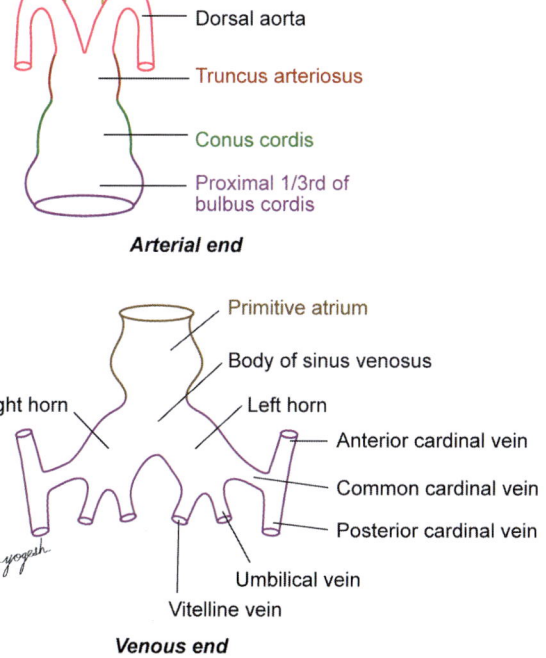

Practice Fig. 18.2: Arterial and venous end of heart tube

FATE OF HEART TUBE^{VIVA, MCQ}

The fate of the heart tube is summarized in Table 18.1 and Practice Fig. 18.1.

Q. Enumerate derivatives of different parts of the heart tube.

Table 18.1	Fate of components of heart tube
Components of heart tube	**Fate or derivative**
Truncus arteriosus	• Ascending aorta • Pulmonary trunk
Bulbus cordis	• Conus arteriosus (smooth part of right ventricle) • Aortic vestibule (smooth part of left ventricle)
Primitive ventricle	• Trabeculated part of right and left ventricles
Primitive atrium	• Trabeculated part of right and left atria
Sinus venosus^{NEXT}	• Right horn: Sinus venarum (smooth part of right atrium)^{NEXT} • Left horn: Coronary sinus and oblique vein of left atrium^{NEXT}

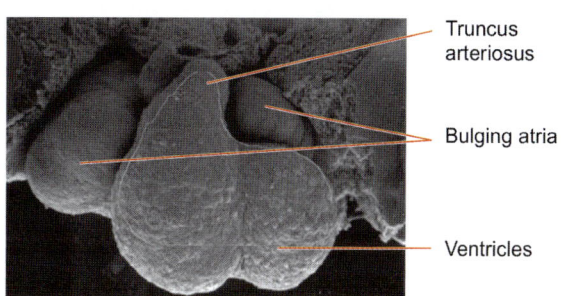

Scanning electron micrograph 18.4: External view of heart at 6 weeks [Species: Mouse, approximate human age: 6 weeks, ventral view]

ACQUISITION OF EXTERNAL FEATURES OF THE ADULT HEART

Heart tube undergoes growth and folding to acquire external features of the adult heart as follows (Figs 18.3 to 18.5, Practice Fig. 18.3, Flowchart 18.2):

- Initially, heart tube is placed longitudinally in pericardial cavity (Fig. 18.4B, C).
- Heart tube is suspended from dorsal wall of pericardial cavity by a fold of pericardium called *dorsal mesocardium* (Fig. 18.4C, D).
- *Formation of bulboventricular loop:* Bulbus cordis and primitive ventricle grow ventrally and form bulboventricular loop (U-shaped) (Figs 18.3D, 18.4D).

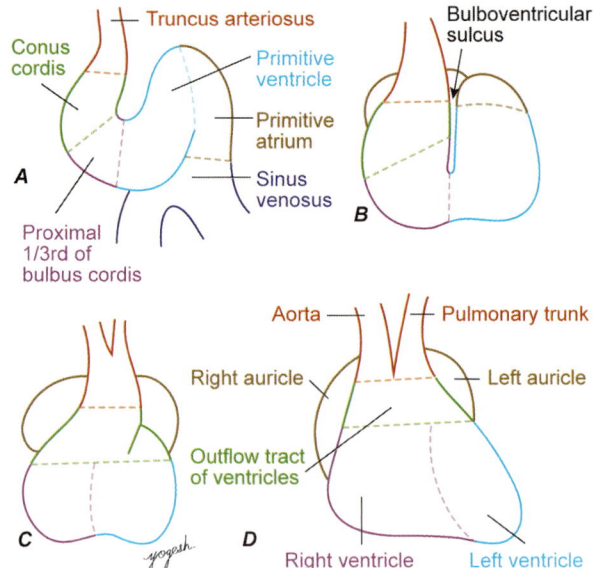

Practice Fig. 18.3: Establishment of external features of heart

Flowchart 18.2: Acquisition of external features of adult heart

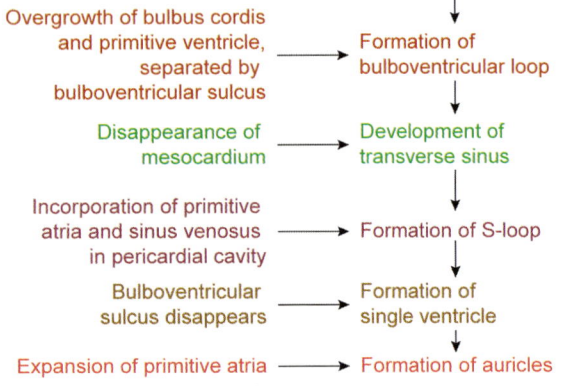

- *Formation of transverse sinus:* The mesocardium connecting bulboventricular loop disappears to form a gap, that later called *transverse sinus* (Fig. 18.4D). NEXT
- *Formation of S-loop:* As primitive atrium and sinus venosus get freed from septum transversum, they come lie in the pericardial cavity dorsocranial to the primitive ventricle and thus, S-shaped cardiac loop is formed (Fig. 18.3E).
- Bulbus cordis and primitive ventricle are separated by *bulboventricular sulcus* (Fig. 18.3D) that later disappears and bulbus cordis and ventricle fuse to form a single chamber (Figs 18.3E, 18.5).

- *Formation of auricles:* Primitive atrium lies dorsal to (behind) the truncus arteriosus. On expansion, primitive atrium projects forward on either side of truncus arteriosus as *auricles* (Fig. 18.3E, SEM 18.4).

DEVELOPMENT OF ATRIA

Atria of heart develop as follows (Practice Fig. 18.4, Flowchart 18.3).

Right Atrium MCQ

Q. Write a short note on development of right atrium.

Summary (Examination Guide)

1. Rough trabeculated part of right atrium and right auricle from right half of primitive atrium.
2. Smooth part of right atrium (sinus venarum) from sinus venosus.
3. Crista terminalis, valve of inferior vena cava, and valve of coronary sinus develop from right venous valve.
4. A small area of most ventral smooth part develops from right half of atrioventricular canal.

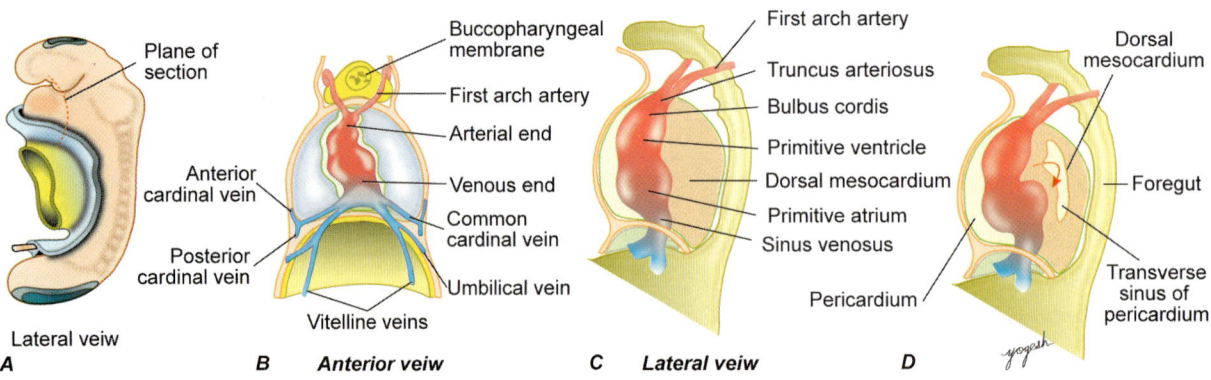

Fig. 18.4: Development of heart tube, truncus arteriosus, conus cordis, bulbar part, and mesocardium

Flowchart 18.3: Formation of atria

	Atria						
Right atrium				**Left atrium**			
Primitive atrium	*Sinus venosus*	*Right venous valve*	*Atrioventricular canal*	*Primitive atrium*	*Pulmonary vein*	*Atrioventricular canal*	
Rough/trabeculated part of right atrium Right auricle	Smooth part of right atrium	Crista terminalis Valve of IVC Valve of coronary sinus	Small ventral smooth part	Rough part of left atrium Left auricle	Posterior smooth part	Small smooth ventral part	

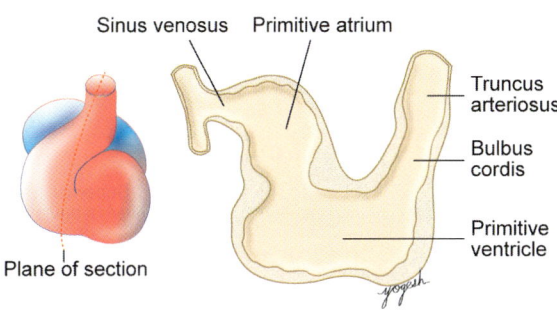

Fig. 18.5: Section of developing heart showing relationship of primitive atria and ventricles

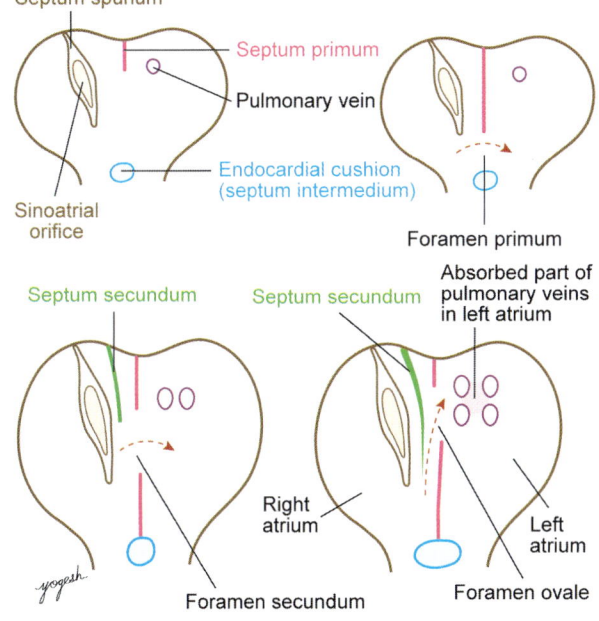

Practice Fig. 18.4: Development of interatrial septum

Left Atrium^{MCQ, Viva}

Q. Write a short note on development of left atrium.

Summary (Examination Guide)

- Anterior rough part of left atrium and left auricle develop from left half of primitive atrium.
- Posterior smooth part (between openings of pulmonary veins) develops from absorption of pulmonary veins.
- Ventral smooth part develops from left half of atrioventricular canal.
  - Details of the development of atria are described in the following sections.

Sinus Venosus

Q. Write a short note on sinus venosus.

Structure of sinus venosus (Figs 18.6, 18.7, Practice Figs 18.5, 18.6, Flowchart 18.4)

- Sinus venosus is a caudal end of heart tube.
- It represents venous end of the developing heart.
- Its unfused part is called *right* and *left horns*.
- Each horn receives blood from various body parts as follows (Figs 18.4B, 18.6A):
  1. Vitelline vein from yolk sac
  2. Umbilical vein from placenta
  3. Common cardinal vein (duct of Cuvier) from body wall.
- Sinoatrial orifice: It is a communication between sinus venosus and primitive atrium (Fig.18.7A).

Changes in left horn (Fig. 18.6)

- At the level of sinoatrial orifice, sickle-shaped sinoatrial fold develops. This fold separates left horn from primitive atrium, and thus left horn becomes just a tributary of the right horn (Fig. 18.6B, C).

Fate of sinoatrial orifice (Fig. 18.7)

- Initially, wide oval-shaped, transversely oriented sinoatrial orifice lies in the centre (Fig. 18.7A).
- On formation of sinoatrial fold, size of the orifice reduces and it becomes a narrow slit. Right margin of sinoatrial orifice is called *right venous valve*, whereas left margin is called *left venous valve* (Fig. 18.7A).
- Cranial fusion of these valves forms a fold called *septum spurium*, whereas caudal fusion forms *sinus septum*.

Fate of tributaries of sinus venous (Flowchart 18.4)

^{MCQ}

- The tributaries of sinus venosus develop to form the following structures (Fig. 18.6):
  1. Right common cardinal vein → part of superior vena cava

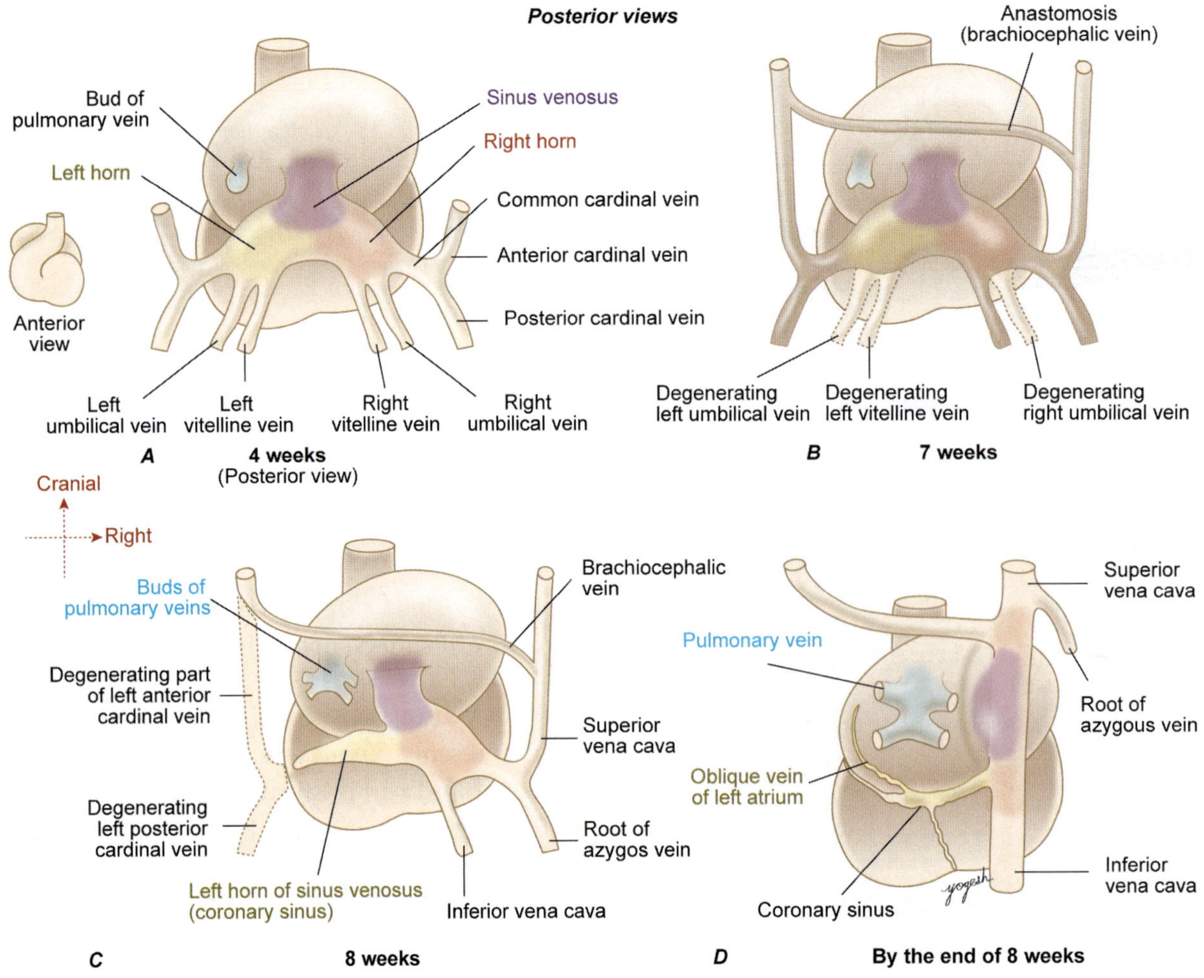

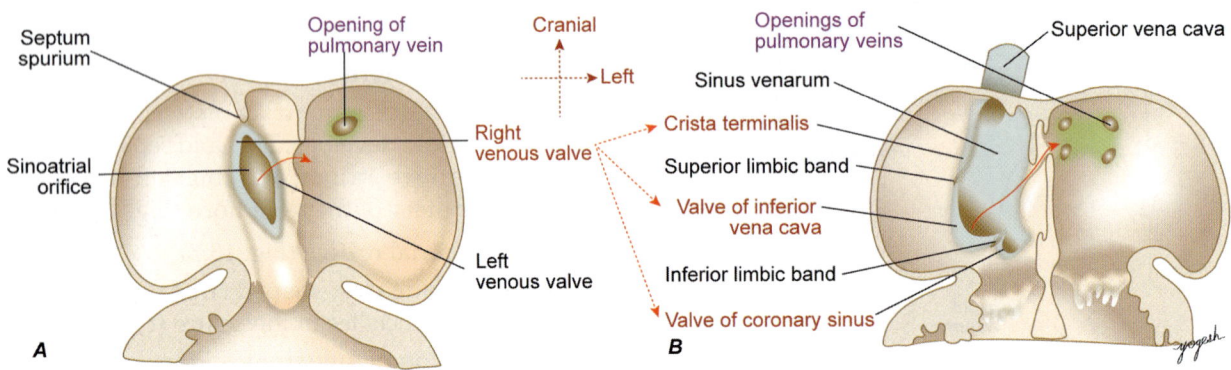

Fig. 18.6: Development of sinus venosus and pulmonary veins

Fig. 18.7: Absorption of sinus venosus in the right atrium. Superior and inferior limbic bands divide right venous valve into three zones. Right venous valve forms crista terminalis, valve of inferior vena cava, and valve of coronary sinus. Left venous valve fuses with the interatrial septum. Absorbed part of sinus venosus forms sinus venarum

2. Right vitelline vein → terminal part of inferior vena cava
3. Left horn of sinus venosus and left common cardinal vein → coronary sinus
4. Left common cardinal vein → oblique vein of left atrium
5. Cephalic part of right posterior cardinal vein → arch of azygos vein
6. Right umbilical vein and left vitelline vein → obliterated by 5th week
7. Left common cardinal vein → obliterated by the 10th week
8. Left umbilical vein → proximal part disappears, distal part drains into inferior vena cava through ductus venosus in fetal life and forms ligamentum teres afterbirth

For details, read Chapter 19. Right umbilical vein and left vitelline vein are obliterated in the fifth week. Left common cardinal vein is obliterated by 10th week.^{MCQ}

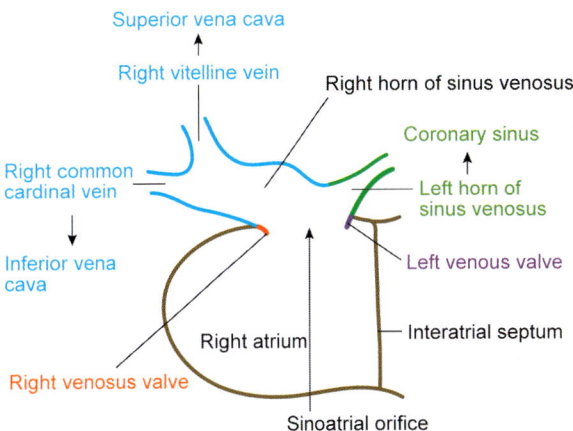

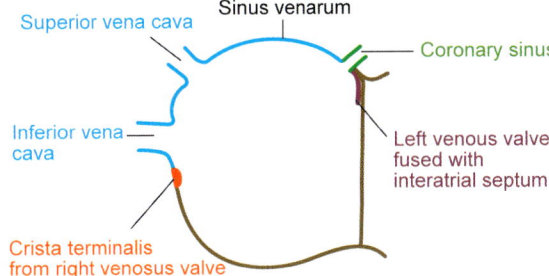

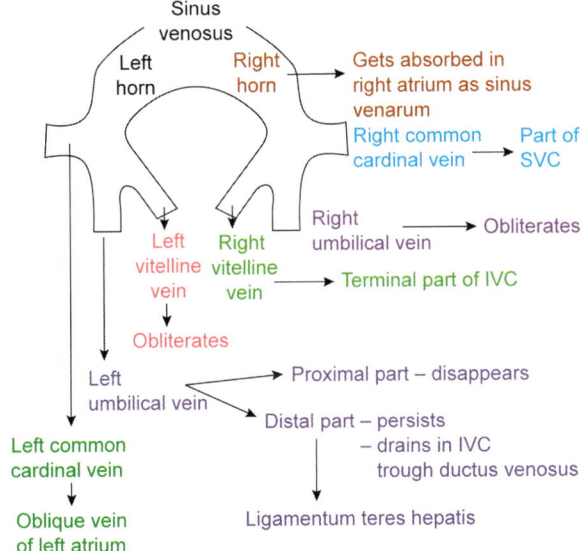

Practice Fig. 18.5: Regression of left horn of sinus venosus

Flowchart 18.4: Sinus venosus and its derivatives

Practice Fig. 18.6: Absorption of sinus venosus into the right atrium

- Major septa of heart are formed between 27th and 37th day of development.^{MCQ}

Development of Interatrial Septum

Q. Write a short note on development of interatrial septum.

Summary (Examination Guide)

- Interatrial septum develops in 5th week of intrauterine life from the following two sources (Practice Fig. 18.4, Flowchart 18.5):
  1. Septum primum
  2. Septum secundum

Flowchart 18.5: Development of interatrial septum

4th Week: Septum primum – grows from root of atria toward sinuatrial openings
↓
Ostium primum: gap between septumprimum and AV cushions
↓
Foramen secundum: gap in septum primum
↓
Closure of foramen primum ← Fusion of septum primum with AV cushions
↓
Septum secundum: Grows downward on the right side of septum primum
↓
Convertion: Foramen secumdum → Foramen ovale
↓
After birth
1. Closure of foramen ovale
2. Septum primum → floor of fossa ovalis
3. Lower margin of septum secundum → annulus fossa ovalis

Changes in Atrioventricular Canal

- The communication between primitive atrium and primitive ventricle is an *atrioventricular canal*.
- AV cushions: Two atrioventricular (AV) cushions appear as thickening of subendocardial mesenchymal cells in ventral and dorsal wall of AV canal. Cardiac jelly forms around the heart tube during early development form endocardial cushion and myocardium (Fig. 18.8A).^{NEXT}
- *Septum intermedium:* AV cushions grow and fuse with each other to form *septum intermedium* and divide the AV canal into right and left halves (Fig. 18.8B).

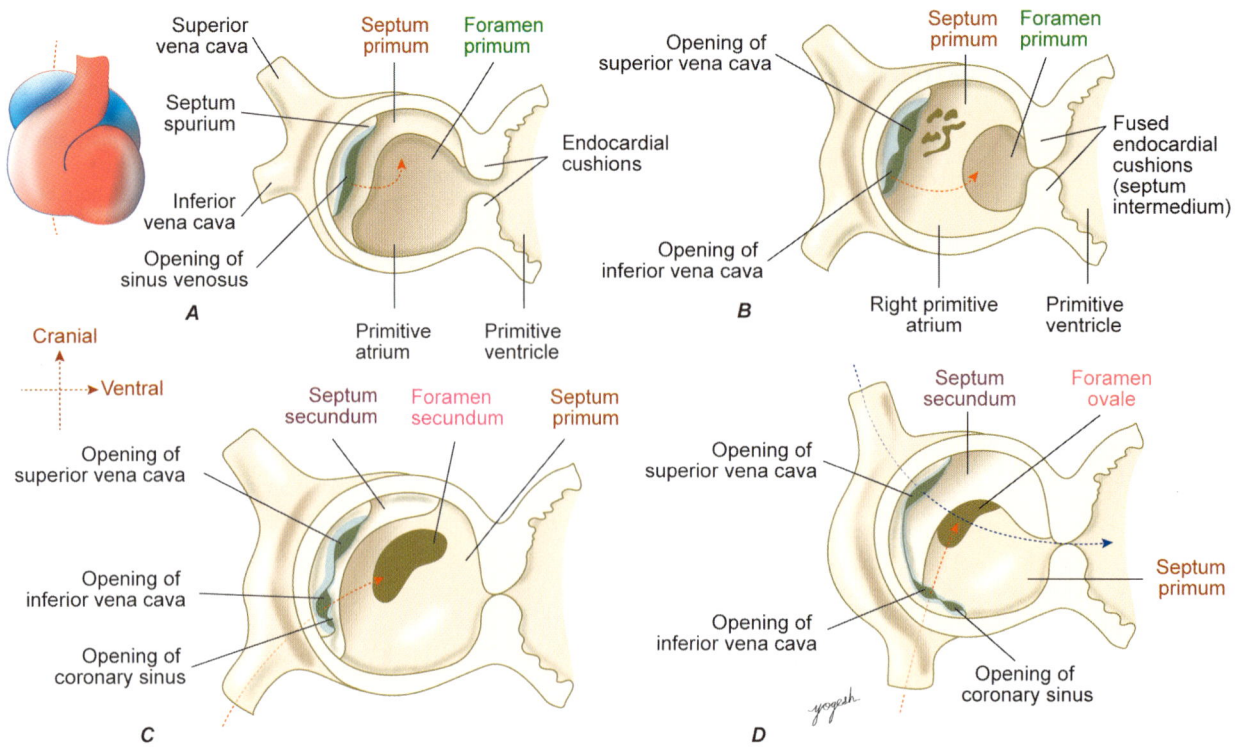

Fig. 18.8: Development of interatrial septum. Sagittal section of the developing heart seen from right side

Stages of Development

1. *Septum primum*: At the end of fourth week, a *septum primum* starts developing from roof of primitive atrium on left side of septum spurium and sinoatrial opening (Figs 18.8A, 18.9A).
2. *Foramen (ostium) primum*: Septum primum grows toward AV cushions (septum intermedium) and becomes sickle-shaped septum. A small gap between the growing septum primum and septum intermedium is called *foramen primum* (Fig. 18.8B).
3. *Foramen secundum:* Finally, septum primum fuses with AV cushions that closes foramen primum. Simultaneously, a small gap as *foramen secundum* appears in the septum primum (Fig. 18.8C).
4. *Septum secundum*: A crescent-shaped *septum secundum* starts growing from roof of the primitive atrium between septum spurium and septum primum (Figs 18.8C, 18.9).
5. *Foramen ovale:* The septum secundum grows toward septum intermedium and overlaps foramen secundum. Overlapping septum secundum converts foramen secundum into an oblique passage called *foramen ovale* (Figs 18.8D, 18.9B).
6. After birth, foramen ovale obliterates. After birth, in the heart, floor of fossa ovalis represents septum primum, whereas the lower free margin of septum secundum forms the *annulus ovalis*.

Function of Foramen Ovale

- Foramen ovale is converted into a valve by opposition of thick-flap of septum secundum over thin mobile flap of septum primum.
- This valve allows transmission of blood from right atrium to left atrium, but blood cannot re-enter the right atrium.
- Thus, foramen ovale allows blood to bypass pulmonary circulation and shunts most of the blood from right atrium to left atrium instead of right ventricle.
- After birth:
  – Immediately after birth, pulmonary circulation begins and volume of blood returning to the left atrium increases. It increases pressure in the left atrium and produces physiological closure of foramen ovale (later it closes anatomically).

Formation of Sinus Venarum (absorption of sinus venosus in the right atrium)

- The right and left horns of sinus venosus are absorbed into right atrium and results in segregation of openings of superior vena cava, inferior vena cava and coronary sinus from each other (Practice Fig. 18.7).
- Superior and inferior limbic bands (muscular bands) divide right venous valve into three zones.
- Right venous valve forms the following structures:
  1. Crista terminalis
  2. Valve of inferior vena cava
  3. Valve of coronary sinus
- Left venous valve fuses with interatrial septum.
- Absorbed part of sinus venosus forms sinus venarum (posterior smooth part of the right atrium).

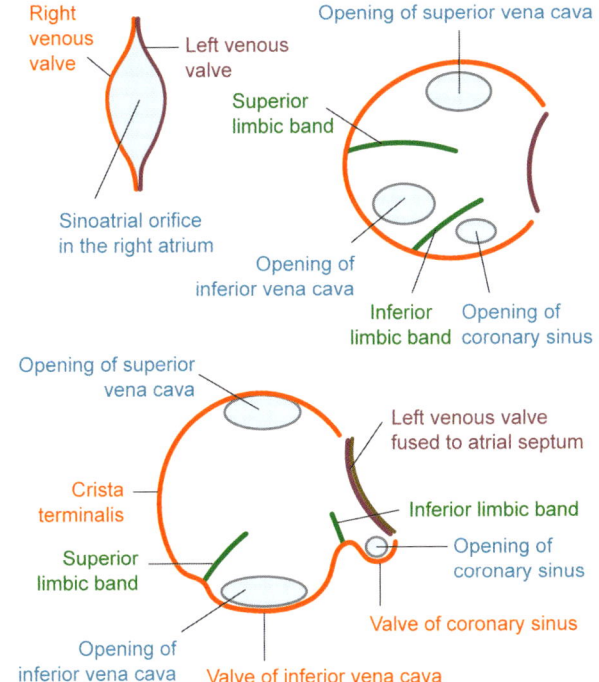

Practice Fig. 18.7: Fate of right and left venous valves

Absorption of Pulmonary Veins into Left Atrium

- The dorsal wall of left atrium outpouches to form a primordial pulmonary vein (Fig. 18.9A).
- Single pulmonary vein divides into two and later into four pulmonary veins (Fig. 18.9A, B).
- Part of pulmonary veins get absorbed into dorsal wall of left atrium and openings of all four pulmonary veins get separated from each other (Fig. 18.9B).
- Absorbed portion of pulmonary veins forms smooth posterior part of left atrium.

Ectopia Cordis
Q. Write a short note on ectopia cordis.
- It is a rare congenital positional anomaly of heart.
- The heart lies exposed on anterior thoracic wall.
- Cause: Nonunion of sternal halves.
- Treatment: Surgical repositioning of heart is not very successful due to high postpartum mortality (deaths).

Box 18.1: Dextrocardia

Definition

It is a congenital condition in that heart points to right side rather than the usual left side.
- *Dexter* in Latin means 'right' and *Kardia* in Greek means 'heart'.
- Dextrocardia is the most common positional anomaly of the heart.

Classification

It is classified as follows:
A. *Isolated dextrocardia:* Only heart is placed on the right side of thorax.
B. *Dextrocardia invertus* (situs invertus): Refers to disposition (reversal) of all thoracic and abdominal viscera including heart.

Incidence: 1 in 7,000 individuals.

Causes: Abnormal left-sided looping of heart tube instead of usual right-sided looping.

Molecular Regulation
- Foregut endoderm secretes bone morphogenic proteins (BMP2 and BMP4) that induce expression of transcription factor NKX2.5 in splanchnic mesoderm and formation of heart tubes in cardiogenic area.
- NKX2.5 is product of master gene for heart development. *MCQ*
- Simultaneously endoderm inhibits secretion of neural tube protein production as WNT proteins inhibit cardiogenic area.
- Laterality inducing genes (nodal and LEFTY-2 genes) are responsible for left sidedness of heart looping.

DEVELOPMENT OF VENTRICLES

Ventricles develop as follows:
A. Rough (inflow) parts: From primitive ventricles.
B. Smooth (outflow) parts (infundibulum of right ventricle and aortic vestibule of left ventricle): From conus cordis or middle one-third of the bulbus cordis.

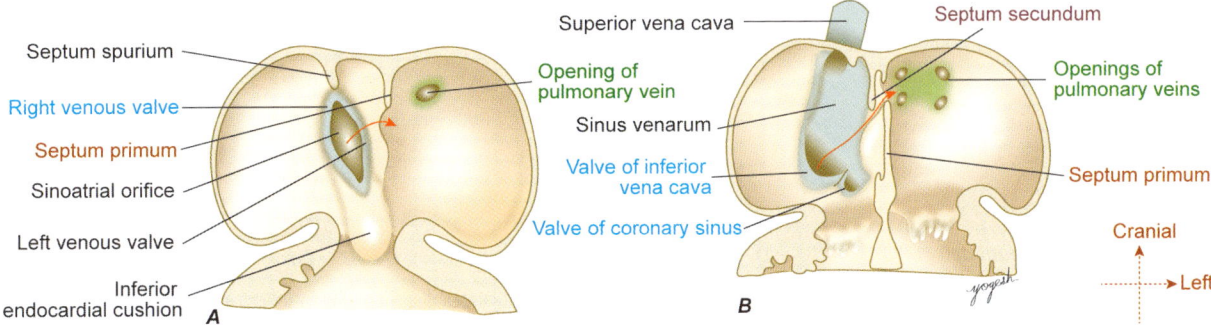

Fig. 18.9: Development of atria, interatrial septum and absorption of sinus venosus and pulmonary veins into the atria: (A) Coronal section passing through the atria at 5 weeks. Blue color indicates the sinus venosus and green shading indicates pulmonary veins; (B) Coronary section of atria at the end of 8th week

Box 18.2: Atrial septal defects (ASD)

Q. Write a short note on atrial septal defects.

- **Definition**
  Atrial septal defects are congenital anomalies that involve defective formation of interatrial septum resulting in an abnormal communication between right and left atria.
- **Incidence**
  6.4 in 10,000 births.
  More common in females (2:1) than in males.
- **Cause**: Mutation of NKX2.5.
- **Types** (Flowchart 18.6)
  1. Ostium secundum defects (Fig. 18.10B)
     Failure of septum secundum to cover septum primum results in ostium secundum defect. It may be due to short septum secundum or more absorption of septum primum. Ostium secundum defect results in formation of large foramen ovale that does not close after birth. It is one of the commonest congenital heart diseases.
  2. Septum primum defect (Fig. 18.10C)
     Failure of septum primum to close foramen primum results in septum primum defect.
  3. Endocardial cushion defect ((Fig. 18.10D)
     Failure of fusion of septum primum with endocardial cushions (septum intermedium) results in persistent foramen primum.
  4. Sinus venosus ASD
     Incomplete absorption of sinus venosus in right atrium results in defective atrial septum near the opening of SVC.
  5. Common atrium/cor triloculare biventriculare (Fig. 18.10E) MCQ
     It is a rare condition with a failure of development of the interatrial septum.

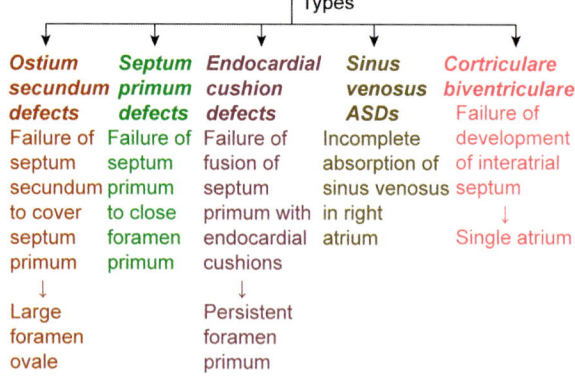

Flowchart 18.6: Atrial septal defects (ASD)

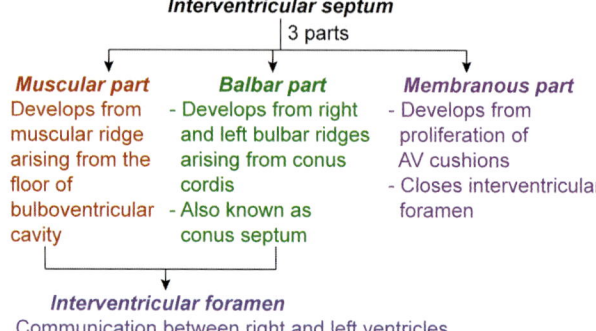

Flowchart 18.7: Development of interventricular septum

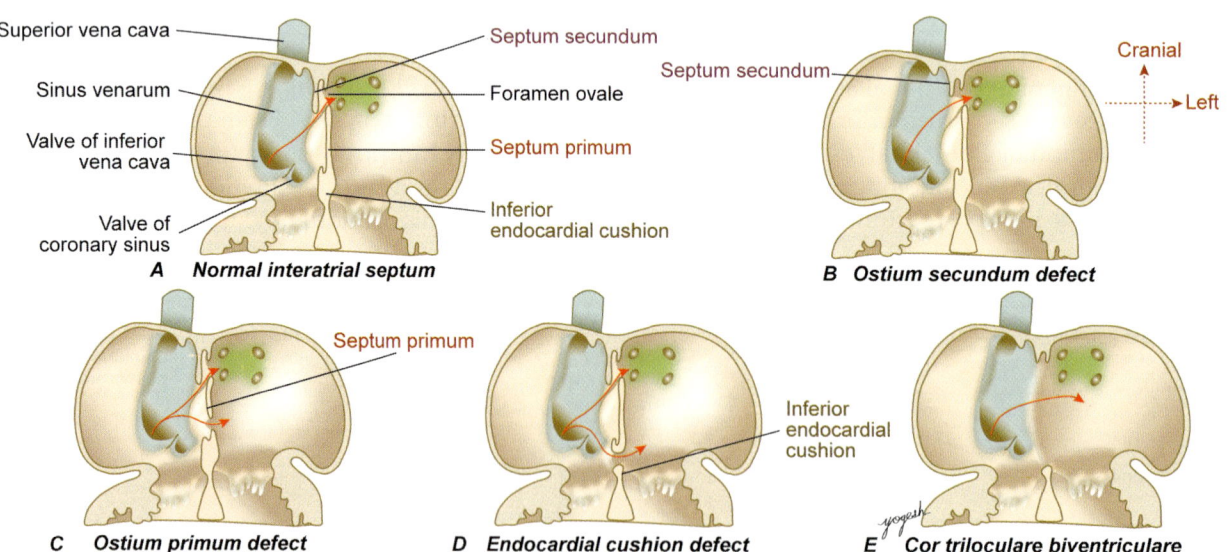

Fig. 18.10: Atrial septal defects involve the defective formation of interatrial septum resulting in an abnormal communication between the right and left atria. Ostium secundum defects are failure of septum secundum to cover septum primum. Ostium primum defect involves incomplete closure of foramen primum. Endocardial cushion defect is the result of failure of fusion of septum primum with endocardial cushions and persistent foramen primum. Common atrium or cor triloculare biventriculare is a failure of development of the interatrial septum

Bulbus Cordis

Q. Write a short note on bulbus cordis.

- The arterial end of developing heart tube shows a dilatation called bulbus cordis.
- There are three parts of bulbus cordis as follows:
  1. **Proximal one-third**: It fuses with primitive ventricle to form *bulboventricular chamber*. Proximal one-third later form the trabeculated part of right ventricle.
  2. **Middle one-third**: It is conical-shaped; hence, called *conus cordis*. It forms outflow parts of both ventricles.
  3. **Distal one-third**: It is called *truncus arteriosus*. A spiral septum divides truncus arteriosus into pulmonary trunk and ascending aorta.

FORMATION OF INTERVENTRICULAR SEPTUM

Q. Write a short note on development of interventricular septum.

- Interventricular septum separates right ventricle from left ventricle (Flowchart 18.7).

Summary (Examination Guide)

- It consists of three parts (Fig. 18.11 and Practice Fig. 18.8):
  - **Muscular part**: Develops from muscular ridge arising on the floor of bulboventricular cavity.
  - **Bulbar part**: Develops from right and left bulbar ridges arising from conus cordis.
  - **Membranous part**: Develops from proliferation of AV cushion that fills the gap between muscular and bulbar parts.

Stages of Development

1. *Muscular part* (Fig. 18.11)
   - A muscular interventricular septum grows from the floor of bulboventricular cavity and divides ventricles into two halves.

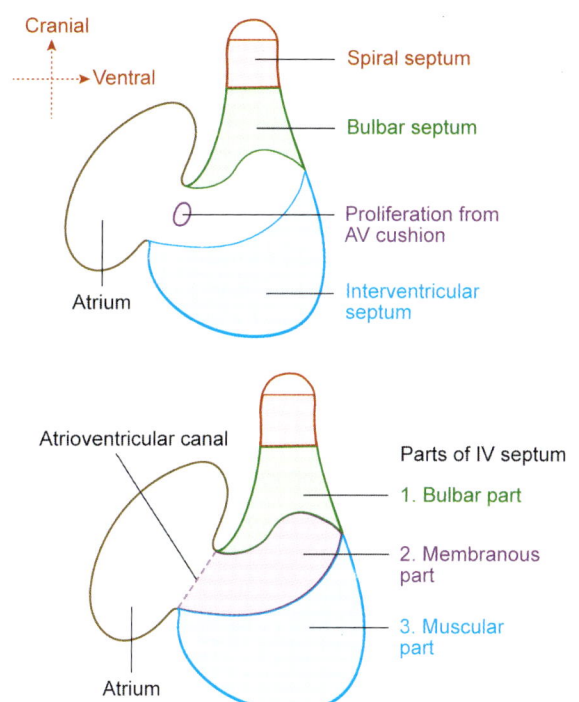

Practice Fig. 18.8: Development of interventricular septum

   - It grows toward septum intermedium (AV cushion) and fuses partially with it.
   - Right and left ventricles communicate with each other through an *interventricular foramen* that lies cranial to the muscular interventricular foramen.

2. *Bulbar part*
   - From conus cordis, the right and left bulbar ridges develop and later fuse to form a bulbar part of the septum.
   - Bulbar part grows caudally toward muscular part of interventricular septum or conus septum.
   - The right and left ventricles communicate with each other through the interventricular foramen that lies between muscular and bulbar parts.

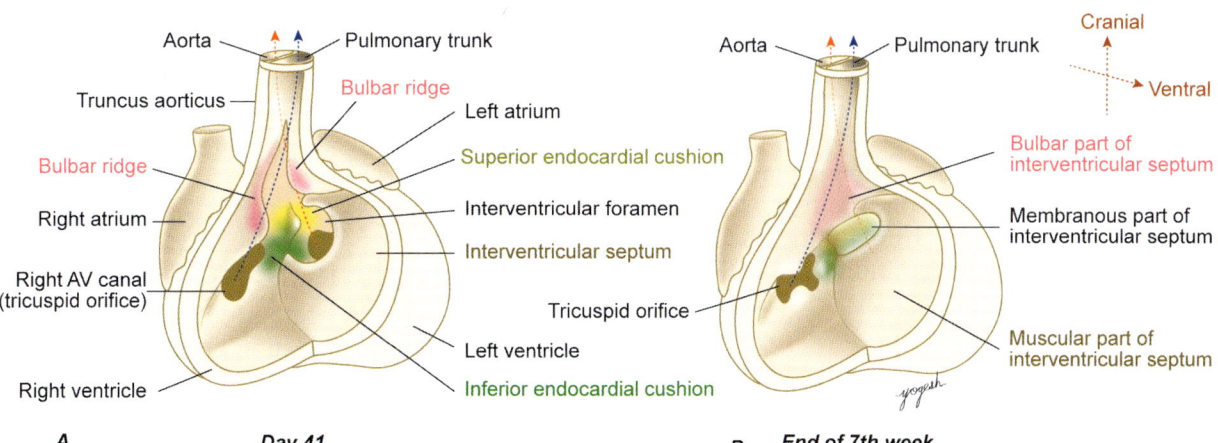

Fig. 18.11: Development of the interventricular septum. Muscular part of the interventricular septum develops from muscular ridge raising from the floor of primitive ventricle. Bulbar part develops from right and left bulbar ridges arising from conus cordis, whereas membranous part develops from the proliferation of AV cushion that fills the gap between muscular and bulbar parts

3. *Membranous part*
   - By 8th week, the gap of interventricular foramen is filled by a tissue that proliferates from right side of AV cushions and right and left bulbar ridges. It forms a membranous part.
   - Presence of interventricular foramen is essential until separation of bulbus cordis and truncus arteriosus.
   - Anterior portion of membranes part of interventricular septum is derived from AV cushions and it separates right and left ventricles.^{NEXT}
   - Posterior portion of membranous part of IV septum is derived from AV cushions and it separates right atrium from left ventricle.^{NEXT}

Formation of Aorticopulmonary Septum

- In the truncus arteriosus, a *spiral septum* called *aorticopulmonary septum* appears (Fig. 18.12).
- This septum divides truncus arteriosus (aorticus) into aorta and pulmonary trunk.

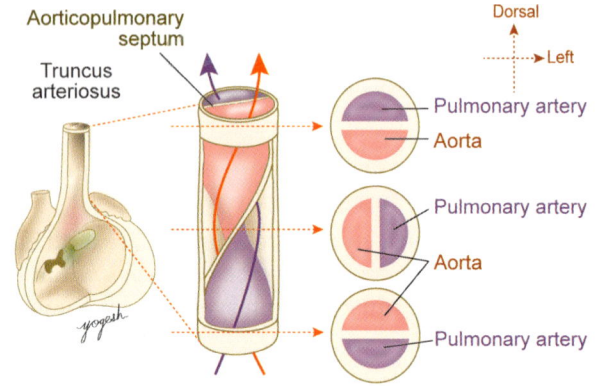

Fig. 18.12: Development of truncus arteriosus. Spiral aorticopulmonary septum divides the truncus arteriosus into aorta and pulmonary trunk. Note the changes in relationship of aorta and pulmonary trunk

Steps

1. *Truncal ridges:* Two truncal ridges appear in truncus arteriosus that grow and fuse to form the *spiral septum* (Fig. 18.11A, B).
2. *Fusion with bulbar septum:* Spiral septum lies in same plane as that of bulbar septum and grows to fuse with bulbar septum. Here, aorta lies behind the pulmonary trunk (Fig. 18.11A, B).
3. *Spiralling of septum:* Spiral septum separates aorta and pulmonary trunk in a spiral course. Aorta that lies behind the pulmonary trunk in the lower part, comes to lie on the right side and finally anterior to the pulmonary trunk (Fig. 18.12).

Clinical Integration

Transposition of great vessels
- Transposition of ascending aorta and pulmonary trunk may occur due to reverse spiral attachment of aortic-pulmonary septum. In this condition, aorta raises from the right ventricle, whereas pulmonary trunk from the left ventricle. Incidence of transposition of great vessels is 4.8 in 10,000 births.

Persistent (Common) Truncus Arteriosus
- Failure of development of spiral septum results in common outflow tract for the right and left ventricles. It is always associated with ventricular septal defect because of failure of contribution of bulbar ridges to the ventricular septum.

DEVELOPMENT OF VALVES OF HEART

Atrioventricular Valves

- Tricuspid valve is present between right atrium and right ventricle, whereas mitral valve is present between left atrium and left ventricle (Fig. 18.13). Initially, atria communicate with ventricles through a single atrioventricular canal (Fig. 18.13B).
- Proliferation of subendocardial mesenchyme forms subendocardial cushions around atrioventricular canals (Fig. 18.13C, D).
- Excavation of these cushions forms cusps of AV valves.
- Free margins of these cusps get connected by thin chordae tendinae with papillary muscles of ventricular wall.
- On the right side, there are three cushions—anterior, posterior and septal, whereas on the left there are two cushions—anterior and posterior. Hence, on right, there is a tricuspid valve and on left, bicuspid (mitral) valve (Fig. 18.13D).

Pulmonary and Aortic Valves

- In truncus arteriosus, at the junction with conus cordis two endocardial cushions appear (right and left) (Fig. 18.14A). Soon two more (ventral and dorsal) cushions also appear (Fig. 18.14B).
- On separation of the pulmonary trunk from aorta by a spiral septum, right and left cushions divide into two parts (Fig. 18.14C, D, E).
- Excavation of these cushions form cusps of aortic and pulmonary valves.
- Aorta and pulmonary trunk undergo spiral rotation and finally, valves show the following cusps (Fig. 18.14F):
  - Aortic valve: One anterior and two posterior
  - Pulmonary valve: One posterior and two anterior

DEVELOPMENT OF CONDUCTING SYSTEM OF HEART

Conducting system of heart is formed during 5th week. The components of conducting system of heart develop as follows:

1. SA node: SA node develops during the fifth week of IUL. After incorporation of sinus venosus into right atrium, SA node comes to lie near opening of SVC.
2. AV node and bundle of His: AV node and bundle of His are derived from interatrial septum near opening

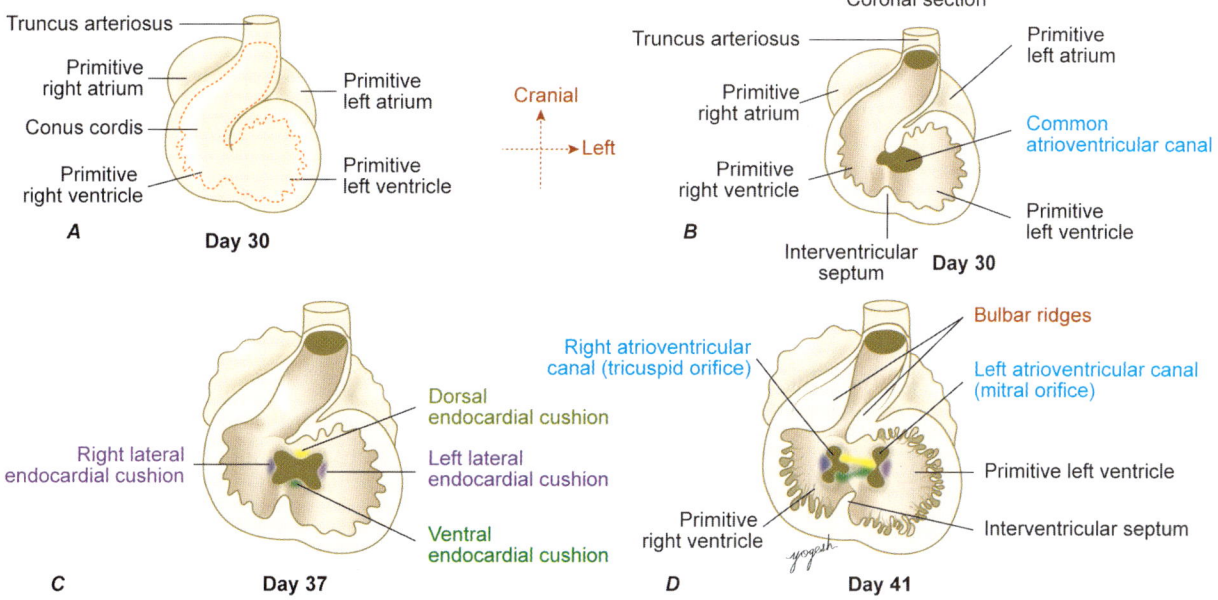

Fig. 18.13: Formation of septum in the atrioventricular canal

of the coronary sinus. It develops from dorsal endocardial cushion of AV canal in 6th week of IUL.

3. **Purkinje fibres:** Fibres from bundle of His form right and left bundle branches that get distributed as Purkinje fibres.

DEVELOPMENT OF PERICARDIUM

Q. Write a short note on development of pericardium.

Summary (Examination Guide)

Pericardium is derived as follows:

- Serous pericardium
  - Visceral layer from splanchnopleuric mesoderm
  - Parietal layer from somatopleuric mesoderm
- Fibrous pericardium from somatopleuric mesoderm and septum transversum.
- Pericardial cavity from intraembryonic coelom.

Stages of Development

1. On head folding, pericardial cavity comes to lie on ventral aspect of foregut.
2. Heart tube with myoepicardial mantle invaginates pericardial cavity.
3. Layer of myoepicardial mantle that lines the pericardial cavity forms visceral layer of pericardium (epicardium).
4. Initially, heart tube is suspended in pericardial cavity by *dorsal mesocardium* (double-layer fold similar to mesentery).
5. On formation of a cardiac loop, arterial and venous ends of heart tube come closer and dorsal mesocardium disappears to form *transverse sinus of pericardium*.
6. On formation of transverse sinus, fibrous and visceral pericardium become continuous with each other at arterial and venous ends of heart tube.

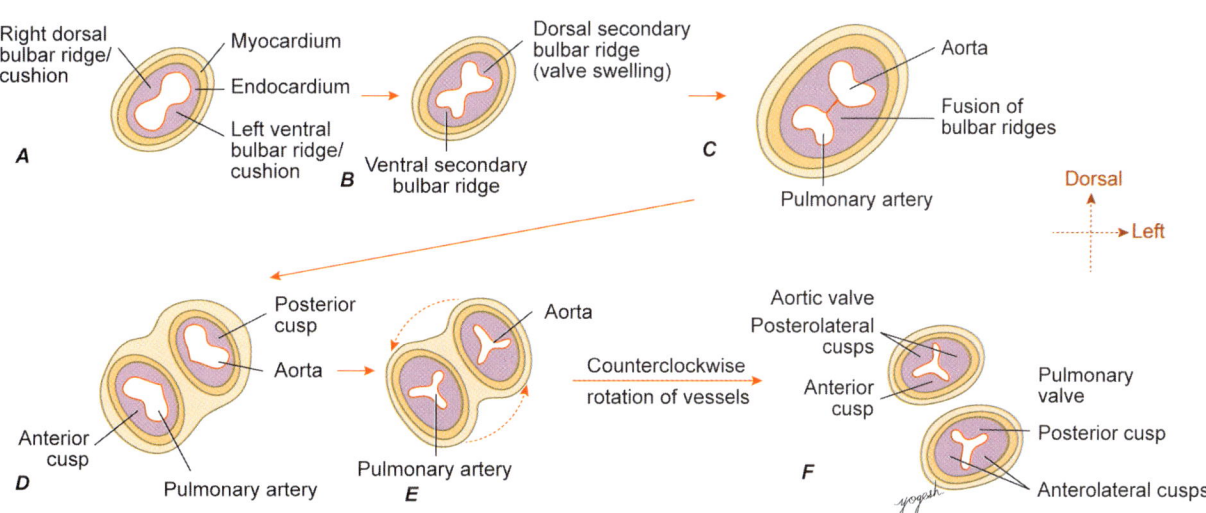

Fig. 18.14: Development of aortic and pulmonary valves (semilunar valves)

7. Somatopleuric layer of mesoderm lining pericardial cavity forms parietal pericardium and fibrous pericardium.
8. Reorientation of SVC, IVC and absorption of pulmonary veins in the left atrium results into formation of *oblique sinus of pericardium*.

Some Interesting Facts

- Appearance of paired angioblastic cords is first sign of development of heart.
- Heart is the first organ of the body to start functioning. Cardiovascular system is the earliest system that start functioning in fetus.^{NEXT}
- Heart tubes are formed in the third week.
- Heart beats begin by 22nd day of IUL.^{NEXT}
- Heart develops completely by 10th week (3rd month).^{NEXT}
- Somatopleuric mesoderm forms myocardium, Purkinje fibres (conduction system of heart).^{NEXT}
- Fallot's tetralogy is the most common congenital cyanotic heart disease.
- Unequal division of conus cordis resulting for anterior displacement of conotruncal septum gives rise to Fallot's tetralogy.^{NEXT}
- Ventricular septal defect is almost common congenital anomaly of the heart (12 in 10,000 births).
- Between 18th and 22nd weeks of IUL, fetal heart echocardiography and Doppler ultrasonography is useful for detecting abnormal fetal heart anomalies.
- Real-time ultrasound can detect fetal heart anomalies even by 16th week.
- Neural crest cells contribute to endocardial endocardia cushion formation in conus cordis and truncus arteriosus. Failure of neural crest cells in the formation of these cushions results in tetralogy of Fallot, pulmonary stenosis, persistent truncus arteriosus and transposition of great vessels.
- In addition to endocardial cushions, the neural crest cells also help in craniofacial development. Hence, facial and cardiac anomalies may be observed together.^{Viva, Clinical fact}

3. Ventricle septal defect (VSD)
4. Overriding of aorta

Incidence
- It is the most common congenital cyanotic heart disease.
- Incidence of TOF is 9.6 in 10,000 births.
- TOF is the most common cyanotic heart disease.
- TOF accounts for 6–10% of all CHDs.

Cause
- Mostly unknown.
- Associates with maternal phenylketonuria.
- Responsible genes: JAG1 (it regulates formation of conotruncal septum by neural crest cells).

Diagnosis
1. Echocardiography.
2. X-ray chest: *Coeur en sabot* (boot-like) appearance of a heart.^{MCQ}

Pathophysiology

Pulmonary stenosis causes concentric right ventricular hypertrophy without cardiac enlargement
↓
Increase in right ventricular pressure
↓
Blood shunts from right ventricle to left ventricle through VSD
↓
Ejection of mixed blood to aorta → *cyanosis*
↓
Overriding of aorta (disposition)

Clinical Manifestation
- Blue-baby: *Cyanotic lips* and nail bed.^{Viva, MCQ}
- Easy fatigability.
- Tet-spells: Acute hypoxic spells characterized by shortness of breath, cyanosis, agitation and loss of consciousness (syncope).

Box 18.3: Tetralogy of Fallot (TOF)

Fallot's tetralogy (Flowchart 18.8)

Q. Write a short note on Fallot's tetralogy.
Q. Give embryological basis of Fallot's tetralogy.

- TOF is a congenital heart defect.
- Components (Fig. 18.15, Practice Fig. 18.9):^{Viva}
  1. Pulmonary stenosis
  2. Right ventricular hypertrophy

Flowchart 18.8: Fallot's tetralogy

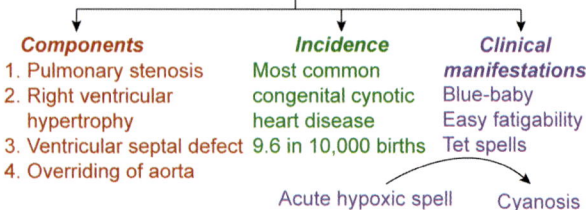

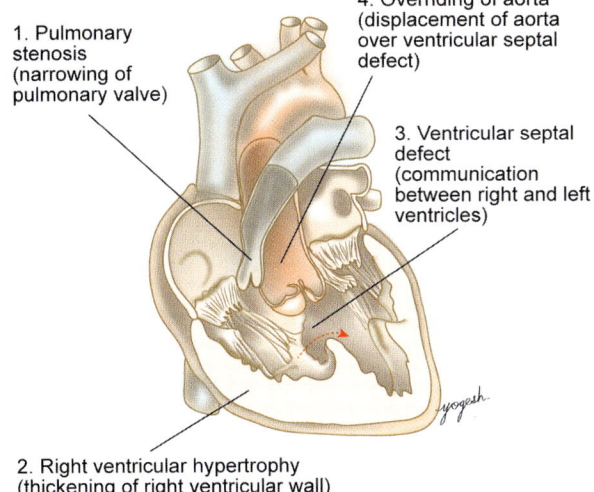

Fig. 18.15: Tetralogy of Fallot. It includes pulmonary stenosis, right ventricular hypertrophy, overriding of aorta and ventricular septal defect

Some Interesting Facts

- **Taussig-Bing syndrome:** It is a ventricular septal defect having a. Double outlet right ventricle, b. Subpulmonic ventricular septal defect (Fig. 18.16).
- **Holt-Oram syndrome:** Preaxial limb abnormalities with ASD. Cause: TBX5 gene mutation (autosomal dominant). *Note:* TBX5 gene is responsible for limb development and septation of heart.
- **Eisenmenger's complex**
  - It includes hypoplasia of pulmonary capillary plexus that causes
    1. Pulmonary hypertension
    2. Dilatation of pulmonary trunk
    3. Hypertrophy of right ventricle.
  - If Eisenmenger's complex is associated with ASD or VSD, then it is called Eisenmenger's syndrome.
- **DiGeorge syndrome**
  In 22q11 deletion syndrome, defective neural crest cells produce children with facial defects, thymic hypoplasia, parathyroid dysfunction, and cardiac anomalies (Fallot's tetralogy, persistent truncus arteriosus).

Ventricular Septal Defects (VSD)

Q. Write a short note on ventricular septal defects.

- VSD is the most common congenital anomaly of the heart.
- VSDs are more common in males than in females.
- VSD commonly involves the membranous part of interventricular septum.
- Incidence isolated VSD is 12 in 10,000 births.

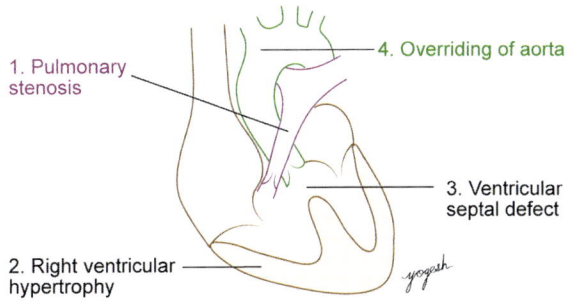

Practice Fig. 18.9: Tetralogy of Fallot

Embryological basis

Failure of fusion of right and left bulbar ridges with AV cushions
↓
Communication between ventricles
↓
Shunting of blood from left ventricle to right ventricle

TIMING OF EMBRYOLOGIC HEART FORMATION

Days 21–22	Umbilical veins, vitelline veins, cardinal veins form
	Single heart tube forms
	Pericardial cavity forms
	Heart begins to beat
Day 23	Heart tube grows rapidly, heart folding begins
Days 25–28	Atrioventriculobulbar loop forms
	Septum primum appears
Days 27–37	Endocardial cushions appear
Days 28	Ventricular septum appears as a small ridge in common ventricle
Days 28–35	Absorption of bulbous cordis and sinus venosus
	Four-chambered heart forms

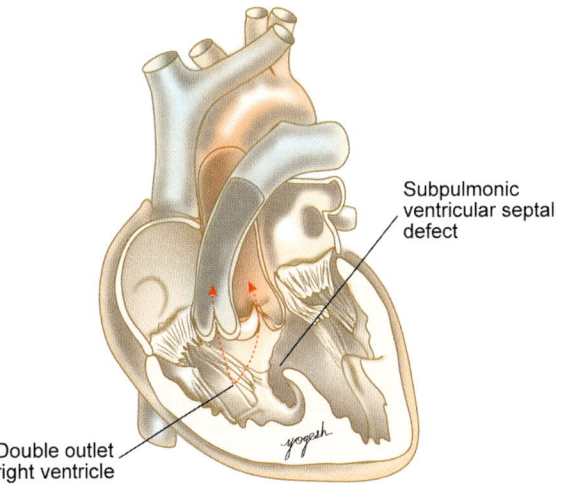

Fig. 18.16: Taussig-Bing syndrome. It is a ventricular septal defect having double outlet right ventricle and subpulmonic ventricular septal defect

Day 29	Pulmonary veins form
Days 31–35	Placental circulation begins
	Atrioventricular node develops
	Ostium secundum forms
	Sinoatrial node develops
Day 33	Tricuspid and mitral valves form
Days 35–42	Coronary arteries form
Days 36–42	Inferior vena cava forms
Days 43–49	Superior vena cava forms
	Coronary sinus forms
Day 49	Muscular interventricular septum forms
Day 56	Aorta and pulmonary arteries form
	Aortic and pulmonic valves form

Box 18.4: Probe patency of foramen ovale ^{Viva, MCQ}

Q. Write a short note on patent foramen ovale.

- Just after birth, foramen ovale closes physiologically by forced opposition of septum primum on septum secundum owing to:
  1. Increased blood return to left atrium from lungs.
  2. Increased pressure in left atrium.
- Anatomical fusion also takes place soon.
- In about 20% cases, anatomical fusion does not occur and a small probe can be passed through the foramen ovale.
- Failure of fusion of septum primum with septum secundum results in patent foramen ovale. ^{NEXT}

Clinical Embryology

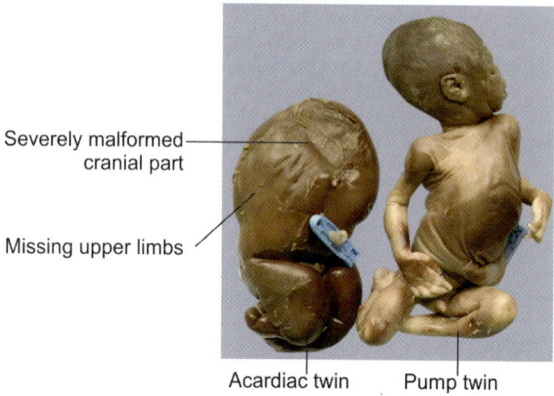

Clinical image 18.1: *Acardiac twins* [twin reversed-arterial perfusion (TRAP) sequence]: It is a rare and serious complication of monochorionic twins. The blood systems of twins are connected. One twin is acardiac and other one is pump twin. Acardiac twin is severely malformed. Its heart may be missing or deformed. The legs may be partially present or missing. Acardiac twin has reversed arterial perfusion because the blood flows in a reversed direction. The pump twin is usually normal and it drives blood through both fetuses (Image courtesy: *Dr Mamatha Gowda, Dr Haritha Sagili*)

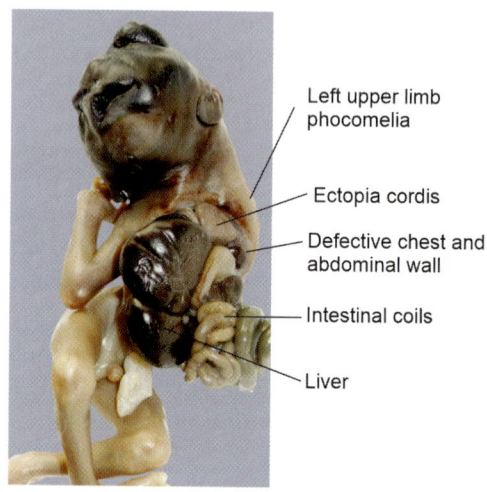

Clinical image 18.2: *Ectopia cordis* with left upper limb phocomelia. Congenital defect of chest wall associated with diaphragmatic hernia with ectopia cordis and omphalocele. Phocomelia is malformations of arms and legs. In the above case, left upper limb is completely absent. Thalidomide intake by mother may give rise to phocomelia (Image courtesy: *Dr Mamatha Gowda*)

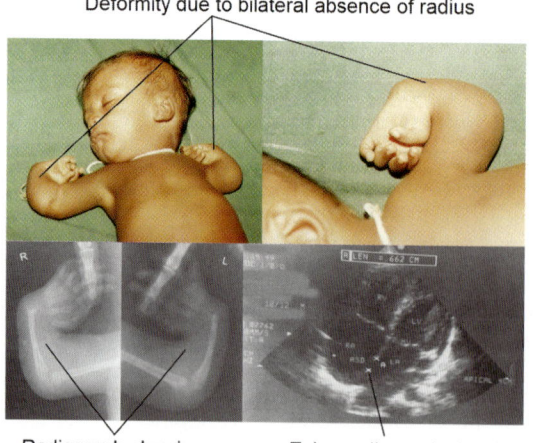

Clinical image 18.3: *Holt-Oram syndrome* (ventriculoradial syndrome): It is an autosomal dominant disorder caused due to TBX5 gene mutation. It includes absence of radius bone and atrial septal defect. Its incidence is 1 in 10,000 people. It may also show absence of carpal bones and heart block. Abbreviations: RA: Right atrium, RV: Right ventricle, LV: Left ventricle, LA: Left atrium, MV: Mitral valve, ASD: Atrial septal defect (Image courtesy: *Dr Kumaravel S*)

Chapter 19

Cardiovascular System II: Blood Vessels and Fetal Circulation

eSmartQuiz

Chapter Outline

- Erythropoiesis
- Development of arterial system
- Pharyngeal arch arteries
  - Derivatives of aortic arch arteries
  - Patent ductus arteriosus
  - Coarctation of aorta
  - Unusual origin of aorta
  - Branches of dorsal aorta
- Umbilical arteries
- Development of vertebral artery
- Development of limb vessels
- Development of venous system
- Vitelline veins
- Umbilical veins
- Somatic veins
  - Primary head vein
  - Cervicothoracic vein
  - Anomalies of superior vena cava
  - Subcardinal veins
  - Supracardinal veins
  - Posterior cardinal veins
  - Azygos venous lines
- Renal collar
- Development of inferior vena cava
  - Anomalies of inferior vena cava
- Development of azygos venous system

Fetal circulation
- Special structures in fetal circulation
- Peculiarities of fetal circulation
- Circulatory changes at birth

Development of lymphatic system

Competencies:

- **AN25.3:** Describe fetal circulation and changes occurring at birth.
- **AN25.5:** Describe development basis of congenital anomalies, transportation of great vessels, dextracardia, patient ductus arteriosus, and coarctation of aorta.
- **AN25.6:** Mention development of aortic arch arteries, SVC, IVC and coronary sinus.

INTRODUCTION

- Development of blood vessels begins in the third week of development.
- It involves vasculogenesis and angiogenesis.
- *Vasculogenesis* is formation of new vessels from mesenchymal tissue in the embryo (Fig. 19.1).

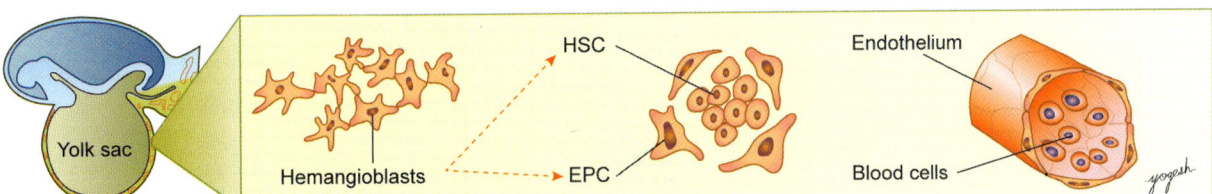

Vasculogenesis begins in the yolk sac, connecting stalk and extra-embryonic mesoderm in tertiary villi

Mesodermal cells form cell masses called blood islands. It consists of hemangioblasts

Hemangioblasts differentiate into primitive hematopoietic stem cells (HSC) and endothelial precursor cells (EPC)

HSC on differentiation form blood cells, whereas EPC differentiate to form vascular endothelium

Fig. 19.1: Vasculogenesis

- *Angiogenesis* is the sprouting of vessels into adjacent area by endothelial budding (Fig. 19.1).
- Formation of vasculature begins in extraembryonic mesoderm of yolk sac, connecting stalk, and chorion.
- Yolk sac is the first supplier of blood cells and it continues up to 60 days as a hematopoietic organ.^MCQ Later liver, spleen, thymus, and bone marrow take over the hematopoietic function.

Box 19.1: Erythropoiesis

- It is a process of formation of new red blood cells.
- It begins in yolk sac wall and continues till death in the following phases.^Viva

Period/Phase^NEXT	Age	Organ
Intravascular	3 weeks to 3rd month of intrauterine life	Wall of yolk sac
Hepatic and extramedullary	2–3 months^NEXT to 5–7 months of IUL	Liver (major organ)^NEXT Spleen, lymph nodes^NEXT
Myeloid (medullary)	8–9 months of IUL and continue in postnatal life	Red bone marrow

Note: After 20 years of age, erythropoiesis occurs mostly in flat bones such as sternum, ribs, ilium, vertebrae, and in proximal ends of humerus, femur, and tibia.

DEVELOPMENT OF ARTERIAL SYSTEM

In the 3rd week, the following vessels are present in embryo (Fig. 19.2):
- A heart tube
- Arteries
  1. Aortic end of heart tube
  2. Aortic arch arteries connecting aortic end of heart to dorsal aortae (Fig. 19.3)
  3. Two dorsal aortae lie in front of notochord
  4. Vitelline arteries supply blood to yolk sac
  5. Umbilical arteries carry blood to placenta
- Veins
  1. Venous end of heart tube
  2. Common cardinal vein brings blood from embryo to heart tube through anterior and posterior cardinal veins
  3. Vitelline veins from the yolk sac
  4. Two umbilical veins from the placenta

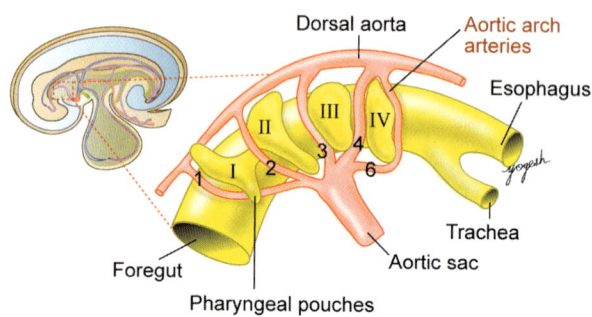

Fig. 19.3: Relation of the pharyngeal arch arteries with foregut

PHARYNGEAL ARCH ARTERIES

- Two primitive aortae arise from arterial end of heart tube (Fig. 19.4).
- These primitive aortae curve to reach near notochord and finally to reach caudal end of the fetus.

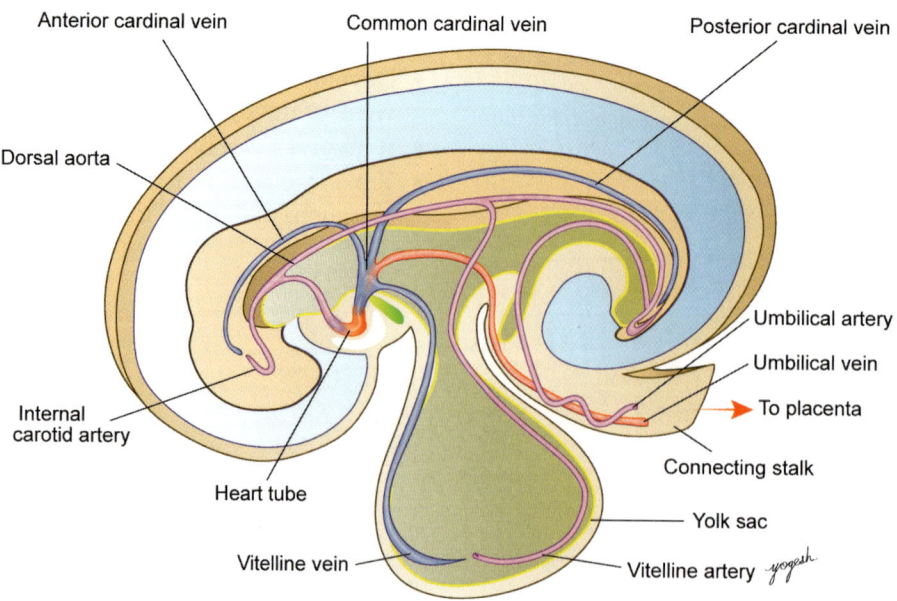

Fig. 19.2: Major vessels of embryo

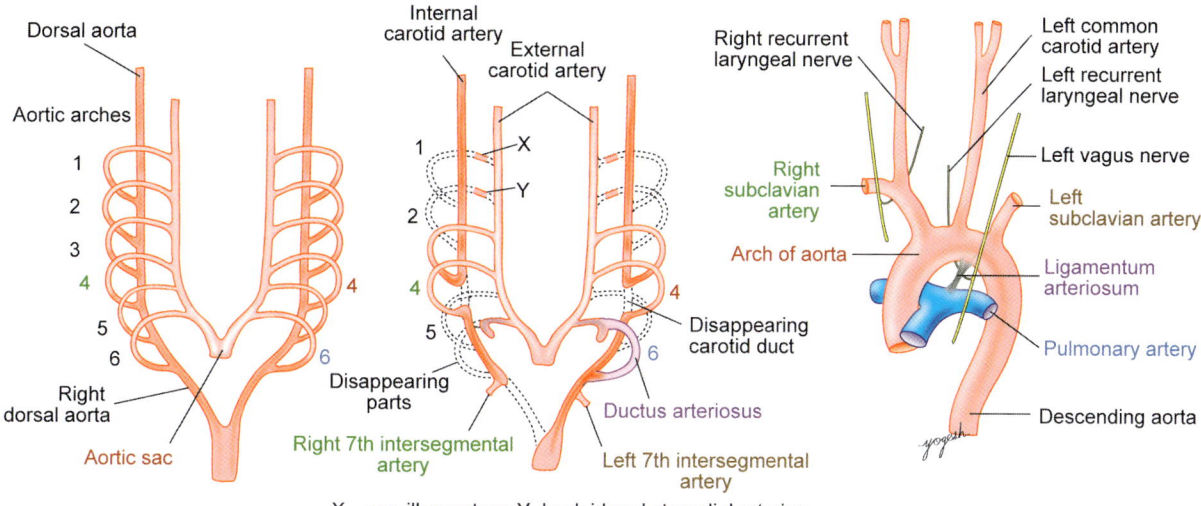

X – maxillary artery; Y–hyaloid and stapedial arteries

Fig. 19.4: Derivatives of pharyngeal arch arteries. First and second arch arteries mostly disappear leaving behind maxillary artery from first pharyngeal arch artery and hyoid and stapedial arteries from second arch artery (not shown in this Fig.). Third arch artery forms common carotid artery, proximal part of internal carotid artery and external carotid artery. Fourth arch artery forms part of arch of aorta on left side and proximal part of right subclavian artery on the right. Fifth arch artery disappears. Sixth arch artery forms left pulmonary artery and ductus arteriosus (ligamentous arteriosum after birth) on the left and right pulmonary artery on the right

- Due to the course, primitive aortae are divided into three parts as follows:
  1. *Ventral aortae* that lies ventral to foregut.
  2. *Dorsal aortae* that lie dorsal to foregut.
  3. *First aortic arch artery* that connects ventral aortae with dorsal aortae and passes through first pharyngeal arch (Figs 19.3, 19.4, Flowchart 19.1).
- Ventral aortae fuse in the midline to form heart tube.
- Near the fused heart tube, part of ventral aortae dilates to form *aortic sac*, whereas an unfused part of ventral aortae forms right and left horn of the sac (Fig. 19.3 and Fig. 18.3 from Chapter 18).
- Pharyngeal arches appear during 4th and 5th weeks.
- Each pharyngeal arch is supplied by an artery called *pharyngeal arch artery*.
- Each pharyngeal arch artery connects aortic sac with dorsal aorta (Fig. 19.4).

- Initially, there are six pairs of aortic arch arteries. Later, fifth pair disappears along with fifth pharyngeal arch. In 50% of embryos, 5th aortic arch is never formed.^{NEXT}
- Pharyngeal arch arteries are numbered craniocaudally as I, II, III, IV and VI.
- All 6 aortic arches are not present simultaneously (Practice Fig. 19.1).^{NEXT}

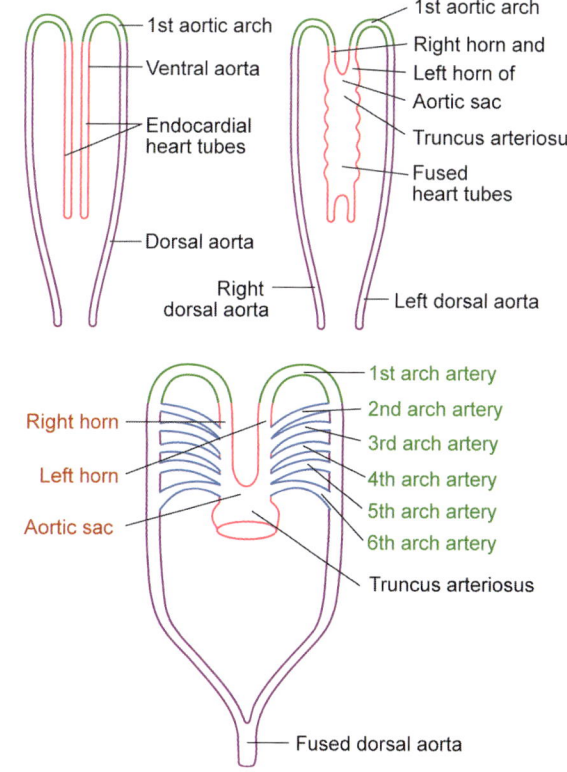

Practice Fig. 19.1: Formation of aortic arches

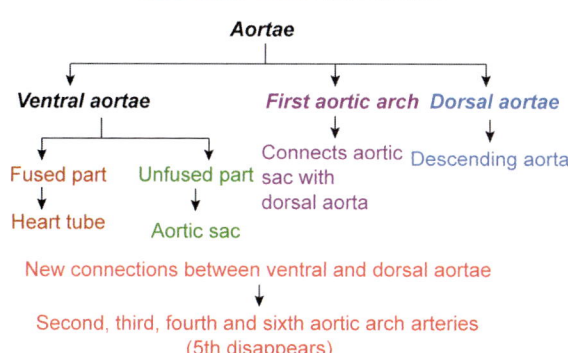

Flowchart 19.1: Arch arteries

Derivatives of Aortic Arch Arteries ^{Viva, High yielding facts}

Q. Write a short note on development of: Arch of aorta, subclavian artery, pulmonary arteries, carotid arteries, coarctation of aorta, ligamentum arteriosum.

Derivatives of aortic arch arteries are as follows (Fig. 19.4, Table 19.1, Flowchart 19.2):

1, 2. First and second arch arteries mostly disappear leaving behind
   – Maxillary artery from first pharyngeal arch artery
   – Hyoid and stapedial arteries from second arch artery
3. Third arch artery forms common carotid artery, proximal part of internal carotid artery, and external carotid artery.^{Viva}
4. Fourth arch artery forms
   – On left: Part of arch of aorta
   – On right: Proximal part of right subclavian artery
5. Fifth arch artery disappears
6. Sixth arch artery:
   – On left: Left pulmonary artery and ductus arteriosus (ligamentous arteriosus after birth)
   – On right: Right pulmonary artery (Practice Fig. 19.2)

Table 19.1	Derivatives of pharyngeal arch arteries. (In 50% of embryos, 5th aortic arch is never formed.)^{High yielding facts, NEXT}
Arch artery	**Fate**
I	Maxillary artery
II	Stapedial artery; hyoid artery
III	Common carotid artery Proximal part of internal carotid artery External carotid artery
IV	Left side: Part of arch of aorta Right side: Proximal part of right subclavian artery^{NEXT}
V	Disappears
VI	Left side: Left pulmonary artery, ductus arteriosus (after birth: Ligamentum arteriosum) Right side: Right pulmonary artery

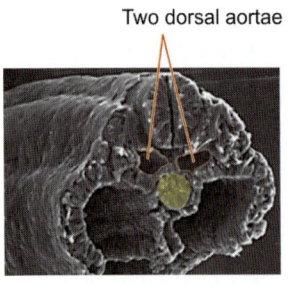
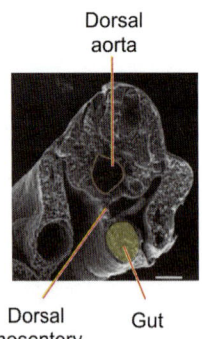

Scanning electron micrograph 19.1: Formation of single dorsal aorta. As development progresses, paired dorsal aortae form a single central vessel [Species: Mouse, approximate human age: 27–28 transverse section]

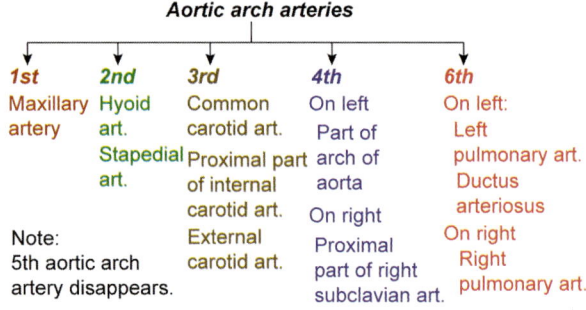

Flowchart 19.2: Derivatives of aortic arch arteries

Note: 5th aortic arch artery disappears.

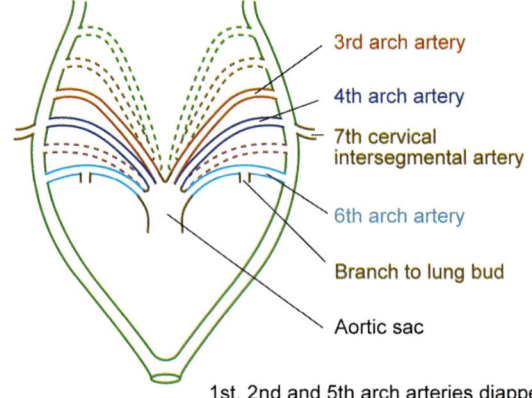

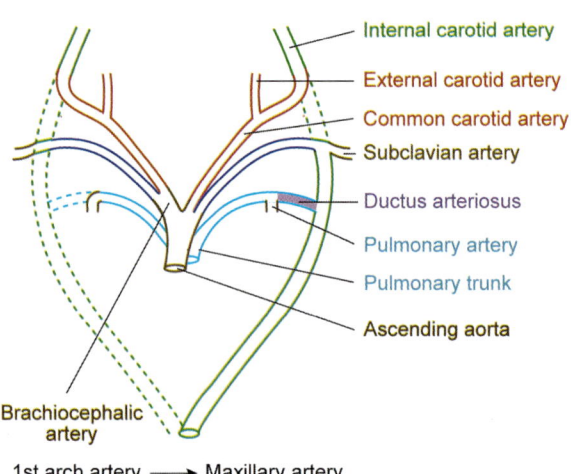

Practice Fig. 19.2: Fate of aortic arch arteries

Changes in Arch Arteries and Aortae

- Dorsal aortae remain separated in the region of pharyngeal arch arteries. Caudal to sixth arch artery, dorsal aortae fuse to form a single dorsal aorta that later forms descending thoracic and abdominal aorta (Table 19.2).
- On development of spiral septum, ascending aorta blood enters third and fourth arch arteries, whereas pulmonary trunk blood is diverted to sixth arch arteries.
- Carotid duct (ductus caroticus): It is portion of dorsal aortae between third and fourth arch arteries. It disappears completely (Table 19.3).

Table 19.2: Development of major arteries^{Viva, MCQ}

Artery	Embryonic source
Arch of aorta	Aortic sac (fused part of ventral aortae)
	Left horn of aortic sac (unfused left ventral aortic arch)
	Left fourth arch artery
Brachiocephalic artery	Right horn of aortic sac (unfused right ventral aortic arch)
Right subclavian artery^{NEXT}	Proximal part: Right fourth arch artery, right dorsal aorta
	Distal part: Right seventh cervical intersegmental artery
Left subclavian artery	Left seventh cervical intersegmental artery
Pulmonary arteries	Proximal part of sixth arch artery
Descending aorta	Proximal part: Left dorsal aorta distal to attachment of fourth arch artery
	Distal part: Fused dorsal aorta

Note: Smooth muscles of dorsal aorta develop from splanchnopleuric layer of lateral plate mesoderm.^{NEXT}

Table 19.3: Development of carotid arteries

Artery	Embryonic source
Common carotid artery	Part of third arch artery proximal to the bud of external carotid artery
External carotid artery	Bud from third arch artery
Internal carotid artery	Part of third arch artery distal to the bud of external carotid artery Cranial extension of dorsal aortae distal to attachment of the third arch artery

Note: Left common carotid artery arising from brachiocephalic trunk is the commonest variation in arteries arising from arch of aorta.^{NEXT}

Following Portions Disappear

1. Most of the part of first and second arch arteries
2. Ductus caroticus
3. Right dorsal aorta caudal to fourth aortic arch artery
4. Fifth aortic arch
5. Distal half of sixth arch artery on right
   – Ductus aorticus: It is distal portion of sixth aortic arch artery that connects left pulmonary artery with left dorsal aorta.

Following Overgrowths Occur

1. Dorsal aortae grow cranially beyond the attachment of first aortic arch artery and form a part of internal carotid artery.
2. Bud form third artery gives rise to external carotid artery.^{MCQ}

3. Communication of seventh intersegmental artery with dorsal aorta at the level of fourth arch artery participate in formation of subclavian arteries.
4. Proximal part of right third and fourth arteries fuse to form brachiocephalic artery that arises from aortic sac.

Patent Ductus Arteriosus (PDA)

Q. Write a short note on patent ductus arteriosus.

Definition

Failure of closure of ductus arteriosus that connects left pulmonary artery with arch of aorta in the fetal life (Flowchart 19.3).

- Normal ductus arteriosus shunts blood between pulmonary trunk and descending aorta to bypass the lungs.^{NEXT}
- Usual closure of ductus arteriosus occurs as follows:
  – Physiological (functional): Immediately after birth due to reflex contraction of muscles of arterial wall. Ductus arteriosus constricts at birth but shunting of blood from aorta to left pulmonary artery may continue up to 4 days after birth.^{NEXT}
  – Anatomical: Within three months (12 weeks)^{NEXT} after birth by proliferation of tunica intima into lumen, under the influence of transforming growth factor β (TGFβ).^{NEXT}
- Patent ductus arteriosus occurs in 8 in 10,000 births.
- PDA leads to shunting of blood from aorta to pulmonary circulation.
- Prostaglandins keep ductus arteriosus open, whereas prostaglandin inhibitors (such as indomethacin) promotes closure of ductus arteriosus.
- Mechanism of closure: After birth, lungs release bradykinin during initial inflation. Bradykinin produces smooth muscle contraction in the wall of ductus arteriosus and closes it physiologically.
- Remnant of ductus arteriosus is called *ligamentum arteriosum*. Left recurrent laryngeal nerve loop around ligamentum arteriosum.

Flowchart 19.3: Patent ductus arteriosus

Patent ductus arteriosus
↓
Shunting of blood from aorta to pulmonary trunk
↓
Pulmonary hypertension

Normal closure	Incidence	Mechanism of closure
Physiological: immediately after birth	8 in 10,000 births	First breathing ↓ Release of bradykinin from lungs ↓ Contraction of smooth muscles ↓ Closure of ductus arteriosus ↓ Ligamentum arteriosum
Anatomical: within 3 months after birth		

Coarctation of Aorta

Q. Write a short note on coarctation of aorta.

Definition: Coarctation of aorta is congenital narrowing of the arch of aorta distal to the origin of left subclavian artery (Fig. 19.5).

- Coarctation of aorta occurs in 3.2 in 10,000 births.
  Types:
  A. Preductal coarctation: It is narrowing of aorta proximal to ductus arteriosus.
  B. Postductal coarctation: It is narrowing of aorta distal to ductus arteriosus
- Coarctation of aorta results in increased blood pressure in upper limb, low blood pressure in lower limb, and left ventricular hypertrophy.

Unusual Origin of Aorta

1. Double aortic arches: It occurs due to *persistence of right dorsal aorta distal* to right seventh intersegmental artery (Fig. 19.6).^NEXT

2. Right aortic arch: It occurs due to regression of left dorsal aorta distal to right seventh intersegmental artery instead of the same segment of right dorsal aorta (Fig. 19.7).

3. Abnormal (aberrant) origin of right subclavian artery: Right subclavian artery may arise from descending aorta. It occurs due to regression of right fourth arch artery (Fig. 19.8).^NEXT It results in: (1) absence of brachiocephalic artery, (2) origin of right common carotid artery from arch of aorta and (3) absence of recurrent course of right recurrent laryngeal nerve.

Branches of Dorsal Aorta (Fig. 19.9, Practice Fig. 19.3)

Dorsal aorta gives three sets of arteries as follows:

1. Dorsolateral branches
   - These are also called *somatic intersegmental vessels*.
   - These arteries form
     - Arteries of limbs
     - Intercostal arteries
     - Lumbar arteries
     - Lateral sacral arteries
2. Lateral splanchnic branches
   - These branches develop
     - Phrenic arteries
     - Suprarenal arteries
     - Renal arteries
     - Gonadal vessels
3. Ventral splanchnic branches
   - These are of two groups:
     A. Vitelline arteries that form coeliac, superior, and inferior mesenteric arteries.
     B. Umbilical arteries form superior vesical arteries and medial umbilical ligament.

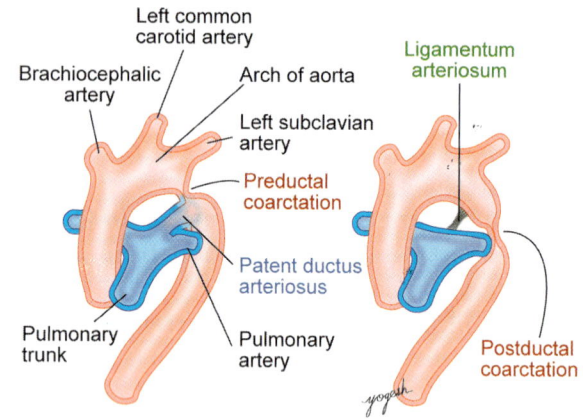

Fig. 19.5: Coarctation of aorta. Coarctation of aorta is a congenital narrowing of arch of aorta distal to the origin of left subclavian artery. Preductal coarctation is narrowing proximal to the ductus arteriosus, whereas postductal coarctation is a narrowing distal to the ductus arteriosus.

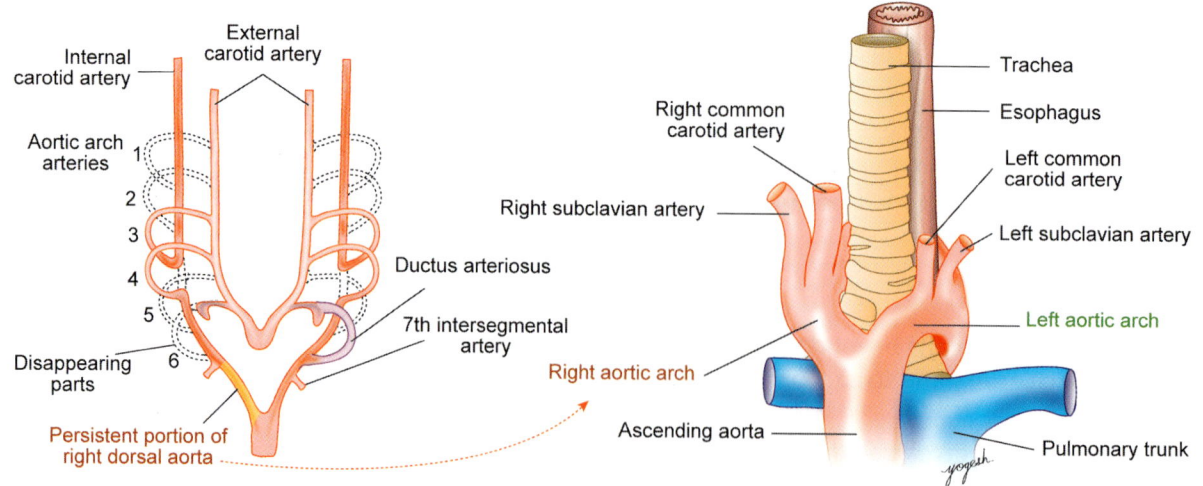

Fig. 19.6: Double aortic arches owing to persistence of right dorsal aorta distal to the right seventh intersegmental artery

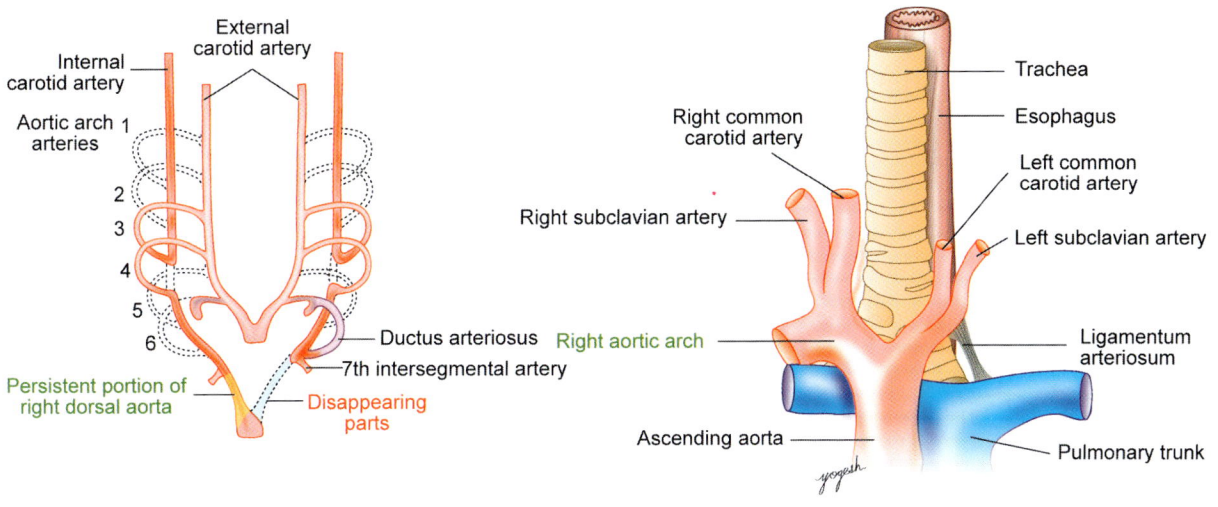

Fig. 19.7: Right aortic arch. Owing to regression of left dorsal aorta distal to the right seventh intersegmental artery instead of same segment of the right dorsal aorta results in right aortic arch

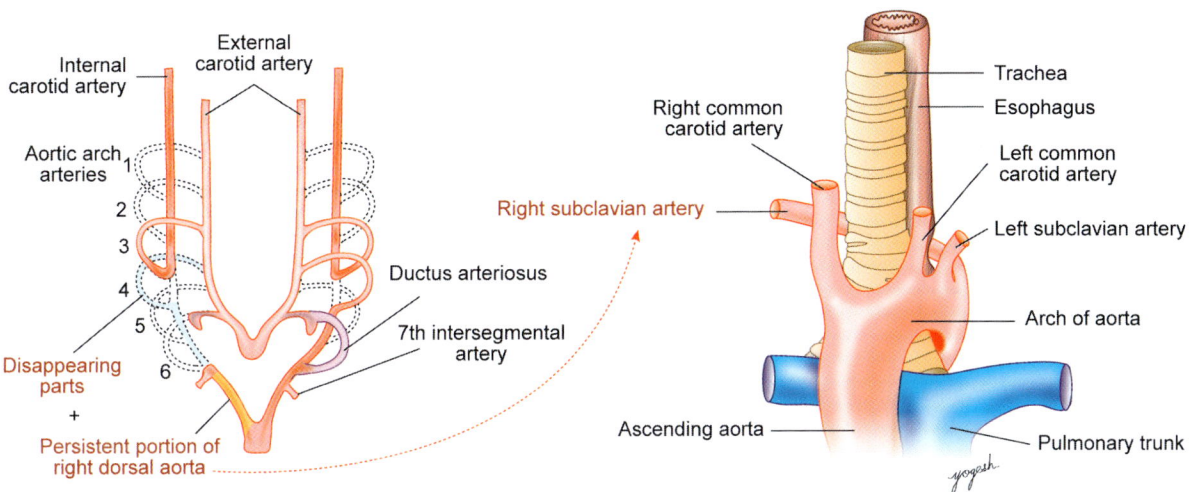

Fig. 19.8: Abnormal origin of right subclavian artery. Right subclavian artery may arise from the descending aorta. It occurs due to regression of right fourth arch artery. It results in absence of brachiocephalic artery, origin of right common carotid artery from arch of aorta and absence of recurrent course of right recurrent laryngeal nerve. This aberrant right subclavian artery may compress esophagus

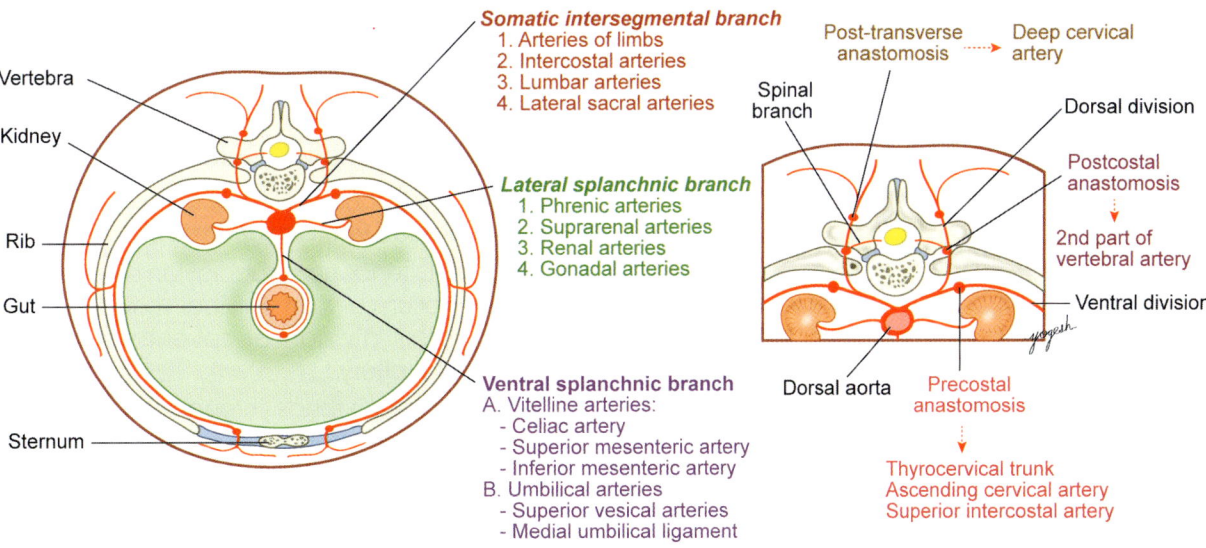

Fig. 19.9: Branching pattern of dorsal aorta and its anastomoses

Cardiovascular System II: Blood Vessels and Fetal Circulation

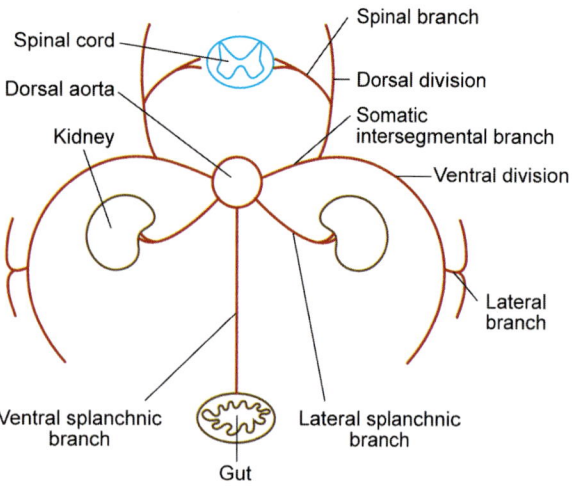

Practice Fig. 19.3: Main branches of dorsal aorta

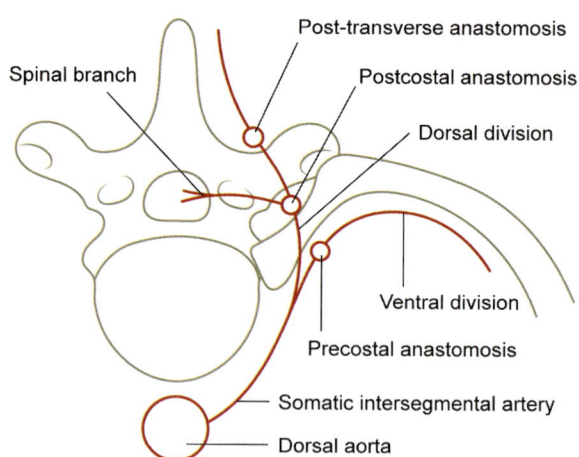

Practice Fig. 19.4: Sites of vertical anastomosis between branches of dorsal aorta

4. Remnant of dorsal aorta below sacral segment forms median sacral artery.

Box 19.2: Umbilical arteries

- Umbilical arteries are ventral splanchnic branches of dorsal aorta (Practice Fig. 19.6).
- Each umbilical artery supplies
  – Mesoderm of connecting stalk
  – Derivatives of allantois
  – Placenta
- Each umbilical artery gets communicated with part of fifth lumbar artery that forms the internal iliac artery.
- Portion of umbilical arteries between dorsal aorta and communication with internal iliac artery disappears. Thus, umbilical arteries become branches of internal iliac arteries.
- Single umbilical artery is present in 1% of cases and it is more common in twins and babies born to diabetic mothers.^{NEXT} Single umbilical artery is usually associated with renal abnormalities.^{NEXT}
- Postnatal change: After birth, umbilical arteries form
  – Superior vesical artery from proximal part.
  – Medial umbilical ligament from distal obliterated part.

DEVELOPMENT OF VERTEBRAL ARTERY

Q. Write a short note on development of vertebral artery.

- In cervical region, intersegmental arteries form longitudinal anastomotic channels as follows (Fig. 19.9, Practice Fig. 19.4):

  A. *Precostal anastomosis*: Connects intersegmental arteries in front of the neck of the ribs.
  B. *Postcostal anastomosis*: Lies between costal elements (ribs) and transverse processes.

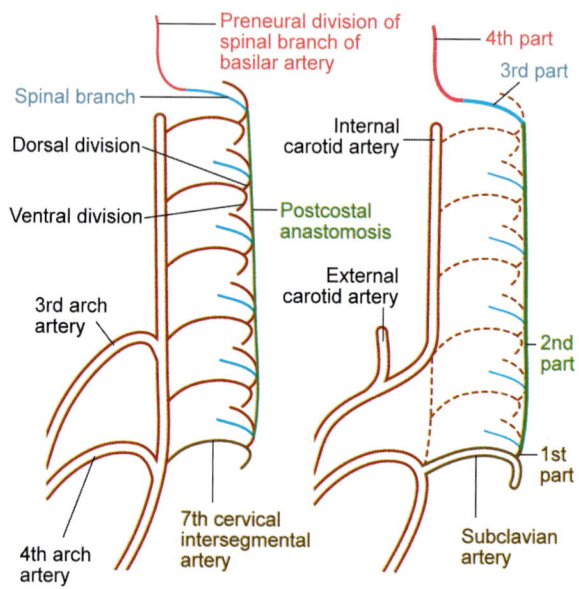

Practice Fig. 19.5: Development of vertebral artery

  C. *Post-transverse anastomosis*: Lies behind the transverse processes.

- Remnants or derivatives of cervical intersegmental arterial anastomosis are given in Table 19.4.

Summary (Examination Guide)

Vertebral artery consists of four parts (Fig. 19.9, Practice Fig. 19.5, Table 19.4, Flowchart 19.4):

1. First part: Extends from subclavian artery to foramen transversarium of sixth cervical vertebra – develops from dorsal division of seventh cervical intersegmental artery.
2. Second part: Extends through foramina transversarium from sixth to first cervical vertebrae – develops from postcostal anastomosis.
3. Third part: Extends from foramina transversarium and rest on posterior arch of the atlas – develops from spinal branch of first cervical intersegmental artery.

Table 19.4	Derivatives of cervical intersegmental arterial anastomosis
Anastomotic channel	Derivative
Precostal	Thyrocervical trunk, ascending cervical, superior intercostal arteries
Postcostal	Part of vertebral artery
Post-transverse	Deep cervical

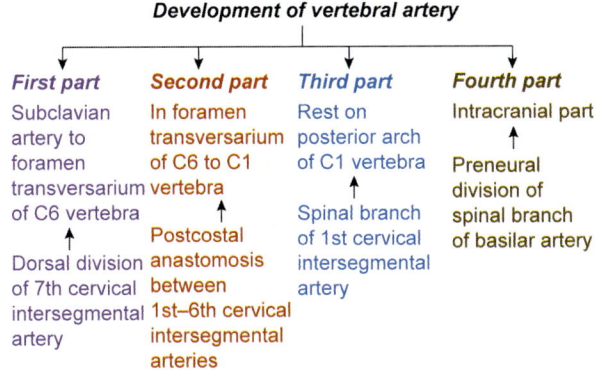

Flowchart 19.4: Development of vertebral artery

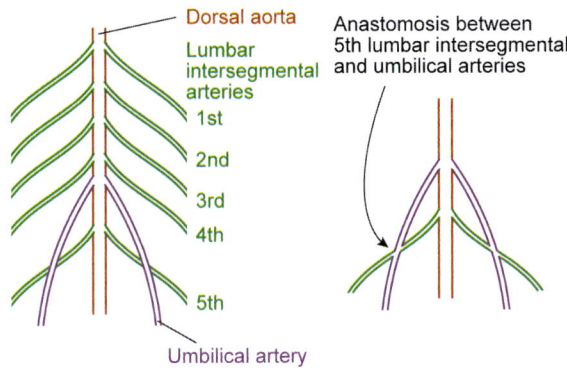

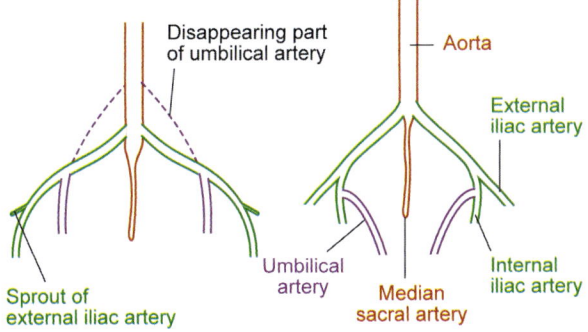

Practice Fig. 19.6: Development of umbilical artery

4. **Fourth part**: Intracranial part – develops from preneural division of spinal branch of basilar artery.

DEVELOPMENT OF LIMB VESSELS

Q. Write a short note on axis artery of upper and lower limbs.

- Each limb is supplied by an axis artery during development that runs along the central axis of limb.
- The axis artery is derived from intersegmental arteries.

Axis Artery of Upper Limb

- It is derivative of seventh cervical intersegmental artery (Fig. 19.10).
- The axis artery of upper limb later forms:^MCQ
  – axillary artery
  – brachial artery
  – anterior interosseous artery^NEXT
  – deep palmar arch
- Radial and ulnar arteries arise as sprouts of the axis artery.

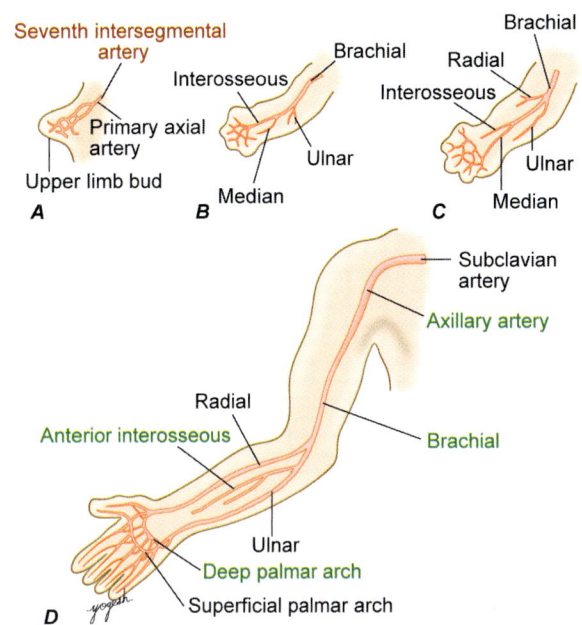

Fig. 19.10: Development of upper limb arteries. Axis artery of upper limb is a derivative of seventh cervical intersegmental artery. The axis artery later forms: Axillary artery, brachial artery, anterior interosseous artery, and deep palmar arch. Radial and ulnar arteries arise as sprouts of the axis artery

Axis Artery of Lower Limb

- It is derivative of *fifth lumbar intersegmental* artery.^NEXT
- The axis artery of lower limb later forms:^MCQ
  – Arteria comitans nervi ischiadici (ischiadic artery that accompanies sciatic nerve)
  – Part of popliteal artery above the popliteus muscle
  – Distal part of peroneal artery
  – Part of plantar arch
- Femoral artery develops from a capillary plexus present on the ventral aspect of the thigh that later forms communication with external iliac artery and popliteal artery (Fig. 19.11).

DEVELOPMENT OF VENOUS SYSTEM

INTRODUCTION

- Veins of developing embryo can be grouped as visceral and somatic veins (Flowchart 19.5, Fig. 19.12).

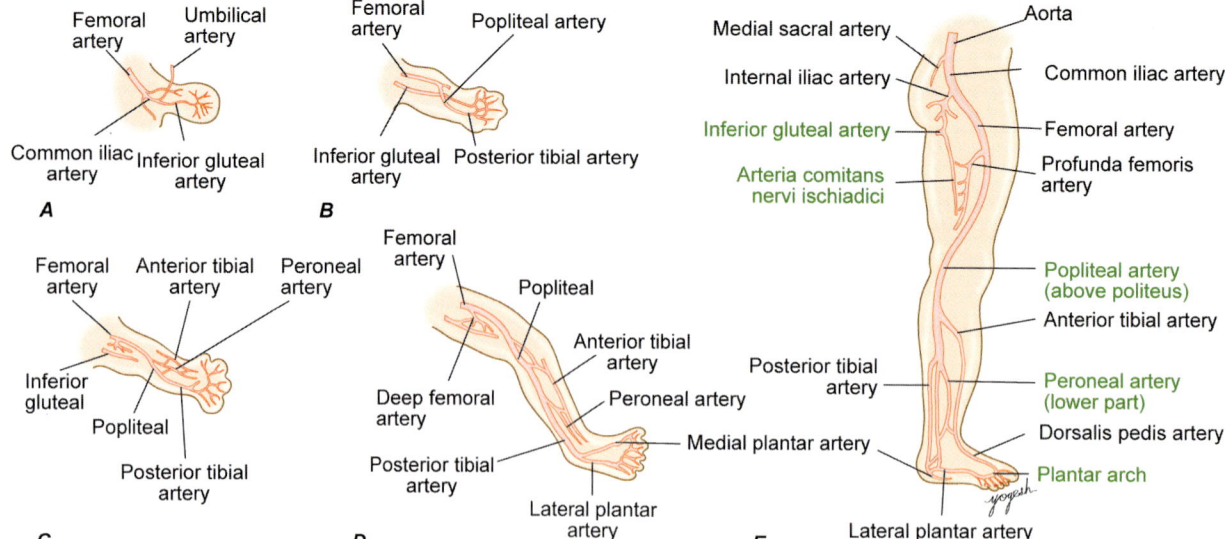

Fig. 19.11: Development of lower limb arteries. Axis artery of lower limb is a derivative of fifth lumbar intersegmental artery. The axis artery of lower limb later forms arteria comitans nervi ischiadici, part of popliteal artery above the popliteus muscle, distal part of peroneal artery, and part of plantar arch. Femoral artery develops from a capillary plexus present on ventral aspect of the thigh that later forms communication with external iliac artery and popliteal artery

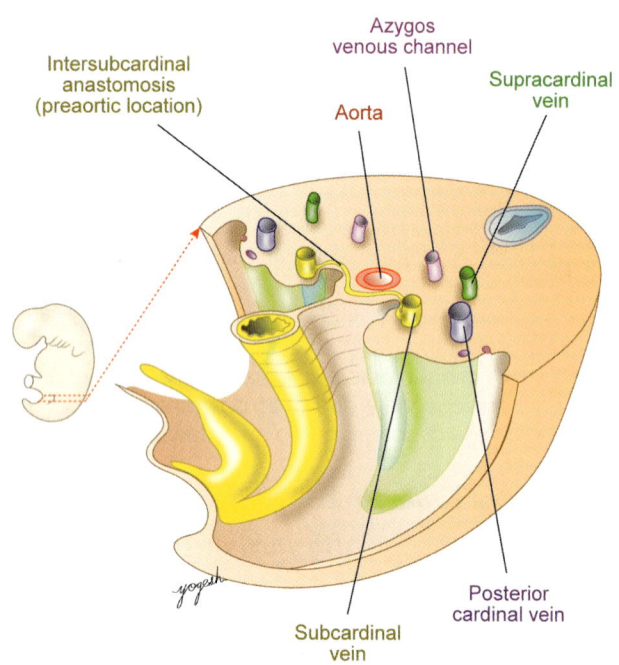

Fig. 19.12: Cross section of the embryo showing major embryonic veins

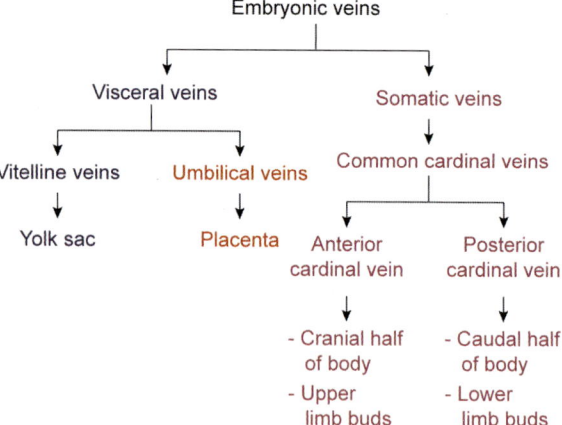

Flowchart 19.5: Embryonic veins

- **Visceral veins**
  These include
  1. Vitelline or omphalomesenteric veins – for draining yolk sac.
  2. Umbilical veins – for placenta.
- **Somatic veins**
  These are cardinal veins for draining body wall (cardinal = important).
  These are
  1. Anterior cardinal veins (right and left)
  2. Posterior cardinal veins (right and left)
  3. Common cardinal veins or *ducts of Cuvier* (right and left)
- Anterior and posterior cardinal veins join to form common cardinal veins.
- Anterior cardinal veins drain:
  – cranial half of embryo
  – upper limb buds
- Posterior cardinal veins drain
  – caudal half of embryo
  – lower limb buds
- Visceral and somatic veins finally drain into the sinus venosus.
- These visceral and somatic veins later form
  – portal veins
  – caval veins
  – azygos veins

VITELLINE VEINS

Q. Write a short note on development of portal vein.

- There are two vitelline (right and left) veins that drain yolk sac.
- On formation of head fold, part of the yolk sac participates in the formation of gut.
- Both vitelline veins pass on either side of gut tube. They pass through septum transversum and finally open in sinus venosus.
- Developing liver in septum transversum divide vitelline veins into three parts: Infrahepatic, intrahepatic and suprahepatic parts (Fig. 19.13, Flowchart 19.6, Practice Fig. 19.7).

A. Infrahepatic part *High yielding facts*

- Infrahepatic parts lie caudal to septum transversum on either side of primitive gut.
- In zone of duodenum, right and left vitelline veins get communicated via three transverse anastomoses: Cranial ventral, middle dorsal and caudal ventral to form a *Figure of 8* (Fig. 19.13A). *MCQ*

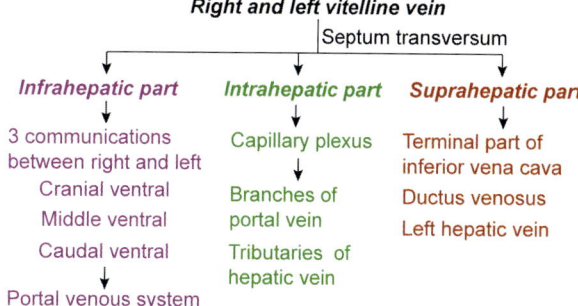

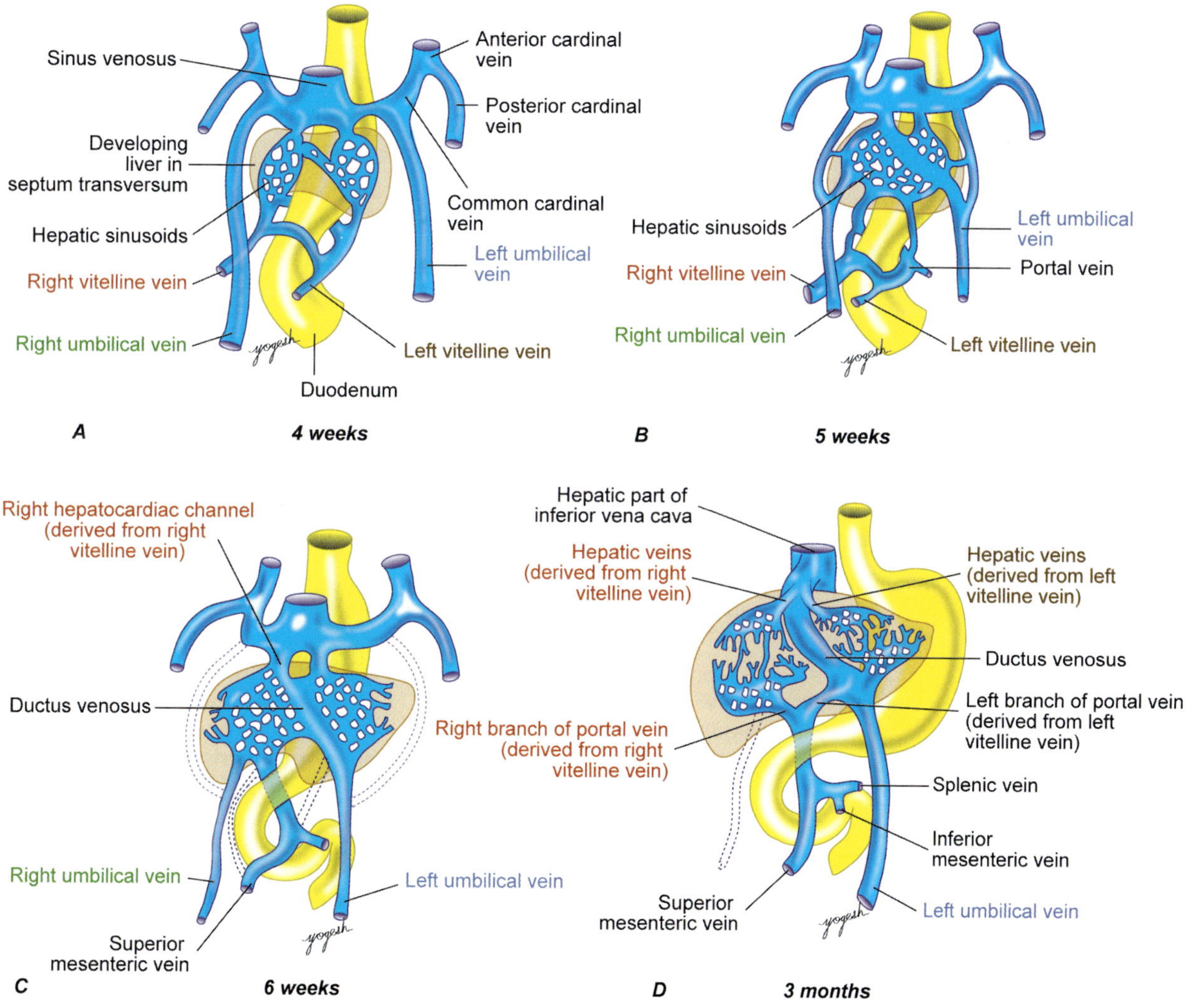

Flowchart 19.6: Development of vitelline veins

Right and left vitelline vein
↓ Septum transversum

- ***Infrahepatic part*** → 3 communications between right and left: Cranial ventral, Middle ventral, Caudal ventral → Portal venous system
- ***Intrahepatic part*** → Capillary plexus → Branches of portal vein; Tributaries of hepatic vein
- ***Suprahepatic part*** → Terminal part of inferior vena cava; Ductus venosus; Left hepatic vein

- Communications:
  – Left umbilical vein develops communications with cranial ventral anastomosis, whereas splenic vein drain spleen into dorsal middle anastomosis.
  – Disappearance of segments of infrahepatic part of vitelline vein results in formation of (Table 19.5, Fig. 19.13):

Fig. 19.13: Development of portal vein. Plexus around the duodenum develops hepatic sinusoid and ductus venosus. Terminal parts of the right and left vitelline veins form right and left hepatocardiac channels respectively. Note the formation of the portal vein, splenic vein, superior mesenteric vein, and hepatic portion of the inferior vena cava

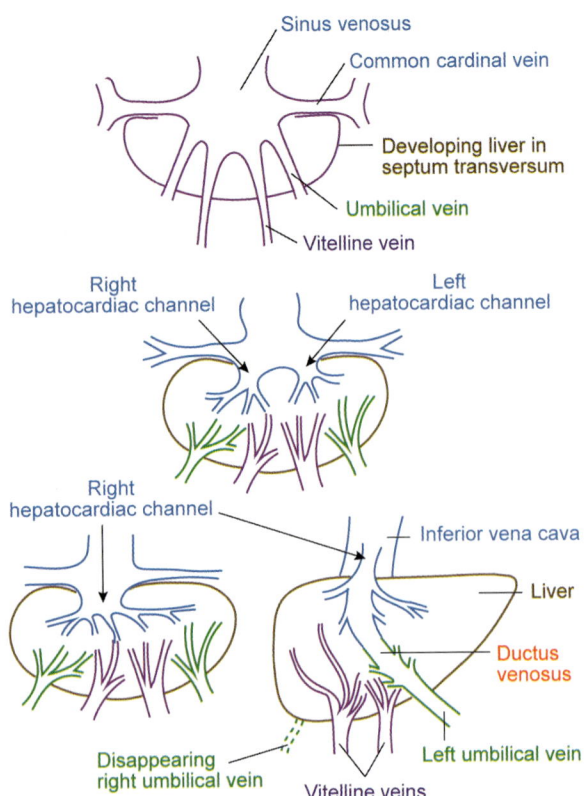

Practice Fig. 19.7: Fate of umbilical and vitelline veins

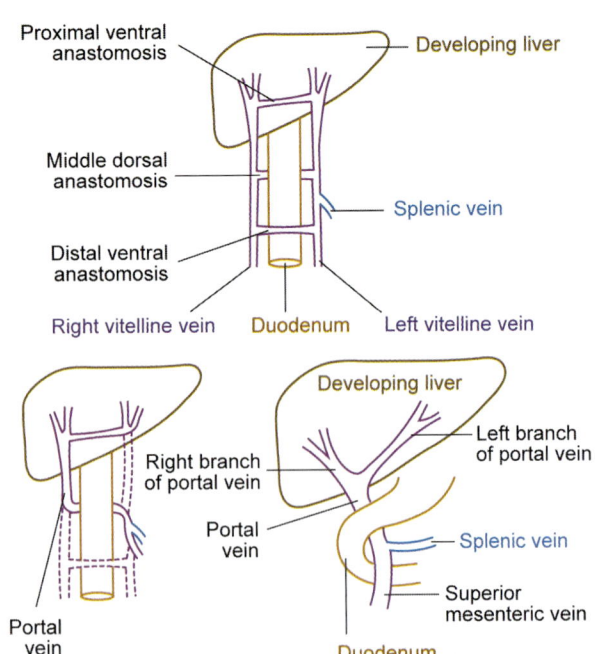

Practice Fig. 19.8: Development of portal vein

- This capillary network forms
  - afferent venae advehentes that develop branches of portal vein.
  - efferent venae revehentes that develop tributaries of hepatic vein.^{NEXT}

C. **Suprahepatic part**
- Subdiaphragmatic anastomosis develops that connects right and left vitelline veins.
- Subdiaphragmatic anastomosis gets connected with cranial ventral intervitelline anastomosis.
- Left vitelline vein regresses (disappears).^{MCQ}
- Remaining portion of suprahepatic vitelline veins forms:
  1. Common hepatic vein that later forms terminal part of inferior vena cava (Fig. 19.14D)^{NEXT}
  2. Ductus venosus (Fig. 19.14C, D)
  3. Left hepatic vein (Fig. 19.14D)^{NEXT}

UMBILICAL VEINS

- Umbilical vein drains blood from placenta into sinus venosus.
- Umbilical veins pass through somatopleuric mesoderm and septum transversum.
- Right umbilical vein regresses, whereas left umbilical vein is left behind.^{MCQ, Viva}
- Left umbilical vein develop communication with left vitelline vein (that later form left branch of portal vein).
- A portion of left umbilical vein cranial to septum transversum disappears.
- Thus, blood from left umbilical vein pass through:
  1. Hepatic circulation via left branch of portal vein
  2. To inferior vena cava through ductus venosus.

Table 19.5	Development of portal venous system (Practice Fig. 19.8)
Derivative	**Embryonic source**
Superior mesenteric vein^{NEXT}	– Infrahepatic part of right vitelline vein distal to caudal ventral anastomosis – Caudal ventral anastomosis – Left vitelline vein between middle dorsal and caudal ventral anastomoses
Trunk of portal vein^{NEXT}	– Middle dorsal anastomosis – Right vitelline vein between cranial ventral and middle dorsal anastomoses
Right branch of portal vein^{NEXT}	– Infrahepatic part of right vitelline vein up to cranial ventral anastomosis
Left branch of portal vein^{NEXT}	– Cranial ventral anastomosis – Infrahepatic left vitelline vein up to cranial ventral anastomosis

1. Superior mesenteric vein^{NEXT}
2. Trunk of portal vein^{NEXT}
3. Right branch of portal vein^{NEXT}
4. Left branch of portal vein^{NEXT}

B. **Intrahepatic part**
- Intrahepatic plexus forms a capillary network that joins with developing hepatic sinusoids (Fig. 19.14A).

Note: Ductus venosus after birth forms ligamentum venosus, whereas left umbilical vein forms ligamentum teres hepatis.

SOMATIC VEINS

- There are two pairs of somatic veins (Fig. 19.14):
  1. *Anterior cardinal veins* (right and left)
  2. *Posterior cardinal veins* (right and left)
- On each side, anterior and posterior cardinal veins join to form the *common cardinal vein* (duct of Cuvier) (Fig. 19.14).
- The common cardinal veins open into corresponding horns of sinus venosus.
- Anterior cardinal vein has two segments: Primary head vein and cervicothoracic vein.

Primary Head Vein

- It lies on side of cranial end of neural tube (or brain vesicles).
- It forms
  1. *Superficial venous plexus* that develops dural venous sinuses.
  2. *Deep venous plexus* that develops cerebral veins.
- Dural venous sinuses form three stems that terminate into primary head vein as follows:
  - cranial (ventral) dural stem for forebrain and midbrain
  - middle dural stem for metencephalon
  - caudal dural stem for myelencephalon
- Most of the part of primary head vein disappears and its small remnant develops ***cavernous sinus***.
- Communicating channels between dural stems form:
  - *Transverse sinus*: Channel between cranial and middle dural stem.
  - *Sigmoid sinus*: Channel between middle and caudal dural stem.
  - *Inferior petrosal sinus*: Channel between primary head vein and cavernous sinus.
  - *Superior petrosal sinus:* Middle dural stem
- *Primary maxillary vein* opens into primary head vein and later it forms superior ophthalmic vein.^{MCQ}
- *Sagittal plexus* develops on superolateral surface of the forebrain that forms:
  1. Superior sagittal sinus
  2. Straight sinus
  3. Great cerebral vein

Cervicothoracic Vein

Q. Write a short note on development of coronary sinus.

Cervicothoracic vein forms the following veins:
1. Internal jugular vein: From part of anterior cardinal vein cranial to opening of subclavian vein.
2. Subclavian vein: From seventh intersegmental vein.^{MCQ}
3. Right brachiocephalic vein: From part of right anterior cardinal vein between right subclavian vein and oblique intercardinal anastomosis.
4. Left brachiocephalic vein: From
   a. part of left anterior cardinal vein between left subclavian vein and oblique intercardinal anastomosis
   b. oblique intercardinal anastomosis (Practice Fig. 19.1B)
5. Superior vena cava:
   It has two parts:
   - Extra-pericardial part: Develops from part of right anterior cardinal vein caudal to oblique intercardinal channel.^{MCQ}
   - Intrapericardial part: Develops from right common cardinal vein.^{MCQ}
6. Left superior intercostals vein: A part of left anterior cardinal vein disappears. A small part of left common cardinal vein near oblique intercardinal channel form superior intercostal vein and ligament of left vena cava.^{MCQ}
7. Oblique vein of left atrium (*oblique vein of Marshall*): From left common cardinal vein.^{MCQ}
8. Coronary sinus: Develops from left horn of sinus venosus.

Note: Normal SVC and IVC develop from right embryonic veins.^{NEXT}

Anomalies of Superior Vena Cava

1. Double superior vena cava
   - It may occur due to failure of development of communicating channel between two anterior cardinal veins.
   - Usually, this channel forms left brachiocephalic vein.
   - In double superior vena cava cases, left superior vena cava develops from left anterior cardinal vein and left common cardinal vein. Left superior vena cava drains into coronary sinus (develops from left horn of sinus venosus).^{NEXT}
2. Left superior vena cava
   - It occurs due to regression of caudal part of right anterior cardinal vein and right common cardinal vein.
   - Left superior vena cava develops from left anterior cardinal vein and left common cardinal vein.
   - Left superior vena cava drains into coronary sinus.^{NEXT}

Subcardinal Veins

- These develop in relation to mesonephric ridge (future site of kidney formation) (Table 19.6).

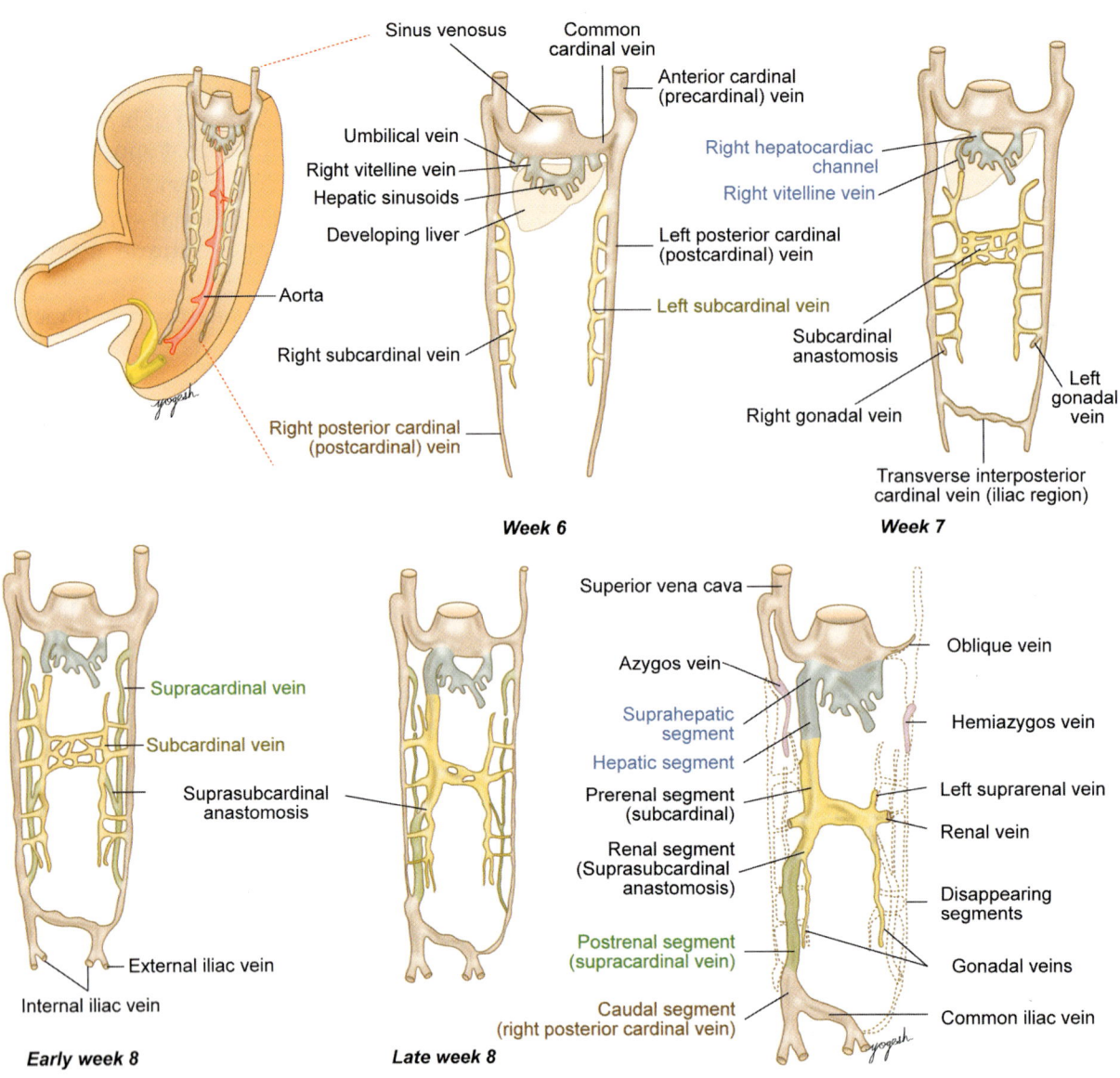

Fig. 19.14: Development of inferior vena cava. Segments of inferior vena cava develops by anastomosis channels of cardinal veins. Caudal segment of IVC develops from caudal part of the right posterior cardinal vein. Postrenal segment of IVC develops from right supracardinal vein. Renal segment develops from right supra-subcardinal anastomosis, prerenal segment from right subcardinal vein, and hepatic segment from anastomosis between right subcardinal vein and right vitelline veins (common hepatic veins), suprahepatic segment from right hepatocardiac channel

- Preaortic anastomosis gets developed between two subcardinal veins.
- Subcardinal veins anastomose cranially and caudally with posterior cardinal vein on the same side.
- A communicating channel develops between right subcardinal vein and common hepatic vein. This channel is called *right hepatocardiac channel*.

Supracardinal Veins (Thoracolumbar Veins)

- These veins develop longitudinally and lie dorsolateral to posterior cardinal veins (Table 19.6).
- Supracardinal veins develop later than subcardinal veins.
- Cranially and caudally supracardinal veins develop communications with corresponding posterior cardinal veins.
- Supracardinal vein anastomoses with corresponding subcardinal vein through suprasubcardinal anastomosis.

Posterior Cardinal Veins

- Posterior cardinal vein joins with anterior cardinal vein to form common cardinal vein (Table 19.7).
- Posterior cardinal veins (right and left) join with each other by *iliac anastomosis* (transverse anastomosis).
- Tributaries of each posterior cardinal vein include:
  - 12 thoracic intersegmental veins
  - 5 lumbar intersegmental veins
  - Iliac veins—internal iliac vein from pelvic cavity and external iliac vein from lower limb bud

- Subset of veins in abdomen:
  - In the abdomen, pairs of subcardinal and supracardinal veins appear.

Azygos Venous Lines

- Longitudinal venous channels appear on medial side of sympathetic trunk.
- Cranially these channels communicate with corresponding posterior cardinal vein.
- Caudally, these channels communicate with corresponding subcardinal veins.

Table 19.6 Subcardinal and supracardinal veins

	Subcardinal vein	Supracardinal vein
Site	Ventrolateral to abdominal aorta	Dorsolateral to abdominal aorta
Communication (cranially and caudally)	Posterior cardinal veins	Posterior cardinal veins
Anastomosis	Intersubcardinal veins	Suprasubcardinal anastomosis
Derivatives on right side	Right gonadal vein Right suprarenal vein Part of inferior vena cava	Postrenal segment of inferior vena cava
Derivatives on left side	Left gonadal vein Left suprarenal vein	Disappears

Box 19.3: Renal collar

Definition: The ring of venous channels around aorta below origin of superior mesenteric artery is called *renal collar*.

Components: The renal collar is formed by the following communications:

1. Anastomosis between two subcardinal veins (preaortic)
2. Anastomosis between supracardinal and subcardinal veins.
3. Anastomosis between supracardinal and azygos veins
4. Anastomosis between azygos venous lines and subcentral veins.
5. Anastomosis between two subcentral veins (postaortic). *Note:* During embryonic period, right and left azygos lines are connected by subcentral vein that develops dorsal to the aorta.

Table 19.7 Right and left posterior cardinal veins

Part	Derivatives of	
	Right posterior cardinal vein	Left posterior cardinal vein
Caudal to anastomosis	• Right common iliac vein • Right internal iliac vein	• Left internal iliac vein
Cranial to anastomosis	• Mostly degenerates • Cranial portion: Arch of azygos vein • Caudal portion: Most caudal part of IVC	• Mostly degenerates • Cranial portion: Part of left superior intercostal vein

- *Intercommunicating channel* develops between azygos veins. This channel runs dorsal to aorta.
- Azygos venous channel develops numerous venous channels with supracardinal vein. On disappearance of part of supracardinal vein, these communicating venous channels develop intersegmental veins and later intercostals and lumbar veins.

DEVELOPMENT OF INFERIOR VENA CAVA ^{High yielding facts}

Q. Write a short note on development of inferior vena cava.

Summary (Examination Guide)

Inferior vena cava develops from the following components (Figs 19.14, 19.15, Practice Fig. 19.9, Flowchart 19.7):^{NEXT}

- **Caudal segment of IVC:** From caudal part of right posterior cardinal vein (between transverse interposterior cardinal veins and caudal to junction of right supracardinal vein with right posterior cardinal vein).^{MCQ}
- **Postrenal segment of IVC:** From right supracardinal vein
- **Renal segment:** From right supra-subcardinal anastomosis
- **Prerenal segment:** From right subcardinal vein
- **Hepatic segment:** From anastomosis between right subcardinal vein and right vitelline veins (common hepatic veins)
- **Suprahepatic segment:** From *right vitelline vein* or right hepatocardiac channel (left hepatocardiac channel disappears due to regression of left horn of sinus venosus).^{NEXT}

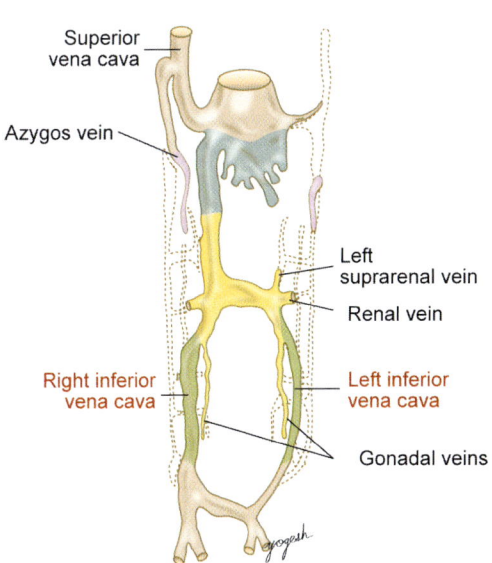

Fig. 19.15: Double inferior vena cava

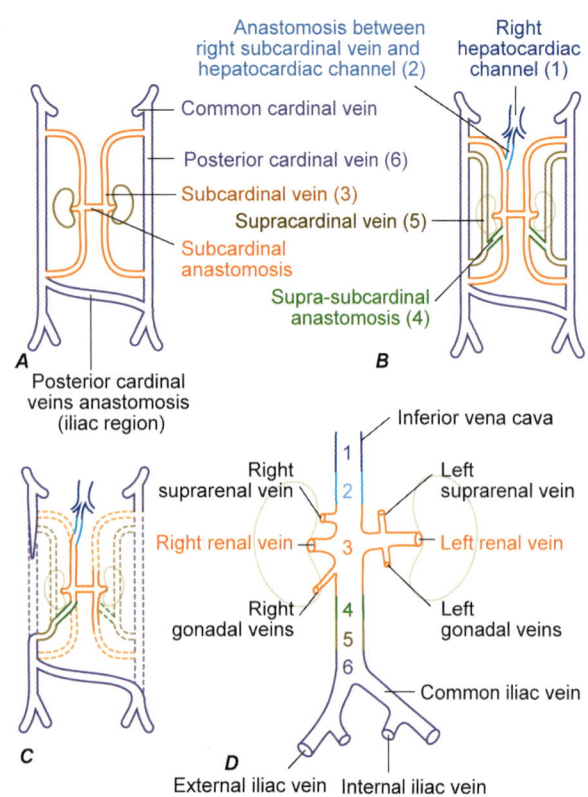

Flowchart 19.7: Development of inferior vena cava

Segment of IVC	Embryological source
Suprahepatic segment	← Right hepatocardiac channel
Hepatic segment	← Anastomosis between right subcardinal & hepatocardiac channel
Prerenal segment	← Right subcardinal vein
Renal segment	← Right supra-subcardinal anastomosis
Postrenal segment	← Right supracardinal vein
Caudal segment	← Right posterior cardinal vein

Practice Fig. 19.9: Development of inferior vena cava

Anomalies of IVC

Owing to complex development of inferior vena cava, its anomalies may be present. These include:

1. **Double IVC:** It occurs due to failure of formation of anastomosis between two posterior cardinal veins or persistence of left subcardianal and supracardinal veins. Left IVC develops from left posterior cardinal vein (below the level of renal veins).
2. **Absence of IVC:** It occurs due to failure of development of communication between right subcardinal vein and right hepatocardiac channel.
3. **Preuretic IVC:** If infrarenal part of IVC develops from subcardinal vein (that lies anterior to ureter) instead of supracardinal vein (that lies posterior to ureter), preureteric IVC develops (anterior to right ureter).
4. **Azygos continuation of IVC:** If a hepatic segment of IVC fails to develop, IVC opens in SVC via the route of azygos vein.

DEVELOPMENT OF AZYGOS VENOUS SYSTEM

The azygos system of veins consists of three major veins: Azygos vein, hemizygos vein and accessory hemiazygos vein (Fig. 19.16).

Azygos Vein

Azygos vein develops from the following sources:
1. Vein of right azygos line
2. Cranial most part of right posterior cardinal vein

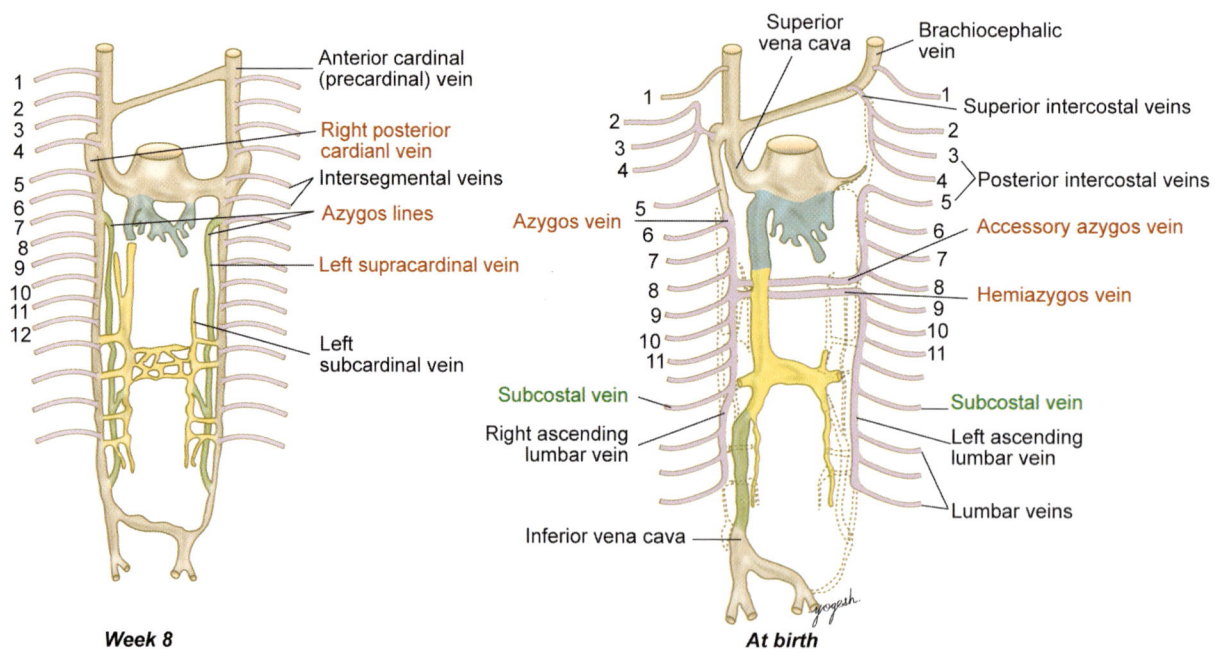

Fig. 19.16: Development of azygos vein and its tributaries

Hemizygos Vein

It is derived from the following sources:
1. Lower part of vein of left azygos line
2. Caudal postaortic anastomosis between veins of right and left azygos lines

Accessory Hemizygos Vein

It is derived from the following sources:
1. Upper part of vein of left azygos line
2. Cranial postaortic anastomosis between veins of right and left azygos lines

FETAL CIRCULATION

Q. Describe fetal circulation.

Developing fetus receives nutrition from placenta. The fetus is dependent on mother for:
1. Nutrients and oxygen intake
2. Carbon dioxide and waste product excretion

SPECIAL STRUCTURES IN FETAL CIRCULATION
(Fig. 19.17, Flowchart 19.8)

1. *Placenta*: It is a site of exchange of substances between mother and fetus.
2. *Umbilical vein*: Carries nutrients and oxygen to fetus.
3. *Umbilical arteries*: Carry waste products and carbon dioxide away from fetus. Oxygen saturation in umbilical arteries is approximately 58%.^MCQ
4. *Foramen ovale*: Helps blood to bypass lungs. It transmits most of the blood from right atrium to left atrium.
5. *Ductus venosus*: Transmits oxygenated blood from umbilical vein and left branch of portal vein to inferior vena cava and thus blood bypasses liver.^NEXT
6. *Ductus arteriosus*: Helps blood to bypass fetal lungs. It transmits the blood from left pulmonary artery to aorta.

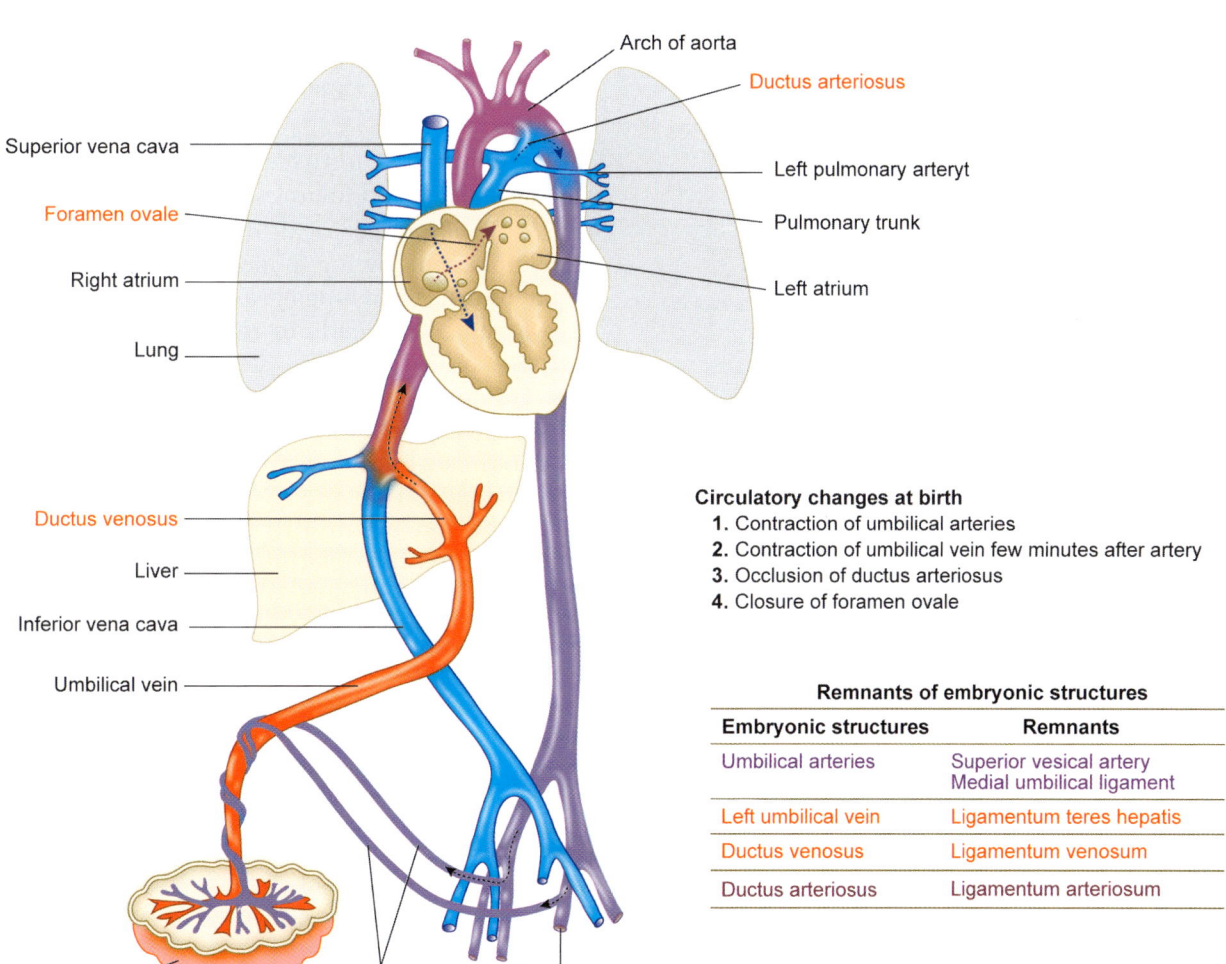

Fig. 19.17: Fetal circulation. Blood shunts three times in fetus at following places: Ductus arteriosus from left pulmonary artery to aorta, foramen ovale from right atrium to left atrium and ductus venosus from left umbilical vein to inferior vena cava. The purpose of these shunts is to bypass lungs and liver

Flowchart 19.8: Fetal circulation (Acknowledgement: Dr G Dhivya Lakshmi)

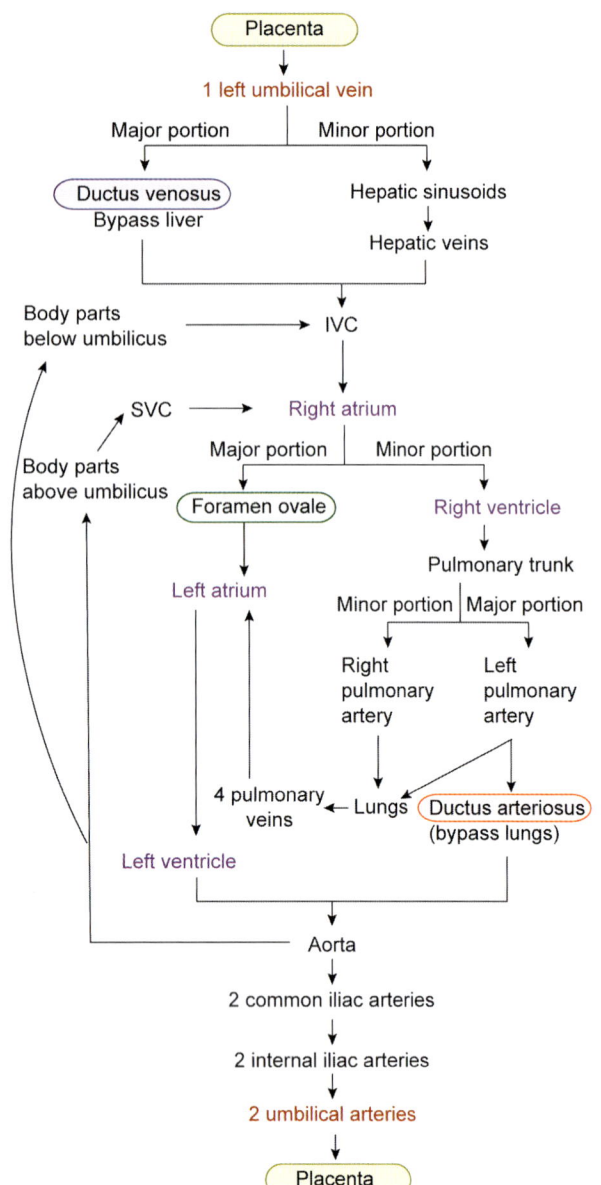

PECULIARITIES OF FETAL CIRCULATION

Q. Write a short note on peculiarities of fetal circulation.

Following are the peculiarities of the fetal circulation:

1. **Blood shunts three times** in fetus at following places: Ductus arteriosus, foramen ovale and ductus venosus to bypass lungs and liver.^{MCQ}
2. **Regulation** of oxygenated blood in fetal circulation: Sphincter at junction of left umbilical vein and ductus venosus regulates flow of oxygenated blood to the fetus.
3. **Mixing** of oxygenated and venous blood takes place at the following places: Liver, both atria, distal part of arch of aorta and terminal part of inferior vena cava.^{MCQ}
4. **Trans septal blood circulation**: Through foramen ovale blood enters from right atria into left atria.
5. **Length** of the upper limb is more in fetus as upper limb bud receives more blood than lower limb bud.

CIRCULATORY CHANGES AT BIRTH

Q. Write a short note on circulatory changes after the birth.

At birth, newborn starts respiration and lungs takeover functions of placenta. This produces the following changes (Table 19.8):

1. Muscle contraction in umbilical arteries occludes their lumen and prevents blood loss.
2. Umbilical vein contracts a few minutes after the umbilical arteries. This mechanism allows the newborn to receive more blood from placenta.^{MCQ}

Table 19.8 Remnants of embryonic vessels *High yielding facts, NEXT*

Embryonic vessel	Remnant
Umbilical arteries	Superior vesical artery
	Medial umbilical ligament
Left umbilical vein	Ligamentum teres hepatis
Ductus venosus	Ligamentum venosum
Ductus arteriosus	Ligamentum arteriosum

3. Occlusion of ductus arteriosus diverts right ventricular blood to lungs.
4. Closure of foramen ovale due to increased pressure in left atrium (owing to increased volume of blood that returns from lungs). *Note:* Premature closure of foramen ovale leads to right ventricular hypertrophy.^{NEXT}
    - The embryonic communications close by vasoconstriction (physiologically) soon after the birth and later by proliferation of intima (anatomical closure).^{MCQ} Completed obliteration of lumen of umbilical arteries and ductus arteriosus take place in 2–3 months after birth. Anatomical closure of foramen ovale takes at about 1 year.^{MCQ}

Fetal heartbeat

- Fetal heartbeat can be heard using a **stethoscope** and Doppler auscultation (**Doppler fetoscope**) (Table 19.9).^{MCQ}

Table 19.9 Fetal heart rate

Gestational age	Heart rate (beats per minute)
5 weeks	80–103
6 weeks	103–126
7 weeks	126–149
8 weeks	149–172
9 weeks	155–195
12 weeks	120–160

DEVELOPMENT OF LYMPHATIC SYSTEM

- At the end of sixth week, lymphatic system begins to develop.
- Lymphatic capillary plexuses join to form endothelium-lined lymph sacs.
- There are six primary lymph sacs as follows (Figs 19.18, 19.19):
  - 1–2: Right and left jugular lymph sacs: Lie near junction of subclavian veins with anterior cardinal veins.
  - 3–4: Right and left posterior (iliac) sacs: Lie near junction of iliac veins with posterior cardinal veins.
  - 5: Single retroperitoneal sac: Lies in root of mesentery on posterior abdominal wall.
  - 6: Single cisterna chyli: Lies dorsal to retroperitoneal sac.
- Two large channels (right and left thoracic ducts) connect jugular sac with cisterna chyli.
- Thoracic ducts get communicated by a large anastomosing channel.
- Thoracic duct develops from
  - caudal part of primitive right thoracic duct
  - anastomosing channel
  - cranial part of primitive left thoracic duct
- Right lymphatic duct develops from cranial part of primitive right thoracic duct.

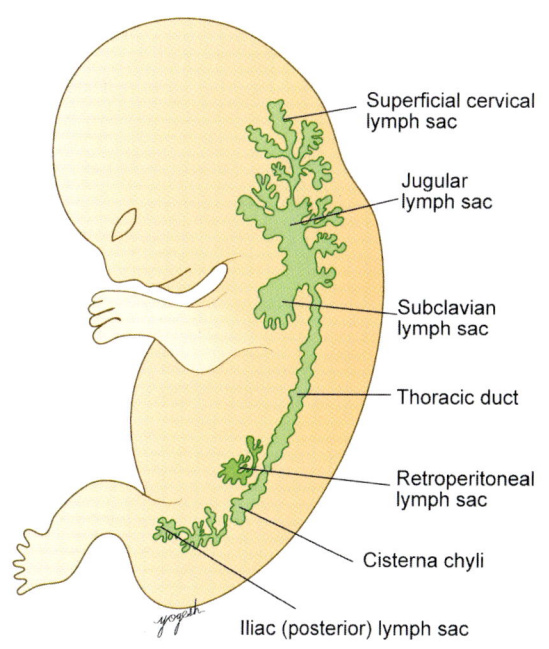

Fig. 19.18: Development of the lymphatic system

- Jugular lymphatic sac forms communication with venous junction of internal jugular and subclavian vein.
- Small lymphatic vessels drain body parts into lymph sac in the following manner:
  - head, neck, upper limb to jugular sacs

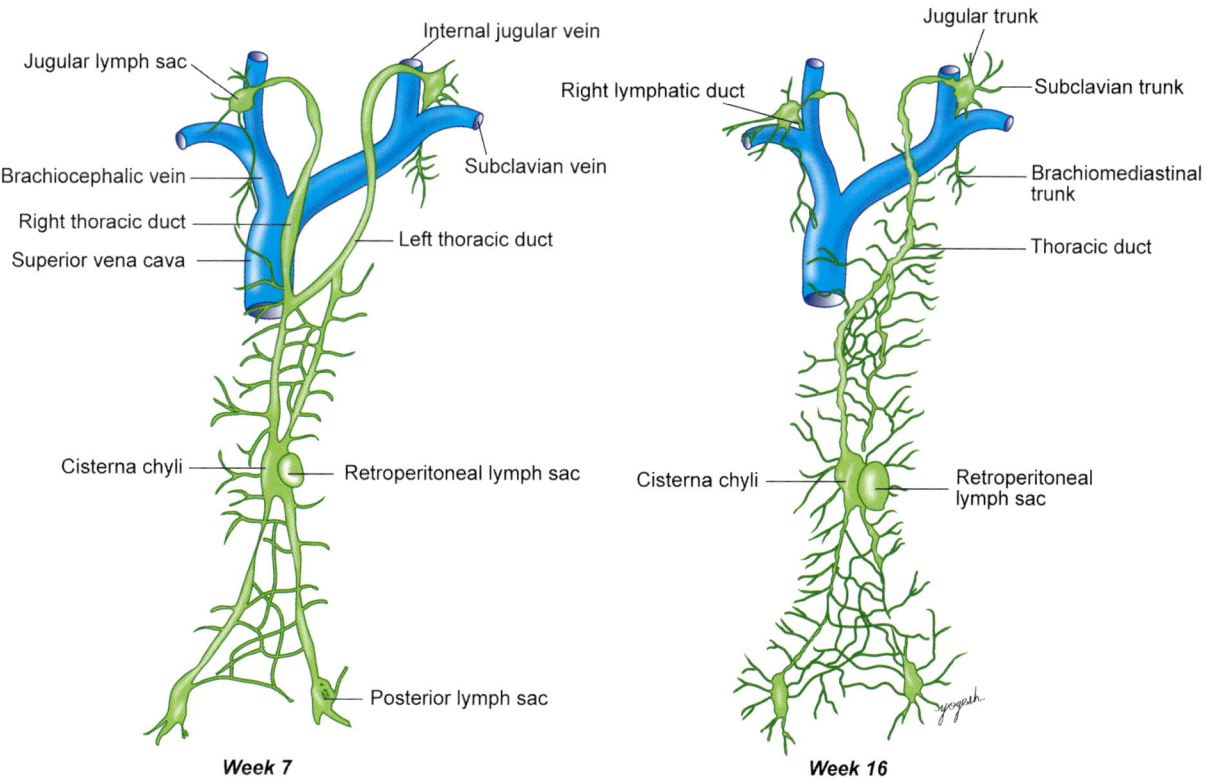

Fig. 19.19: Development of lymphatic system

- lower trunk and lower limb to iliac lymph sacs
- primitive gut to retroperitoneal sac

Clinical Conditions

- Congenital lymph edema: It occurs due to dilation of primordial lymphatic channels.
- Cystic hygromas (cystic lymphangioma/macrocystic lymphatic malformation): It is a congenital multiloculated lymphatic lesion mostly present in left posterior triangle of neck and armpits. Hygromas arise from jugular lymph sac or from lymphatic spaces that fail to establish connections with primary lymphatic channels.

TIMING OF AORTIC ARCH FORMATION

Table 19.10 Timing of aortic arch formation

Timing	Event
Days 19–20	First pair of aortic arch forms
Days 20–23	Second pair of aortic arch forms
Days 24–25	Third pair of aortic arch forms Third pair of aortic arches becomes internal carotid arteries
Days 26–30	First and second pairs of aortic arches disappear Fourth pair of aortic arches forms Fourth left arch becomes definitive aorta Fourth right arch becomes right subclavian artery Fifth pair of aortic arches never fully develop
Day 30	Sixth pair of aortic arches forms Sixth right arch becomes right pulmonary artery Sixth left arch becomes left pulmonary artery (ductus arteriosus)

Chapter 20

Urinary System: Kidney, Ureter, Urinary Bladder, Urethra

eSmartQuiz

Chapter Outline

- Introduction
  - Intermediate mesoderm
  - Cloaca
  - Mesonephric duct
  - Paramesonephric duct
- Development of kidneys
  - Evolutionary history of kidney
  - Stages of kidney development
  - Congenital anomalies of kidney
- Development of ureter
  - Anomalies of ureter
- Development of urinary bladder
  - Stages of development
- Ectopia vesicae
- Development of urethra
  - Development of female urethra
  - Development of male urethra

Competency:
- **AN52.7:** Describe the development of urinary system.

INTRODUCTION

- Urinary and genital systems develop from the common sources: Intermediate mesoderm and cloaca.

Intermediate Mesoderm

- On formation of the somites and intraembryonic coelom, the intraembryonic mesoderm is divided into three segments as follows (Fig. 20.1, Flowchart 20.1):
  - *paraxial mesoderm* that forms somites.
  - *intermediate mesoderm* that forms genitourinary system.
  - *lateral plate mesoderm* that forms somatopleuric and splanchnopleuric layers.
- Intermediate mesoderm forms bulging urogenital ridge on dorsal body wall just lateral to attachment of dorsal mesentery (Fig. 20.2).
- Urogenital ridge has two parts: Medial *genital ridge* and lateral *nephrogenic cord*.

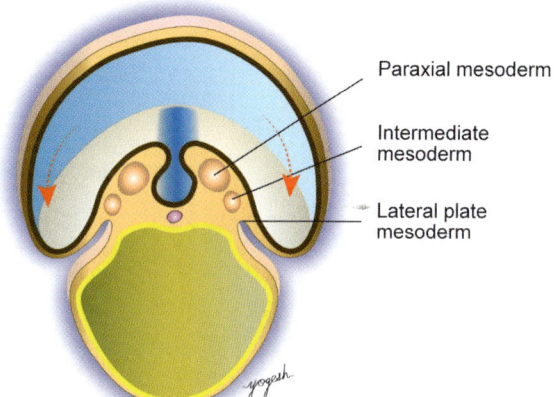

Fig. 20.1: Intraembryonic mesoderm. It is divided into three segments: Paraxial mesoderm, intermediate mesoderm (forms genitourinary system) and lateral plate mesoderm

- Nephrogenic cord extends from cervical to sacral segments of embryo.
- The nephrogenic cord passes through pronephric, mesonephric, and metanephric phases that show formation of renal tubules and mesonephric ducts, paramesonephric duct, and gonads (Fig. 20.3, Practice Fig. 20.1).

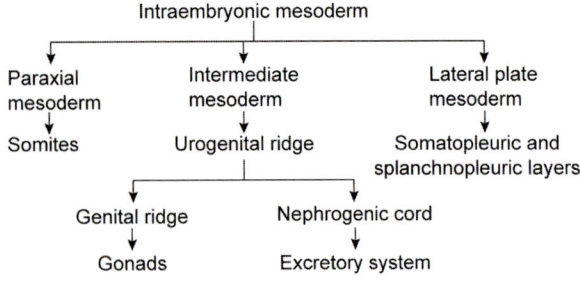

Flowchart 20.1: Intermediate mesoderm

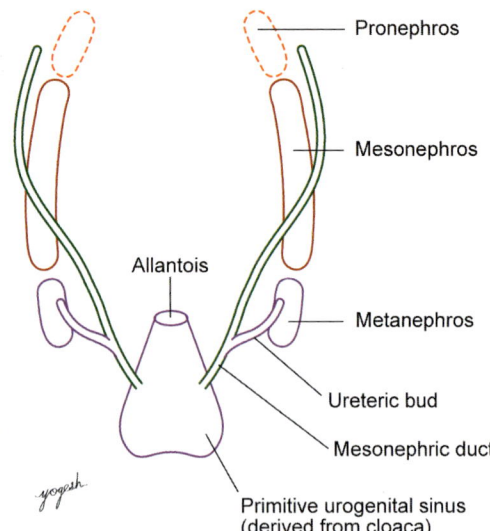

Practice Fig. 20.1: Pronephros, mesonephros, metanephros, and mesonephric duct

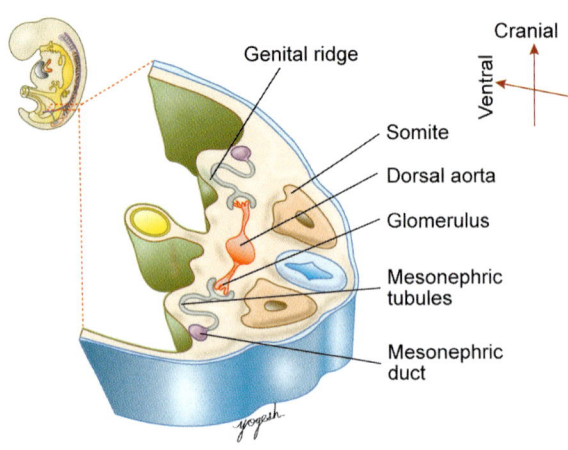

Fig. 20.2: Section of embryo with genital ridge and mesonephric duct and mesonephric tubules

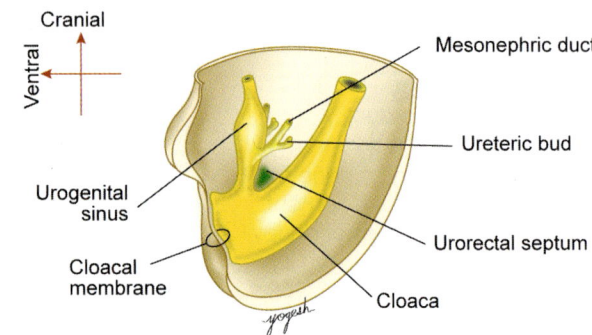

Fig. 20.4: Endodermal cloaca and allantois

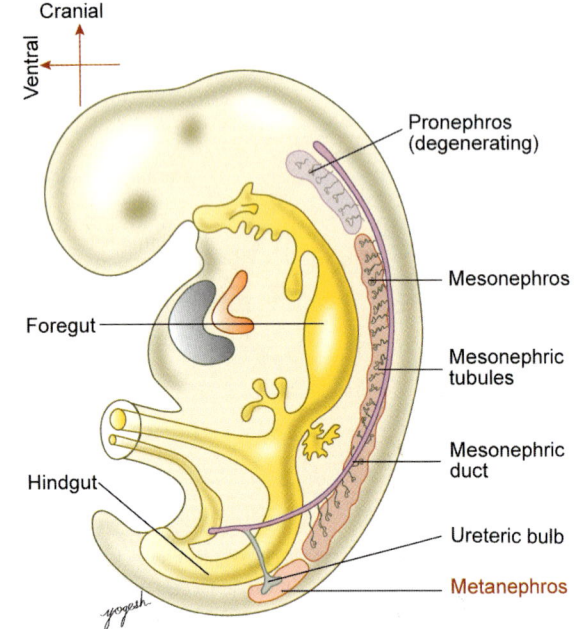

Fig. 20.3: A 28 days fetus showing pronephros, mesonephros, and metanephros. Pronephric tubules appear in the cervical region and they soon disappear. Ureteric bud aises from mesonephric duct and grows toward metanephros

Cloaca

- Cloaca is part of hindgut shared by genitourinary and digestive system (Fig. 20.4, Practice Fig. 20.2, Flowchart 20.2).

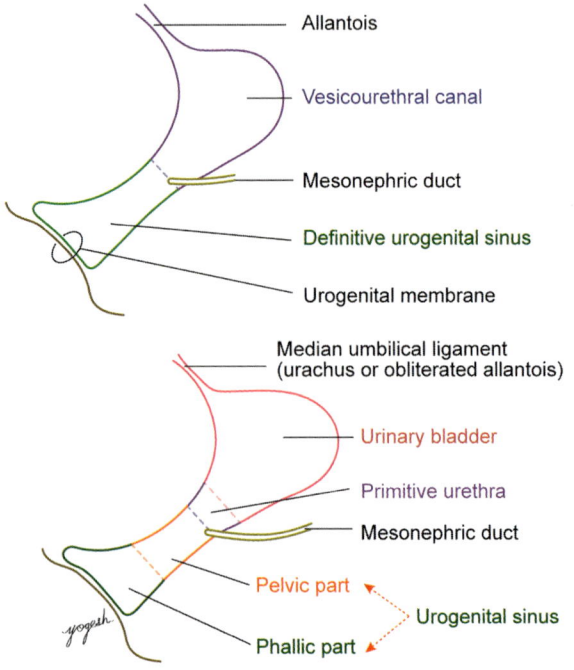

Practice Fig. 20.2: Primitive urogenital sinus

Flowchart 20.2: Subdivisions of cloaca and development of urinary bladder

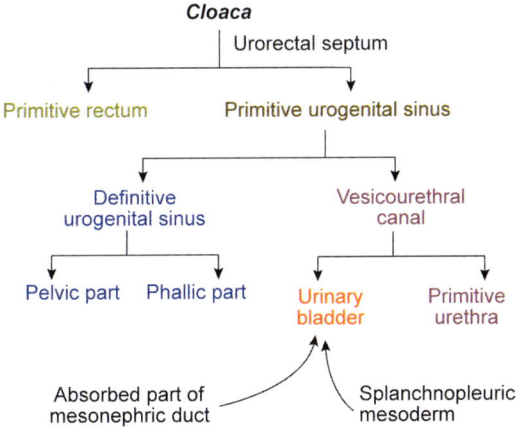

- The cloaca is divided into *primitive urogenital sinus* and dorsal *primitive rectum* by *urorectal septum*.
- Later, openings of mesonephric ducts divide primitive urogenital sinus into cranial *vesicourethral canal* and caudal *definitive urogenital sinus*.

Mesonephric Duct (Wolffian Duct) High yielding facts
(*see* Fig. 21.8)

Q. Write a short note on mesonephric duct.

- A mesonephric duct is a paired duct that develops in the intermediate mesoderm that later communicates with primitive urogenital sinus.
- The mesonephric duct is also called Wolffian duct, Leydig's duct, archinephric, or nephric duct.
- Casper Fredrich Wolf has first described the mesonephros (1759).
- Anti-müllerian hormone of Sertoli cells is absent in females. Hence, mesonephric duct regresses.

Derivatives (Flowchart 20.3) Viva, MCQ
- Mesonephric duct forms the following structures:

In male
- Trigone of urinary bladder (in both sexes) MCQ
- Efferent ducts of testis, epididymis
- Vas deferens NEXT
- Posterior wall of prostatic urethra, appendix of epididymis. NEXT (*Note*: Hydatid of Morgagni is appendix of testis in male or paratubal cyst in female.) NEXT
- Seminal vesicles, ejaculatory ducts NEXT

In female
- Trigone of urinary bladder
- Epoöphoron
- Paroöphoron
- Gartner's duct or cyst
- Skene's glands

Ureteric bud *arises from* Wolffian duct and it gives rise to ureter, renal pelvis, major and minor calyces, ampulla, and 1–3 million collecting tubules. NEXT

Paramesonephric Duct (Müllerian Ducts) High yielding facts
(*see* Fig. 21.8)

Q. Write a short note on paramesonephric ducts.

- Paramesonephric ducts are paired ducts that develop in urogenital ridge of intermediate mesoderm lateral to the mesonephric ducts.
- In 6th week of IUL, lining epithelium of peritoneal cavity (*coelomic epithelium*) invaginates intermediate mesoderm and forms paramesonephric ducts.
- These ducts cross ventrally to mesonephric ducts (from lateral to the medial) and fuse with each other to form *uterovaginal canal* (uterine canal).
- Later, uterovaginal canal gets communicated with definitive urogenital sinus.
- Absence of anti-Müllerian factor results in development of paramesonephric ducts in females, whereas in male, anti-Müllerian factor secretion by Sertoli cells inhibits the development of paramesonephric ducts.

Derivatives (Flowchart 20.4) Viva, MCQ

In females
- Uterine tube
- Uterus
- Upper part of vagina

In males
- Appendix of testis
- Prostatic utricle (vagina musculina/vesicula-prostatica)

- *Note:* Prostatic utricle in male is homologous to uterus and vagina in female.

Flowchart 20.3: Mesonephric (Wolffian) duct

Mesonephric (Wolffian) duct
Paired ducts, develops in intermediate mesoderm
Derivatives

In male	In female
Trigone of urinary bladder	Trigone of urinary bladder
Efferent ducts of testis	Epoöphoron
Epididymis	Paroöphoron
Vas deferens	Gartner's duct
Posterior wall of prostatic urethra	Skene's gland
Appendix of epididymis	
Seminal vesicles	
Ejaculatory ducts	

Flowchart 20.4: Paramesonephric duct

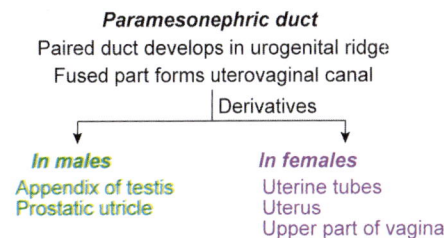

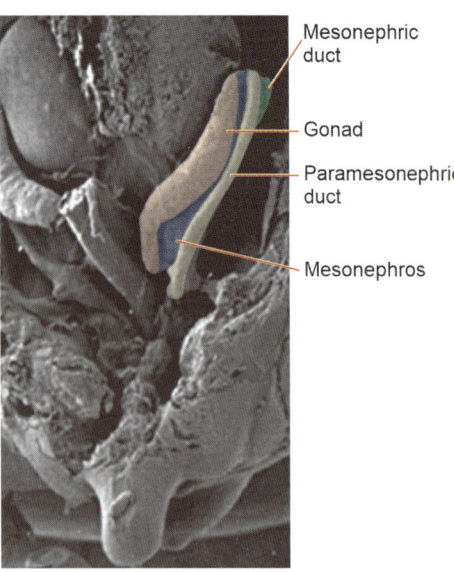

Scanning electron micrograph 20.1: Genital ducts and developing internal genitalia. The intact mesonephric and paramesonephric ducts, mesonephros, and gonad of a 7-week human embryo are shown. [Species: Human, gestation: 7 weeks]

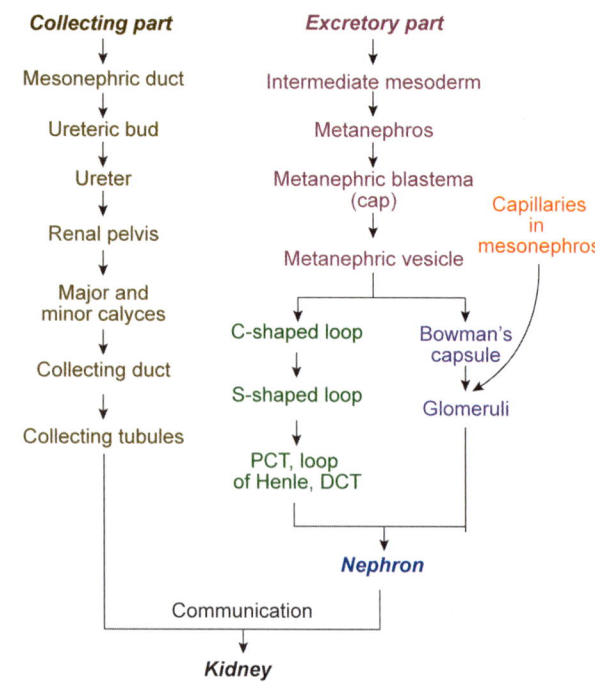

20 DEVELOPMENT OF KIDNEYS

Q. Write a short note on development of kidney.

Summary (Examination Guide) (Practice Fig. 20.3, Fig. 20.7, Flowchart 20.5)^{High yielding facts}

- Human kidney shows two developmental parts as:
  A. *Collecting part:* It consists of collecting tubules, collecting ducts, minor and major calyces, renal pelvis and ureter. ^{NEXT}
  B. *Secretory part:* It consists of glomeruli, Bowman's capsule, proximal and distal convoluted tubules and loop of Henle.
- Embryological sources:
  – Ureteric bud forms collecting part of kidney.
  – Metanephric blastema forms secretory part of kidney.
- Kidney ascends from sacral region to thoracolumbar region to get better blood supply.
- Primitive kidney initially gets supply from median sacral artery via renal artery. Later receives from common iliac artery.^{NEXT} On ascent, kidney receives supply from lateral splanchnic branches of the aorta as renal artery.
- On rotation of kidney by 90° medially, hilum turns from ventral to medial side.
- Fetal kidney starts functioning by 12th week of IUL and excretes urine into amniotic cavity.^{MCQ}

Evolutionary History of Kidney

- Kidney develops from nephrogenic cord of intermediate mesoderm that extends from cervical to sacral region.
- Ontogeny repeats phylogeny in kidney development: Evolutionary history is repeated during the development of kidney.
- Pronephric kidney is present in some cyclostomes and some teleost fish.
- Mesonephric kidney is present in amphibians and most of fishes.
- Metanephric kidney is present in primates including human.^{MCQ}
- Thus, evolutionary stages are pronephric kidney → mesonephric kidney → metanephric kidney^{Viva}
- During the development of human kidney, nephrogenic cord forms three sets of successive kidneys as follows:
  1. *Pronephros* appears in cervical region at the beginning of 4th week and later it regresses and pronephric duct continues as mesonephric duct.
  2. *Mesonephros* appears in thoracolumbar region at the end of 4th week. It also completely regresses. Mesonephric tubules mostly regress (some form vasa efferentia of testis). The mesonephric duct forms collecting part of the kidney and other parts in the male reproductive tract.
  3. *Metanephros* appears in lumbosacral region in the beginning of 3rd month. It forms secretory part of the human kidney.

Stages of Kidney Development

1. Development of collecting system

- *Ureteric buds* arise from caudal region of mesonephric duct and grow towards metanephros (nephrogenic cord) (Practice Fig. 20.1).
- *Metanephric blastema* caps growing dilated end (ampulla) of ureteric bud.

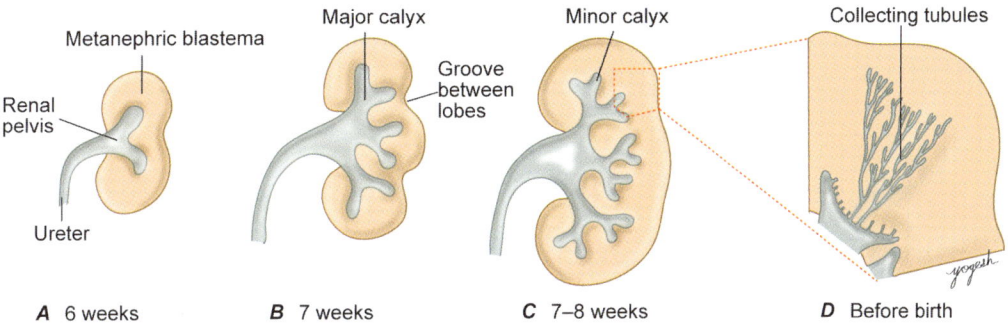

Fig. 20.5: Development of kidney. Ureteric bud divides dichotomously to form renal pelvis, major calyces, minor calyces, and collecting tubules

- *Ampulla* divides dichotomously for 12–14 generations to form renal pelvis, major calyces, minor calyces, collecting ducts, and collecting tubules (Fig. 20.5A to D).

2. Development of secretory (excretory) part

- Cells of the *metanephros* form metanephric blastema that caps dividing ureteric bud (Fig. 20.6).
- *Metanephric cap* dilates to form a pear-shaped *metanephric vesicle* that later forms S-shaped *primitive renal tubule* (Fig. 20.6B, Practice Fig. 20.3).
- One end of the primitive tubule dilates to form Bowman's capsule, whereas the other end communicates with collecting tubules (derived from ureteric bud) (Fig. 20.6E).
- Primitive tubule finally forms Bowman's capsule proximal convoluted tubule, loop of Henle and distal convoluted tubule.
- Bowman's capsule is invaginated by a tuft of capillaries from adjacent mesoderm to form *renal corpuscles* (Fig. 20.6E).
- Thus, metanephros give rise to secretory unit or nephron up to collecting tubule that includes renal vesicle, glomeruli, Bowman's capsule, proximal convoluted tubule, loop of Henle, and distal convoluted tubule (Fig. 20.6).^{NEXT}

3. Ascent of kidney

Q. Write a short note on ascent of kidney.

- Metanephric kidney develops in metanephros of nephrogenic cord that lies in pelvic cavity at sacral level (Fig. 20.8).

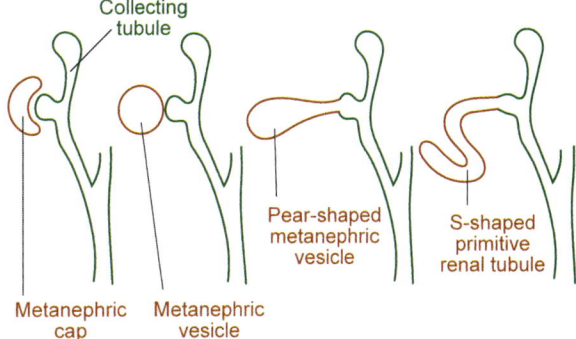
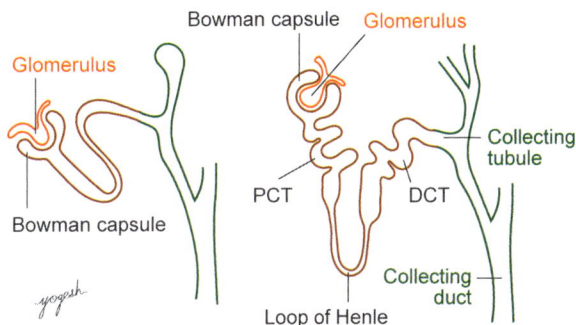

Practice Fig. 20.3: Development of nephron

- Kidney ascends from its initial sacral position to thoracolumbar region (in 9th week).
- Cause for ascent of kidney^{MCQ, Viva}
  - In search of better blood supply
  - Due to smaller pelvic cavity that fails to accommodate enlarging kidney

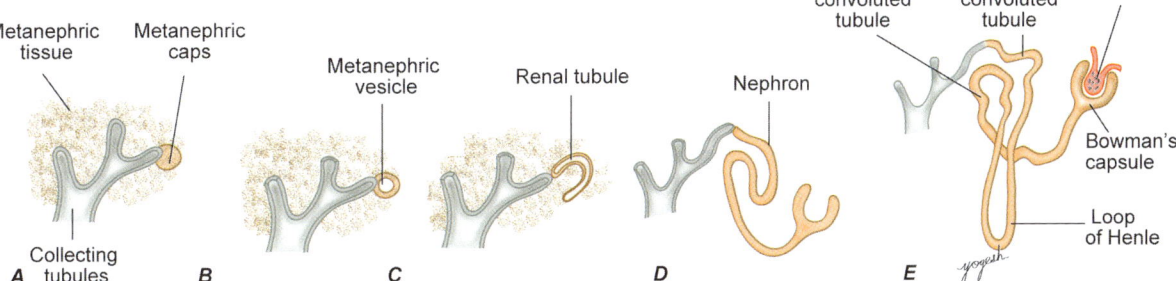

Fig. 20.6: Development of nephron from metanephric blastema. Excretory part of kidney develops from metanephric blastema (brown-colored structure) and establishes communication with collecting tubules (ash-colored structure) that develop from ureteric bud (mesonephric duct)

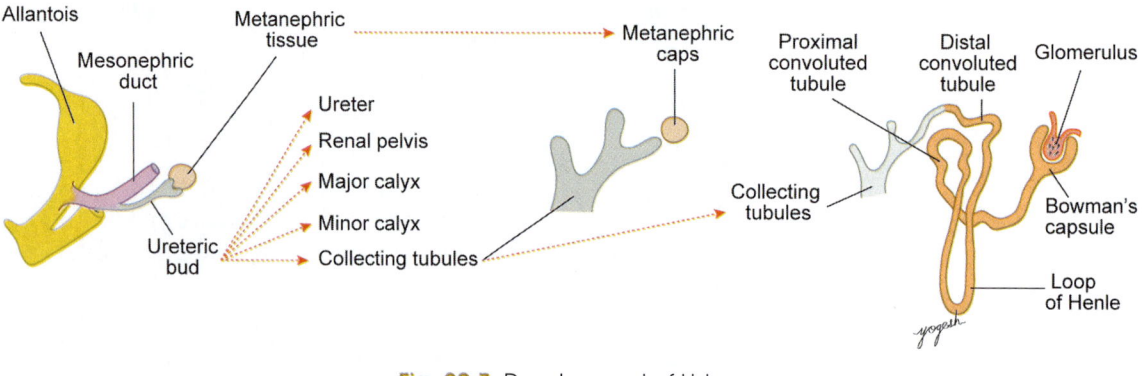

Fig. 20.7: Development of kidney

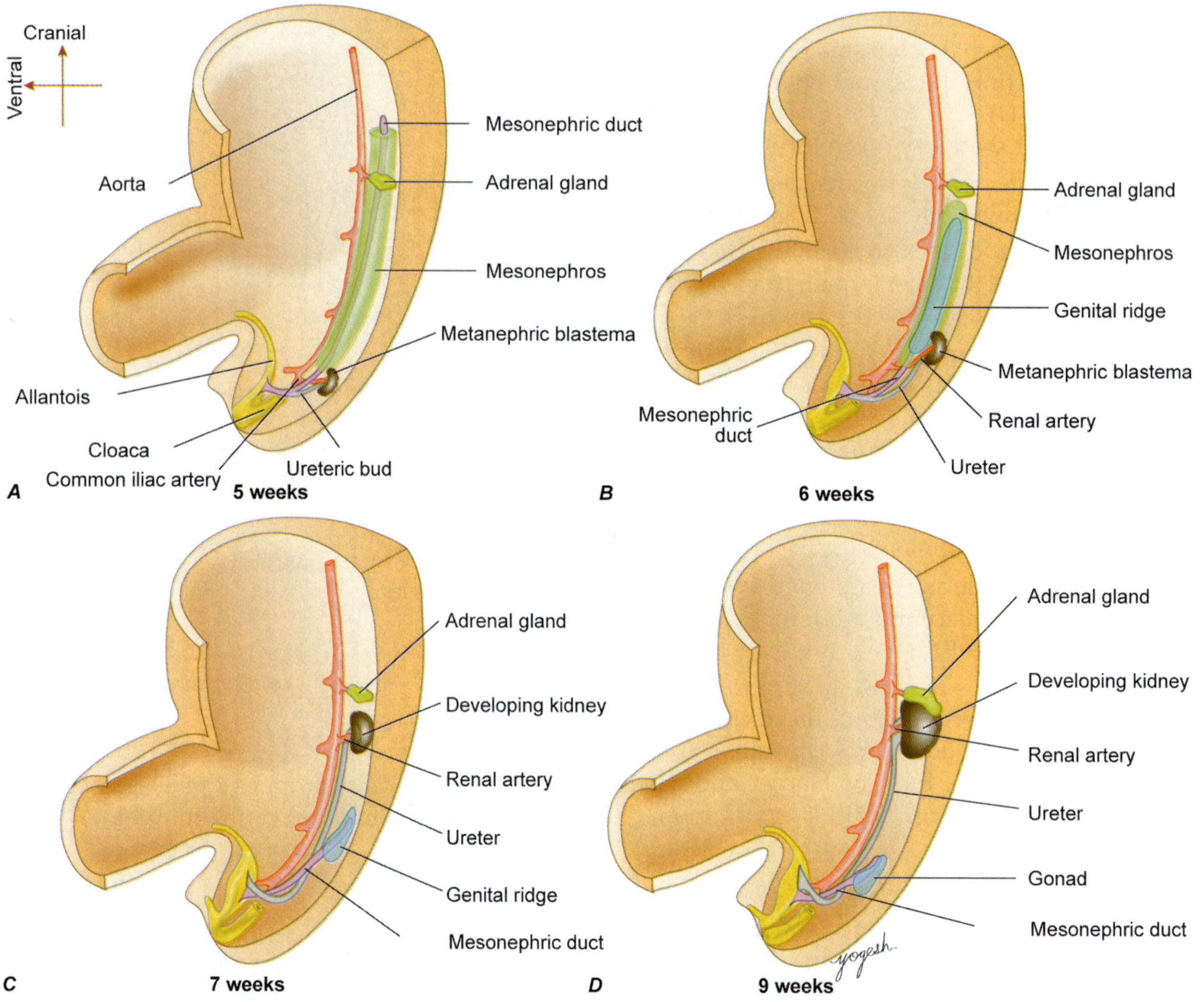

Fig. 20.8: Ascent of kidney. Kidney ascends from its sacral position to thoracolumbar region between 5th and 9th weeks of IUL. Simultaneously, size of mesonephros reduces

- Differential growth of posterior abdominal wall
- Reduction of fetal curvature
- Duration
  - Metanephros appears by 5th week of IUL
  - By 9th week, kidneys ascend to their adult position within the abdomen.^{MCQ}

4. Blood supply of kidney

- In initial phase, kidney is supplied by *median sacral artery* (continuation of the aorta).
- During ascent of kidney, lateral splanchnic branches of aorta supply it.
- Finally, one of the lateral splanchnic branches of aorta corresponding to L2 vertebra forms *definitive renal artery*.

5. Rotation of kidney

- On reaching thoracolumbar region, kidney rotates medially around the vertical axis. Hence, hilus changes its position from ventral to medial aspect of kidney.

Congenital Anomalies of Kidney (Flowchart 20.6)

Q. Write a short note on congenital anomalies of kidney, horseshoe kidney, and unilateral renal agenesis.

1. Renal agenesis (Fig. 20.9A)
   - Unilateral or bilateral, complete failure of kidney development is called renal agenesis.
   - Cause: Failure of ureteric bud formation.^{NEXT}
   - Genetic basis: Metanephros produces glial-derived neurotrophic factor (GDNF) that stimulates branching and growth of ureteric bud. Mutation in genes regulating GDNF production may cause renal agenesis (for example, SALL, PAX2, EYA1). SALL1 causes Townes-Brock syndrome. PAX2 causes coloboma syndrome. EYA1 causes branchio-otorenal syndrome.
2. Duplication: Early division of ureteric bud may produce extra kidney. There may be a separate or fused kidney. The ureters may be separate or partially fused with duplicate kidney (Fig. 20.9B).
3. Horseshoe kidney: Kidneys may be connected by an isthmus at lower poles. In this condition, kidney lies at the level of lower lumbar vertebrae as *inferior mesenteric artery* blocks the ascent of isthmus of horseshoe kidney (Fig. 20.10A).^{NEXT}
4. Pancake kidney: In this condition both the kidneys fuse to form a single mass (Fig. 20.10B).
5. Lobulated kidney: During development, kidney is lobulated. The lobulation disappears in the first year of life. If it persists, it forms lobulated kidney (Fig. 20.11).
6. Anomalies of ascent of kidney (Fig. 20.12)
   - Pelvic kidney: Kidney lies in pelvic cavity.
   - Lower lumbar kidneys: Kidney lies against lower lumbar vertebrae.
   - Thoracic kidneys: Abnormally high ascent of kidneys in thoracic cavity.
7. Congenital polycystic kidney
   - Failure to establish communication between secretory/excretory and collecting part of kidney results in polycystic kidney.
   - These cysts are filled with urine.
   - The congenital polycystic kidney is usually bilateral.
   - Newer concept: This condition occurs due to abnormal dilation of uriniferous tubules.
   - It has two presentations:
     - Autosomal recessive polycystic kidney disease (ARPKD) (childhood): It is less common and symptoms appear shortly after birth.
     - Autosomal dominant polycystic kidney disease (ADPKD) (adult): It is more common and develops in adulthood (30–40 years).
   - Incidence of
     ARPKD: 1 in 5000 births
     ADPKD: 1 in 500–1000 births
   - Treatment: Kidney transplantation and dialysis.

Flowchart 20.6: Congenital anomalies of kidney

Congenital anomalies of kidney
1. Renal agnesis – absence of kidney ← Failure of ureteric bud formation
2. Duplication – additional kidney ← Early division of ureteric bud
3. Horseshoe kidney ← Fusion of lower poles of kidneys
4. Pancake kidney – fused kidneys
5. Lobulated kidney
6. Anomalies of ascent – Pelvic, lumbar or thoracic kidney
7. Congenital polycystic kidney ← Failure of communication between excretory and secretory part
8. Accessory renal artery ← Persistent fetal renal artery
9. Wilm's tumor ← Mutation of WT1 gene

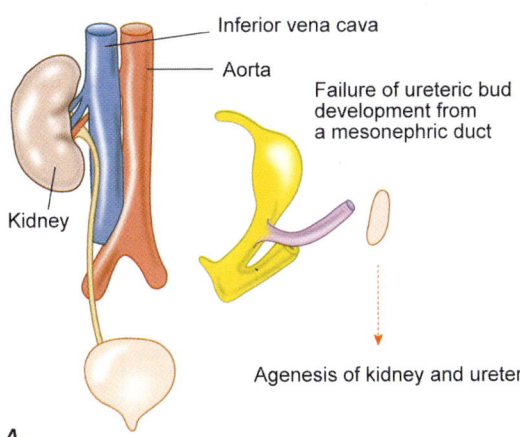
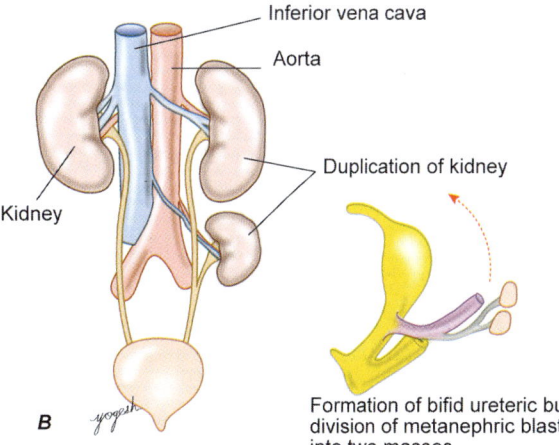

Fig. 20.9: Agenesis (A) and duplication (B) of kidney

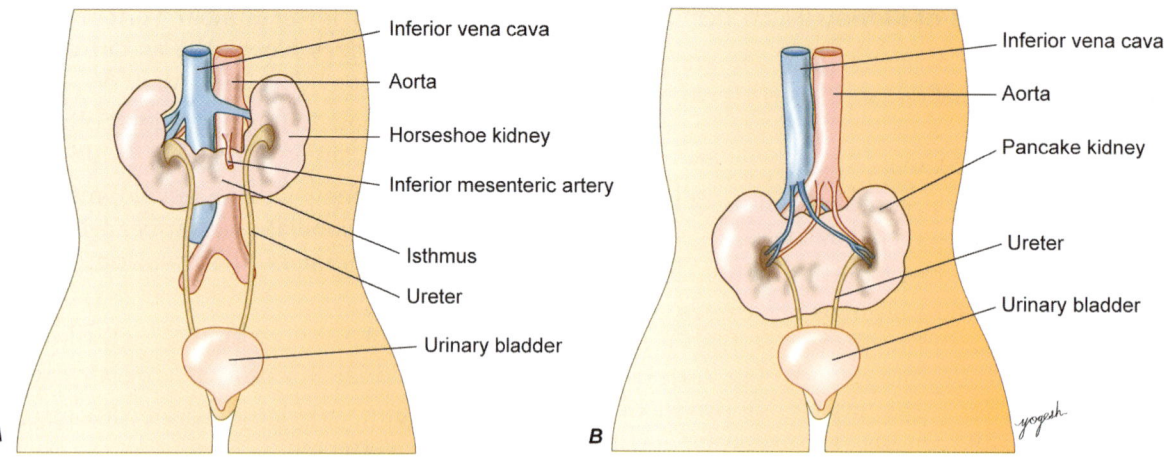

Fig. 20.10: Horseshoe kidney (A) and pancake kidney (B). Horseshoe kidney lies at the level of lower lumbar vertebrae as inferior mesenteric artery blocks ascent of isthmus of horseshoe kidney

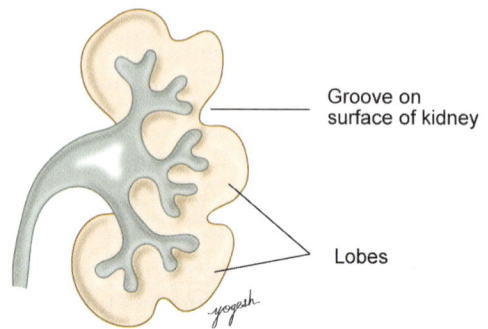

Fig. 20.11: Lobulated kidney. Usually, lobulation disappears in the first year of life. If it persists, it forms lobulated kidney

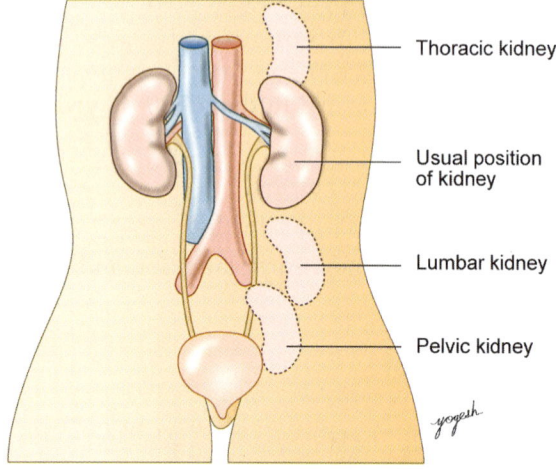

Fig. 20.12: Anomalies of ascent of kidney. Pelvic kidney lies in pelvic cavity, lumbar kidney lies against lower lumbar vertebrae, and thoracic kidney lies in thoracic cavity

- ADPKD: Etiology – mutation in short arm of chromosome 4 or chromosome 16.
8. Accessory renal artery (Fig. 20.13)
   - Persisting fetal renal arteries give rise to accessory or supernumerary renal arteries.^{MCQ}
   - Accessory renal artery is the most common renal vascular anomaly.^{NEXT} It may cause ureter compression resulting in hydronephrosis.

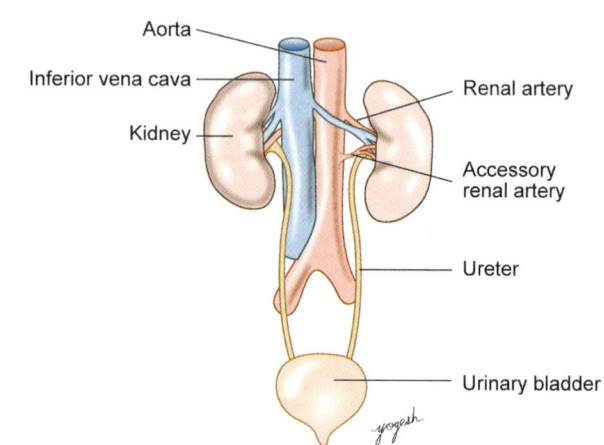

Fig. 20.13: Accessory renal artery represents persistent fetal renal artery

9. Wilms' tumor is the most common primary renal tumor of the childhood that is produced due to mutation of WT1 gene (location – chromosome 11p13).

DEVELOPMENT OF URETER

- Ureter develops from ureteric bud that raises from Wolffian duct (mesonephric duct).
- The part of ureteric bud that lies between renal pelvis and vesicourethral canal (a portion of cloaca) forms ureter.

Anomalies of Ureter

1. *Ectopic ureter*
   - If ureter does not open into bladder at its usual site, it is called *ectopic ureter*.
   - Abnormal sites of ectopic ureteric openings are as follows:
     a. In male: Lower part of bladder, prostatic urethra, seminal vesicles, rectum (Fig. 20.14A).
     b. In female: Urethra, vagina, vestibule, rectum (Fig. 20.14B).

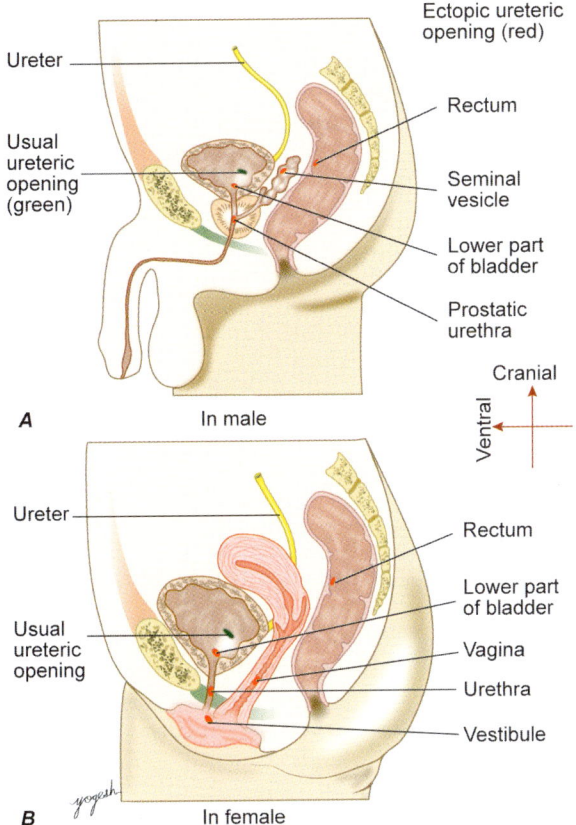

Fig. 20.14: Ectopic ureter. If ureter does not open into bladder at its usual site, it is called ectopic ureter. In male, ectopic ureter opens in lower part of urinary bladder, prostatic urethra, seminal vesicles, or rectum, whereas in female in urethra, vagina, vestibule, or rectum

2. *Ureteric obstruction (hydroureter):* Congenital ureteric obstruction may result in dilation of ureter (hydroureter). Postcaval ureter (right ureter hooks around left side of inferior vena cava) may cause ureteric obstruction (Fig. 20.15).

3. *Duplication:* Ureter may be partially or completely duplicated. Duplication of ureter may or may not be associated with duplication of kidney. Duplicated ureter may open into bladder together or separately (Fig. 20.16A).

4. *Blind ureter:* It is a rare anomaly and can be diagnosed using intravenous urography. Blind ureter is not connected to kidney (Fig. 20.16B).

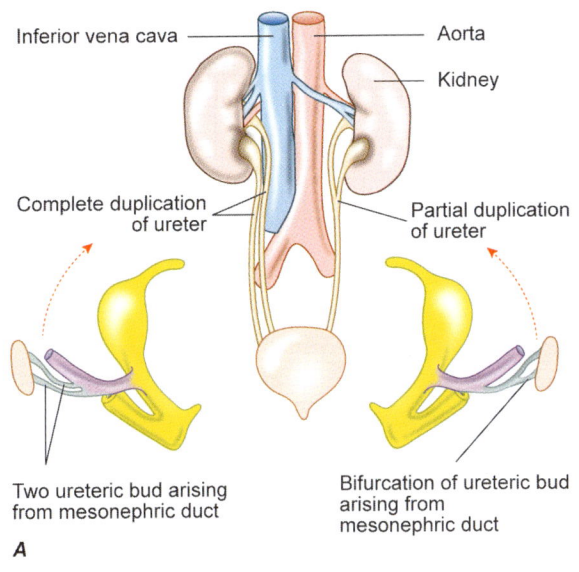

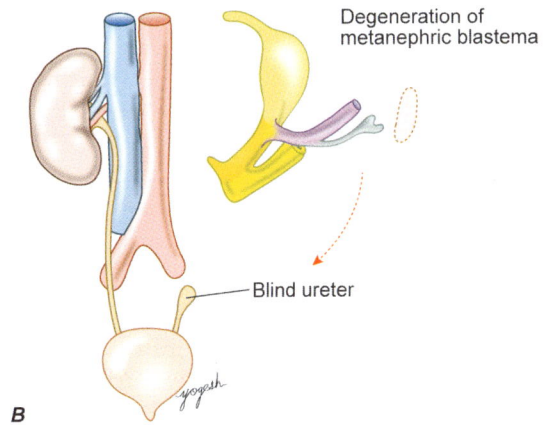

Fig. 20.16: Anomalies of ureter include partial or complete duplication of ureter (A) and blind ureter (B)

DEVELOPMENT OF URINARY BLADDER

Q. Write a short note on development of urinary bladder.

Q. Write a short note on primitive urogenital sinus.

- Urinary bladder shows three layers as inner lining (transitional) epithelium, middle connective tissue and smooth muscle layer and outer serous (connective tissue) layer.
- Interior of bladder shows a smooth triangular region called *trigone* of bladder. Ureters open at the superolateral angles of trigone, whereas its apex has a urethral orifice.

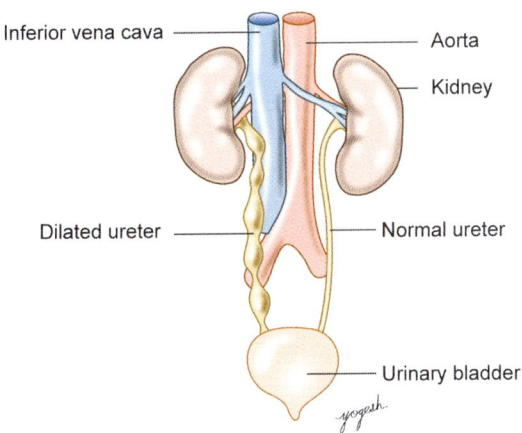

Fig. 20.15: Hydroureter (megaloureter). Congenital ureteric obstruction may result into dilation of ureter

Summary (Examination Guide) (Table 20.1, Fig. 20.17, Practice Fig. 20.4, Flowchart 20.7)^{High yielding facts}

Developmentally bladder shows following sources:

- **Lining epithelium of bladder except for trigone:** It is derived from cranial dilated part of vesicourethral canal (endoderm).
- **Lining epithelium of trigone:** It develops from mesoderm by absorption of mesonephric ducts in dorsal wall of vesicourethral canal.
- **Muscles and connective tissue coats:** They develop from mesoderm – splanchnopleuric intraembryonic mesoderm surrounding vesicourethral canal.
- **Urachus (median umbilical ligament)** is derived from allantois.^{NEXT}

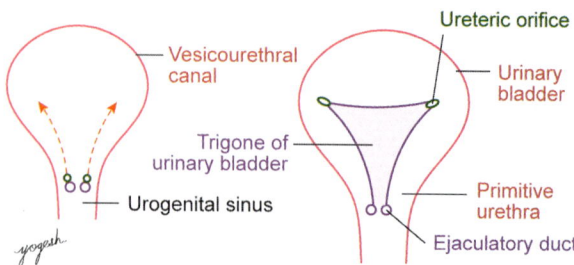

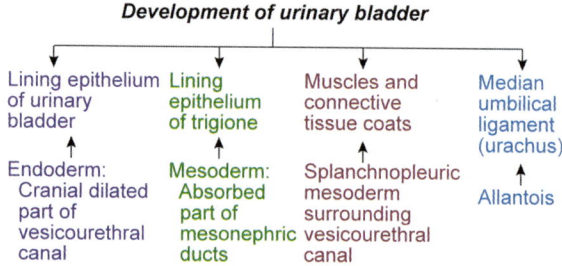

Practice Fig. 20.4: Development of urinary bladder

Table 20.1	Development of urinary bladder^{NEXT}
Part of urinary bladder	*Embryological source*
Lining epithelium (transitional epithelium) of urinary bladder except for trigone	Endoderm: Cranial dilated part of vesicourethral canal^{NEXT}
Lining epithelium of trigone	Mesoderm: Absorbed part of mesonephric ducts in vesicourethral canal
Connective tissue and muscles	Splanchnopleuric intraembryonic mesoderm surrounding vesicourethral canal
Urachus (median umbilical ligament), apex of urinary bladder	Allantois

Flowchart 20.7: Development of urinary bladder

Development of urinary bladder

- Lining epithelium of urinary bladder ← Endoderm: Cranial dilated part of vesicourethral canal
- Lining epithelium of trigone ← Mesoderm: Absorbed part of mesonephric ducts
- Muscles and connective tissue coats ← Splanchnopleuric mesoderm surrounding vesicourethral canal
- Median umbilical ligament (urachus) ← Allantois

Congenital anomalies

1. Rectovesical fistula
2. Vesicovaginal fistula
3. Urachal fistula
4. Urachal cyst
5. Urachal sinus
6. Hourglass bladder

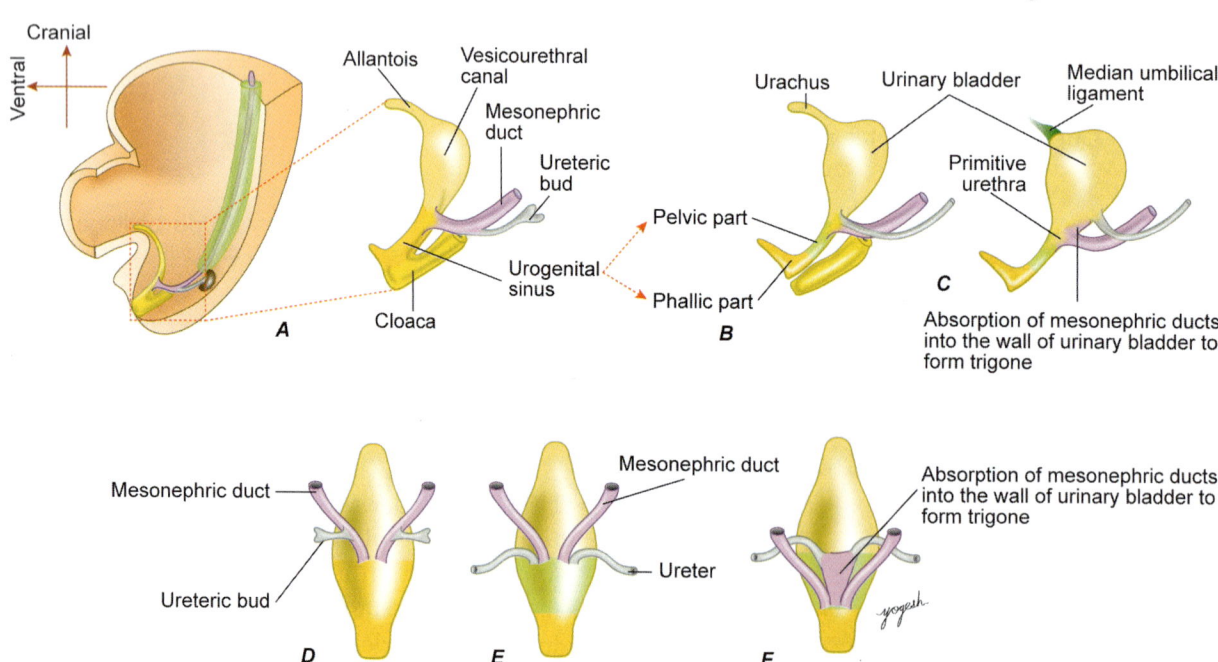

Fig. 20.17: Development of urinary bladder. A–C: Side view of developing urinary bladder; D–F: Dorsal view of the developing bladder showing changing relationship of ureter and mesonephric duct

Stages of Urinary Bladder Development

1. Cloacal division:
   - Cloaca is divided by urorectal septum into ventral *urogenital sinus* and dorsal *primitive rectum*.
   - Urorectal septum establishes contact with cloacal membrane to divide it into ventral *urogenital membrane* and dorsal *anal membrane*.
   - Urorectal septum forms *perineal body*. ^MCQ
   - Urorectal septum contains four ducts, a pair of mesonephric ducts and a pair of paramesonephric ducts.
   - In the 5th week, mesonephric ducts open into the urogenital sinus.
   - The opening of mesonephric duct divides the urogenital sinus in cranial *vesicourethral canal* and caudal *definitive urogenital sinus*.
   - Definitive urogenital sinus is subdivided into cranial *pelvic part* and caudal *phallic part*.
2. Absorption of mesonephric ducts into vesicourethral canal
   - Initially, ureteric bud (future ureters) and mesonephric ducts have a common opening in the vesicourethral canal.
   - Slow absorption (incorporation) of mesonephric duct in dorsal wall of vesicourethral canal separates openings of mesonephric ducts from ureteric buds.
   - Gradually absorption continues, and openings of ureteric buds move laterally and cranially.
   - Incorporated mesonephric ducts form a triangular zone on the dorsal wall of vesicourethral canal. This triangular part (trigone of urinary bladder) lies between the openings of ureters (ureteric bud) and mesonephric ducts.
   - *Note:* Terminal parts of mesonephric ducts disappear in female and in male they form ejaculatory ducts (for details, read Chapter 21).
3. Development of muscular and connective tissue coats
   - Muscular and connective tissue coats (serous) of urinary bladder are derived from a splanchnopleuric layer of intraembryonic mesoderm that surrounds vesicourethral canal.

Congenital Anomalies

Q. Write a short note on congenital anomalies of urinary bladder.

1. Fistulas:
   a. Congenital rectovesical fistula: It develops due to incomplete urorectal septum.
   b. Congenital vesicovaginal fistula: Müllerian eminence is elevation in dorsal wall of the phallic part of the urogenital sinus formed by fused caudal ends of paramesonephric ducts. If Müllerian eminence projects into the vesicourethral part of cloaca, it results in *vesicovaginal fistula*.
   c. Urachal fistula: It is persistent allantois.^NEXT In this condition, urinary bladder communicates with exterior at the umbilicus (Fig. 20.18A).
2. *Urachal cyst*: Urachal cyst develops from non-obliterated middle part of allantois.^NEXT It forms palpable midline cystic part of anterior abdominal wall (Fig. 20.18B).
3. *Urachal sinus*: It develops from nonobliterated distal part of allantois that shows opening at umbilicus (Fig. 20.18C).
4. Hourglass bladder: In this condition, urinary bladder is divided into upper and lower compartments by a constriction in middle zone (Fig. 20.19).

DEVELOPMENT OF URETHRA

Q. Write a short note on development of urethra.

Development of Female Urethra

- Female urethra is short (4 cm).
- Female urethra is derived as follows (Practice Fig. 20.5):
  – Mostly from narrow caudal part of the vesicourethral canal.

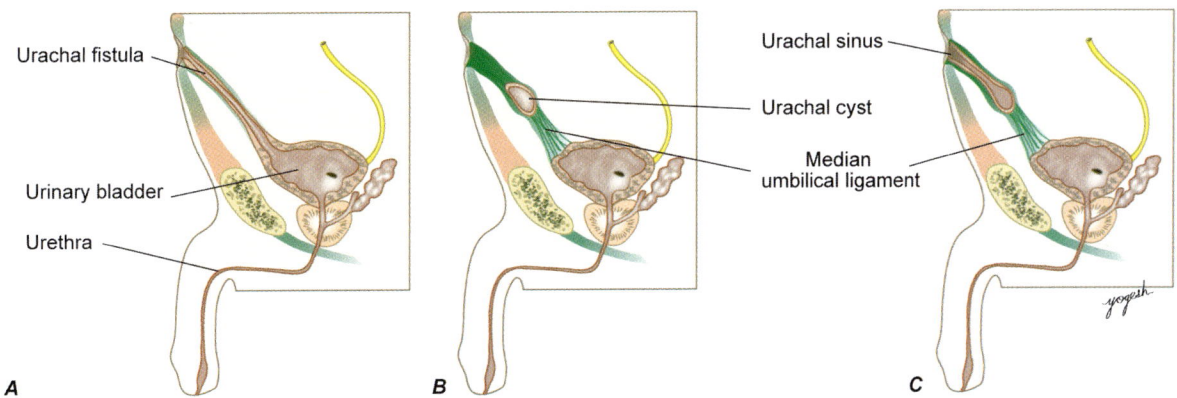

Fig. 20.18: Anomalies arising due to persistent urachus: (A) Urachal fistula; (B) Urachal cyst; (C) Urachal sinus

Box 20.1: Ectopia vesicae

Q. Write a short note on ectopia vesicae.
- It is also called *extrophy of urinary bladder*.
- Abnormality:
  - Deficient midline infraumbilical part of anterior abdominal wall
  - Deficient anterior wall of urinary bladder
  - Interior of bladder exposed
  - Urine dribbles from exposed bladder
- Embryological basis:
  - Failure of complete formation of lateral fold of embryo.
  - Failure of migration of mesoderm in lateral folds.
- Incidence: 1:10,000 births.
- Constant association: Ectopia vesicae is always associated with epispadias.

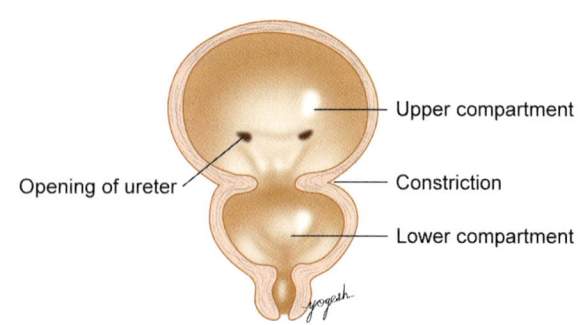

Fig. 20.19: Hourglass bladder is divided into upper and lower compartments by a constriction in middle zone

- Terminal part of urethra from pelvic part of definitive urogenital sinus (endodermal derivative).
- A small part of dorsal wall from absorbed part of mesonephric ducts (mesodermal derivative) in vesicourethral canal.
- Female urethra corresponds to prostatic part of male urethra.^{MCQ}

Development of Male Urethra

Q. Write a short note on development of male urethra.
- Male urethra has
  a. Prostatic part
  b. Membranous part
  c. Spongy part
  d. Glandular part

Summary (Examination Guide)

Male urethra develops as follows (Table 20.2, Practice Fig. 20.5):
- Caudal part of vesicourethral canal (primitive urethra) forms prostatic part of urethra, above level of openings of ejaculatory ducts.

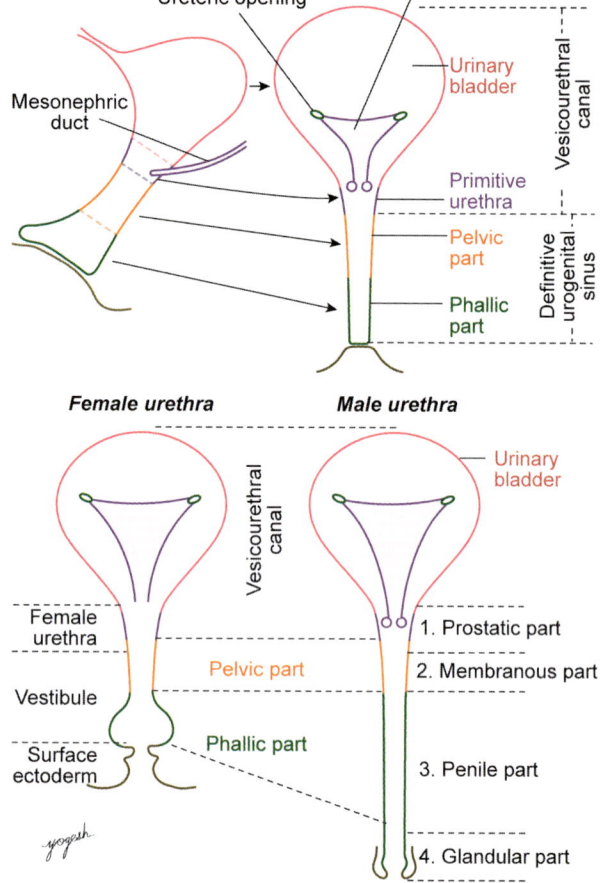

Practice Fig. 20.5: Development of urethra

Table 20.2	Development of urethra
Part	Embryonic source
Prostatic part – Above opening of ejaculatory ducts – Below opening of ejaculatory ducts	 Caudal part of vesicourethral canal, primitive urethra Pelvic part of definitive urogenital sinus
Membranous part	Pelvic part of definitive urogenital sinus
Spongy (penile) part	Phallic part of definitive urogenital sinus
Glandular part (terminal part of glans penis)	Surface ectoderm

- Pelvic part of definitive urogenital sinus forms:
  a. Prostatic part of urethra below level of opening of ejaculatory ducts
  b. Membranous part of urethra
- Phallic part of definitive urogenital sinus forms spongy part except near terminal opening that develops from surface ectoderm.

For further details, read the development of male external genitalia (Chapter 21).

Clinical Embryology

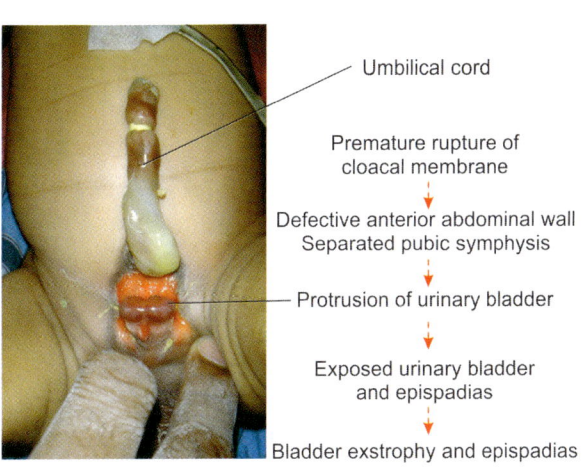

Clinical image 20.1: Bladder extrophy (ectopia vesicae) is a congenital anomaly that includes extrophy and epispadias with protrusion of the urinary bladder through a defect in the anterior abdominal wall. In this condition, posterior wall of the bladder is seen externally just below the umbilicus. Incidence is 1:10,000–50,000 live births with male preponderance (3:1) (Image courtesy: *Dr Kumaravel S*)

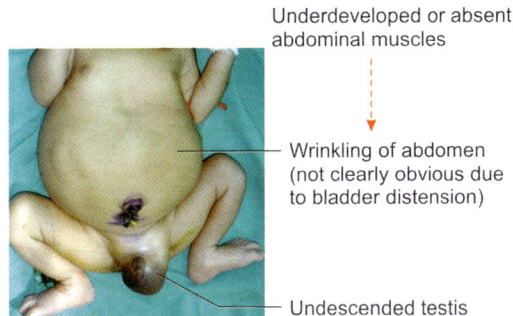

Clinical image 20.2: Prune-belly syndrome (Eagle-Barrett syndrome). It is a disorder of urinary tract that is characterized by the triad of anomalies: (1) Wrinkling of abdominal skin (due to underdeveloped or absent abdominal muscles, (2) cryptorchidism (undescended testis), (3) urinary tract malformations (megaloureter, hydronephrosis, vesicoureteral reflux of urine → renal failure). It has incidence of 1 in 40,000 births and affects male babies commonly (97%) (Image courtesy: *Dr Kumaravel S*)

Chapter 21

Reproductive System: Male and Female Reproductive Organs

eSmartQuiz
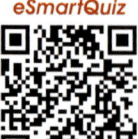

Chapter Outline

- Formation of primitive gonads
  - Genital ridge
  - Migration of primordial germ cells
  - Differentiation into definitive gonad
- Development of testis
  - Stages of development
  - Descent of testis
  - Anomalies of testis
- Cryptorchidism
- Development of ovary
  - Stages of development
  - Descent of ovary
  - Anomalies of ovary
- Genital ducts
  - Mesonephric ducts
  - Paramesonephric ducts
- Development of uterus
  - Anomalies of uterus
- Development of vagina
  - Congenital anomalies of vagina
- Development of prostate
- Development of external genitalia
  - Male external genitalia
  - Female external genitalia
- Hypospadias
- Epispadias

Competency:
- **AN52.8:** Describe the development of male and female reproductive system.

INTRODUCTION

- The genital system consists of gonads and genital (sex) ducts.
- *Gonads* include testes in male and ovaries in females.
- Gonads develop from the genital ridge with incorporation of primordial germ cells.
- Genital ducts in male include efferent ductules of testis, epididymis, vas deferens, seminal vesicle, and ejaculatory duct.
- Genital ducts in female include uterine tubes, uterus, and vagina.
- *Accessory sex glands* in male include prostate and bulbourethral glands, whereas in female include greater vestibular glands (Bartholin's glands).
- During early embryonic period, two paired ducts, namely mesonephric (Wolffian) and paramesonephric (Müllerian) are present. These ducts undergo further differentiation or regression depending on sex differentiation and finally form the genital duct system.

Primordial germ cells

- Primordial germ cells arise from epiblasts (primary ectoderm) in the second week.^NEXT
- These primordial germ cells remain within extra-embryonic mesoderm of connecting stalk and wall of the yolk sac (Fig. 21.1, Practice Fig. 21.1).^NEXT
- On formation of the tail fold, the primordial germ cells come to lie in splanchnopleuric mesoderm that surrounds hindgut.
- In **5th week**, coelomic epithelium covering mesonephric ridges proliferates to form genital ridges (Fig. 21.2). Formation of genital ridge is the first sign of gonad formation.^NEXT
- By 5th week, primordial germ cells migrate bilaterally through dorsal mesentery to the region of genital ridges (by amoeboid movements).

218

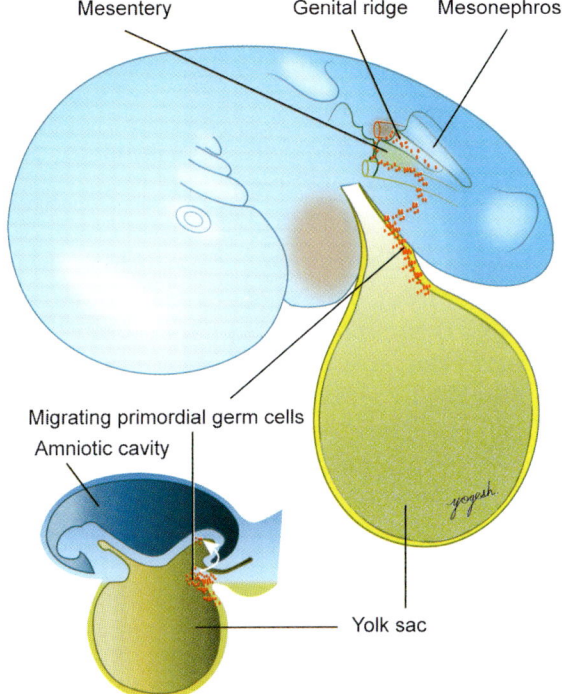

Fig. 21.1: Primordial germ cells (PGC). PGC reside in the yolk sac and migrate to wall of gut during fourth to sixth weeks. Later, these cells migrate through mesentery of gut to dorsal body wall and colonies to form gonadal ridge and subsequently gonads (testes or ovaries)

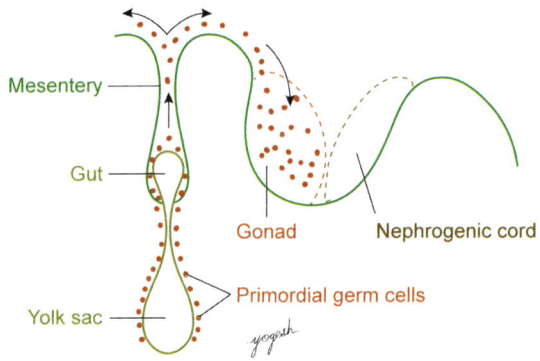

Practice Fig. 21.1: Migration of primordial germ cells

FORMATION OF PRIMITIVE GONADS

Genital Ridge (Gonadal Ridge)

- In the fifth week of intrauterine life, coelomic epithelium (lining epithelium of primitive peritoneal cavity) covering medial surface of mesonephros proliferates to form a *genital ridge*. Genitourinary system develops from genital ridge of intermediate mesoderm.^{NEXT}
- Genital ridge is an elevation of posterior abdominal wall, in between dorsal aorta and mesonephros (Fig. 21.2).
- Genital ridge consists of inner medulla and outer cortex.
- Testis or ovary arises from genital ridge (intermediate mesoderm) retroperitoneally, on the posterior abdominal wall in lumbar region (at T10 level).^{NEXT}

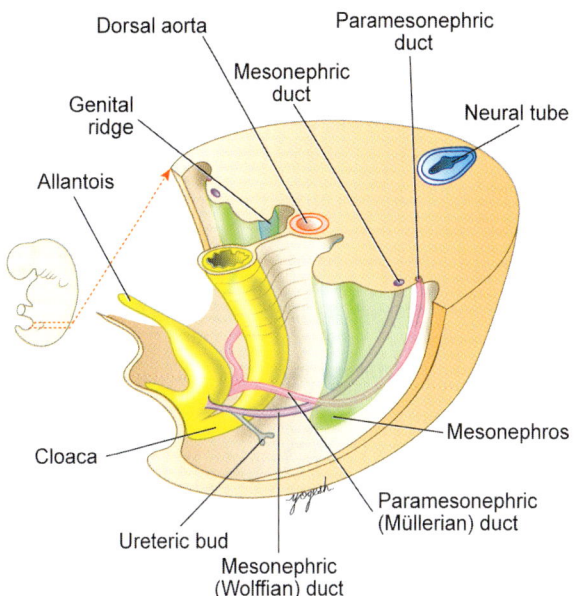

Fig. 21.2: Cross-section of embryo showing mesonephric and paramesonephric ducts

Migration of Primordial Germ Cells

- In the fourth week, primordial germ cells migrate to genital ridge along dorsal mesentery (Fig. 21.1).
- *Formation of primitive sex cords:* From surface (coelomic) epithelium, numerous cord-like processes develop and enter the genital ridge to form finger-like cords called *primitive sex cords* (Practice Fig. 21.2).

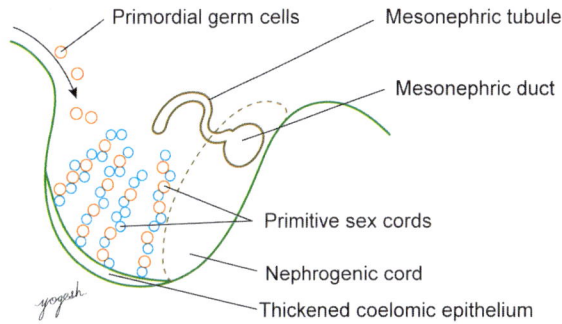

Practice Fig. 21.2: Indifferent gonad

Differentiation into Definitive Gonad

- *Up to 7th week* of IUL, gonad is ambisexual or indifferent.^{NEXT}
- Differentiation of genital ridge (undifferentiated gonad) into testis or ovary (definitive gonad) entirely depends on chromosomal constitution of the individual (Flowcharts 21.1, 21.2).
- Y-chromosome determines testis formation as *testis-determining factor* (TDF) is located on short arm of chromosome Y. TDF is controlled by *SRY gene* (sex-determining region of Y chromosome).^{MCQ}
- TDF induces differentiation of Sertoli cells.
- In the absence of TDF, cells of sex cords differentiate into follicular cells of ovary. Both X chromosomes

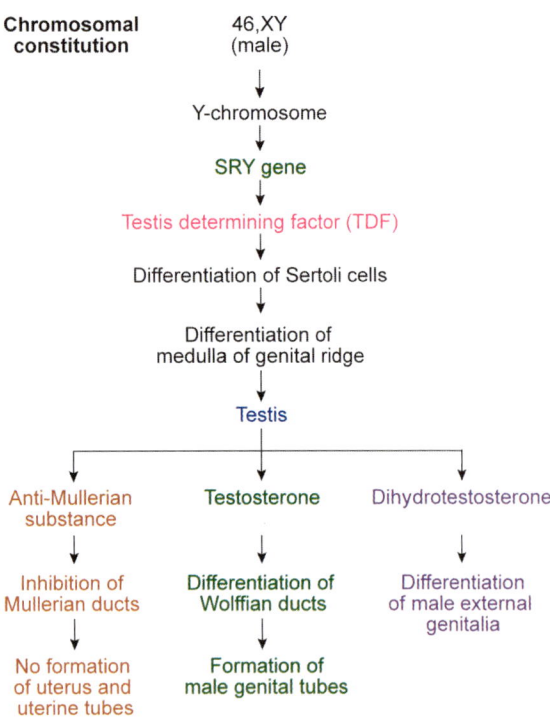

Flowchart 21.1: Sex differentiation in male

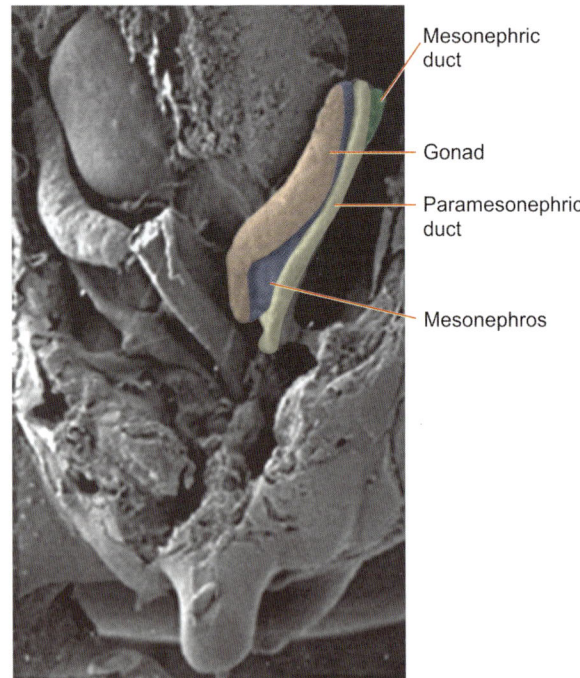

Scanning electron micrograph 21.1: Genital ducts and developing internal genitalia [Species: Human, gestational age: 7 weeks]

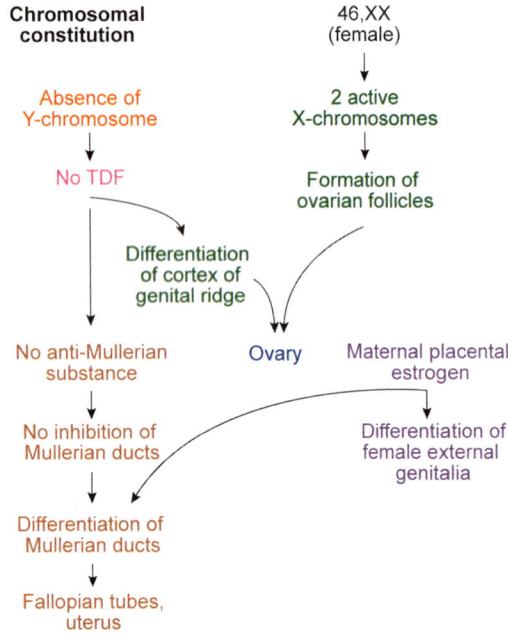

Flowchart 21.2: Sex differentiation in female

should be genetically active to form primary ovarian follicles. After formation of definitive female gonad, only one X chromosome remains active, whereas the other X chromosome becomes inactive to form the *Barr body*.^{NEXT} Barr body appears soon after the beginning of embryonic period, after 2nd–3rd week.^{NEXT}

- Genital ridge has an outer cortex and inner medulla.
- In female fetus, cortex differentiates to form ovary and medulla regresses.
- In male fetus, medulla differentiates to form testis and cortex regresses.

- TDF differentiate Sertoli cells that start producing *anti-Müllerian substance* (AMS) or hormone. Anti-Müllerian substance inhibits development of the Müllerian ducts.^{MCQ}
- Thus, absence of Y-chromosome (SRY gene) or TDF results in the formation of ovary.^{NEXT}
- TDF also helps in differentiation of Leydig cells from mesoderm of gonadal ridge.^{NEXT} Leydig cells start secreting testosterone and dihydrotestosterone 8 weeks onward.^{NEXT} Testosterone stimulates growth of mesonephric duct that forms male genital duct system. Dihydrotestosterone helps in formation of penis, penile urethra, prostate and scrotum.
- The absence of androgens (testosterone and dihydrotestosterone) allows differentiation of Müllerian ducts into uterine tubes and uterus under influence of maternal and placental estrogen. This estrogen also differentiates genital swellings into female external genitalia.
- Differentiation of gonad starts after 7th week (2 months).^{NEXT}

DEVELOPMENT OF TESTIS

Q. Write a short note on development of testis.

Summary (Examination Guide)^{High yielding facts}

- Testis is the male gonad. Various parts of the testis develop as follows (Flowchart 21.3, Table 21.1, Practice Figs 21.3, 21.4):

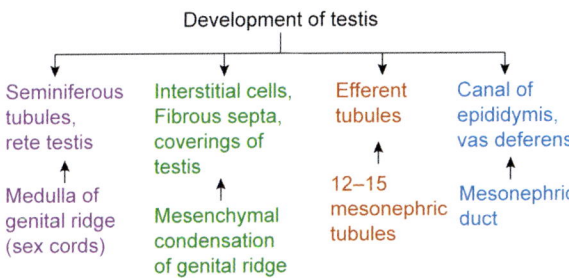

Flowchart 21.3: Development of testis

Remnant of paramesonephric duct → Appendix of testis
Remnant of mesonephros → Appendix of epididymis

Table 21.1 Development of testis

Part of testis	Embryological source
1. Seminiferous tubules, rete testis	Medulla of genital ridge (sex cords)
2. Interstitial cells of Leydig, fibrous septa and coverings of testis	Mesenchymal condensation of genital ridge
3. Efferent tubules	12–15 mesonephric tubules
4. Canal of epididymis and vas deferens	Mesonephric duct
5. Appendix of testis[NEXT]	Remnant of paramesonephric duct
6. Appendix of epididymis	Remnant of mesonephros

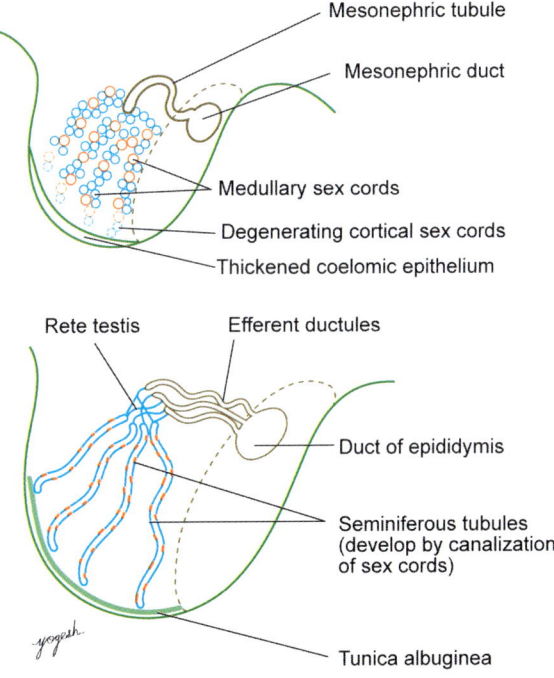

Practice Fig. 21.3: Development of testis

1. **Medulla of genital ridge:** It forms seminiferous tubules, rete testis, interstitial cells, fibrous septa, and intrinsic coverings of testis.
2. **Mesonephric tubules:** 12–15 mesonephric tubules form efferent ductules.
3. **Mesonephric duct:** It forms canal of epididymis and vas deferens.

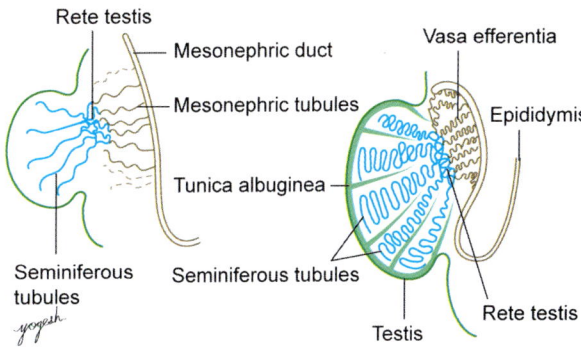

Practice Fig. 21.4: Development of testis

4. **Paramesonephric (Müllerian) duct:** It gets degenerated (remnants – appendix of testis).
5. **Mesonephros:** It degenerates (remnants – appendix of epididymis).

Stages of Development

- Testis-determining factor (TDF) produced by SRY gene located on short arm of chromosome Y influence development of testis.[MCQ]
- Testis develops from medulla of genital ridge of primary gonads.
- In the genital ridge, primitive sex cords extend to form *medullary cords* that converge towards hilus of the developing testis (Fig. 21.3A).
- Near hilus, medullary cords anastomose with each other to form a network (Fig. 21.3B).
- Later, medullary cords get canalized to form *seminiferous tubules*, whereas anastomotic network forms the *rete testis* (Fig. 21.3B to E).
- Communication between rete testis and seminiferous tubules develop by fourth month of IUL.
- Sex cord cells derived from coelomic epithelium form *Sertoli cells*, whereas primordial germ cells form *spermatogonia*.
- In seventh week, mesenchymal tissue separates sex cords from coelomic epithelium and forms a fibrous layer of *tunica albuginea*; *mediastinal septa* and *interstitial cells of Leydig* (Fig. 21.3D to E).
- The tubules of rete testis develop communication with adjacent 12–15 mesonephric tubules. These mesonephric tubules form *efferent ductules of testis*.
- Later, mesonephric duct form duct of *epididymis, vas deferens, seminal vesicles,* and *ejaculatory duct*.

Descent of Testis

Q. Write a short note on descent of testis and its applied aspects.

Q. List the factors responsible for descent of testis.

- Testis develops in dorsal abdominal wall at the level of upper lumbar vertebrae.
- During development, the testis descends slowly from lumbar region to the scrotum. After birth, testis lies outside the body (within the scrotal sac).

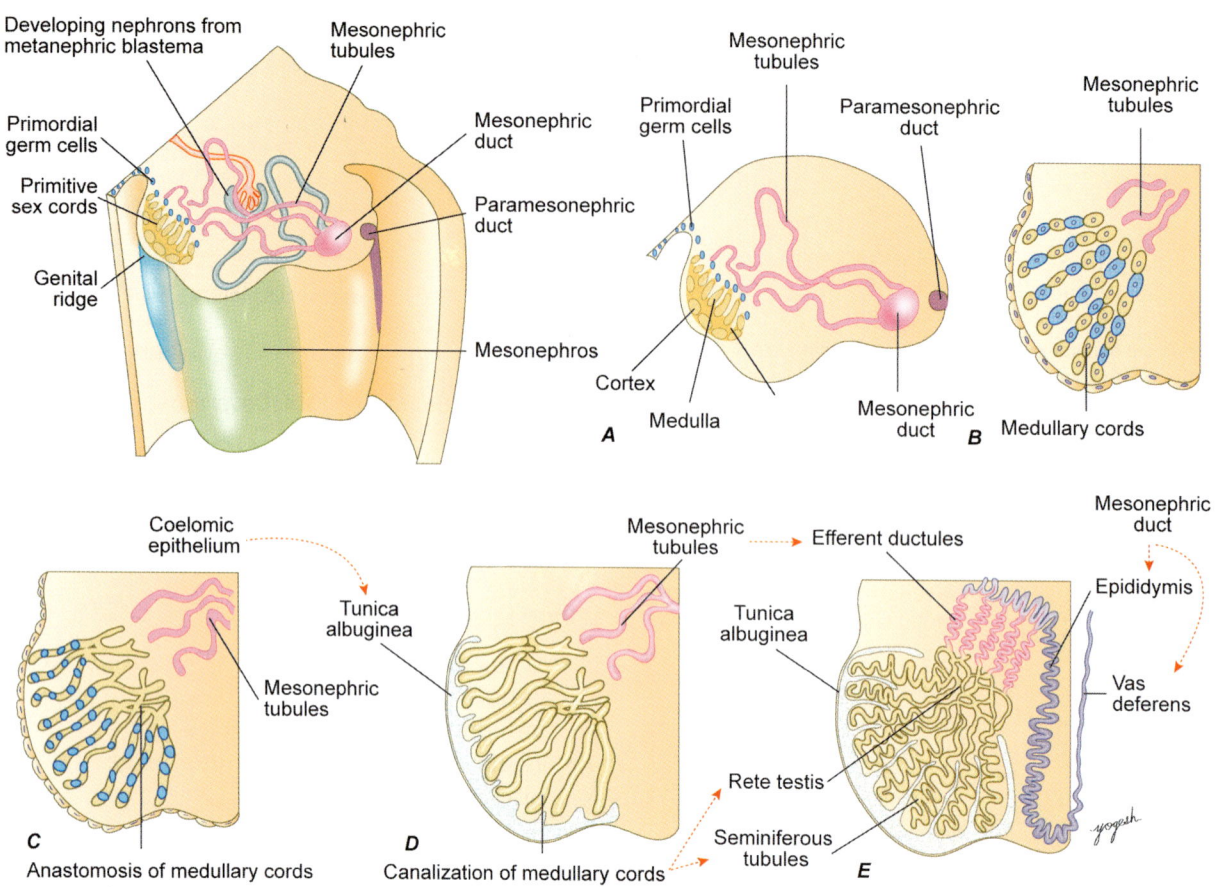

Fig. 21.3: Development of male gonad (testis). Medulla of genital ridge forms seminiferous tubules, rete testis, and interstitial cells. Mesonephric tubules form efferent ductules. Mesonephric duct forms canal of epididymis and vas deferens. Paramesonephric (Müllerian) duct gets degenerated except at appendix of testis. Mesonephros also degenerates, but its small remnant form appendix of epididymis

Summary (Examination Guide) *High yielding facts, NEXT*

Testis descends slowly with the following schedule (Fig. 21.4, Practice Fig. 21.5, Flowchart 21.4):
1. During 3rd month: Testis reaches to iliac fossa (Fig. 21.4A).
2. At the end of 6th month: It reaches to deep inguinal ring (Fig. 21.4B). *NEXT*
3. In 7th month: It travels through inguinal canal. *NEXT*
4. At the end of 8th month: It reaches to superficial inguinal ring (Fig. 21.4C).
5. By the end of 9th month: It reaches to scrotum (Fig. 21.4D). *NEXT*

Factors Responsible for Descent of Testis

The descent of the testis is influenced and assisted by the following factors (Table 21.2):
1. *Differential growth* of the posterior body wall.
2. *Formation of inguinal bursa*: Anterior abdominal wall forms an outpouching called *inguinal bursa*. Passage of inguinal bursa through anterior abdominal wall is given rise to the *inguinal canal*, whereas surface elevation forms the *scrotum*.
3. *Gubernaculum testis*: It is the mesenchymal band that connects *lower pole* of testis to bottom of scrotum (initially, to *anterior abdominal wall*). *NEXT* Body wall and embryo continue to grow rapidly but gubernaculum grows very slowly. Thus, testis progressively shifts to lower position. Gubernaculum also helps to dilate inguinal bursa and guides testis to scrotum.
4. *Processus vaginalis:* It is a diverticulum of the peritoneal cavity that extends into scrotum through inguinal canal. Processus vaginalis guides testis to the scrotum during descent and later it forms a covering of the testis called *tunica vaginalis*. Proximal part of processus vaginalis is obliterated by androgens (via calcitonin gene-related peptide, CGRP, released from genitofemoral nerve) and by hepatocyte growth factor. *NEXT* Distal portion of processus vaginalis forms tunica vaginalis. *NEXT*
5. Other factors:
   - Increased abdominal pressure due to growing abdominal viscera
   - Male sex hormones
   - High abdominal temperature than scrotal temperature (4°C higher)
   - Neurotransmitter (calcitonin gene-related peptide) secreted by the genitofemoral nerve causes contraction of the cremaster muscle.

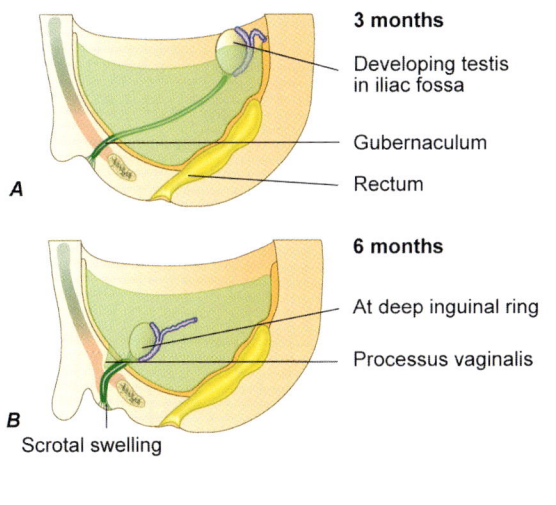

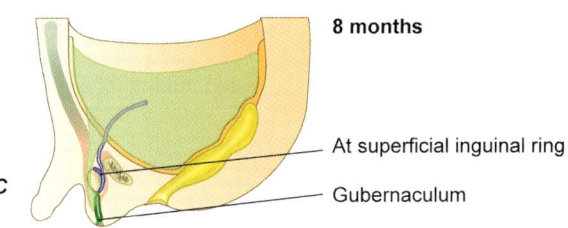

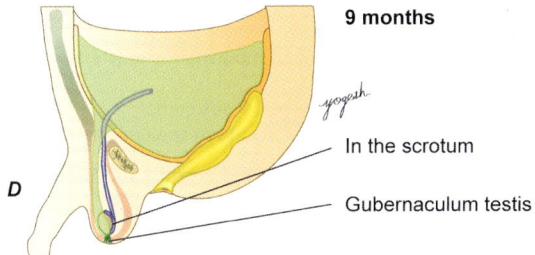

Fig. 21.4: Descent of testis

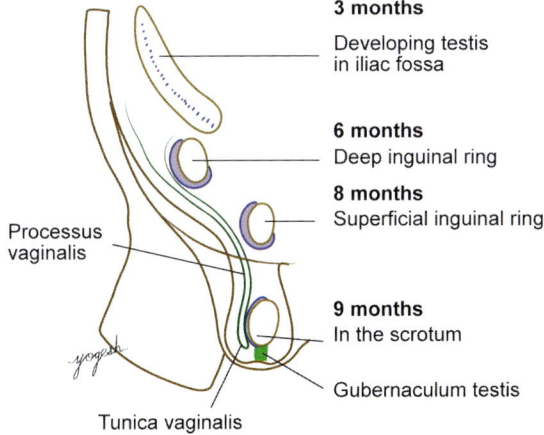

Practice Fig. 21.5: Descent of testis

Anomalies of Testis

1. Cryptorchidism (Box 21.1)
2. *Anorchism:* Both the testis are absent or present as rudimentary gonads in abdomen.
3. *Monorchism:* Only one testis is descended, whereas another one remains intra-abdominal.

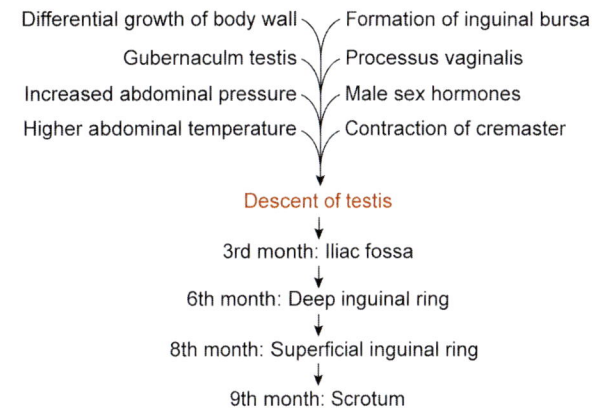

Flowchart 21.4: Descent of testis

Table 21.2	Factors assisting descent of testis

1. Differential body wall growth
2. Formation of inguinal bursa
3. Gubernaculum testis
4. Processus vaginalis
5. Other factors
   – Increased abdominal pressure
   – Male sex hormones
   – Higher abdominal temperature
   – Contraction of the cremaster muscle

Box 21.1: Cryptorchidism (undescended testis)

Q. Write a short note on cryptorchidism.

Definition
- Cryptorchidism is a failure of descent of testis that results in absence of one or both the testes from scrotum.

Incidence
- 3% of full-term and about 30% of premature infant boys show undescended testis. Out of these in about 80% cases, testis descent during the first year of life.

Locations of testis in cryptorchidism
- In case of cryptorchidism, testis may be located at one of the following positions:
  1. High up in scrotum
  2. At superficial inguinal ring
  3. Within inguinal canal
  4. At deep inguinal ring
  5. In iliac fossa or lumbar region.

Signs and symptoms
1. Infertility: Exposure of undescended testis to higher temperature than scrotal temperature results in failure of spermatogenesis.
2. Undescended testis may result in malignancy or atrophy.

Treatment
1. Watchful waiting: Most of the times, testis descent within the first year of life.
2. Orchidopexy: Testis can be surgically moved to the scrotum.

4. *Ectopic testis:* Testis deviated from its usual course of descent becomes ectopic testis (Fig. 21.5).

The ectopic positions of testis are as follows:
- In superficial perineal pouch (perineal)
- In front of pubic symphysis
- In femoral canal (femoral)
- In skin of the penis (penile)
- Under skin in front of thigh

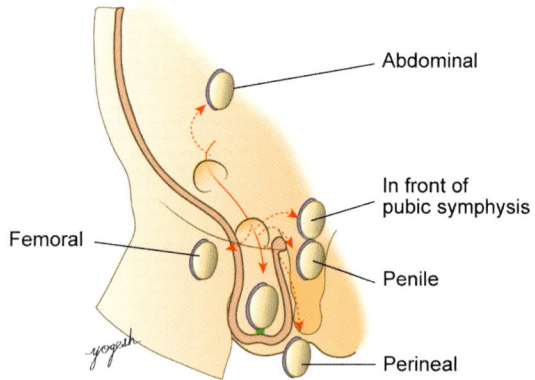

Fig. 21.5: Ectopic testis

5. *Congenital hydrocoele* and *congenital inguinal hernia* (Fig. 21.6):
- Processus vaginalis normally obliterates by one year.
- Persistent processus vaginalis forms a passage through which coils of intestine protrude and form *congenital inguinal hernia.*
- Accumulation of fluid in part of processus vaginalis results in *congenital hydrocoele.*

DEVELOPMENT OF OVARY

Q. Write a short note on development of ovary.

Summary (Examination Guide)
- Ovaries are female gonads.
- The components of ovary are derived as follows (Flowchart 21.5, Table 21.3, Practice Fig. 21.6):

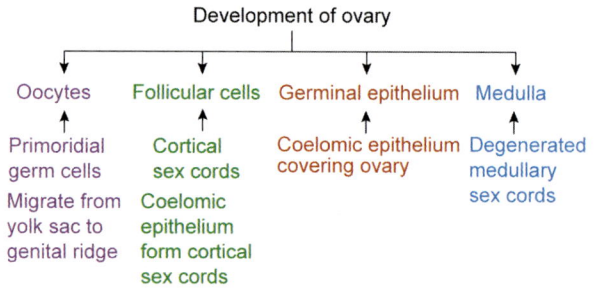

Flowchart 21.5: Development of ovary

Table 21.3	Development of ovary
Part of ovary	*Embryological source*
Oocytes	Primordial germ cells
Follicular cells	Cortical sex cords
Germinal epithelium	Coelomic epithelium
Medulla	Degenerated medullary sex cords

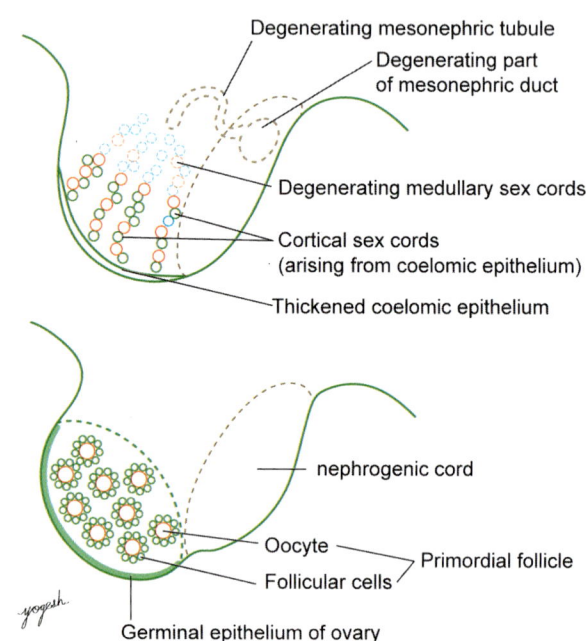

Practice Fig. 21.6: Development of ovary

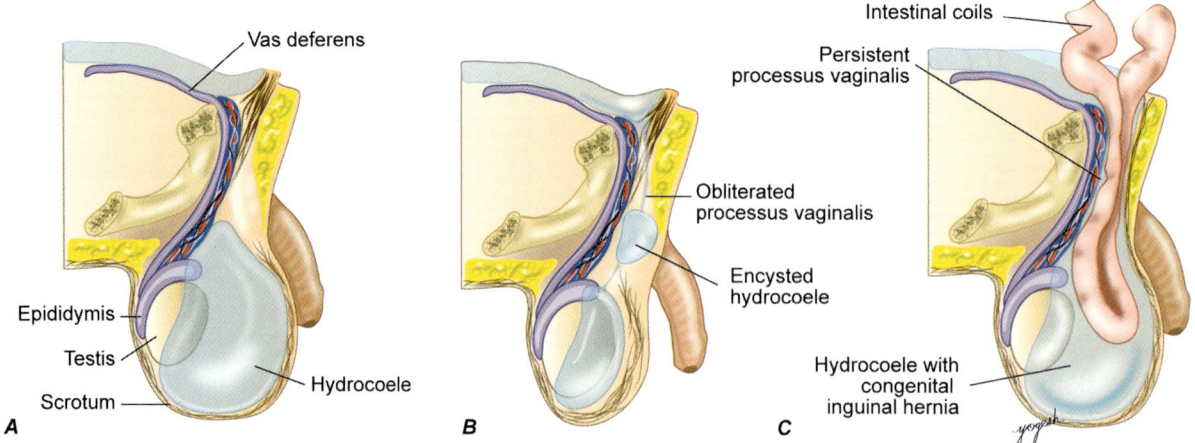

Fig. 21.6: Anomalies of processus vaginalis: (A) Hydrocoele; (B) Encysted hydrocoele; (C) Hydrocoele with congenital inguinal hernia

1. Oocytes develop from *primordial germ cells* that migrate from yolk sac.
2. Follicular cells are derived from *cortical sex cords* that are raised from the coelomic epithelium.
3. Germinal epithelium (cuboidal epithelium covering the ovaries) is derived from *coelomic epithelium* that covers genital ridge.
4. Medulla of ovary is derived from degenerated *medullary sex cords*.

Stages of Development

1. Primordial germ cells migrate from yolk sac in the genital ridge (Fig. 21.7).
2. Primitive medullary sex cords degenerate and form ovarian medulla.
3. In the seventh week, coelomic epithelium gives rise to second generation of sex cords called *cortical cords*. Cortical cords do not extend in the medulla.
4. In the third month, cortical cord forms clusters of cells that surround each primordial cell.
5. Thus, primordial germ cell forms *oogonia* and surrounding cortical cell cluster forms *follicular cells* to develop *primordial follicle*.
6. The coelomic epithelium forms a single-layered epithelial covering of the ovary called *germinal epithelium* (it is misnomer as it does not give rise to germ cells).
7. The ovary is suspended by a fold of peritoneum called *mesovarium*.

Descent of Ovary

- Ovaries develop in the posterior abdominal wall and descent to true pelvis.

Factors affecting descent of ovary

1. Gubernaculum ovarii: It is a fibromuscular band that extends from caudal end of ovary to genital swelling (future labium majus).
2. Developing uterus and broad ligament: They arrest the descent of ovary in true pelvis as the gubernaculum gets attached to the angle of uterus. Gubernaculum forms two derivatives:

Some Interesting Facts

1. Absence of Y chromosome (SRY gene, TDF proteins) and presence of two active X chromosomes are required for the formation of ovary.
2. Mesoderm does not form tunica albuginea (fibrous layer) during the development of ovary.
3. Processus vaginalis or canal of Nuck: It is a tubular prolongation of peritoneum that extends into inguinal canal is also present in females but get obliterated before birth.

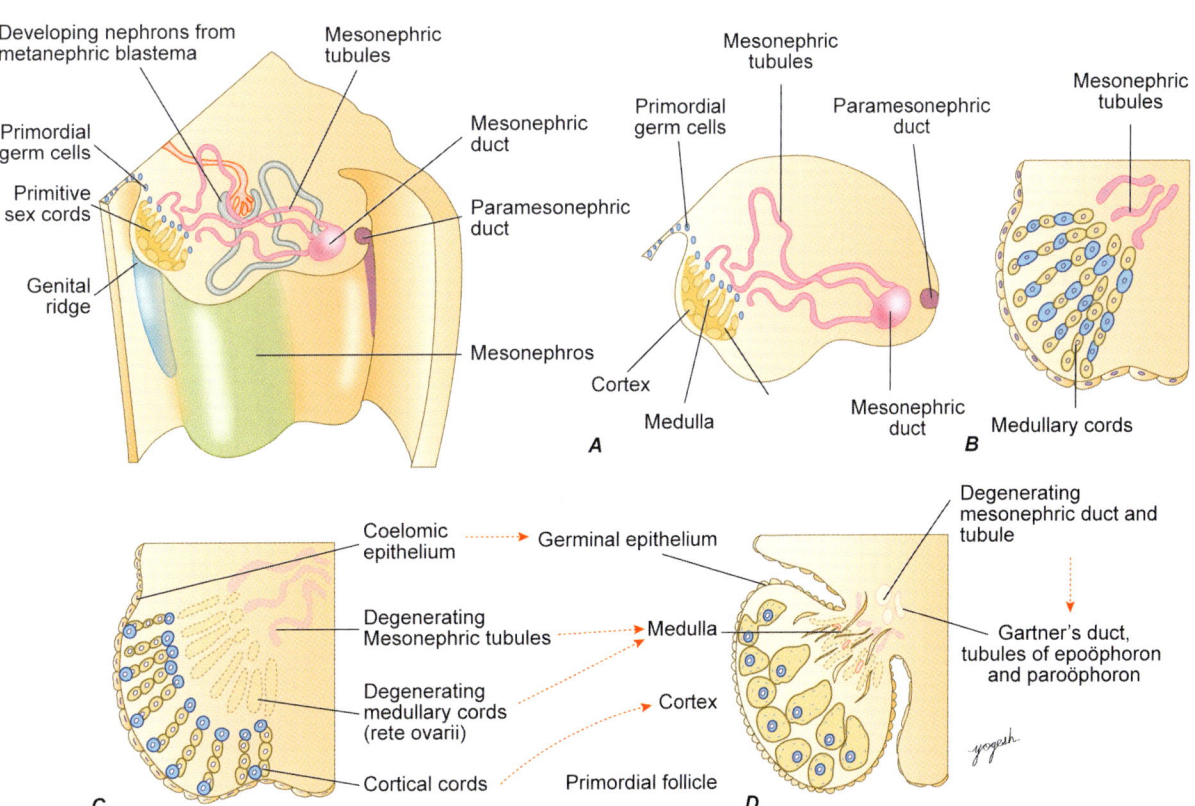

Fig. 21.7: Development of female gonad (ovary). Oocyte develops from primordial germ cells of cortical cords. Follicular cells are derived from cortical sex cords. Germinal epithelium is derived from coelomic epithelium that covers genital ridge. Medulla of ovary is derived from the degenerated medullary sex cords

a. Ligament of ovary: It extends between ovary and uterus.
b. Round ligament of uterus: It passes from uterus to labium majus through inguinal canal. NEXT

Anomalies of Ovary

1. Ovary may be
   a. absent on one or both sides
   b. duplicated
   c. present in inguinal canal or labium majus.
2. Ovarian teratoma: It is a teratoma that may consist of derivatives of all germ layers such as adrenal or thyroid tissue, bone, cartilage, hair, and so on.

GENITAL DUCTS

- In embryonic life, two pairs of ducts form primitive genital ducts. They are mesonephric (Wolffian) and paramesonephric (Müllerian) ducts (Practice Fig. 21.7).
- Mesonephric ducts form genital duct system in males, whereas paramesonephric ducts form genital duct system in females.

Mesonephric Tubules and Ducts in Male NEXT

Q. Name the derivatives of mesonephric duct in male and female.

- Persistent mesonephric tubules form efferent ductules of the testis (Fig. 21.8) [also refer Chapter 20].
- Remaining some mesonephric tubules form:
   a. superior aberrant ductules
   b. inferior aberrant ductules and
   c. tubules of paradidymis
- Mesonephric duct forms:
   a. canal of epididymis
   b. ductus deferens and
   c. ejaculatory duct
- Ductus deferens gives rise to seminal vesicles.

Mesonephric Tubules and Ducts in Female

- Mesonephric tubules form vestigial remnants such as tubules of epoöphoron and tubules of paroöphoron (Fig. 21.8). MCQ
- Mesonephric duct in female forms the duct of epoöphoron (Gartner's duct) that joins with tubules of epoöphoron. MCQ Thus, organ of Rosenmüller (epoöphoron) is derivative of mesonephric tubules and duct. NEXT

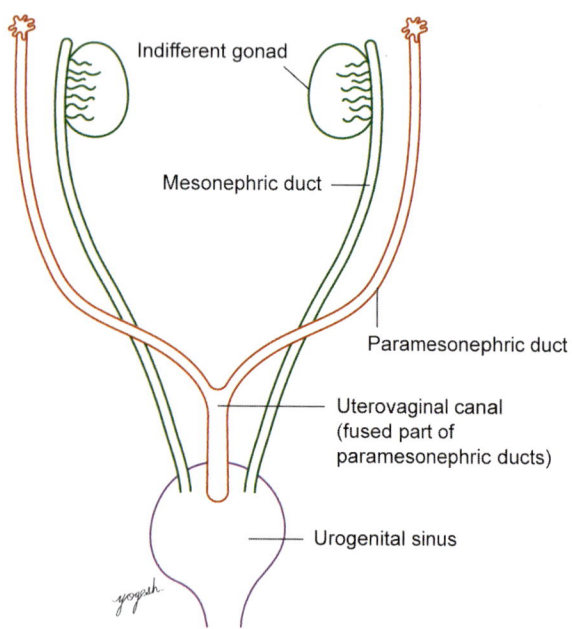

Practice Fig. 21.7: Genital ducts and formation of uterovaginal canal

Mesonephric Ducts High yielding facts, MCQ

- Mesonephric duct develops in mesonephros and runs up to urogenital sinus through urorectal septum.
- Mesonephric duct gives rise to *ureteric bud* that later forms the collecting part of urinary system.
- Part of the mesonephric duct gets absorbed in *trigone* of urinary bladder.

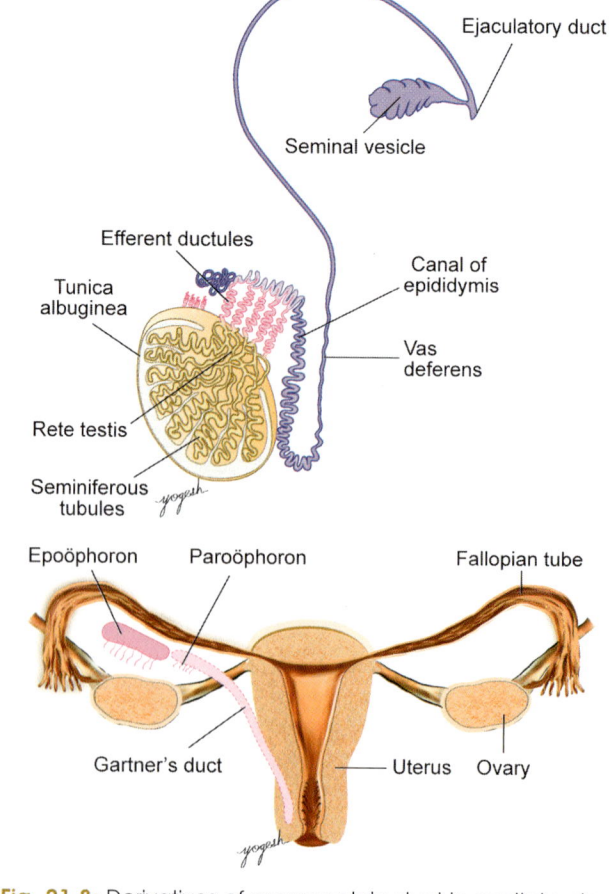

Fig. 21.8: Derivatives of mesonephric duct in genital system

- All these structures (tubules of epoöphoron, paroöphoron, and Gartner's duct) are present in the broad ligament of uterus (fold of peritoneum attached to uterus).

Paramesonephric Ducts
(Müllerian Ducts) *High yielding facts, MCQ*

Q. Name the derivatives of paramesonephric duct in male and female.

- In 6th week, paramesonephric ducts develop from coelomic epithelial invagination into mesonephric ridge.
- Cranial ends of paramesonephric ducts open into peritoneal (coelomic) cavity.
- In the 8th week, caudal ends grow caudally and cross mesonephric ducts ventrally to enter urorectal septum.
- By the 3rd month, caudal ends of both (right and left) paramesonephric ducts meet and fuse to form *uterovaginal canal*.
- Fused uterovaginal canal bulges into dorsal wall of urogenital sinus to form bulging called *Müllerian tubercle*.

Paramesonephric Ducts in Female

- Cephalic unfused part of each of paramesonephric duct forms the *uterine tube* (fallopian tube) (Fig. 21.9).
- Cranial opening of paramesonephric ducts in coelomic cavity forms the *pelvic ostium* of fallopian tubes.
- Degeneration of mesonephros develop *fimbriae* around pelvic ostium of fallopian tube.
- Fused caudal part of paramesonephric ducts forms *uterovaginal canal*.
- Cranial part of uterovaginal canal forms *uterus*.
- Blind caudal end of uterovaginal canal projects into dorsal wall of urogenital sinus as an elevation called *Müllerian tubercle*.

- Part of the uterovaginal canal adjacent to the Müllerian tubercle proliferates and forms solid bar of tissue (*vaginal cord*).
- Endodermal urogenital sinus develops two cellular cord-like outgrows as *sinovaginal bulbs*.
- Sinovaginal bulbs later fuse and form a plate-like structure called *vaginal plate*; that pushes vaginal cord (part of uterovaginal canal away from urogenital sinus).
- By the 5th month, vaginal cord and vaginal plate get canalized to form *vaginal canal*.
- Expansion of sinovaginal bulbs around the cervix of uterus forms *fornix of vagina*.
- Central part of Müllerian eminence degenerates to form *orifice of hymen* and remnant of peripheral part of Müllerian eminence forms *hymenal membrane*.
- Thus, paramesonephric duct in female forms fallopian tube, upper part of vagina, and vaginal fornices.^{NEXT}

Paramesonephric Ducts in Male

- Due to the presence of anti-Müllerian hormone, paramesonephric ducts (Müllerian ducts) in male degenerate.
- Remnant of paramesonephric ducts in male forms appendix of testis and prostatic utricle. *MCQ*

DEVELOPMENT OF UTERUS

Write a short note on development of uterus.

Uterus develops from the following sources (Fig. 21.9, Practice Fig. 21.8, Flowchart 21.6):

1. Epithelium from uterovaginal canal (fused part of paramesonephric ducts).
2. Myometrium from mesoderm surrounding paramesonephric ducts.
3. Fallopian tubes from unfused part of paramesonephric ducts.

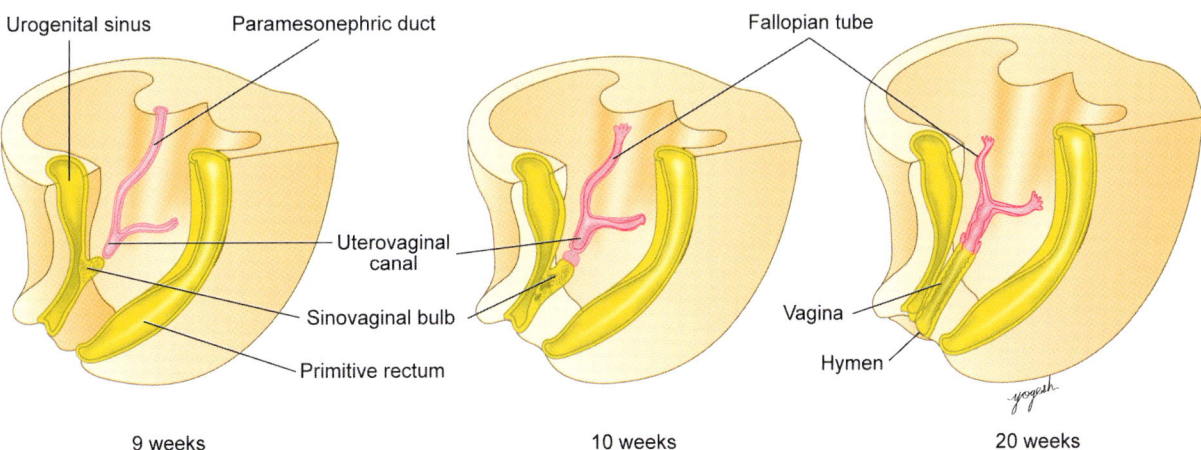

Fig. 21.9: Development of uterus and vagina. Paramesonephric ducts (Müllerian ducts) grow caudally, fuse and form uterovaginal canal. The uterovaginal canal forms solid vaginal cord. Endodermal urogenital sinus develops two sinovaginal bulbs that later fuse and form vaginal plate. By the 5th month, vaginal cord and vaginal plate get canalized to form vaginal canal. Central part of Müllerian eminence degenerates to form orifice of hymen and remnant of peripheral part of Müllerian eminence forms hymenal membrane

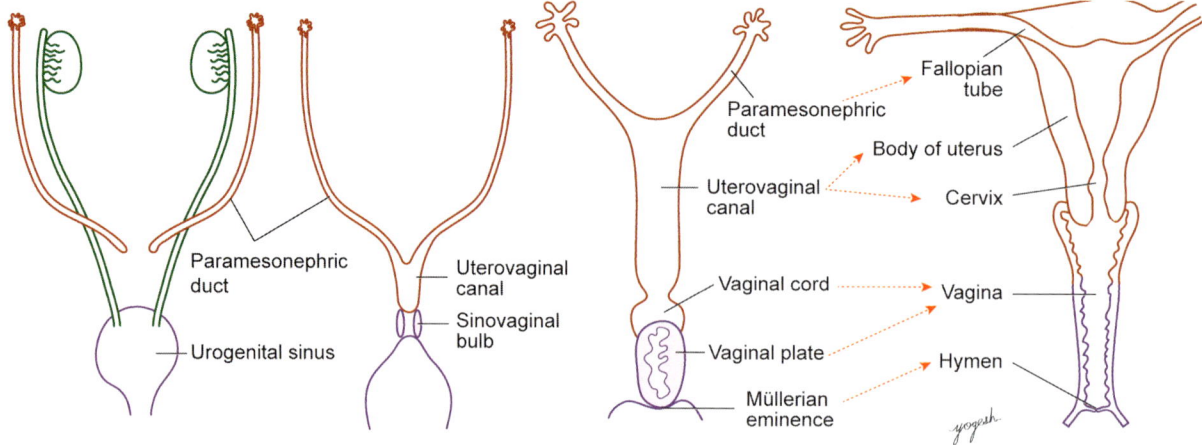

Practice Fig. 21.8: Development of uterus and vagina

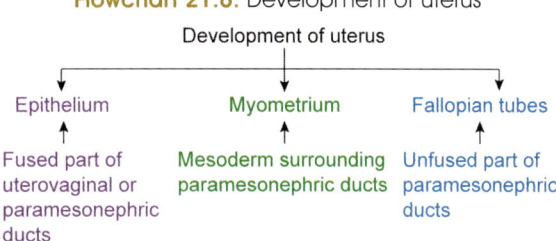

Flowchart 21.6: Development of uterus

At birth: Cervix length is double than uterine body
After puberty: Body of uterus elongates
Anomalies of uterus: Bicornuate uterus, septate uterus, absence of uterus, double uterus with double vagina

4. At birth, cervix is twice in length than body of uterus. After puberty, the body of uterus elongates and becomes longer than the cervix.

Anomalies of Uterus

1. *Bicornuate uterus:* In this condition, body of uterus is duplicated and it forms horn or cornua of uterus. Each horn communicates with one fallopian tube. It occurs due to partial nonfusion of caudal part of paramesonephric ducts (Fig. 21.10A).
2. *Unicornuate uterus:* Due to failure of development of one paramesonephric duct, half of uterus and one fallopian tube are absent (Fig. 21.10B).
3. *Septate uterus:* In this condition, two paramesonephric ducts fuse but portion between them does not disintegrate (Fig. 21.10C).
4. *Absence of uterus:* Complete failure of uterus development is a rare condition.
5. *Double uterus:* In this condition, no fusion of paramesonephric ducts results in formation of two separate half of uteruses (*uterus didelphys*) (Fig. 21.10D).
6. *Double uterus with double vagina:* In this condition, failure of fusion of right and left sinovaginal bulbs and right and left paramesonephric ducts result in double uterus with double vagina.

DEVELOPMENT OF VAGINA

Summary (Examination Guide)

Various parts of vagina develops as follows:
- Above hymen (upper 3/4ths):
  – Mucous membrane derives from sinovaginal bulbs (*endoderm*).*NEXT*
  – Muscles and connective tissue derive from *mesoderm* surrounding paramesonephric ducts.*NEXTJ*
- Below hymen (lower 1/4th): Derives from urogenital sinus (endoderm).
- External vaginal orifice derives from genital folds after rupture of urogenital membrane.
- Hymenal membrane derives from Müllerian eminence.

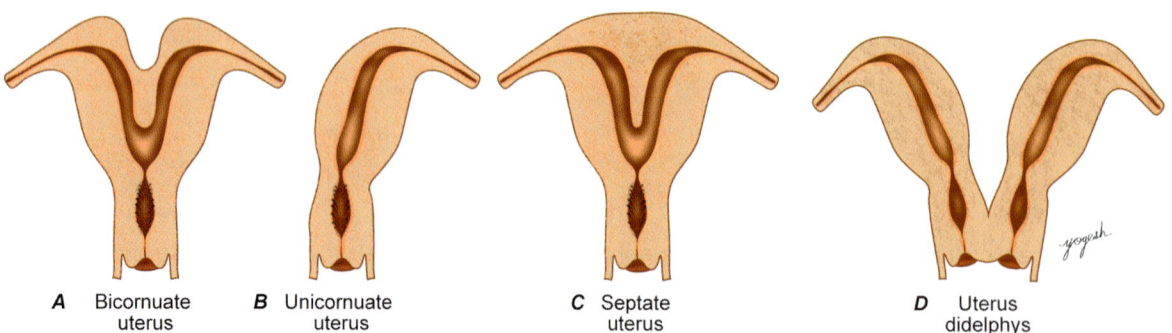

A Bicornuate uterus B Unicornuate uterus C Septate uterus D Uterus didelphys

Fig. 21.10: Congenital anomalies of uterus

Congenital Anomalies of Vagina

1. *Imperforate hymen:* It occurs due to failure of canalization of the central part of Müllerian eminence.
2. *Atresia of the vagina:* It occurs due to failure of canalization of vaginal plate.
3. *Agenesis of vagina:* It is absence of vagina due to failure of formation of vaginal plate by sinovaginal bulb.
4. *Septate vagina:* It occurs due to patchy disintegration of central part of sinovaginal bulb.
5. *Rectovaginal or vesicovaginal fistula:* It occurs if Müllerian eminence projects into vesicourethral part of cloaca or primitive rectum.

DEVELOPMENT OF PROSTATE

Summary (Examination Guide)

Prostate develops from the following sources (Fig. 21.11):

A. *Outer glandular zone:* It develops from buds arising from prostatic urethra (endodermal in origin).

B. Inner glandular zone: It develops from buds arising from mesodermal posterior wall of urethra above the openings of ejaculatory ducts.
 - There are total five buds arising from the prostatic urethra, namely one anterior, two posterior and two lateral.

C. Muscle, connective tissue, and capsule: They develop from surrounding mesoderm of urethra.

DEVELOPMENT OF EXTERNAL GENITALIA

- In initial stages, the development of male and female external genitalia is same.
- In 4th week, somatopleuric lateral plate mesoderm thickens on the side of cloacal membrane. This thickening produces surface elevation called *cloacal folds* (Fig. 21.12).^{NEXT}
- Urorectal septum divides the cloacal membrane into ventral *urogenital membrane* and dorsal *anal membrane*.

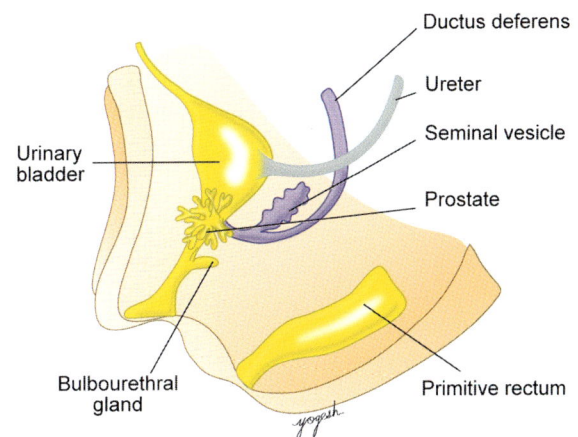

Fig. 21.11: Development of seminal vesicle, prostate and bulbourethral gland

- Along with the division of cloacal membrane, cloacal fold is also divided into cranial larger *urethral folds* and caudal *anal folds* (Fig. 21.12).
- Lateral to urethral folds, another swelling called *genital swellings* appears (Fig. 21.12).
- Genital swelling forms scrotum in males and labia majora in females, whereas *genital tubercle* forms clitoris/glans penis.^{NEXT}

Development of Male External Genitalia

Stages of Development

- Development of male external genitalia can be divided into three stages as follows (Practice Fig. 21.9):
  1. Development of penile urethra
  2. Development of prepuce of the penis and
  3. Development of scrotum

1. Development of penile urethra
   - Genital tubercle elongates to form *phallus* or *primitive penis* (Fig. 21.13).
   - Primitive urethral groove (ectoderm) appears on surface of urogenital membrane and it extends to tip of primitive penis.
   - Simultaneously, urethral folds and *primitive urethral groove* also elongate on the undersurface of primitive penis.

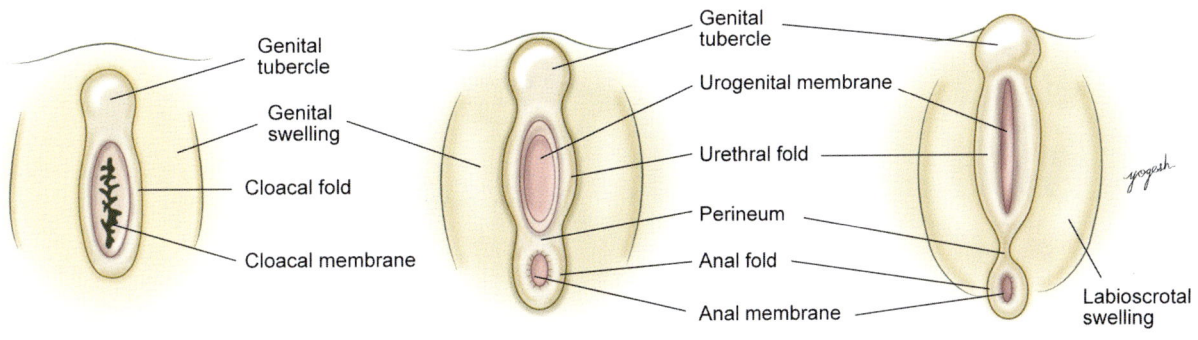

Fig. 21.12: Development of external genitalia: Indefinitive stage

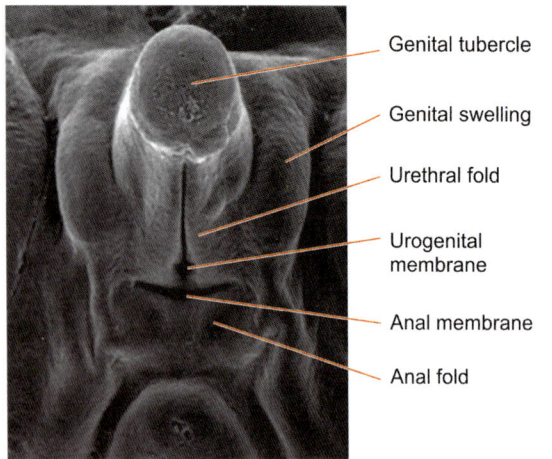

Scanning electron micrograph 21.2: Undifferentiated external genitalia. In 8th week of human development, male and female external genitalia appear the same. [Species: Human, gestational age: 52 days]

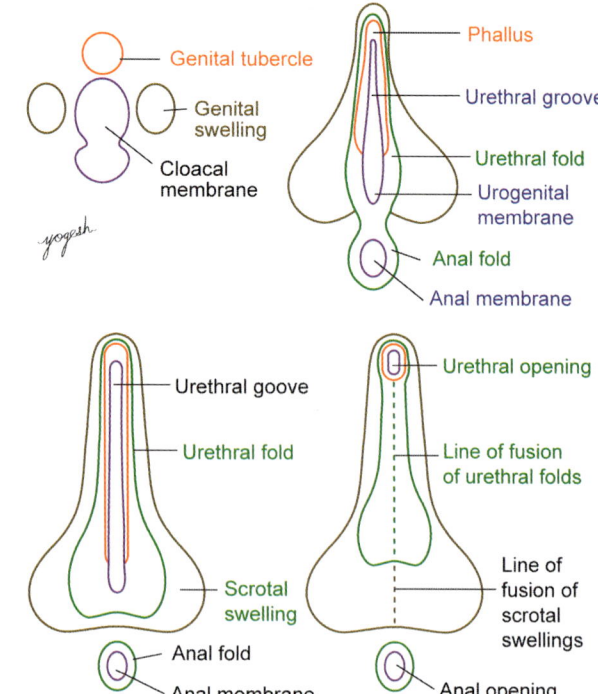

Practice Fig. 21.9: Development of male external genitalia

- Endoderm of phallic part of *urogenital sinus* proliferates into phallus (primitive penis) and forms solid plate called *urethral plate*.^{NEXT}
- Soon solid urethral plate gets canalized and forms a tube (endodermal) that is closely attached to a urethral groove (ectoderm).
- Urethral groove (urogenital membrane) ruptures and a deep groove called *definitive urethral groove* under the surface of phallus.
- Through definitive urethral groove, urogenital sinus communicate with the exterior. Margins of this groove are called *definitive urethral folds*.
- Definitive urethral folds fuse with each other in caudocranial direction (from base to the tip of primitive penis) to form *penile urethra*.
- Midline ectodermal fusion forms *penile raphe*.
- The terminal part of urethra develops from the solid ectodermal mass that later gets canalized (Fig. 21.14).

2. Development of prepuce of the penis (Fig. 21.14)
   - Near the tip of the primitive penis (phallus), a circular sulcus appears that separate glans penis from the rest of the penis.
   - Surface ectoderm proliferates and forms a fold called *prepuce* or foreskin.
3. Development of scrotum (Fig. 21.15)
   - On fusion of urethral folds, both the genital swellings enlarge to form scrotal swellings.
   - Scrotal swellings enlarge and fuse in the midline to form scrotum.

Development of Female External Genitalia
(Fig. 21.16, Practice Fig. 21.10)

Female external genitalia develops as follows:
1. Clitoris develops from genital tubercle (phallus).
2. Labia minora develops from primitive urethral folds.

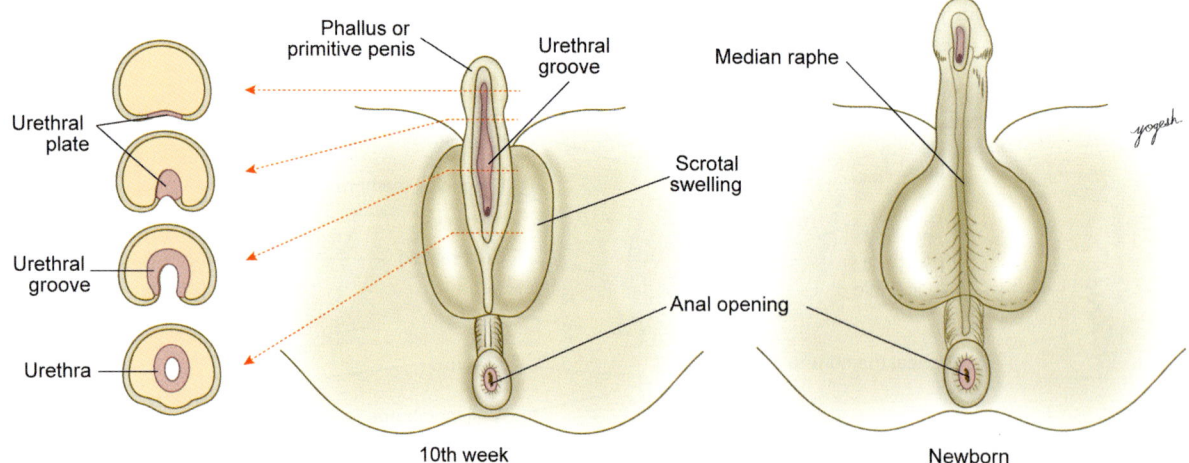

Fig. 21.13: Development of male external genitalia

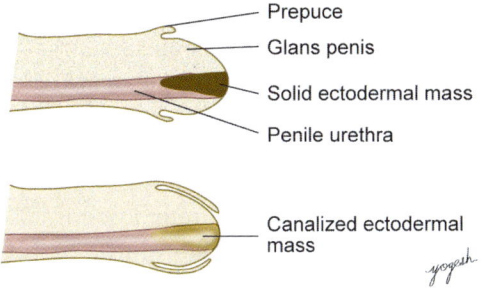

Fig. 21.14: Development of glandular portion of penile urethra

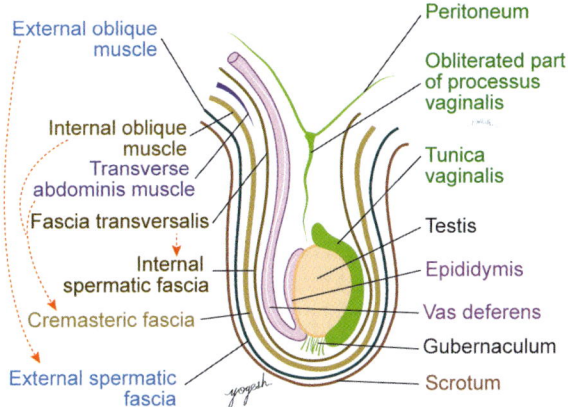

Fig. 21.15: Development of layers of scrotum from layers of anterior abdominal wall

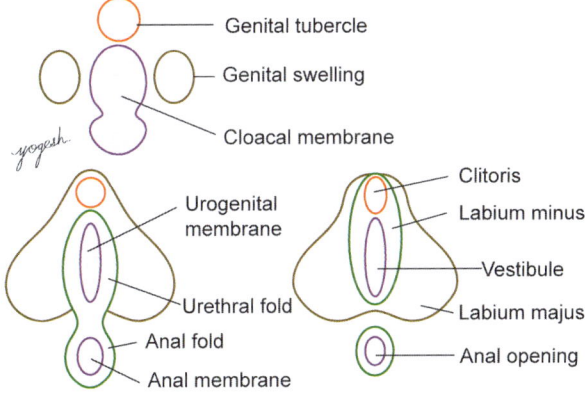

Practice Fig. 21.10: Development of female external genitalia

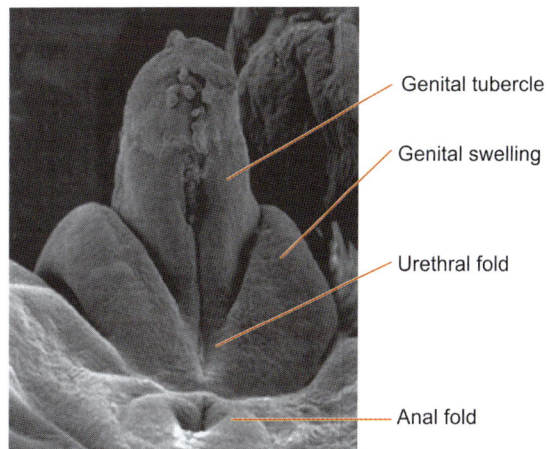

Scanning electron micrograph 21.3: Female external genitalia. In the female, urethral folds remain unfused and form labia minora, while genital swellings become labia majora. [Species: Human, gestational age: 72 days]

3. Labia majora develops from genital swellings. Labia majora fuse posteriorly to form posterior labial commissure and anteriorly to form mons pubis and anterior labial commissure.
4. Vestibule of vagina develops by rupture of urogenital membrane.

Box 21.2: Hypospadias

Q. Write a short note on hypospadias.

Definition
- It is a congenital anomaly of urethra; in that external urethral orifice is located on ventral aspect of penis, instead of at tip of penis.

Incidence: One in every 300 male births.

Embryological basis
- Hypospadias results due to
  1. Failure of canalization of ectodermal cord that forms the terminal part of urethra in glans penis.
  2. Failure of fusion of urethral folds that completes formation of penile urethra.

Contd.

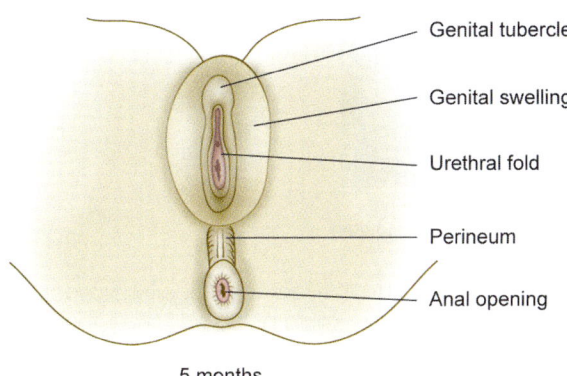
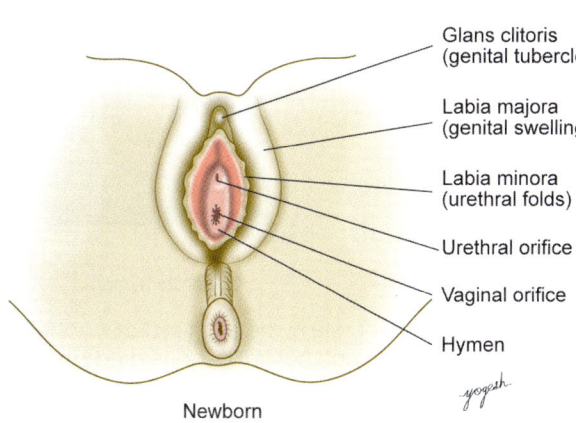

Fig. 21.16: Development of female external genitalia

231

Contd.

Classification (Fig. 21.17)
- Hypospadias is classified according to location of external urethral opening into the following types:
  1. Glandular hypospadias: Urethra opens on ventral surface of glans penis.
  2. Balanic hypospadias: Urethra opens at the base of glans penis.
  3. Penile hypospadias: Urethra opens on ventral surface of penis in between glans and scrotum.
  4. Penoscrotal hypospadias: Urethra opens at the junction of penis and scrotum.
  5. Perineal hypospadias: Urethra opens at unfused part of scrotum due to failure of fusion of labioscrotal folds.

Treatment
- Surgical correction is the treatment of choice.
- Hypospadias usually produces a condition called chordee. In this condition, head of penis curves downward that shows resistance during erection.

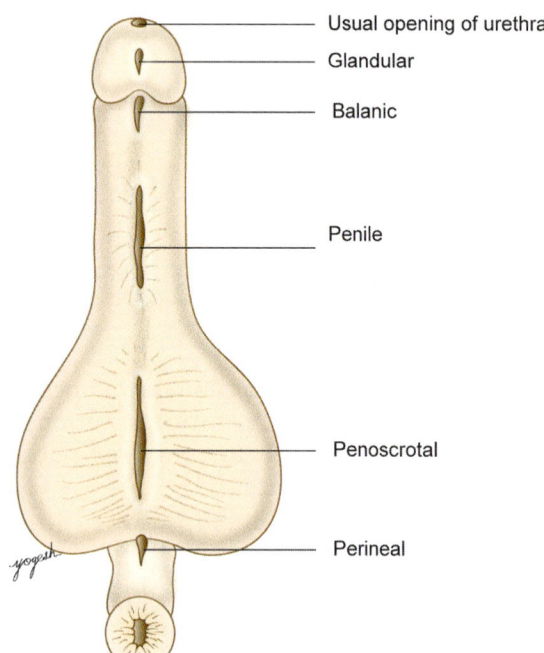

Fig. 21.17: Hypospadias. External urethral orifice is located on ventral aspect of the penis or scrotum, instead of at tip of the penis. It may be glandular (on ventral surface of glans), balanic (at base of glans), penile (on ventral surface of penis), penoscrotal (at junction of penis and scrotum), perineal (at unfused part of scrotum)

Box 21.3: Epispadias

Definition
It is congenital anomaly of penis in that external urethral orifice is located on dorsal (upper) surface of penis.

Incidence: 1 in 30,000 births.

Embryological basis
- Embryological basis is not clear.
- Probably due to the formation of genital tubercle caudally.

Association
- Mostly epispadias is associated with bladder exstrophy (ectopia vesicae).

Treatment
- Comprehensive surgical correction is the treatment of choice.

Clinical Embryology

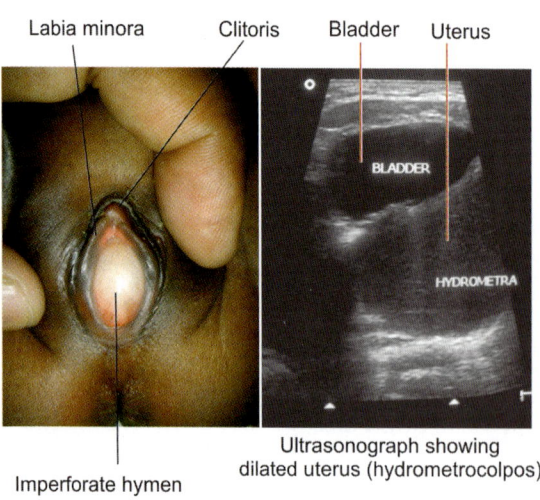

Clinical image 21.1: Imperforate hymen with hydrometrocolpos. During embryonic life, the remnant of peripheral part Müllerian eminence forms the hymen and central degenerated part forms orifice of the hymen. Failure of the degeneration of Müllerian eminence or failure of the sinovaginal bulb canalization causes imperforate hymen. Its incidence is 1:1000–1:10,000 females. In the infant babies, there may be hydrocolpos due to the accumulation of secretions in uterus and vagina or during puberty, there may be hematocolpos (Image courtesy: *Dr Kumaravel S*)

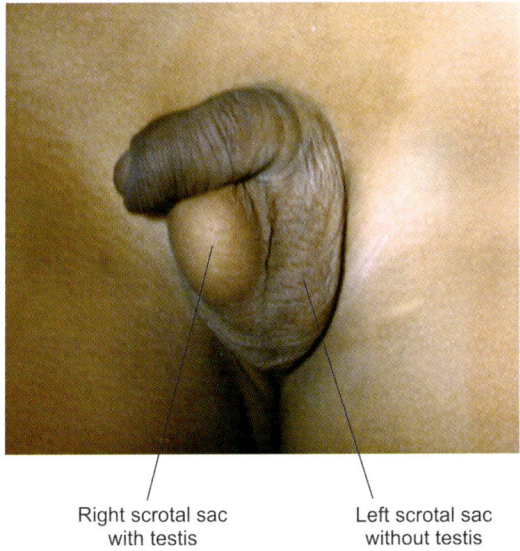

Right scrotal sac with testis | Left scrotal sac without testis

Clinical image 21.2: Undescended testis (left). Cryptorchidism is the failure of descent of testis. Undescended testis may descend on its own during the first year of life. If it does not have descend, then it can be surgically placed in the scrotum (orchidopexy). Undescended testis cannot produce sperms (male infertility), but produces testosterone (normal secondary sexual characters) (Image courtesy: *Dr Kumaravel S*)

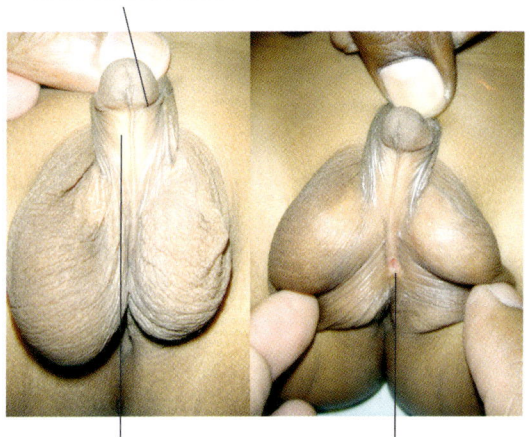

Under developed prepuce

Ventral deviation of penis | Perineal urethral meatus

Failure of fusion of labioscrotal (urogenital) folds

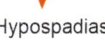

Hypospadias

Clinical image 21.4: Perineal hypospadias: It is a congenital anomaly of the urethra in that external urethral orifice is located on the ventral aspect of penis instead of at the tip of penis. In perineal hypospadias, urethra opens at the unfused part of scrotum due to failure of fusion of labioscrotal swelling. (Image courtesy: *Dr Kumaravel S*)

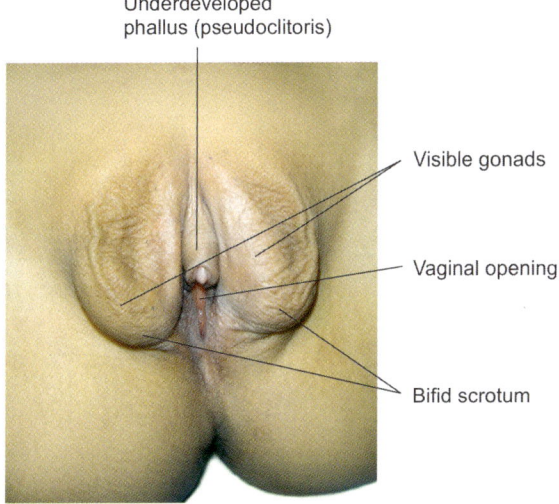

Underdeveloped phallus (pseudoclitoris)

Visible gonads

Vaginal opening

Bifid scrotum

Clinical image 21.3: Male pseudohermaphrodite. Pseudohermaphrodite is the condition in which the individual has gonad of one sex and external genitalia of the other sex. Male pseudohermaphrodite shows testes with external genitalia that resembles female. These patients may have **androgen insensitivity** or they may not have Leydig cells in testis (no secretion of testosterone). Hence, they do not have secondary sexual characters → feminine appearance. The above case shows underdeveloped phallus (pseudoclitoris), vaginal opening, bifid scrotum with testis. Unfused scrotal swellings give appearance of labia majora (Image courtesy: *Dr Kumaravel S*)

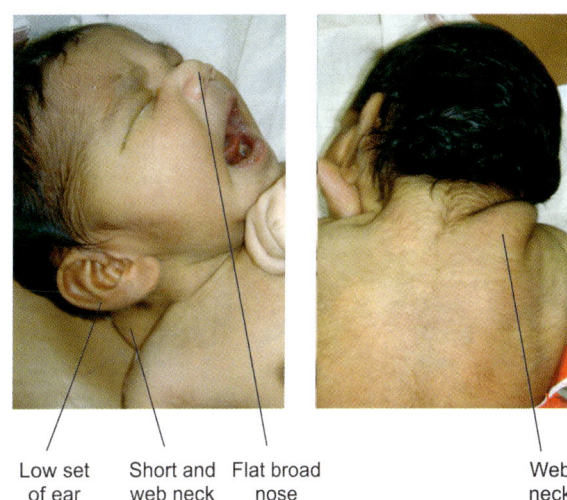

Low set of ear | Short and web neck | Flat broad nose | Web neck

Clinical image 21.5: Webbed neck in Turner syndrome or 45,X0 syndrome. Turner syndrome (karyotype: 45,X) occurs due to the absence of one X chromosome in female. The absence of second X chromosome results in ovarian dysgenesis. Incidence is 1 in 2500–3000 newborn girls. Female mainly has ovarian dysgenesis, infertility, webbing of neck, short stature, low set of ears and cubitus valgus (For details, refer *Principles of Clinical Genetics*, by Dr Yogesh Sontakke). *Note:* Webbed neck is associated with Turner syndrome, Noonan Syndrome (mutations pathways) in RAS/mitogen activated protein kinase), Klippel-Feil syndrome (fused spinal vertebrae). (Image courtesy: *Dr Kumaravel S*)

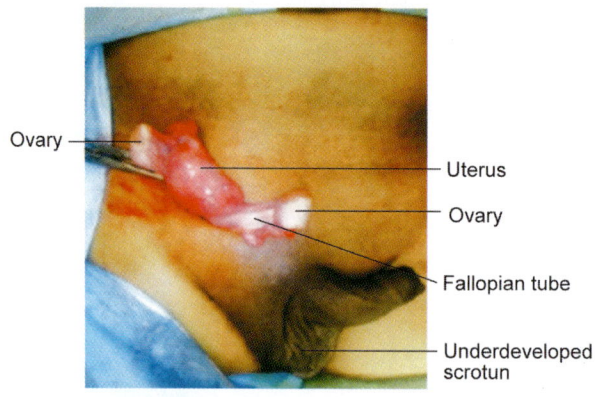

Clinical image 21.6: Persistent Mullerian Duct Syndrome (PMDS) or Hernia-utero inguinalis. Intraoperative image during right inguinal hernia surgery. Hernial sac containing uterus with bilateral ovaries and fallopian tubes. Scrotum is undeveloped with absent testes. Karyotype: 46X,inv(Y)(P11q11) [Image courtesy: *Dr. Uday Kumbhar*].

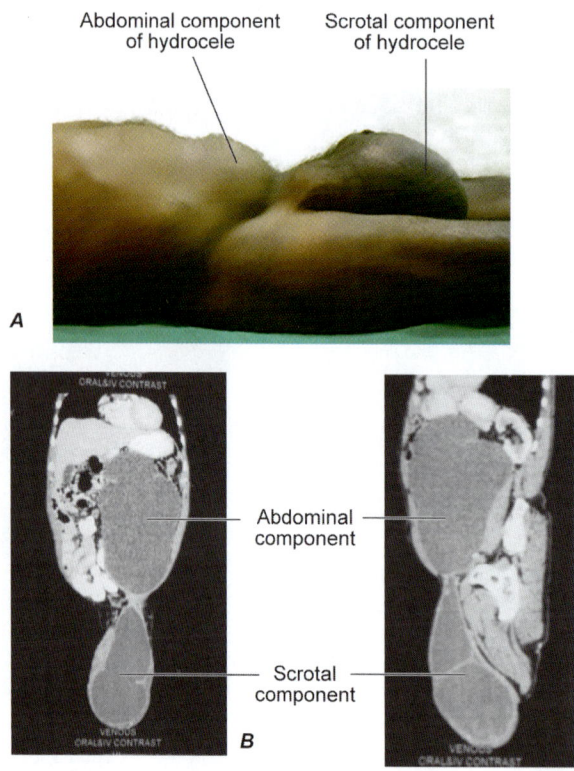

Clinical image 21.7: Hydrocele en bisac: adult presentation. A. Scrotal and abdominal components of the hydrocele. B. High-dose contrast-enhanced computed tomography (CECT) abdomen with retroperitoneal cyst and primary vaginal hydrocele [Image courtesy: *Dr. Uday Kumbhar*]

Chapter 22

Nervous System

eSmartQuiz

Chapter Outline

- Neurulation
- Differentiation of neural tube
  - Flexures of neural tube
  - Cavity of neural tube
- Neural crest cells
- Spinal cord
  - Phases of development
  - Functional columns of spinal cord
- Myelination
- Neural tube defects
  - Spina bifida
- Hydrocephalus
- Functional columns of brainstem
- Development of medulla oblongata
- Development of pons
- Development of midbrain
- Development of cerebellum
- Evolutionary aspect of cerebellum
- Development of diencephalon
- Development of cerebrum

Competencies:

- **AN63.2:** Describe anatomical basis of congenital hydrocephalus.
- **AN64.2:** Describe the development of neural tube, spinal cord, medulla oblongata, pons, midbrain, cerebral hemisphere, and cerebellum.
- **AN64.3:** Describe various types of open neural tube defects with its embryological basis.
- **AN79.3:** Describe the process of neurulation.
- **AN79.5:** Explain embryological basis of neural tube defects.
- **AN79.6:** Describe the diagnosis of pregnancy in first trimester and role of teratogens, alpha-fetoproteins. (This chapter includes alpha-fetoproteins).

INTRODUCTION

- Nervous system includes brain, spinal cord, peripheral nerves and ganglia.
- Whole nervous system is derived from a part of surface ectoderm, called *neuroectoderm.*
- Neuroectoderm extends between primitive node to prechordal plate (Practice Fig. 22.1).
- Neural plate gets folded to form *neural tube* that later forms central nervous system (Practice Fig. 22.2).

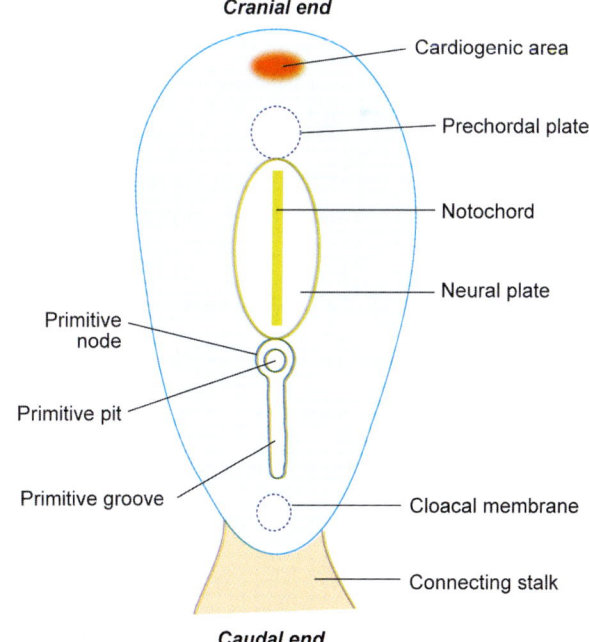

Practice Fig. 22.1: Germ disc showing notochord, primitive pit, primitive node, primitive groove, and cloacal membrane

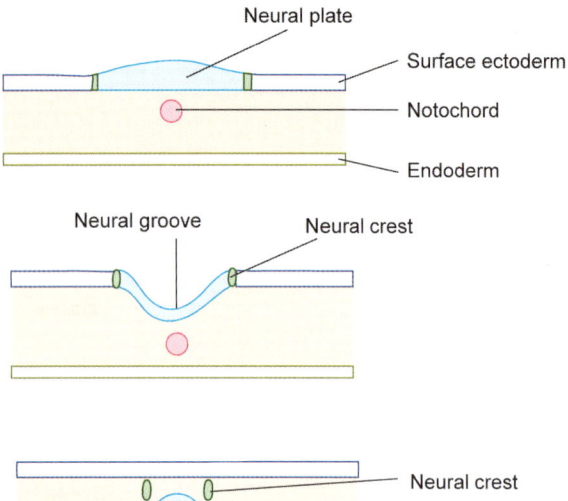

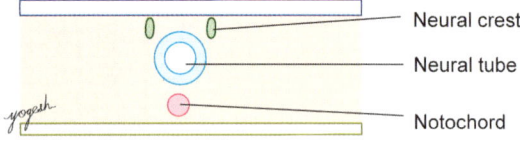

Practice Fig. 22.2: Formation of neural plate and neural crest

NEURULATION

Q. Write a short note on neurulation.

Definition: The process of formation of neural tube from neural plate is called neurulation.

Stages of neurulation (Flowchart 22.1)

1. Neuroectoderm and neural plate stage
   - In presomitic period (16th–19th day), surface ectoderm differentiates and thickens in the centre (between the prechordal plate and primitive node). This thickened zone is *neural plate* or *medullary plate*.
   - Notochord acts as a primary inducer for neural plate formation and differentiation (Practice Fig. 22.2).[NEXT]
   - Neural plate grows rapidly and elongates craniocaudally in the length.
2. Neural folding stage
   - Continuous growth of neural plate makes it depressed in the midline. This linear depression is called *neural groove*.

Flowchart 22.1: Formation of neural tube

```
3rd week: thickening of central part of the ectoderm
                        ↓
       Formation of neural plate/medullary plate
                        ↓
              Folding of neural plate
                        ↓
       Formation of neural folds and neural crest
                        ↓
      Fusion of neural folds in craniocaudal direction
                        ↓
        25th day: closer of cranial neuropore
     27th–28th day: closer of caudal neuropore
                        ↓
                Formation of neural tube
                        ↓
           Separation of neural tube and
        neural crest from surface ectodem
```

- Elevated margins of neural groove form *neural folds*.
- At the junctional zone of neural plate and surface ectoderm, the cells differentiate to form *neural crest*.
- Neural crest forms peripheral and autonomic nerves.

3. Stage of neural tube formation
   - Due to rapid proliferation of neural plate, the neural folds come closer to each other and start fusion in the midline.
   - On fusion, it forms neural tube.
   - Fusion begins in cervical region and extends in craniocaudal direction.[NEXT]
   - Neural tube forms central nervous system.

4. Stage of neural tube closure
   - Neural tube remains open at cranial end as ***cranial (anterior) neuropore*** and at caudal end as ***caudal (posterior) neuropore*** (Fig. 22.1A, B).
   - Open neural tube facilitates circulation of amniotic fluid through the lumen of neural tube. It provides nutrition to rapidly developing neuroectodermal cells before the establishment of sufficient uteroplacental circulation.
   - Cranial neuropore closes by 25th day of IUL, whereas caudal neuropore closes by 27th day of IUL, at the age of aproximately 29 somites (Fig. 22.1C).[MCQ]
   - Closure of cranial neuropore occurs at the 20 somite stage, whereas closure of posterior neuropore occurs at 29 somite stage (Fig. 22.1C).
   - Nonclosure of neuropore results in neural tube defects.
   - In later life, the location of anterior neuropore is represented by lamina terminalis, whereas posterior neuropore by terminal ventricle (lies in caudal end of spinal cord).[MCQ]

DIFFERENTIATION OF NEURAL TUBE

- Neural tube has a central cavity that forms ventricles of brain and central canal of spinal cord and a peripheral wall forms tissue of nervous system.
- Neural tube elongates craniocaudally.
- Cranial part of the cavity of neural tube dilates to form brain vesicles, whereas the caudal part of central cavity remains tubular.
- Dilated cranial part of neural tube forms 3 primary brain vesicles (Fig. 22.2, Practice Figs 22.3, 22.4, Flowchart 22.2, Scanning electron micrograph 22.1, 22.2):
  1. Prosencephalon (cranial most)
  2. Mesencephalon (middle)
  3. Rhombencephalon (caudal most)
- Prosencephalon, mesencephalon, and rhombencephalon are also called forebrain, midbrain, and hindbrain, respectively.

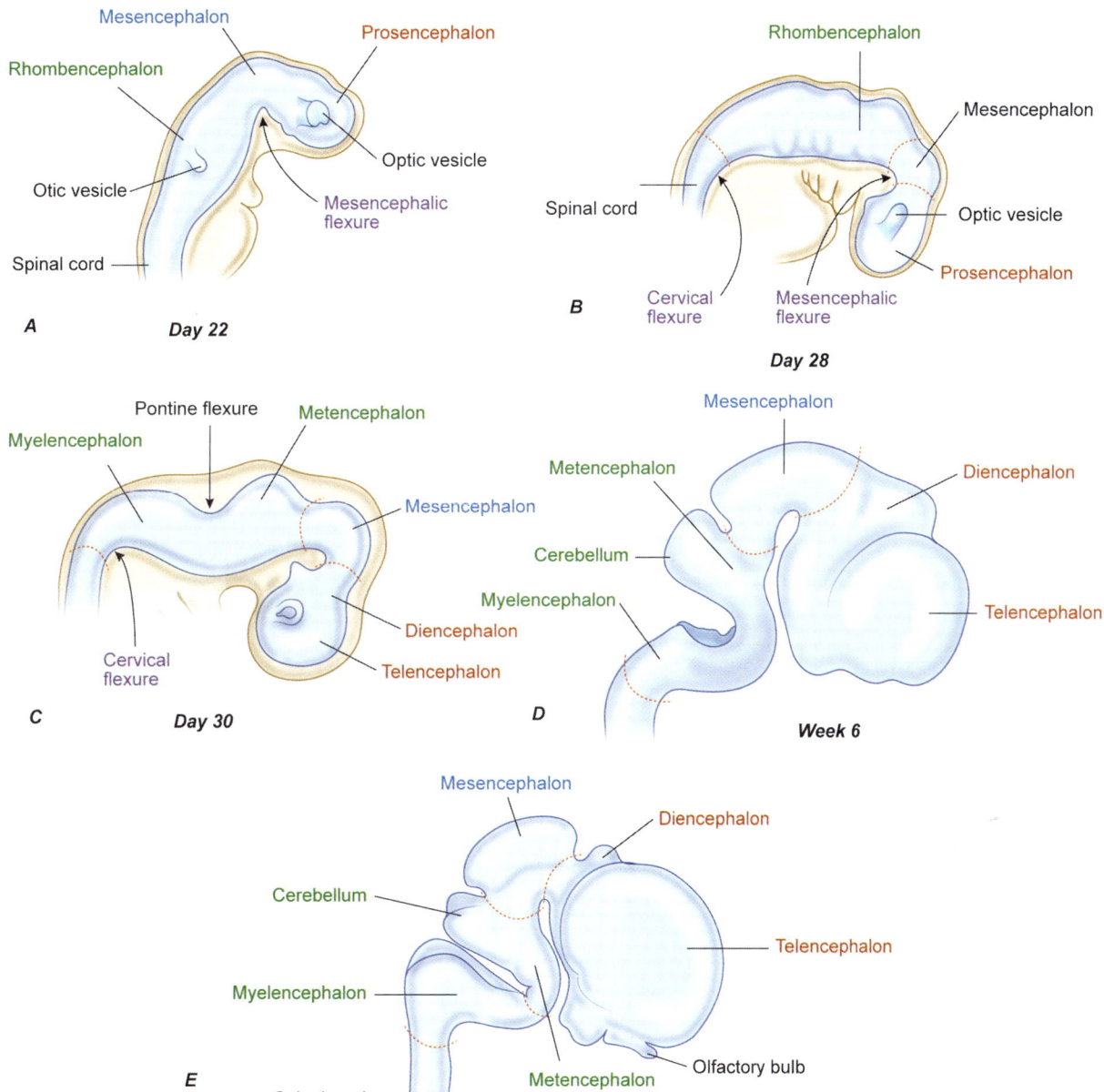

Fig. 22.1: Folding of neural plate and closure of anterior and posterior neuropores

Fig. 22.2: Developing brain vesicles

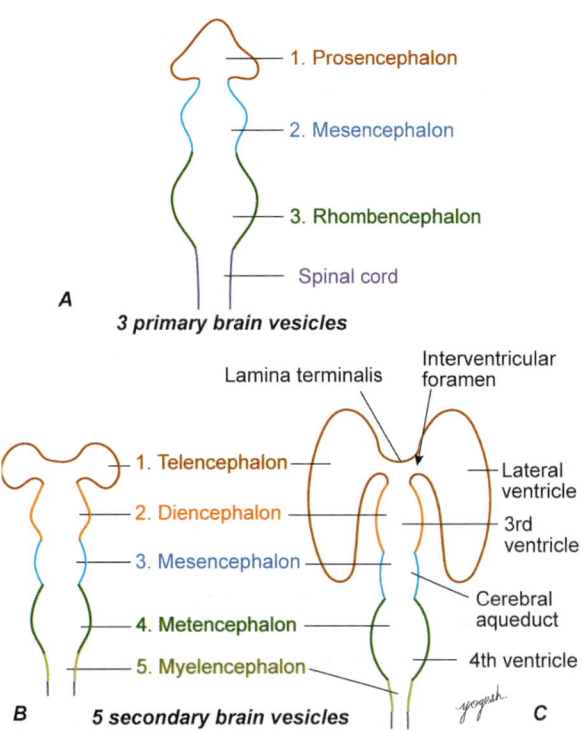
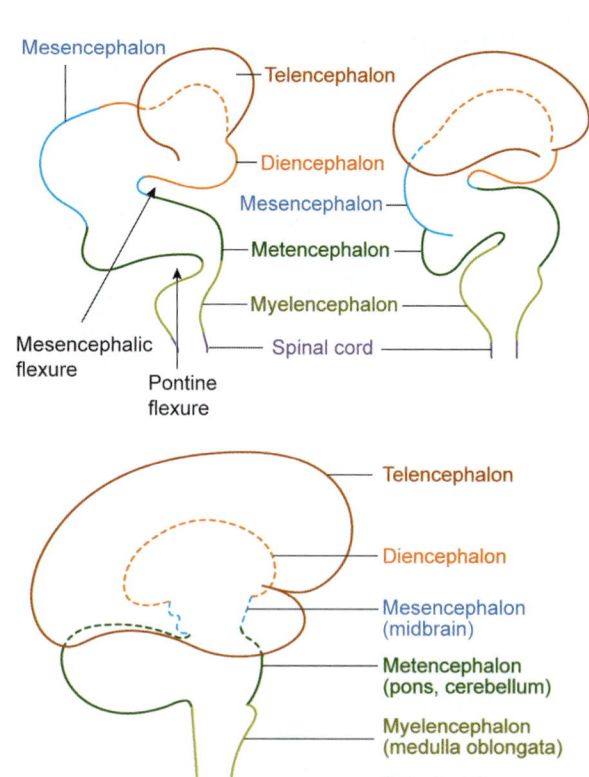

Practice Fig. 22.3: Developing brain vesicles

Practice Fig. 22.4: Further developing brain vesicles

Flowchart 22.2: Vesicles of neural tube

```
                        Vesicles of neural tube
         ┌──────────────────┬──────────────┬──────────────┐
   Prosencephalon       Mesencephalon   Rhombencephalon   Spinal cord
         │                 Midbrain           │
   ┌─────┴─────┐                       ┌──────┴──────┐
Telencephalon  Diencephalon        Metencephalon   Myelencephalon
Cerebral       Optic vesicle,      Pons            Medulla oblongata
hemisphere     pineal gland        Cerebellum
               thalamus, hypothalamus,
               posterior pituitary
```

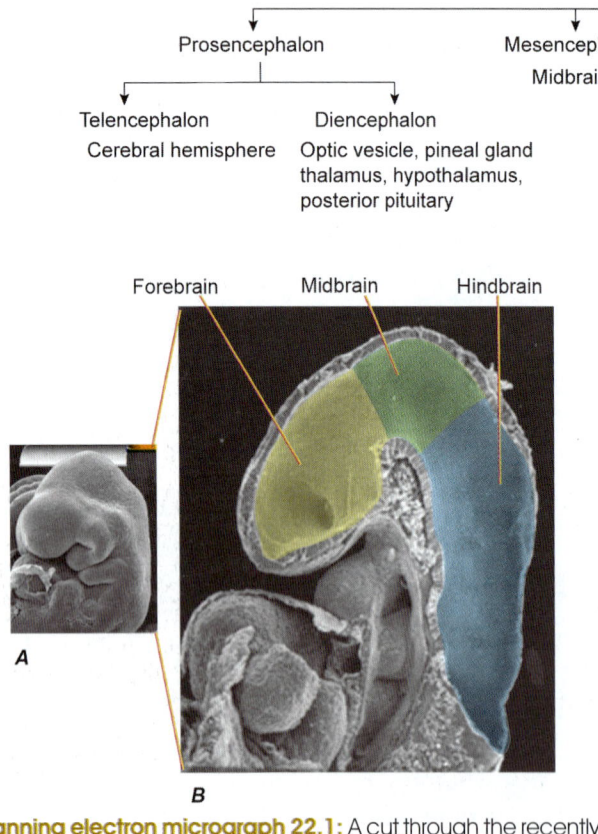

Scanning electron micrograph 22.1: A cut through the recently closed cranial neural tube illustrates the forebrain (prosencephalon), midbrain (mesencephalon), and hindbrain (rhombencephalon) [Species: Mouse, approximate human age: 5 weeks, lateral view in A and sagittal section in B]

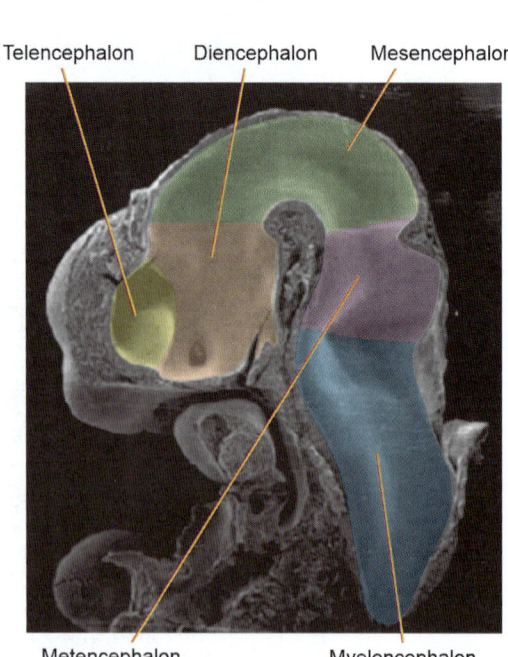

Scanning electron micrograph 22.2: Formation of brain vesicles [Species: Mouse, approximate human age: 6 weeks, sagittal section]

- On further growth, 5 brain vesicles develop as follows (Fig. 22.2C to E):
  1. Prosencephalon divides into
     - Cranial telencephalon – gives rise to two cerebral hemispheres
     - Diencephalon – gives rise to optic vesicle, pineal gland, thalami and hypothalami, posterior hypophysis
  2. Mesencephalon – gives rise to midbrain
  3. Rhombencephalon divides into
     - Cranial metencephalon – gives rise to pons and cerebellum
     - Caudal myelencephalon – gives rise to medulla oblongata

Flexures of Neural Tube

- Unequal growth rates of various components of neural tube result in flexions, constrictions, thickenings, invaginations, and evaginations of neural tube (Fig. 22.2).

Major Flexures of Neural Tube

- Flexion of embryo (folding) and differential growth of nervous tissue forms the following 4 basic flexures of neural tube:
  1. *Cervical flexure* at the junction of spinal cord and hindbrain. It makes 90° angle (Fig. 22.2B).
  2. *Cephalic flexure* (mesencephalic flexure): It occurs in the region of midbrain. It is concave ventrally (Fig. 22.2B).
  3. *Pontine flexure* at the junction of myelencephalon and metencephalon. It is convex ventrally (Fig. 22.2C).
  4. *Telencephalic flexure* at the junction of telencephalon and diencephalon (Fig. 22.2D).

Cavity of Neural Tube

- Cavity of neural tube gives passage to amniotic fluid till the closure of anterior and posterior neuropores. Flowing amniotic fluid nourishes rapidly growing brain and spinal cord.
- On the formation of brain vesicles, cavity of neural tube gets converted into ventricles and communications as follows:
  1. Cavity of telencephalon develops lateral ventricles.
  2. Communication between cavities of telencephalon and diencephalon develops interventricular foramina of Monro.
  3. Cavity of diencephalon forms 3rd ventricle.
  4. Cavity of mesencephalon forms cerebral aqueduct of Sylvius that connects the 3rd and 4th ventricle.^{MCQ}
  5. Cavity of rhombencephalon forms *4th ventricle*.
  6. Cavity of spinal cord forms central canal of spinal cord and its terminal ventricle (5th ventricle or ampulla caudalis). Terminal ventricle lies in conus medullaris (terminal part of spinal cord).
  7. Due to rupture of roof, the 4th ventricle communicates with subarachnoid space through (two lateral) foramina of Luschka and one central foramen Magendie.

NEURAL CREST CELLS ^{High yielding facts}

Q. List the derivatives of neural crest cells.

Q. Write a short note on neural crest.

- During invagination of neural plate, a distinct group of ectodermal cells appears along the edges of neural groove. This group of cells is called *neural crest cells*.
- On the formation of neural tube, neural crest cells come to lie in zone between the neural tube and surface ectoderm.
- Neural crest cells get divided into *dorsal mass* and *ventral mass* that migrates freely and forms various derivatives (Fig. 22.3).

Derivatives of Neural Crest Cells ^{High yielding facts}
(Fig. 22.3)

Dorsal Mass

A. Neuroblast cells
  - Dorsal root ganglia
  - Sensory ganglia of V, VII, IX and X cranial nerves
  - Skeletal elements of pharyngeal arches
  - Odontoblast of teeth
  - Parafollicular cells of thyroid gland

B. Spongioblast cells
  - Satellite cell in ganglion
  - Schwann cells

C. Pluripotent cells
  - Melanocytes

Ventral Mass

A. Sympatho-chromaffin organ

B. Sympathoblasts
  - Sympathetic ganglionic neurons
  - Parasympathetic ganglionic neurons (ciliary, pterygopalatine, submandibular and otic)

C. Chromaffin cells
  - Chromaffin cells of medulla of adrenal gland
  - Para-aortic body
  - Argentaffin cells in respiratory system
  - Enterochromaffin cells in gut

Other Derivatives

- Facial bones and vault of skull
- Dermis of face and neck
- Muscles of ciliary body
- Smooth muscle to blood vessels of face and forebrain
- Sclera and choroids of eyeball

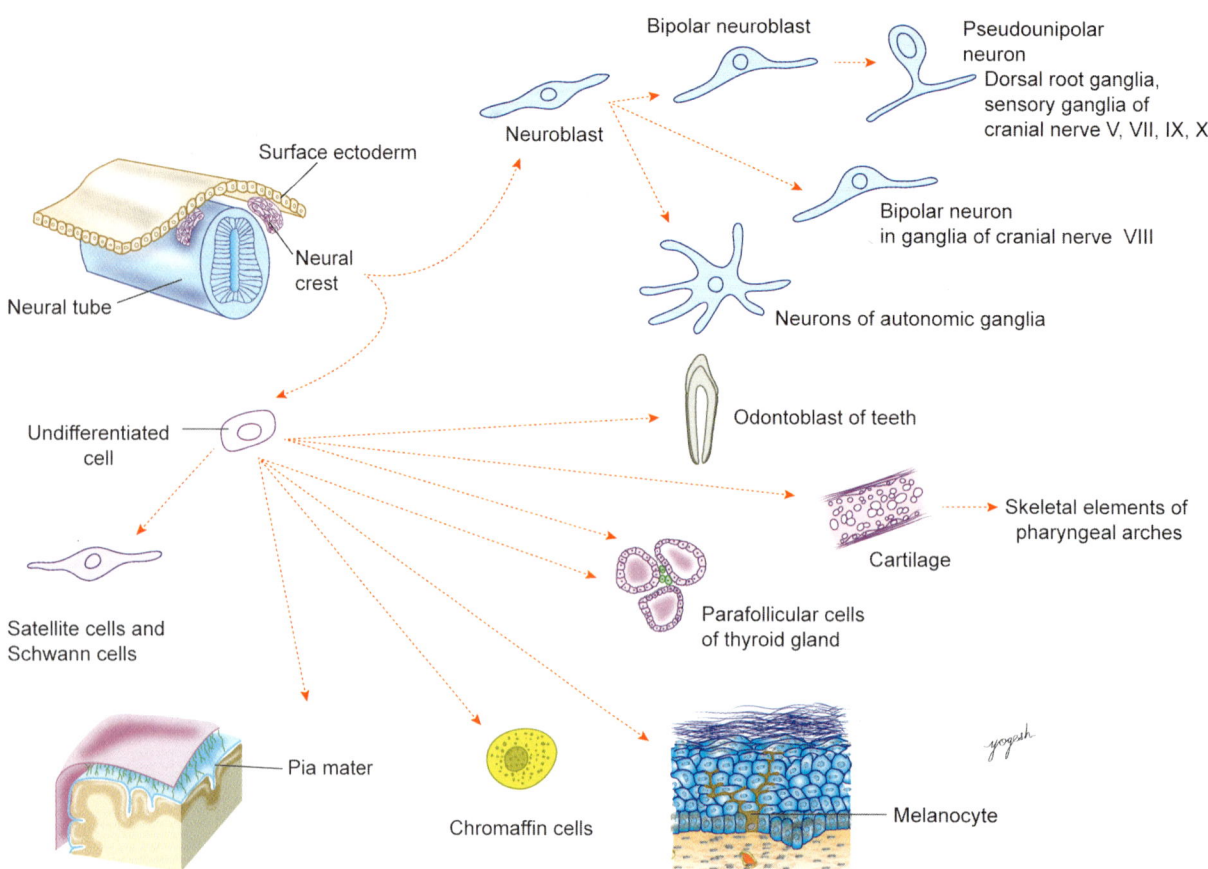

Fig. 22.3: Derivatives of neural crest cells

- Substantia propria and posterior epithelium of cornea
- Pharyngeal arch cartilages
- Semilunar valves in heart
- Pia mater
- Spiral and bulbar septum in heart

SPINAL CORD

- Parts of neural tube caudal to the hindbrain (rhombencephalon) form the spinal cord.
- Formation of spinal cord occurs in 4 phases as follows (Practice Fig. 22.5, Flowchart 22.3):
  1. Formation of mantle and marginal layers
  2. Formation of basal and alar plates
  3. Histogenesis of cells and
  4. Positional changes of spinal cord.

Some Interesting Facts

- Role of bone morphogenic proteins (BMPs)
  – Fibroblast growth factors (FGF) inhibit BMPs and transforming growth factor β (TGF-β).
  – Notochord produces noggin, chordin, follistatin that inactivate BMPs and causes neurulation.
  – Ectodermal cells
    1. that have high level of BMP get converted into surface ectoderm
    2. that have low level of BMP get converted into neural crest cells and
    3. that have absence of BMP form neural plate (neuroectoderm).
- Glomus (type I) cells are chemoreceptors that are located in carotid body and aortic body. They are derived from neural crest cells. Glomus (type II) cells are derived from neuroectoderm and they lie in arterial chemoreceptors.^{NEXT}

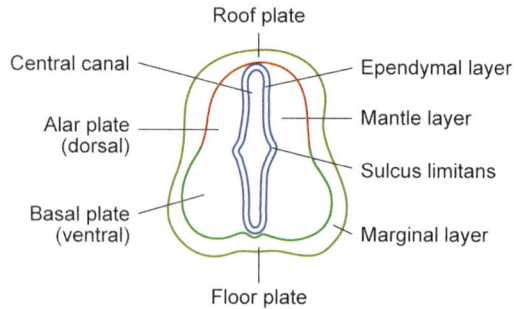

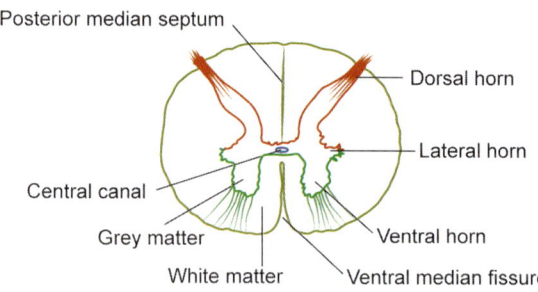

Practice Fig. 22.5: Development of spinal cord.

Flowchart 22.3: Development of spinal cord

Phase 1: Formation of mantle and marginal layers
Proliferation of neuroepithelial cells
↓ Differentiation
Innermost ependymal cell layer
Middle mantle layer
Outer marginal layer

Phase 2: Formation of basal and alar laminae
Rapid growth of mantle and marginal zones
↓ Sulcus limitans
Formation of basal lamina
Formation of alar lamina
↓
Growth of alar lamina → obliterates canal of neural tube → dorsal median septum
Growth of basal lamina → bulgings separated by ventral median fissure

Phase 3: Histogenesis of cells in neural tube
Proliferation of neuroepithelial cells
↓ Differentiation

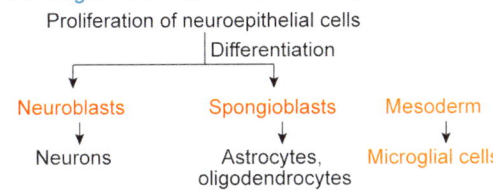

Neuroblasts → Neurons
Spongioblasts → Astrocytes, oligodendrocytes
Mesoderm → Microglial cells

Phase 4. Positional changes in spinal cord
3rd month: cord extends entire length of vertebral canal
↓ Differential growth
At birth: up to L3 vertebra
↓
Adult: up to lower border of L1 (or upper border of L2 vertebra)

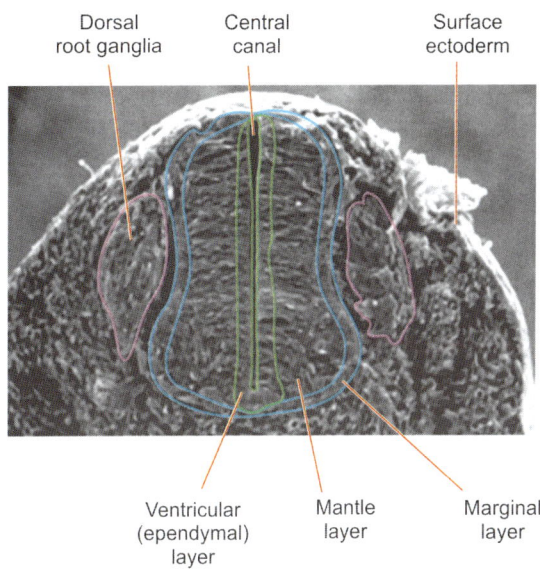

Scanning electron micrograph 22.3: Development of spinal cord. The cells of the neural tube form three layers, a ventricular ependymal layer of undifferentiated, proliferating cells, a mantle layer of differentiating neurons that will form the grey matter of the spinal cord, and a marginal layer that contains nerve fibres and will be the white matter [Species: Mouse, approximate human age: 6 weeks, transverse section]

Phases of Development

Phase 1: Formation of mantle and marginal layers

- Neural tube is lined by a single layer called neuroepithelial cells.
- Neuroepithelial cells lining the lateral wall of central canal proliferate and differentiate into three zones as follows:
  Innermost – primitive *ependymal cell layer*.
  Middle *mantle layer* that later forms neurons and neuroglial cells.
  Outermost *marginal layer* that later forms supporting neuroglial cells and contains processes of neurons of mantle layer.

Phase 2: Formation of basal and alar laminae (Fig. 22.4, Scanning electron micrograph 22.3)

- The cells in mantle zone proliferate rapidly.
- Rapid growth in the mantle zone of ventral portion of the neural tube forms *basal plate* or lamina, whereas rapid growth in the dorsal portion forms *alar lamina* or plate.
- Dorsal and ventral portion of the neural tube are now called *roof* and *floor plates,* respectively.
- A longitudinal groove called *sulcus limitans* appears in the canal of spinal cord. Sulcus limitans separates alar lamina from basal lamina.
- Continued growth of the alar lamina obliterates dorsal part of canal of neural tube that results in the formation of *dorsal median septum* of spinal cord.
- Continuous growth of the basal laminae produces bulging separated by *ventral median fissure.*
- A small remaining part of the central canal of neural tube forms *central canal of spinal cord*.

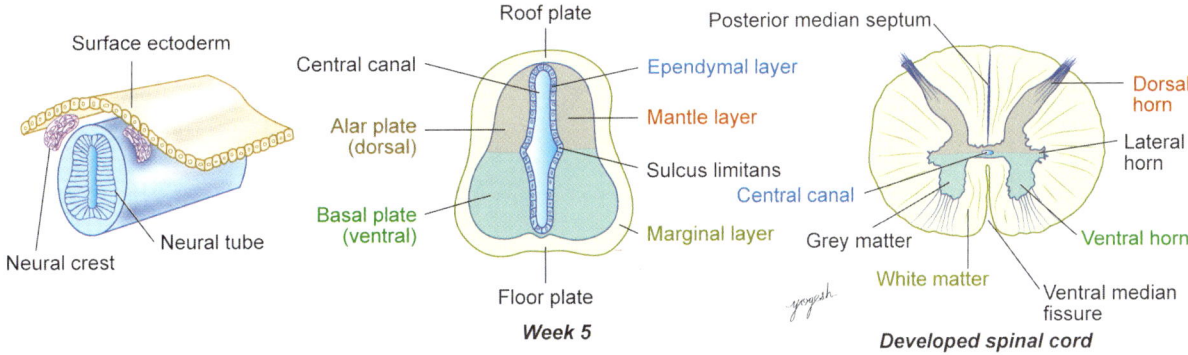

Fig. 22.4: Development of spinal cord

Phase 3: Histogenesis of cells in neural tube
(Figs 22.5, 22.6)

- The neuroepithelial cells of mantle and marginal laminae proliferate rapidly and get differentiated into two types of cells:
  A. Neuroblasts (form neurons) and
  B. Spongioblast (forms astrocytes, oligodendrocytes).
- **Histogenesis of neurons:**
  - *Neuroblast cells* in the mantle layer lose their cell processes to form *apolar neuroblasts*. From apolar neuroblasts, two processes develop at opposite pole and convert it into *bipolar neuroblast*.
  - Bipolar neuroblast loses one process to form *unipolar neuroblast*. Remaining single process of unipolar neuroblast elongates to develop *axon*.
  - Multiple small processes (primitive dendrites) appear on the surface of unipolar neuroblast to form *multipolar neuroblast*. These multipolar neuroblasts later form *mature neurons*.
  - Neuroblast loses mitotic activity. Motor neurons differentiate earlier than sensory neurons.[MCQ]
- Formation of grey and white columns
  - Neurons that develop in the mantle zone of basal lamina form neurons of anterior grey horn. Axons of these anterior grey horn neurons grow out at ventrolateral angle of spinal cord to form *ventral motor roots* of spinal nerves.
  - Nerve cells that develop in the mantle zone of alar lamina form neurons of *posterior grey horn*. Axons of these cells travel through marginal zone and form *ascending tracts*.
  - Many neurons of mantle zone form interneurons.
  - Neural crest cells form pseudounipolar neurons of *dorsal root ganglia* (spinal ganglia). Central processes of these pseudounipolar neurons enter the spinal cord at dorsolateral angle to form dorsal *sensory roots* of spinal nerve. Peripheral processes of these neurons run laterally as sensory fibres of spinal nerve.
  - Both sensory and motor roots join to form a typical spinal nerve.
  - Axons of neurons from various parts of the brain enter the marginal zone of spinal cord to form *descending tracts*.
  - Thus, mantle layer forms *grey matter*, whereas marginal layer forms *white matter* of spinal cord.
  - Cells at the junction of alar and basal laminae in the mantle zone proliferate to form *lateral horn* of spinal cord.
- Glial cells
  - Spongioblasts (glioblasts) differentiate into astrocytoblast and oligodendroblast.
  - Astrocytoblasts differentiate into *protoplasmic and fibrous astrocytes*, whereas oligodendroblasts differentiate into *oligodendrocytes*.

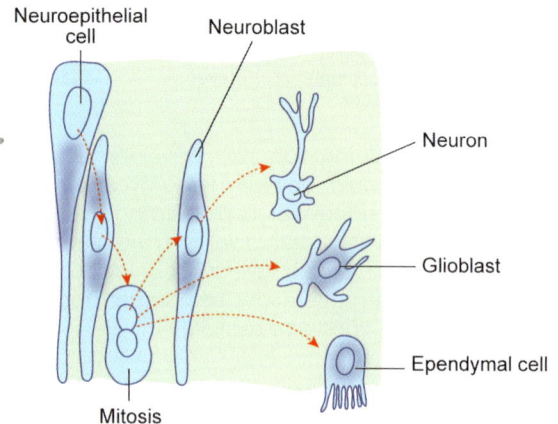

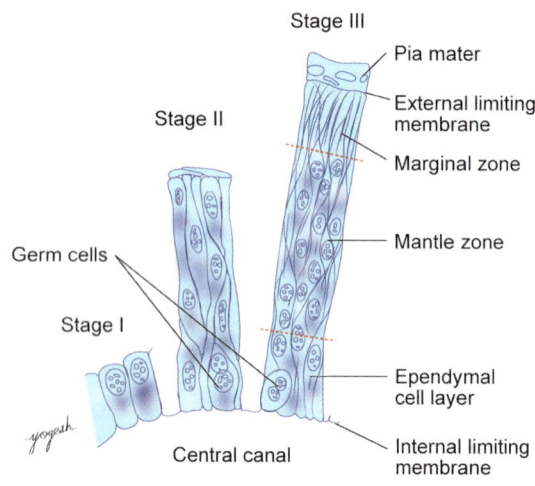

Fig. 22.5: Histogenesis of spinal cord

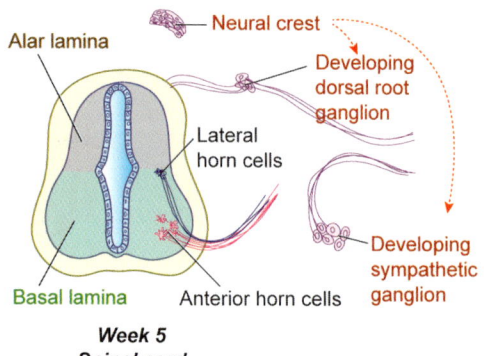

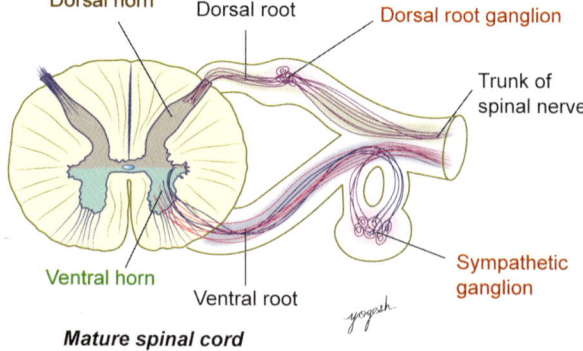

Fig. 22.6: Development of spinal nerve

- *Microglial cells* (phagocytes) are derived from mesenchymal tissues.^{NEXT}
- Lining epithelium of neural tube cavity differentiates to form *ependymal cells* and lining epithelium of choroid plexuses.

Phase 4. Positional changes in spinal cord (Fig. 22.7)
Q. Write a short note on positional changes of spinal cord.

- Spinal cord extends through the entire length of vertebral canal up to 3rd month of IUL. Spinal nerves run horizontally and emerge from corresponding intervertebral foramina.^{MCQ}
- Due to differential growth, vertebral column elongates faster than spinal cord and terminal end of spinal cord shifts to a higher level.
- At birth, lower end of spinal cord is located at the level of 3rd lumbar vertebra.^{MCQ}
- The process of differential growth continues up to the adult life, hence, in adult, lower end of spinal cord is located at the level of lower border of first lumbar vertebra (or upper border of L2 vertebra).^{MCQ}
- Cauda equina is a derivative of neural tube.^{NEXT}

Result of spinal cord recession
1. Spinal nerves do not arise at the level of corresponding intervertebral foramen.
2. Spinal nerves run obliquely downloads to reach corresponding intervertebral foramen.
3. Lower portion of pia mater forms fibrous band called *filum terminale*, that extends from lower end of spinal cord up to the first coccygeal vertebra.^{MCQ}
4. Dura mater extends up to second sacral vertebra.^{MCQ}

Note: Pia mater is derived from neural crest cells, whereas arachnoid mater and dura mater are derived from condensation of mesenchyme that surrounds the neural tube.^{NEXT}

Functional Columns of Spinal Cord
- The neurons of basal and alar lamina are arranged according to the designated function in the form of functional columns as follows:

Box 22.1: Myelination (Fig. 22.8)
- Myelination (myelinogenesis) is the process of formation of myelin around the axons.
- Myelination in the central nervous system is the function of oligodendrocytes, whereas in the peripheral nervous system, it is the function of Schwann cells.^{NEXT}
- Myelination begins when the nerve fibres start functioning.
- It begins during the 4th month of IUL and continues after the birth up to 2–3 years.
- Motor fibres myelinate earlier than sensory fibres.^{MCQ}
- Myelination of corticospinal tract begins at 9 months of IUL and continues up to 2 years after birth.^{Clinical fact}

Columns in basal lamina
1. *General somatic efferent column* – provides innervations for skeletal muscles.
2. *General visceral efferent column* – presents only in the thoracolumbar region and sacral region as lateral-horn of the spinal cord. It provides preganglionic sympathetic and parasympathetic fibres.

Columns in alar lamina
1. *General visceral afferent column*: It is present only in thoracolumbar and sacral regions of spinal cord and receives sensory inputs form viscera (organs).
2. *General somatic afferent column*: It receives exteroceptive and proprioceptive information.

NEURAL TUBE DEFECTS ^{High yielding facts}

Q. Write a short note on spina bifida and neural tube defects.

Definition: Neural tube defects (NTDs) are a group of conditions formed owing to nonclosure of neural tube.

- Closure of the neural tube begins in the third week of IUL. Cranial neuropore closes by 25th day and caudal neuropore by 27th day of IUL.

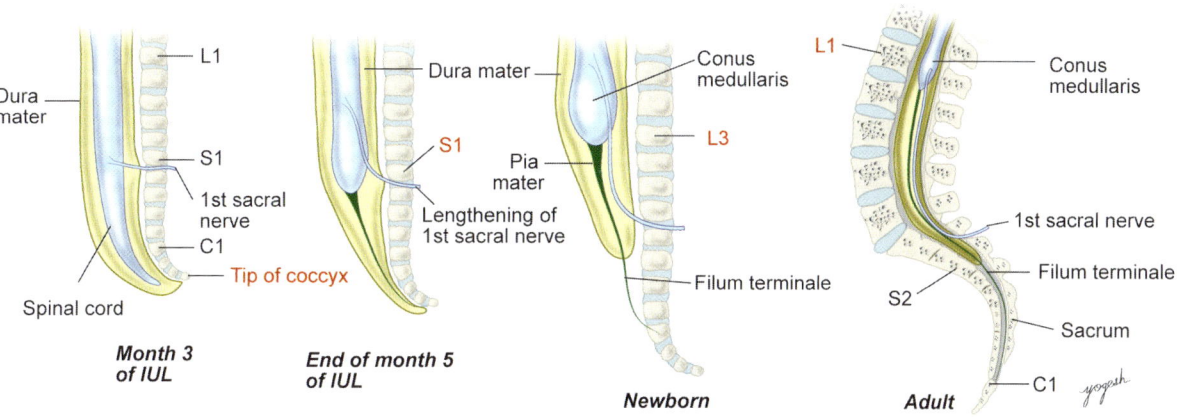

Fig. 22.7: Developing spinal cord – positional changes. Abbreviation: IUL, intrauterine life

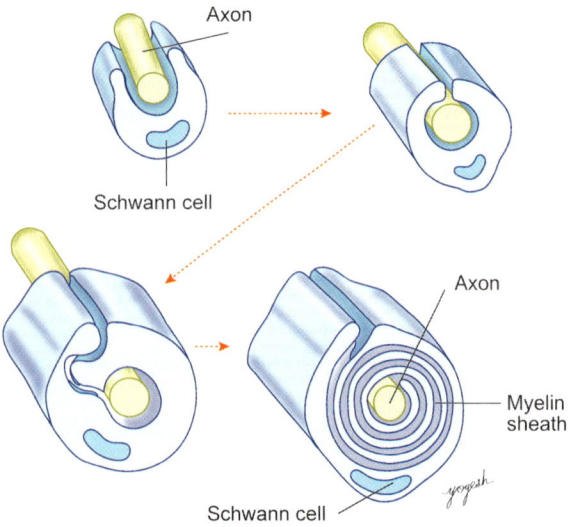

Fig. 22.8: Process of myelination of peripheral nerve fibres

- NTDs are the commonest birth defect.
- Most common cause for NTDs is folic acid (vitamin B9) deficiency.^MCQ Folate is essential for DNA/RNA synthesis, cell division and myelination.
- Folic acid supplements to the mother reduce chances of NTDs.
- Methylenetetrahydrofolate reductase (MTHFR) enzyme deficiency due to MTHFR gene mutation is also associated with neural tube defects.^NEXT, Clinical fact
- NTDs are listed in Table 22.1.

Table 22.1 Neural tube defects

1. Spina bifida
   – Spina bifida occulta
   – Meningocele
   – Myelomeningocele
2. Anencephaly
3. Encephalocele
4. Iniencephaly
5. Rachischisis

Spina Bifida (Fig. 22.9, Practice Fig. 22.6)

Q. Write a short note on spina bifida.

- **Definition**
  Spina bifida is a neural tube defect that occurs within the first four weeks of pregnancy due to the incomplete closure of neural tube.
- **Pathology**
  Folic acid deficiency or MTHFR gene defect → incomplete closure of neural tube → incomplete formation of vertebrae → bifid spines of vertebrae (spina bifida)

Types

A. *Spina bifida occulta*
   – In this condition, spine is bifid but not visible on the surface (occulta means hidden).
   – It commonly occurs in lumbosacral region.
   – Its location is marked by dimple on the skin and hairy skin.
   – Spinal cord and meninges are normal in position.

B. *Spina bifida cystica*
   It is of two types:
   1. Meningocele
      It is the protrusion of arachnoid and pia mater (only meninges) through the bifid spine.
      It produces cystic swelling covered with skin.
   2. Myelomeningocele (meningomyelocele)
      It is the protrusion of spinal cord through bifid spine.
      It also produces cystic swelling covered with skin.

Prevention

- Supplementation of 0.4 mg/day folic acid from three months prior to conception up to the first 12 weeks of the pregnancy can prevent neural tube defects.

Screening

- Neural tube defects can be detected by
  1. Ultrasonography
  2. Increased maternal serum α-fetoprotein.^NEXT

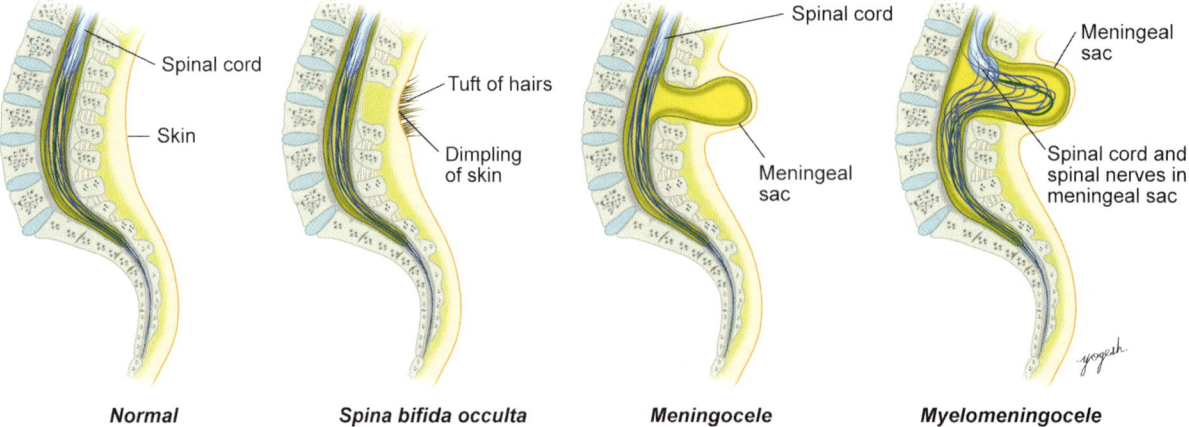

Fig. 22.9: Spina bifida

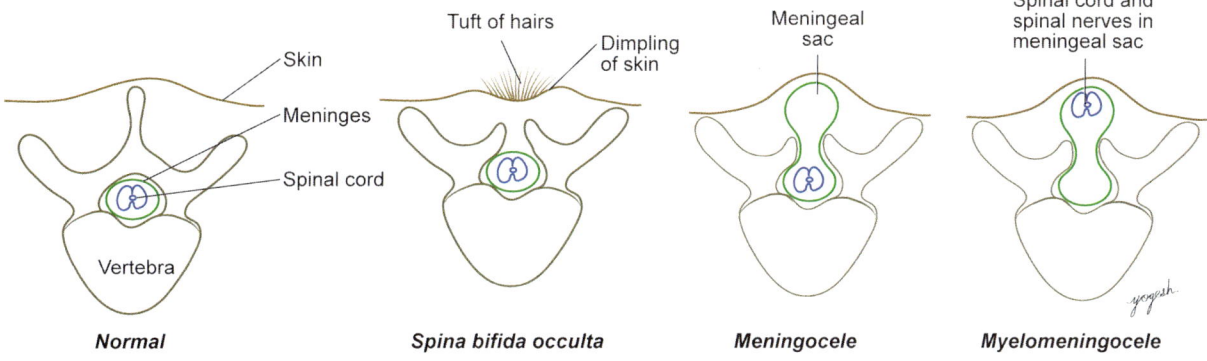

Practice Fig. 22.6: Spina bifida

Treatment
- Spina bifida can be treated by surgery after delivery.

Other Defects

1. *Anterior spina bifida*: In this condition, two halves of vertebral body fail to fuse and result in a gap. Through this gap, spinal meninges protrude ventrally.
2. *Anencephaly*: It occurs due to the failure of closure of anterior neuropore. It shows irregular degenerated brain mass.
3. *Encephalocele*: Due to failure of formation of skull vault bones, brain tissue and meninges protrude outside the skull cavity and form encephalocele.
4. *Iniencephaly* (inion = nape of neck in Greek): It involves defective occipital bone, spina bifida of cervical vertebrae and retroflexion of head (backward bending).
5. *Rachischisis* (myeloschisis): It is the failure of closure of neural folds to form neural tube. It results in the exposure of flattened neural tissue onto the surface (Flowcharts 22.4, 22.5).

FUNCTIONAL COLUMNS OF BRAINSTEM

- Medulla oblongata, pons, and midbrain together constitute the brainstem.
- Sulcus limitans divide lateral part of the brainstem into dorsal *alar lamina* and ventral *basal lamina*.
- Cells of basal lamina form the efferent group of neurons (*efferent columns*), whereas cells of alar lamina form afferent group of neurons (*afferent columns*).

Box 22.2: Hydrocephalus

Q. *Write a short note on hydrocephalus.*
- Hydrocephalus is the excess of CSF in the ventricular system.
- **Causes**
  - Obstruction of CSF passage
  - Excess production of CSF
  - Impaired communication between ventricles and subarachnoid space
- **Pathology**
  Dilatation of ventricular system results in separation of cranial bones. It produces large head size and degeneration of nervous tissue.
- Enlargement of central canal of spinal cord is called **syringomyelia**.NEXT

- These columns show group of neurons that perform specific function via cranial nerves. Such group of neurons in the brainstem forms *cranial nerve nuclei*.

Division of Functional Columns (Fig. 22.10)

- According to functions, nuclear columns are divided as follows:
  1. *General somatic efferent* (GSE): For striated muscles of head that are not originated from the pharyngeal arches.
  2. *Special visceral efferent* (SVE) or branchial efferent: For striated muscles of pharyngeal arches, trapezius, and sternocleidomastoid muscles.
  3. *General visceral efferent* (GVE) as preganglionic parasympathetic fibres.

Flowchart 22.4: Neural tube defects

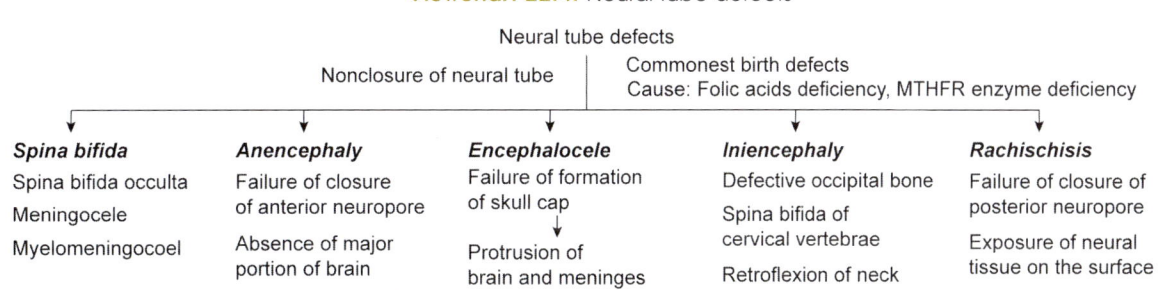

Flowchart 22.5: Spina bifida

```
                    Spina bifida
        Incomplete closure of neural tube in first 4 weeks
        Cause: MTHFR gene defect or folic acid deficiency
                         │
         ┌───────────────┴───────────────┐
   Spina bifida occulta            Spina bifida cystica
   Bifid spine                             │
   Not visible on          ┌───────────────┴───────────────┐
   surface             Meningocele                  Myelomeningocele
   Site covered by     Bifid spine                  Bifid spine
   hairy skin          Protrusion of                Protrusion of spinal
                       meninges                     cord with meninges

   Prevention
        Folic acid supplementation
        Increased maternal serum fetoprotein
```

4. *General visceral afferent* (GVA) for visceral sensation via vagus nerve.
5. *Special visceral afferent* (SVA) for taste sensation.
6. *General somatic afferent* (GSA) for proprioception, tactile sensation from face and oral, nasal and pharyngeal mucosa via trigeminal nerve.
7. *Special somatic afferent* (SSA) for auditory and vestibular impulses.

For further details, refer Tables 22.2 and 22.3 and read cranial nerves from Gross Anatomy book.

DEVELOPMENT OF MEDULLA OBLONGATA

- Rhombencephalon (hindbrain) is divided into two parts:
  - *Myelencephalon* (caudal part) that forms medulla oblongata.
  - *Metencephalon* (cranial part) that forms pons and cerebellum.
- Cavity of rhombencephalon forms the 4th ventricle.^NEXT
- Fusion between mesencephalon and rhombencephalon is marked by a construction called *rhombencephalic isthmus*.
- On appearance of the fifth vesicle of brain, external appearance of myelencephalon changes markedly.
- Cavity of myelencephalon forms lower part of the 4th ventricle.

Developmental Stages

- *Sulcus limitans* divide alar and basal lamina.
- Roof plate of cranial part of medulla widens to form *roof* of the 4th ventricle.
- Widening of the roof plate brings alar lamina dorsolateral to the basal lamina and thus, both the laminae form *floor* of 4th ventricle.

Differentiation of Basal Lamina (Fig. 22.11)

- Basal lamina of myelencephalon differentiates into the following columns:
  1. General somatic efferent (GSE): It includes hypoglossal nuclei (XII) for the muscles of tongue.
  2. Special visceral efferent (SVE): It includes nucleus ambiguus for the muscles of third arch (glossopharyngeal nerve), muscles of fourth arch (superior laryngeal branch of vagus), and sixth

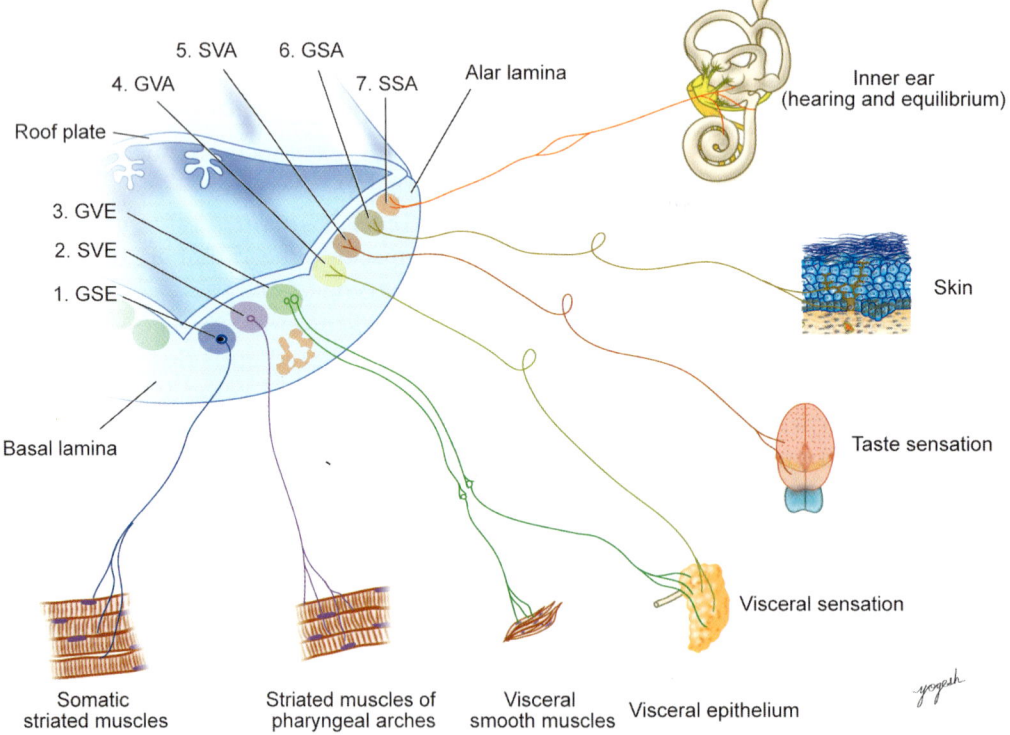

Fig. 22.10: Organisation of functional columns of cranial nerve nuclei in brainstem. GSE: General somatic efferent, SVE: Special visceral efferent, GVE: General visceral efferent, GVA: General visceral afferent, SVA: Special visceral afferent, GSA: General somatic afferent, SSA: Special somatic afferent

Q. List the functional columns of basal lamina of brainstem.

Table 22.2 Functional columns of brainstem – part I: Efferent columns

Component	Function	Nucleus	Location	Cranial nerve	Remark
General somatic efferent (GSE)	Striated muscles of head which are not of pharyngeal arch origin	Third cranial nerve nucleus	Midbrain	3rd nerve	Extraocular muscles except lateral rectus and superior oblique muscles
		Fourth cranial nerve nucleus	Midbrain	4th nerve	Superior oblique muscle
		Sixth cranial nerve nucleus	Pons	6th nerve	Lateral rectus muscle
		Twelfth cranial nerve nucleus	Medulla	12th nerve	Muscles of tongue except palatoglossus
Special visceral efferent (SVE) (branchial efferent)	Striated muscles of pharyngeal arch origin as well as trapezius and sternocleidomastoid	Motor nucleus of trigeminal nerve	Pons	5th nerve	Muscles of the first arch via mandibular nerve
		Motor nucleus of facial nerve	Pons	7th nerve	Muscles of the second arch
		Nucleus ambiguus	Medulla	9th nerve	Muscle of the third arch—stylopharyngeus
		Nucleus ambiguus	Medulla	10th nerve	Muscles of 4th arch via superior laryngeal nerve
		Nucleus ambiguus	Medulla	11th nerve	Muscles of sixth arch (fibres of 11th nerve via recurrent laryngeal branch of vagus)
General visceral efferent (GVE)	Preganglionic autonomic fibres	Edinger-Westphal nucleus	Midbrain	3rd nerve	Sphincter pupillae, ciliaris
		Superior salivatory nuclei	Pons	7th nerve	Submandibular and sublingual gland
		Lacrimatory nucleus	Pons	7th nerve	Lacrimal gland
		Inferior salivatory nucleus	Medulla	9th nerve	Parotid gland
		Dorsal nucleus of vagus	Medulla	10th nerve	

Q. List the functional columns of alar lamina of brainstem.

Table 22.3 Functional columns of brainstem – part II: Afferent columns

Component	Function	Nucleus	Location	Cranial nerve	Remark
General visceral afferent (GVA)	Visceral sensation	Dorsal nucleus of vagus	Medulla	10th nerve	
Special visceral afferent (SVA)	Taste	Nucleus tractus solitarious	Pons and medulla	7th, 9th, 10th nerve	Taste sensation
General somatic afferent (GSA)	Proprioception, tactile sensation from face, and oral, nasal and pharyngeal mucosa	Mesencephalic nucleus of trigeminal nerve	Midbrain	5th nerve	
	General sensation from face, and oral, nasal and pharyngeal mucosa	Spinal nucleus of trigeminal nerve	Pons and medulla	5th nerve	
Special somatic afferent (SSA)	Auditory (hearing) and vestibular (equilibrium) impulses from inner ear (sight is also SSA)	Cochlear and vestibular nuclei	Pons and medulla	8th nerve	Hearing and equilibrium

arch (recurrent laryngeal branch) of vagus via spinal accessory nerve.

3. General visceral efferent (GVE): It includes dorsal nucleus of vagus and inferior salivatory nucleus for parotid gland (glossopharyngeal nerve).

Differentiation of Alar Lamina (Fig. 22.11)

- Cells from each alar lamina migrate ventrally in the marginal layer to form **bulbopontine extension** and finally develop into olivary group of nuclei.[MCQ]

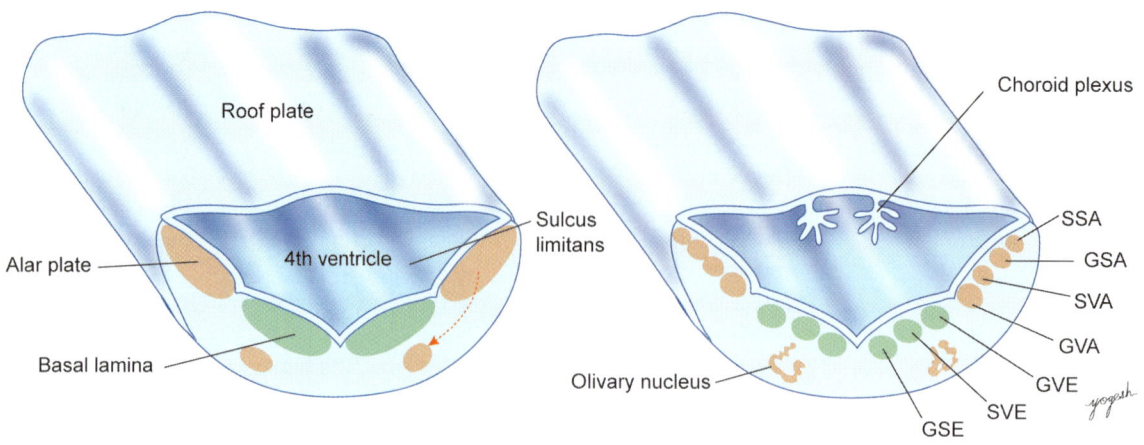

Fig. 22.11: Section of myelencephalon (medulla). Basal and alar lamina of myelencephalon. Roof plate connects alar laminae and forms the roof of the 4th ventricle. Cells of the alar laminae migrate in marginal zone that later forms olivary group of nuclei. GSE: General somatic efferent, SVE: Special visceral efferent, GVE: General visceral efferent, GVA: General visceral afferent, SVA: Special visceral afferent, GSA: General somatic afferent, SSA: Special somatic afferent.

- Due to growth and appearance of white matter, the nuclei shift from their initial positions to the definitive positions.
- Remaining cells of the alar lamina differentiate to form the following columns:
  1. General visceral afferent (GVA): It includes dorsal nucleus of vagus.
  2. Special visceral afferent (SVA): It includes nucleus tractus solitarious to receive taste sensation via IX and X nerves.
  3. General somatic afferent (GSA): It includes spinal nucleus of trigeminal (for V nerve), nucleus gracilis and cuneatus (for tract of Goll and Burdach).
  4. Special somatic afferent (SSA): It includes cochlear and vestibular nuclei (for VIII nerve).
- White matter of medulla oblongata is mostly derived from ascending and descending tracts.

Formation of Tela Choroidea and Choroid Plexus

- Widening of roof plate of the myelencephalon results into formation of single cell layered ependymal roof plate of the 4th ventricle. This roof plate is surrounded by vascular pia mater called *tela choroidea*.
- The vascular proliferation of pia mater invaginates underlying ependyma. Thus, formed vascular tuft covered with ependyma called *choroid plexus*.
- Choroid plexus produces cerebrospinal fluid (CSF).
- Tela choroidea ruptures to form *foramina of Luschka* that communicates the 4th ventricle with subarachnoid space.

DEVELOPMENT OF PONS (Fig. 22.12)

- Rhombencephalon (hindbrain) is divided into cranial *metencephalon* and caudal *myelencephalon*.
- Metencephalon is divided into ventromedial part that forms *pons* and dorsolateral part called *rhombic lip* that forms cerebellum.^{MCQ}
- Roof plate of metencephalon also becomes thin and broad (similar to myelencephalon) to form roof of the 4th ventricle. The alar lamina becomes dorsolateral to the basal lamina.

External Features

- *Pontine flexure* separates pons from the medulla oblongata at pontomedullary junction.
- Bulging basilar part of pons shows midline groove (basilar sulcus).
- Pontocerebellar fibres form *middle cerebellar peduncles*.
- Dorsal surface shows elevation in the floor of 4th ventricle as *facial colliculus*.

Formation of Pontine Nuclei

- Cells of alar lamina of medulla oblongata (myelencephalon) migrate ventrally to form **bulbopontine extension**.
- This bulbopontine extension forms *olivary group of nuclei* and cranial migration of bulbopontine extension forms *pontine nuclei* in the ventral basilar part of pons.^{NEXT}
- Axons of pontine nuclei form *middle cerebellar peduncle*.

Differentiation of Basal Lamina

- Basal lamina of pons differentiates into the following columns:
  1. General somatic efferent (GSE): It includes motor nucleus of VI nerve for the lateral rectus muscle.
  2. Special visceral efferent (SVE): It includes motor nucleus of V nerve for muscles of 1st pharyngeal arch and facial nucleus for muscles of 2nd arch.

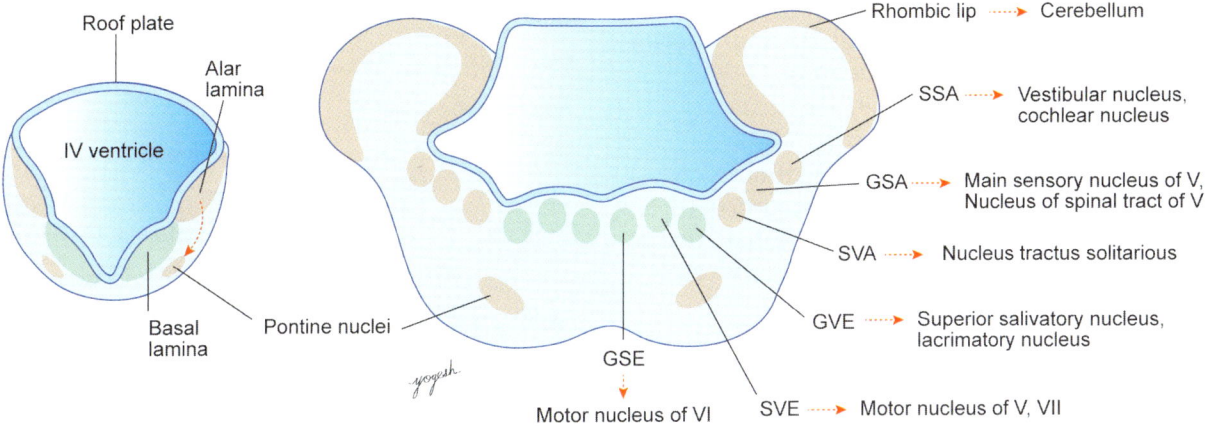

Fig. 22.12: Development of pons

3. **General visceral efferent (GVE):** It includes superior salivatory nucleus for submandibular and sublingual gland (via VII nerve) and lacrimatory nucleus for lacrimal gland (via VII nerve).

Differentiation of Alar Lamina

- Alar lamina of pons differentiates to form the following columns:
  1. **Special visceral afferent (SVA):** It includes nucleus tractus solitarious for taste sensation via VII nerve.
  2. **General somatic afferent (GSA):** It includes the main sensory nucleus of V nerve and nucleus of spinal tract of trigeminal nerve.
  3. **Special somatic afferent (SSA):** It includes vestibular and cochlear nuclei.
  4. Rhombic lip is the dorsolateral expansion of alar lamina of metencephalon. Rhombic lip forms cerebellum.

DEVELOPMENT OF MIDBRAIN (Fig. 22.13)

- Midbrain develops from mesencephalon.

Stages of Development

- Sulcus limitans divides the mantle layer into dorsal alar lamina and ventral basal lamina.

Differentiation of Basal Lamina

- Basal lamina along with floor plate of mesencephalon forms tegmentum of midbrain.
- Basal lamina of midbrain differentiates into the following columns:
  1. **General somatic efferent (GSE) column:** It includes oculomotor nucleus (III nerve) and trochlear nucleus (IV nerve) for extraocular muscles.
  2. **General visceral efferent (GVE):** It includes Edinger-Westphal nucleus (III nerve).

Differentiation of Alar Lamina

- Alar lamina gives rise to stratified zones of colliculi (superior and inferior) and pretectal nuclei.

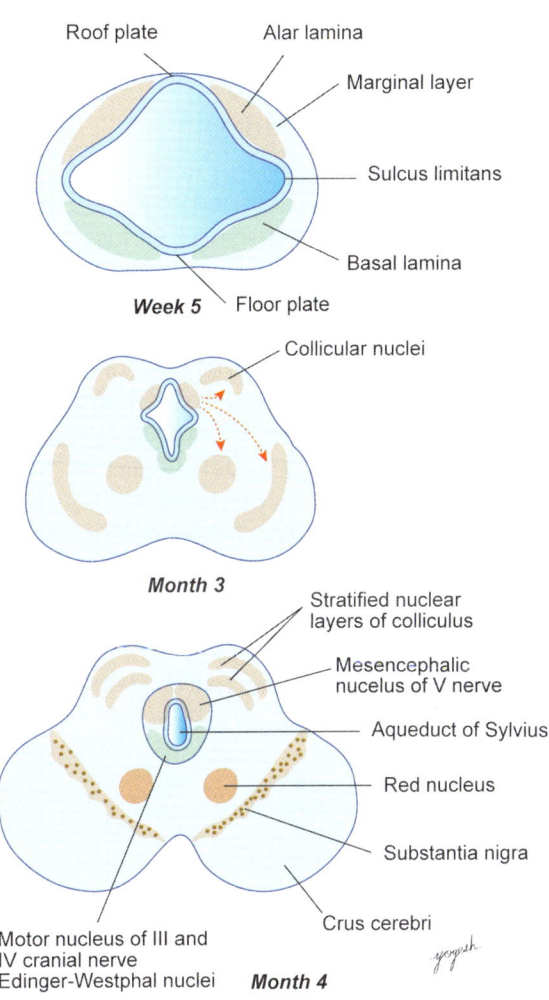

Fig. 22.13: Development of mesencephalon

- Cells of the alar lamina migrate ventrally to form *red nucleus* and *substantia nigra*.
- Remaining cells of alar lamina along with basal lamina form periaqueductal grey matter.
- Alar lamina of midbrain differentiates to form the following columns:
  1. **General somatic afferent:** It includes mesencephalic nucleus of trigeminal nerve.

2. **Special somatic afferent:** It includes superior colliculus (reflex centre for light) and inferior colliculus (reflex centre for hearing).

White Matter of Midbrain

- Formation of crus cerebri (cerebral peduncles): Most of the descending fibres (corticospinal, corticobulbar, corticopontine) pass through the marginal zone of ventral part of midbrain that forms the crus cerebri.

Cerebral Aqueduct

- The cavity of mesencephalon forms *cerebral aqueduct of Sylvius* that connects the 3rd ventricle with 4th ventricle.^MCQ

DEVELOPMENT OF CEREBELLUM

Q. Write a short note of development of cerebellum.

Summary (Examination Guide)

- Bilateral rhombic lips arising from alar lamina of metencephalon form cerebellum (Flowchart 22.6).
- Rhombic lips produce bulging that fuse in midline to form *cerebellar plate*.
- Cerebellar plate differentiates to form *vermis* and *cerebellar hemispheres*.
- Some cells of mantle layer migrate outward to form *external granular layer*, whereas remaining cells of mantle layer form *cerebellar nuclei*.
- External granular layer differentiates to form *cerebellar cortex*.
- Axons of dentate nucleus form superior cerebellar peduncles, axons of pontine nuclei form middle and axons of olivary nuclei form inferior cerebellar peduncles.

Flowchart 22.6: Development of cerebellum

External differentiation of cerebellum

Metencephalon
↓
Proliferation of cells of *rhombic lip*
↓
Fusion of rhombic lips in midline
↓
Formation of cerebellar plate
↓ *Proliferation*
Primitive cerebellum
↓ *Differentiation*
Central vermis and bilateral cerebellar hemispheres
↓ *Development of fissures*
Separation of lobes and lobules

Cellular differentiation of cerebellum

3 layers of rhombic lips (ependymal, mantle, marginal)
↓ ↓ Outward migration
Cerebellar nuclei (dentate, emboliformis, globosus and fastigius)   Formation of external granular layer
↓ *Differentiation*
Astrocytes, oligodendrocytes

Table 22.4 Parts of cerebellum

Lobe	Components
Anterior lobe	Lingula
	Central lobule
	Culmen
	Ala of central lobule
	Quadrangular lobule
Middle lobe	Declive
	Folium
	Tuber
	Pyramid
	Uvula
	Lobulus simplex
	Biventral lobule
	Semilunar lobule
	Tonsil
Flocculonodular lobe	Nodule
	Flocculus

Box 22.3: Evolutionary aspect of cerebellum

- Phylogenetically cerebellum is divided into archicerebellum (older part), paleocerebellum, and neocerebellum (newest part).
- Their functions and components are given in Table 22.5.

Stages of Development (Fig. 22.14)

- Development of cerebellum begins on 40–45 days of IUL.
- Two rhombic lips (right and left) appear in the caudal part of metencephalon.
- Initially, rhombic lips are separated by roof plate of metencephalon.
- Later, both the rhombic lips fuse across the midline to form *cerebellar plate*.
- In 12 weeks, cerebellar plate shows a small midline swelling called *vermis* and two lateral swellings called lateral *cerebellar lobes*.
- A transverse sulcus separates flocculus from lateral lobes and nodule from vermis and thus, *flocculonodular lobe* arises.
- Many transverse fissures appear and give cerebellum its characteristic adult appearance.
- Primary fissure separates anterior lobe from middle lobe (Table 22.4).

Histogenesis of Cerebellum (Fig. 22.15)

- Initially, *cerebellar primordium* consists of outer marginal and inner mantle zone of neuroepithelial cells.
- Cells from mantle zone migrate through the marginal zone to form *external granular layer*.

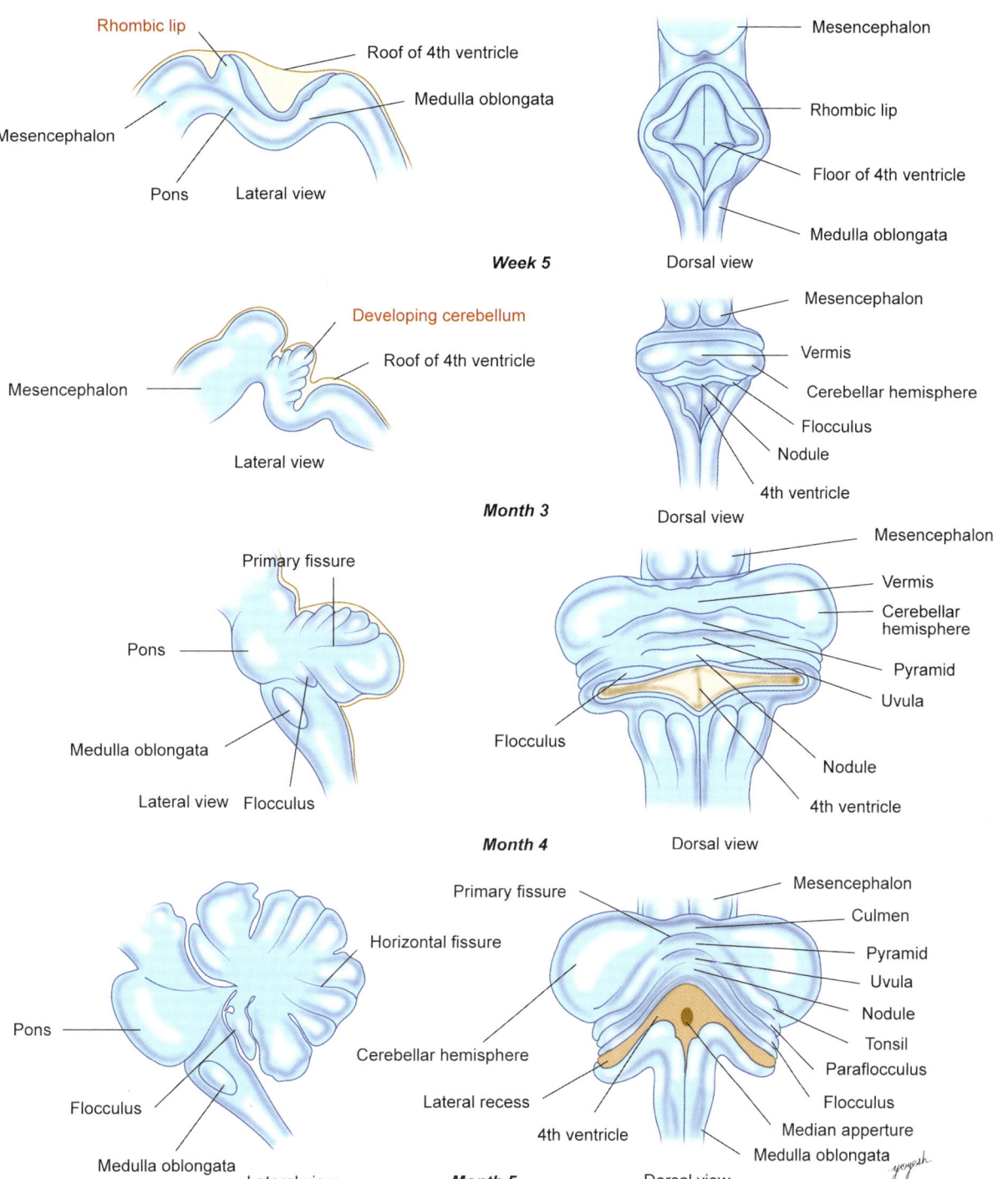

Fig. 22.14: Development of cerebellum

- Cells of external granular layer proliferate and migrate inward to form *cerebellar cortex*.
- It consists of outer molecular layer (stellate cells and basket cells), middle single cells layer (Purkinje cell layer) and inner granular layer (granule cells and Golgi cells).
- Formation of cerebellar cortex continues from 6th month of IUL till 1 ½ years after birth. *MCQ Note*: DNA synthesis inhibitors (antiviral drugs) given up to the age of 2 years may cause cerebellar damage.
- Remaining cells of mantle layer (nonmigrated cells) form dentate, emboliform, globosus and fastigial nuclei.
- The part of the roof plate of 4th ventricle (with pia mater) that do not participate in the formation of cerebellum forms *superior* and *inferior medullary velum*.

Cerebellar Peduncles

The fibres passing through the marginal layer (white matter) of cerebellum form 3 cerebellar peduncles as follows:

Table 22.5	Phylogenetic parts of cerebellum		
Phylogenetic part	Example	Components	Function
Archicerebellum	Aquatic vertebrates	Flocculonodular lobe, lingula	Maintenance of equilibrium
Paleocerebellum	Terrestrial vertebrates	Anterior lobe except lingula, pyramid and uvula	Controls tone, posture and crude movements of limbs
Neocerebellum	Higher animals	Middle lobe except pyramid and uvula	Regulation of fine movements of body

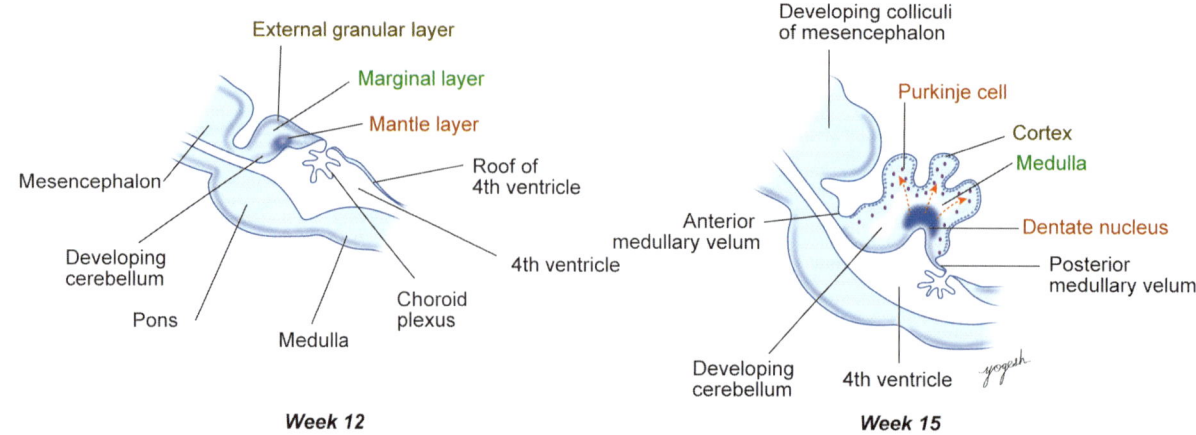

Fig. 22.15: Histogenesis of cerebellum. Cross-sectional view. Mantle layer gives rise to external granular layer that further produces cerebellar cortex and Purkinje cells. Mantle layer cells that left behind form deep cerebellar nuclei (dentate, emboliform, fastigus, globosus)

- Superior cerebellar peduncle mainly consists of outgoing axons from dentate nucleus.^{MCQ}
- Middle cerebellar peduncle mainly consists of ingrowing axons of pontine nuclei.^{MCQ}
- Inferior cerebellar peduncle mainly consists of ingrowing axons of inferior olivary nuclei.^{MCQ}

DEVELOPMENT OF DIENCEPHALON (Fig. 22.16)

- Prosencephalon is divided into cranial *telencephalon* (cerebral hemispheres) and caudal *diencephalon*.
- Diencephalon has a cavity that forms 3rd ventricle.^{MCQ}
- The 3rd ventricle communicates with lateral ventricles through interventricular foramen of Monro and caudally with 4th ventricle through cerebral aqueduct.^{MCQ}
- Diencephalon has a roof plate and alar plates.

Differentiation of Roof Plate

- Roof plate is made up of ependymal cell layer covered by vascular pia mater.
- A portion of ependymal layer with tuft of capillaries from pia mater invaginates 3rd ventricle and forms *choroid plexus of 3rd ventricle*.
- Caudal part of roof plate forms *pineal body*.

Development of epithalamus

- Roof plate of diencephalon gives rise to epithalamus.
- It lies in the form of group of nuclei around the pineal gland.
- It includes habenular nuclei and habenular commissure.
- It is concerned with olfactory pathway.
- A small posterior commissure connecting epithalimi also develops caudal to pineal gland.
- Some authors consider pineal gland in the entity of epithalamus.

Differentiation of Alar Plates

- Alar plates form lateral wall and floor of diencephalon.
- Alar plates are divided into three zones by two sulci (hypothalamic sulcus and epithalamic sulcus) into three zones: Hypothalamus (lower part), thalamus (middle part), and epithalamus (upper part).
- *Thalamus* gradually bulges into the cavity of 3rd ventricle and differentiates to thalamic nuclei.
- *Hypothalamus* gets pushed caudoventrally (anteroinferiorly in adult) due to enlarging thalamus.
- In the floor of cavity of diencephalon, a group of neurons assembles to form *mammillary body*.
- *Note:* On the 22nd day, in the region of hypothalamus, the lateral wall of diencephalon forms *optic sulcus* and later it becomes *optic vesicle* (optic cup). Optic cup forms retina and muscles of iris.
- From the floor of diencephalon, a downward growth develops that forms *infundibular process*. Later, the infundibular process develops posterior pituitary gland (neurohypophysis).

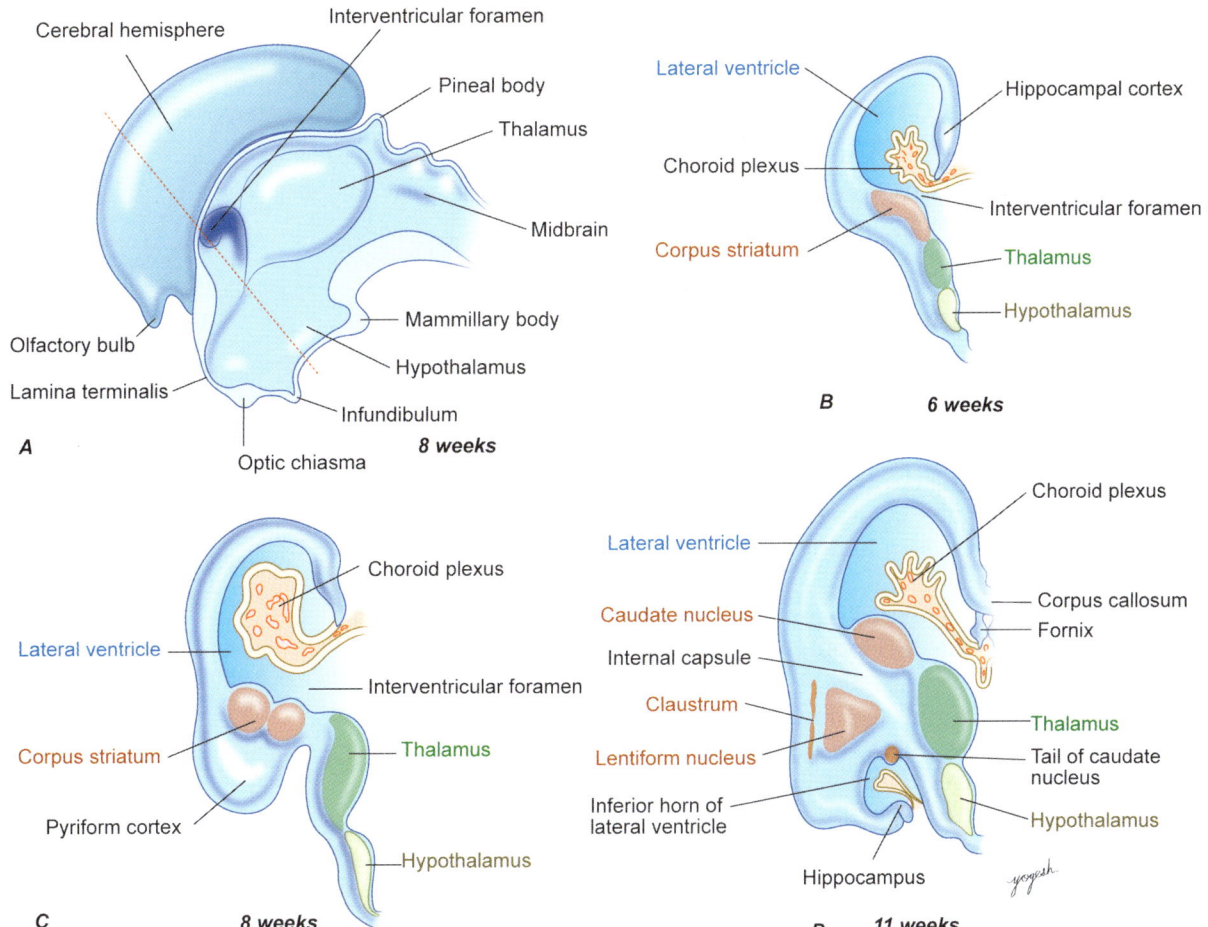

Fig. 22.16: A: In 8-week embryo, section showing medial surface of the right half of the telencephalon and diencephalon (red broken line indicates the plane of the section for B, C and D). B, C and D: Transverse sections through the right half of the telencephalon and diencephalon at the level of the broken line in A

DEVELOPMENT OF CEREBRUM

- Procencephalon is divided into *telencephalon* and *diencephalon*.
- Prosencephalon consists of two lateral outpouchings as *cerebral hemisphere* and a median *lamina terminalis*.
- Cavity of prosencephalon forms *lateral ventricles* (right and left) that communicates with 3rd ventricle through interventricular foramen.^{MCQ}
- The development of cerebral hemisphere can be studied as development during first 2 months and development after 2nd month.

Development during First 2 Months

- Each cerebral hemisphere consists of two parts:
  A. Thin *superior pallium*
  B. Thick *basal part*
- Cells from basal part migrate into the pallium that forms *cerebral cortex*.
- Remaining cells of basal part forms *corpus striatum*.
- The junctional zone of two pallium (cerebral cortex) is very thin and gets invaginated by choroid plexus.
- Pallium grows and gets differentiated into allocortex and neopallium. Human brain consists of 90% of neopallium.
- Allocortex = Archipallium + Paleopallium.
- Efferent and afferent fibres from the cerebral cortex form *internal capsule*.

Development after 2nd Month

- Neopallium overgrows and compresses the allocortex.
- Increase in the cortical mass reduces ventricular cavity.
- In the floor of cerebral hemisphere, group of neurons condenses to form *striated nuclei*.
- These striated nuclei get transversed by fibres (axons) of *internal and external capsule*.
- Striated nuclei differentiate into three groups:
  1. Lateral neostriatal nuclei: They form caudate nucleus, putamen, and claustrum.
  2. Medial paleostriatal nuclei: They form globus pallidum.
  3. Archeostriatal nuclei: They form amygdaloid nucleus below the lenticular nucleus.

Soon, the putamen and globus pallidum fuse to form lentiform nucleus.

Development of Lobes of Cerebral Hemispheres
(Fig. 22.17, Scanning electron micrograph 22.4)

- Cerebral cortex grows in various directions to form various lobes in the following manner:
  - Ventral growth forms *frontal lobe*.
  - Dorsal growth forms *occipital lobe*.
  - Parietal (lateral) growth forms *parietal lobe*.
  - Occipital pole expands ventrally to form *temporal lobe*.

Effects of development of cerebral hemispheres

1. Effect on lateral ventricle: Growth of occipital lobe and temporal lobe results in expansion of lateral ventricle to form *inferior horn* and *posterior horn* of lateral ventricle.
2. Effect on caudate nucleus: Expanding caudate nucleus turns around the developing ventricle and becomes 'C' shaped.
3. Formation of sulci and gyri: Continued growth of cerebral cortex starts formation of fissures. Parietooccipital fissure of Rolando appears by 7th month.^NEXT Lateral sulcus appears during the 4th month.^NEXT
4. Insula: A part of cortex covering the external surface of corpus striatum grows relatively slower. This part forms *insula*. Insula gets buried in the depth of lateral sulcus by overgrown cortex of frontal and temporal lobes.
5. Formation of olfactory bulb and tracts: From the frontal lobe, elongated evagination develops to form *olfactory bulb*. A stem that connects to the frontal lobe forms the *olfactory tract*.

Differentiation of Allocortex (Fig. 22.16)

- Allocortex differentiates to form limbic structures as follows:
  1. Allocortex has two parts: *Archipallium* that initially lies on medial surface of cerebral hemisphere and *paleopallium* that lies on ventral surface of hemisphere (ventrolateral to the corpus striatum).
  2. Allocortex differentiate to form *limbic lobe*. Limbic lobe differentiates into the following structures:
     a. *Hippocampal cortex*: Its *dorsal part* forms a thin band of grey matter called *indusim griseum* on the dorsal surface of corpus callosum.

     Its *ventral part* forms *hippocampus* and *dentate gyrus* that projects into the cavity of inferior horn of lateral ventricle.

     b. *Projection fibres of hippocampal cortex:* The axons from hippocampal cortex forms *fimbria, fornix* and its *commissure*.
  3. Allocortex also forms *olfactory bulb and tract*.

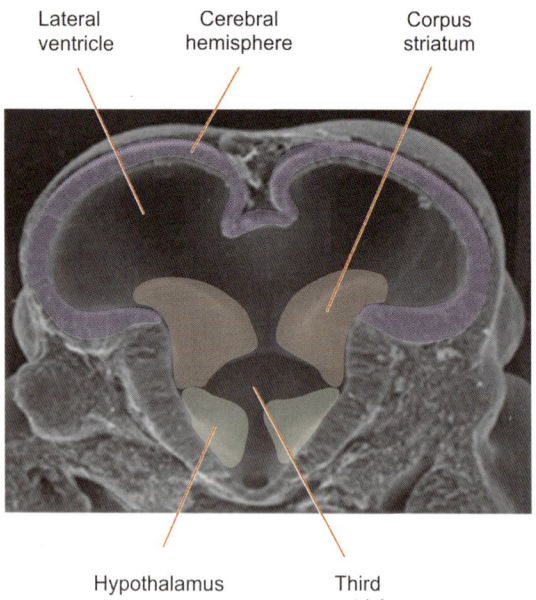

Scanning electron micrograph 22.4: A cut through the forebrain at the level of the line illustrates the expanding cerebral hemispheres surrounding the lateral ventricles, the third ventricle, hypothalamus and corpus striatum [Species: Mouse, approximate human age: 6 weeks, sagittal section]

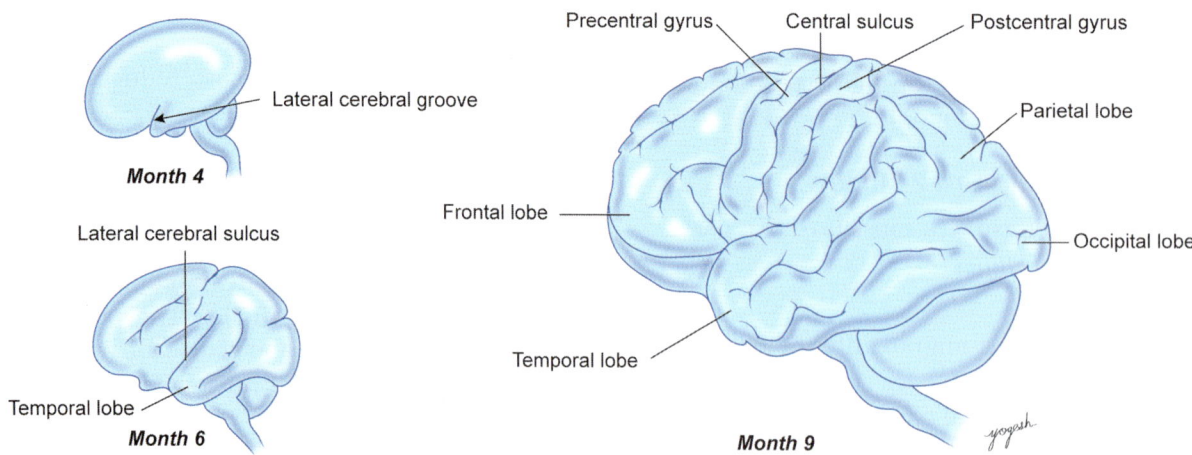

Fig. 22.17: Development of cerebral hemisphere during fetal life

Some Interesting Facts

- Brain of mature infant has 9–14 billion neurons.
- Only neuroglial cells continue to multiply after birth.
- Total surface of adult cerebral cortex is about 285,000 mm^2.

Commissures of Telencephalon (Fig. 22.18)

- Lamina terminalis is the cranial most part of telencephalon and it connects two cerebral hemispheres. Hence, commissural fibres that connect two cerebral hemispheres pass through lamina terminalis.^{MCQ}
- Thickened band of fibres develops in lamina terminalis as follows:
  1. *Anterior commissure* connects two temporal lobes.
  2. *Corpus callosum* connects right and left cerebral hemispheres. With the growth of cerebral hemispheres, the size of corpus callosum also increases and it gets separated from fornix by *septum pellucidum*.
  3. *Hippocampal (fornix) commissure*: Connects right and left hippocampus.
  4. *Posterior commissure* is essential for light reflex (connections not yet discovered fully).
  5. *Habenular commissure* connects habenular nuclei of both sides. Habenular nuclei are part of epithalamus.
  6. Optic chiasma.

Some Interesting Facts

- Neural tube is covered by loose mesenchymal tissue that forms arachnoid and dura mater.
- Neural crest cells form pia mater.
- Pia mater and arachnoid mater together form leptomeninges (soft meninges).
- Leptomeninges coalesce to form subarachnoid space.

Developmental Anomalies

- *Anencephaly* is 4 times more frequent in females and 4 times more frequent in whites.
- Anencephaly in last trimester of pregnancy is associated with hydramnios due to lack of swallowing mechanism in the fetus.
- *Encephalocele* is defective closure of neural groove. It results in the herniation of parts of brain under the skin through a hole in the skull.
- *Dandy-Walker malformation*: Atresia of foramina of Magendie and Luschka (that communicate 4th ventricle with subarachnoid space) result in dilation of 4th ventricle and agenesis of cerebellum.
- *Microcephaly*: It is underdeveloped brain causing gross mental retardation. It is autosomal recessive disorder or may be produced due to antenatal cytomegalovirus infection or exposure to radiation.
- *Arnold-Chiari malformation*: It is downward displacement of cerebellar tonsil through foramen magnum.

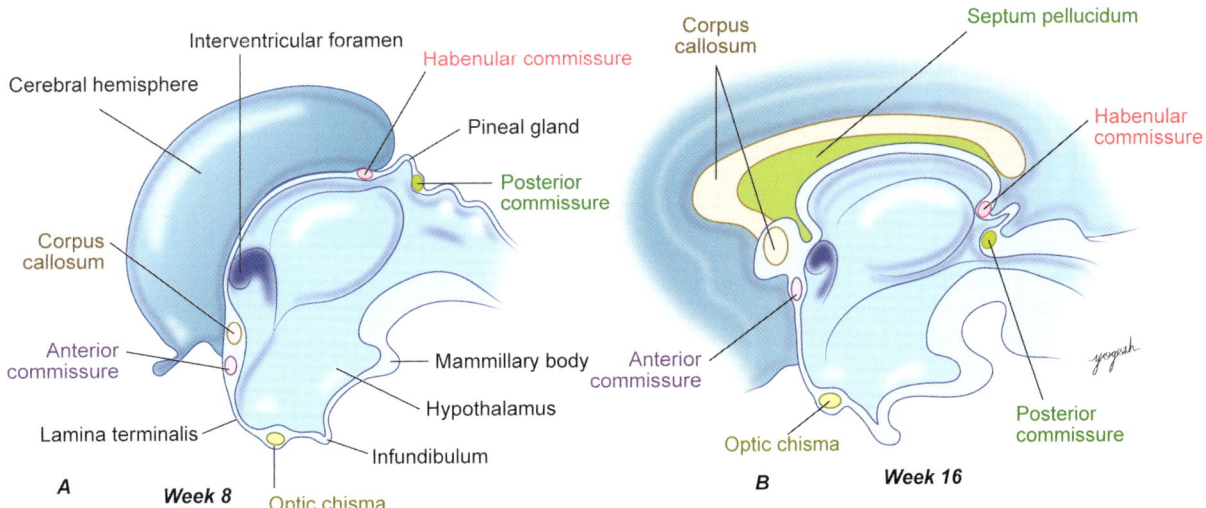

Fig. 22.18: Formation of commissures of telencephalon at 8 weeks: (A) and 16 weeks (B) For integration of the activity of right and left cerebral hemispheres, commissures play a key role

Clinical Embryology

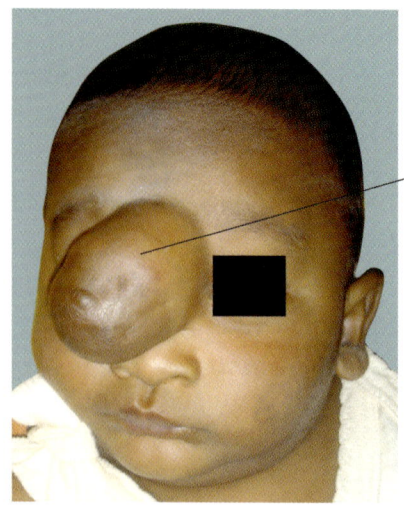

Clinical image 22.1: *Frontonasal (anterior) encephalocele* is a sac-like protrusion of the brain and meninges through a gap in the skull due to the failure of the neural tube closure (Image courtesy: *Dr Kumaravel S*)

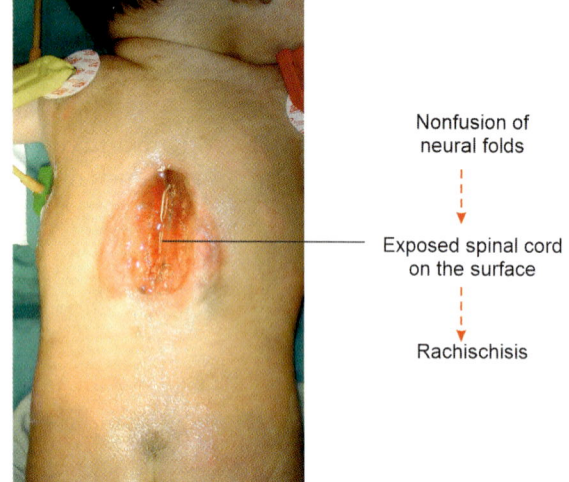

Clinical image 22.2: *Rachischisis.* Rachischisis is the severe neural tube defect that occurs due to failure of neural tube folding. In this defect, a portion of spinal cord is exposed on the surface and there is always failure of fusion of vertebral arches (spina bifida) due to nonfusion of neural folds. If rachischisis involves brain, it is called craniorachischisis or cranioschisis (Image courtesy: *Dr Kumaravel S*)

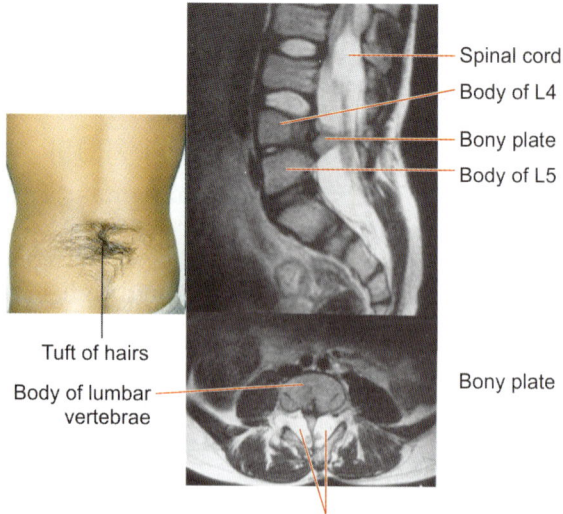

Clinical image 22.3: *Spina bifida occulta* with diastematomyelia. It occurs due to the failure of fusion of vertebral arches (neural arches) dorsally in the midline. Due to nonfusion, the spine becomes bifid and the defect is filled with connective tissue. Site of the defect usually shows a dimple and tuft of hairs. In this case, spina bifida occulta is present in the association of a bony plate arising from posterior surface of the body lumbar vertebrae. This bony plate splits the spinal cord into two halves hence called diastematomyelia or **split cord malformation** (Image courtesy: *Dr Kumaravel S*)

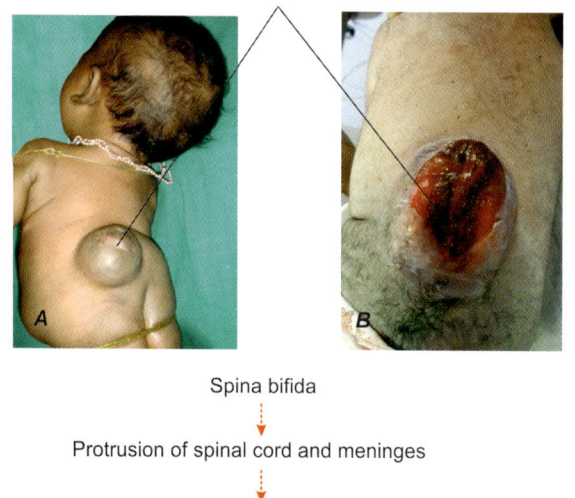

Clinical image 22.4: *Myelomeningocele.* It is a type of spina bifida (form of neural tube defect) in that spinal canal and backbone do not close. The spinal cord and the meninges along with tissue that covers spinal cord protrude through the skin on the back of newborn. Folic acid deficiency before and during early pregnancy may result in neural tube defects (Image courtesy: A: *Dr Adhisivam B*, B: *Dr Prakhar Mohniya*)

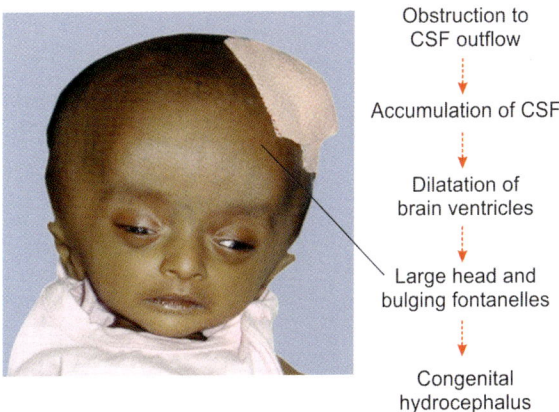

Clinical image 22.5: *Anencephaly with unilateral cleft lip and cleft palate.* A newborn with absence of a large part of brain and skull. Anencephaly occurs due to failure of closure at anterior neuropore of the neural tube. Cleft lip is a congenital split in the upper lip that occurs due to failure of fusion of the maxillary processes with the medial nasal process (part of frontonasal process). Cleft palate is a congenital split defect of the palate that causes communication between oral and nasal cavities. Cleft palate occurs due to the nonfusion of the median and lateral palatine processes (Image courtesy: *Dr Adhisivam B*)

Clinical image 22.7: *Congenital hydrocephalus.* It is caused by excessive cerebrospinal fluid (CSF) accumulation in brain ventricles and subarachnoid space. This causes increased intracranial pressure and increases size of the ventricles. Infants with hydrocephalus show an unusually large head and a bulging fontanelle (Image courtesy: *Dr Adhisivam B*)

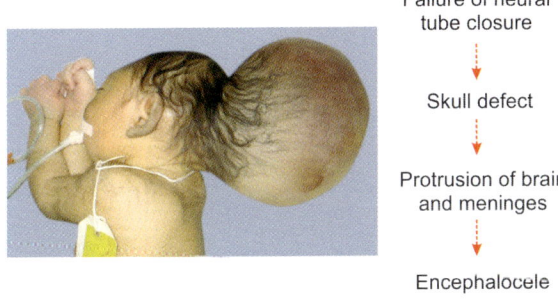

Clinical image 22.6: *Encephalocele* (cranium bifidum). It is neural tube defect having sac-like protrusions of brain with meninges through a defect in skull. It is caused by failure of neural tube to close completely during fetal development (Image courtesy: *Dr Adhisivam B*)

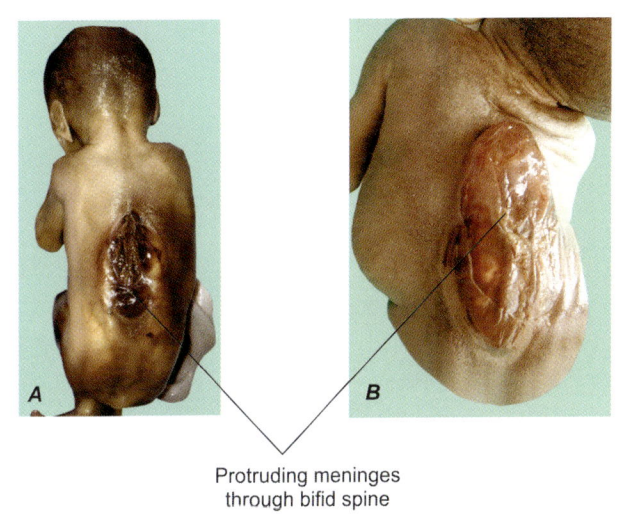

Clinical image 22.8: Meningocele (A and B are two separate cases). It is protruding arachnoid and pia mater (only meninges) through bifid spine that causes cystic swelling partially covered with skin (Image courtesy: *Dr Mamatha Gowda*)

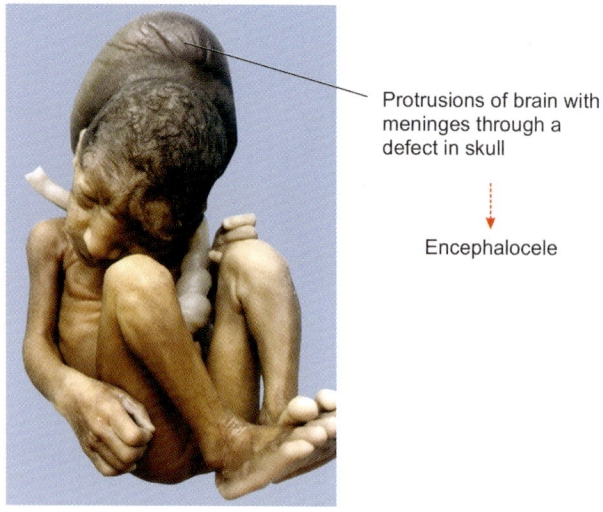

Protrusions of brain with meninges through a defect in skull

↓

Encephalocele

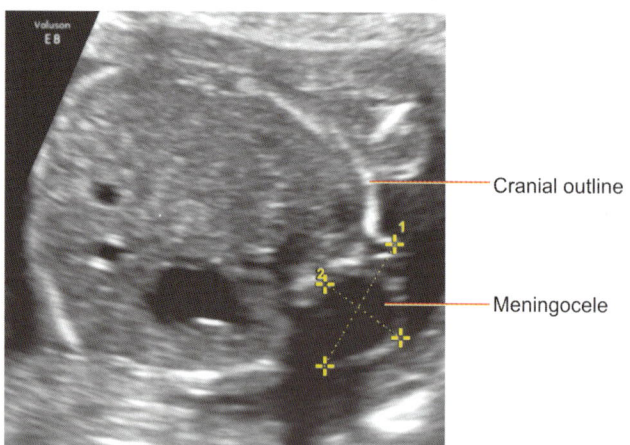

Cranial outline

Meningocele

Clinical image 22.9: Encephalocele (cranium bifidum). It is a neural tube defect having sac-like protrusions of brain with meninges through a defect in skull. It is caused by failure of neural tube to close completely during fetal development. (Image courtesy: *Dr Mamatha Gowda*)

Clinical image 22.10: Ultrasound image of invivo fetus showing encephalocele (cranium bifidum) (marked by yellow dotted line). Skull outline shows defect through that sac of meninges is protruding. Encephalocele/meningocele is protrusion of arachnoid and pia mater (only meninges) through bifid spine or skull defect that cause cystic swelling partially covered with skin. (Image courtesy: *Dr Mamatha Gowda*)

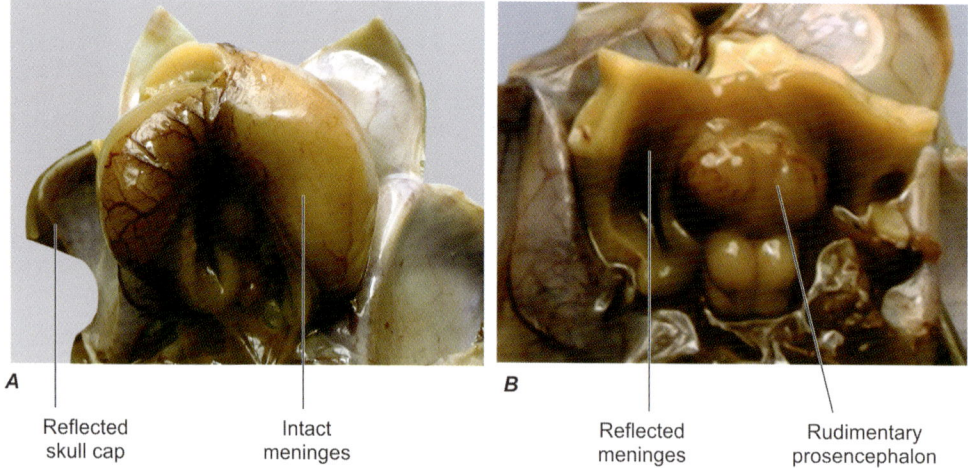

A

Reflected skull cap — Intact meninges

B

Reflected meninges — Rudimentary prosencephalon

Clinical image 22.11: Holoprosencephaly (HPE) is a cephalic disorder with failure of prosencephalon (the forebrain of the embryo) development. Normally, the forebrain is formed and face begins to develop in 5th–6th weeks of intrauterine life; (A) Skull coverings are dissected to show the intact meninges; (B) Meninges are dissected to expose brain – holoprosencephaly (Image courtesy: *Dr Mamatha Gowda*)

Chapter 23

Development of Eye

eSmartQuiz

Chapter Outline

Development of various parts of eyeball
- Cornea
- Lens
- Retina
- Optic nerve
- Sclera and choroid
- Ciliary body
- Iris
- Anterior and posterior chambers
- Vitreous
- Accessory structures of eyeball
  - Extraocular muscles
  - Eyelids and conjunctival sac
  - Lacrimal apparatus

Congenital anomalies of eye

Competency:
- **AN43.4:** Describe the developmental basis of congenital anomalies of face, palate, tongue, branchial apparatus, pituitary gland, thyroid gland, eye.
Development of eye is included in this chapter.

INTRODUCTION

- The eyeball development begins early in the 4th week of intrauterine life with formation of optic vesicle (a diverticulum) from diencephalon.
- Various components of eyeball are derived from the following sources:
  1. Retina, iris and optic nerves are derived from optic vesicle that arises from neuroectoderm of diencephalon.
  2. Lens and corneal epithelium are derived from lens placode that arises from surface ectoderm.
  3. Fibrous and vascular coats of eyeball are derived from mesodermal condensation surrounding the optic vesicle.
  4. Choroid and sclera are derived from migrating neural crest cells.
- The structure of eyeball is shown in Fig. 23.1.

Optic Vesicle and Lens Vesicle

- *Formation of optic sulcus:* On 22nd day, wall of the diencephalon shows thickening and depression to form *optic sulcus*.^{MCQ} Formation of the optic sulcus or groove is the first indication for development of the eye (Fig. 23.2A, Practice Fig. 23.1).^{NEXT}
- *Formation of optic vesicle:* Optic sulcus further invaginates laterally in the surrounding mesoderm and form a bulging called *optic vesicle* (Fig. 23.2B).
- *Formation of optic stalk:* Optic vesicles grow laterally but remain connected to forebrain by a stalk-like structure called *optic stalk* (Fig. 23.2B).
- *Formation of lens placode:* Optic vesicle meets surface ectoderm. In region of contact, the surface ectoderm forms localized thickening called *lens placode* (Fig. 23.2B).
- *Formation of lens vesicle:* Lens placode depresses to form *lens pit* and later, *lens vesicle* (Fig. 23.3A, Practice Fig. 23.2).
- Lens vesicle loses contact with surface ectoderm by 33rd day.
- *Formation of optic cup:* Lens vesicle invaginates the optic vesicle and converts it to a double-layered *optic cup* (Fig. 23.3B).
- By 6th week, margins of the optic cup overgrow and cover lens vesicle except on caudal side of the lens and partly on caudal surface of optic stalk. This gap is called *choroidal fissure* or fetal fissure (Fig. 23.3B).^{MCQ}
- In a mesodermal encroachment along the choroidal fissure, *hyaloid vessels* develop that supply optic and

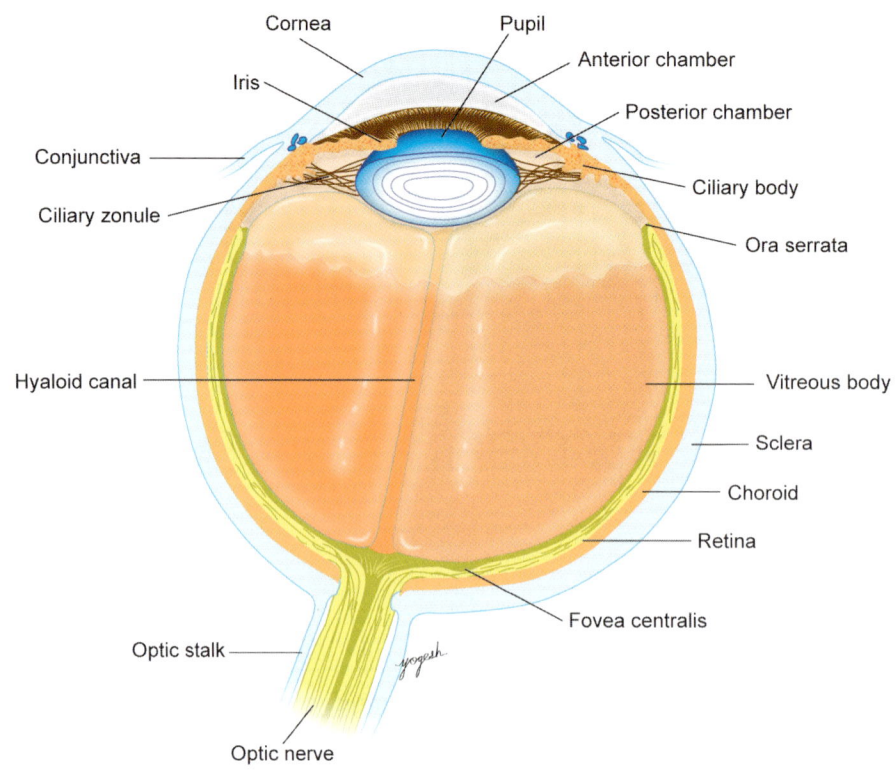

Fig. 23.1: Fully developed eyeball

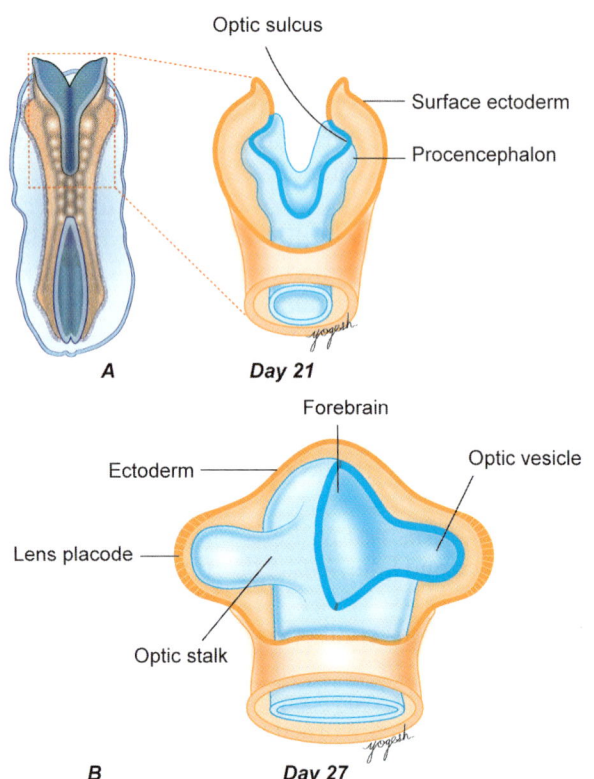

Fig. 23.2: Development of eyeball on day 21 and 27

lens vesicles. The distal part of hyaloid vessels degenerates, whereas the proximal parts from *central artery of retina* and *central vein of retina* (Fig. 23.4).

DEVELOPMENT OF VARIOUS PARTS OF EYEBALL

Cornea

- Cornea consists of outer stratified squamous epithelium resting on basement membrane, lamina propria, Descemet's membrane, and inner corneal epithelium.
- All these layers are derived from the following sources:
  1. Surface ectoderm forms outer stratified squamous epithelium and its basement membrane (Bowman's layer). ^{NEXT}
  2. Lamina propria or stroma is derived from mesoderm.
  3. Neural crest cells form Descemet's membrane and inner corneal epithelium (Practice Figs 23.1, 23.2). ^{NEXT}

Lens

- Lens is a transparent, biconvex structure that lies between aqueous and vitreous of the eyeball.
- Lens has three main parts:
  1. Lens capsule
  2. Lens epithelium (simple cuboidal epithelium)
  3. Lens fibers

Stages of Development

- By 33rd day of IUL, lens vesicle gets separated from surface ectoderm.

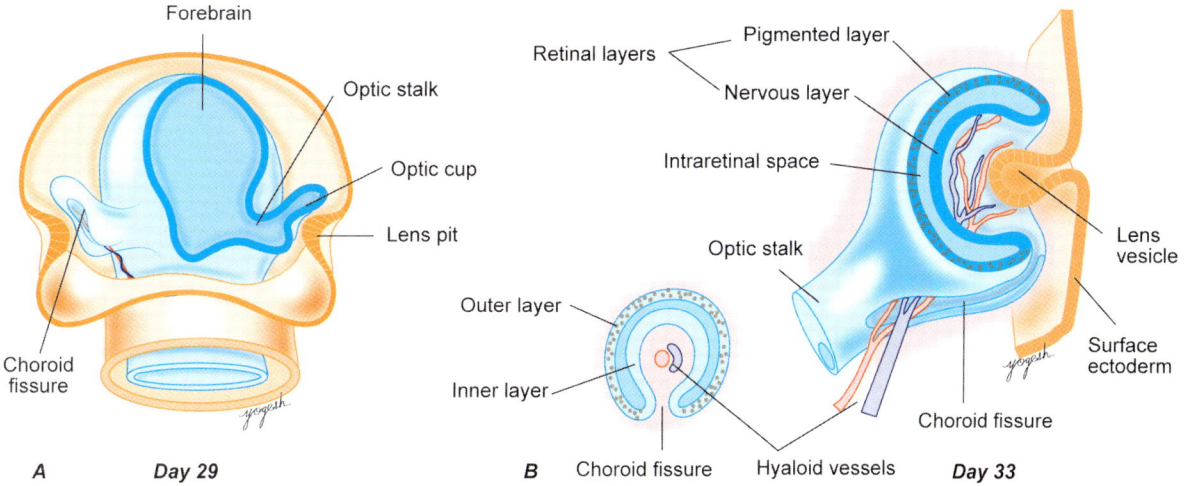

Fig. 23.3: Further development of eyeball (day 29 and day 33)

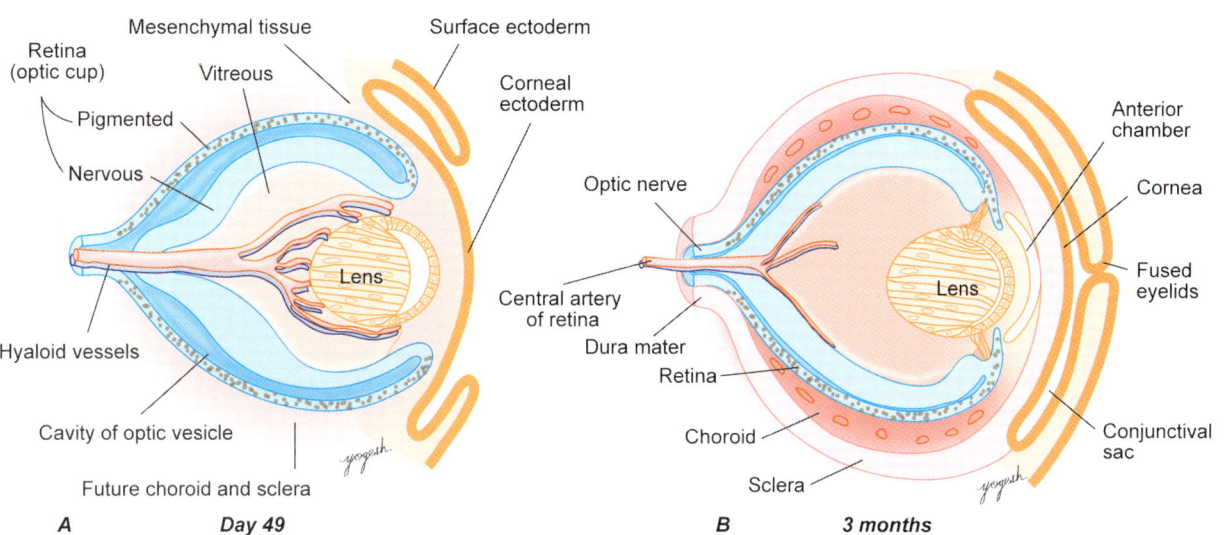

Fig. 23.4: Further development of eyeball (day 49 and 3 months)

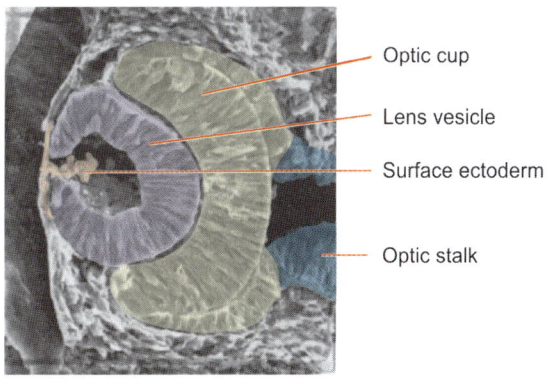

Scanning electron micrograph 23.1: SEM showing developing eye. The invaginating lens placode forms lens vesicle that pinches off surface ectoderm. Invagination of optic vesicle forms bilayer optic cup that remains connected to forebrain via optic stalk [Species: Mouse, approximate human age: 36 days, coronal section]

- Initially lens vesicle is lined by a single layer of cuboidal epithelium (Fig. 23.5D).

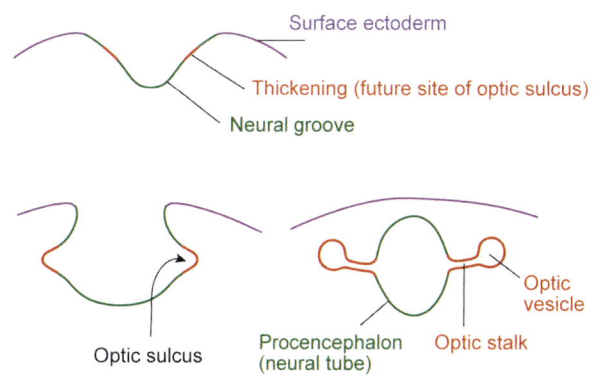

Practice Fig. 23.1: Formation of optic vesicle

- Cells of ventral wall of lens vesicle remain cuboidal. Cells of deep wall of lens vesicle elongate, become columnar, and occupy cavity of the lens vesicle (Fig. 23.5E).
- These elongated cells of posterior wall lose their nuclei and form transparent *primary lens fibers* (Fig. 23.5F).

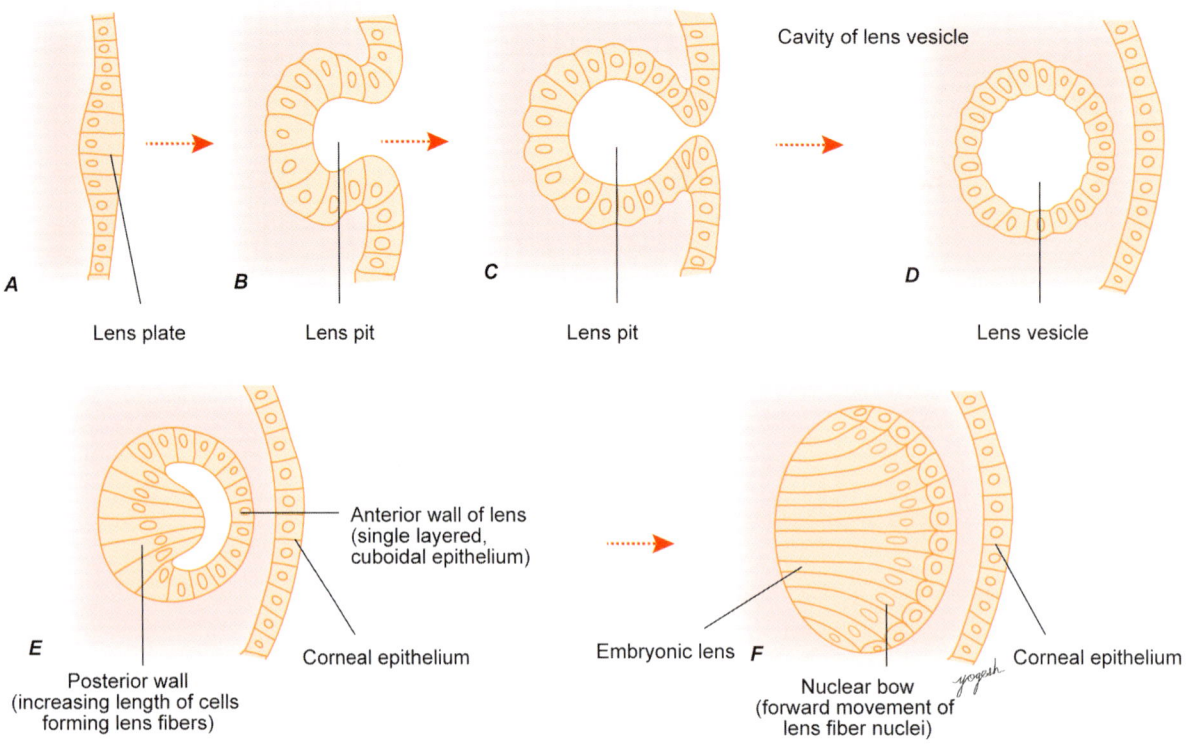

Fig. 23.5: Development of the embryonic lens

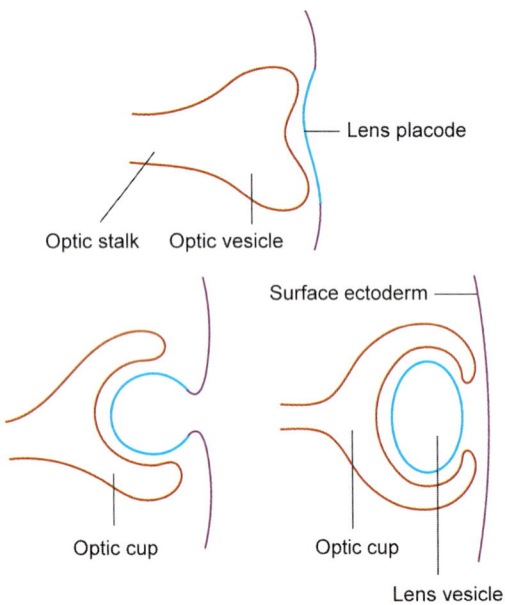

Practice Fig. 23.2: Formation of lens vesicle

- The equatorial cells continue to contribute new lens fibers and lens grow. These fibers later become hard and form *secondary lens fibers*.
- Cells of anterior wall persist and form *epithelium of lens*.
- On degeneration of hyaloid artery (that supplies lens), lens becomes avascular structure.
- In 7th week, solid lens is formed.^MCQ

Congenital Cataract

- Congenital cataract is an opacity of lens that is present at birth.

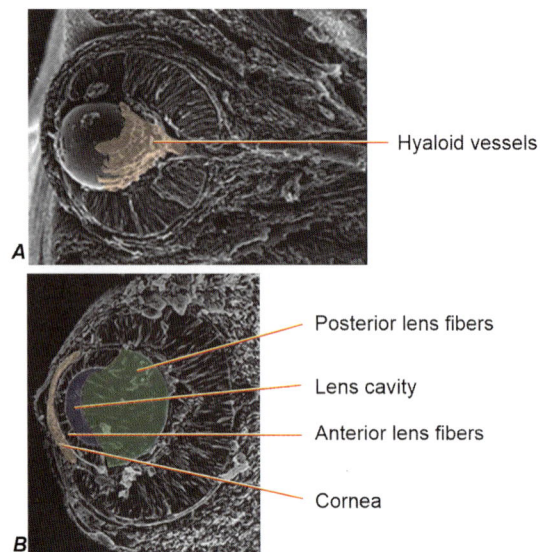

Scanning electron micrograph 23.2: Developing eye: (A) The hyaloid vasculature surrounds the back of the lens; (B) Following separation of the lens from the surface, the posterior lens fibers elongate to obliterate the lens cavity and the cornea begins to differentiate. [Species: Mouse, approximate human age: 7 weeks, coronal section]

- Congenital cataract may be unilateral or bilateral
- Causes: It may be due to rubella virus, toxoplasmosis infection, Down syndrome or inborn error of metabolism such as galactosemia.
- Treatment: Congenital cataract can be treated surgically. Bilateral congenital cataract should be removed before the age of 10 weeks.

Retina

- Cellular layers of retina from outside inwards include:
  1. Pigmented cell layer
  2. Layer of rods and cones
  3. Bipolar neuron layer
  4. Ganglionic cell layer
- All these layers are derived from the optic cup.

Stages of Development

- From wall of diencephalon, optic vesicle arises that grows laterally but remains connected by optic stalk with the diencephalon (Fig. 23.2B).
- Optic vesicle comes in contact with lens vesicle and forms optic cup (Fig. 23.3).
- Optic cup has two parts – anterior and posterior.
- Anterior part of optic cup forms an epithelial covering of ciliary body and iris.
- Posterior part of optic cup forms various layers of retina as follows:
  - Outer wall: Forms pigmented layer of retina.
  - Inner wall: Differentiates into three layers:
    1. Matrix layer – forms rods and cones.
    2. Mantle layer – forms bipolar cells and ganglionic cells as well as other neurons of retina.
    3. Marginal layer – forms optic nerve. Axons of ganglion cells form marginal layer that converges towards optic stalk and finally, forms optic nerve.
- Space between outer and inner wall of the optic cup is called *intraretinal space*. This space gets obliterated by increasing number of retinal neurons.

Optic Nerve

- Optic stalk contains
  1. Hyaloid artery and vein
  2. Axons of ganglionic cell layer
- On inferior (caudal) surface of optic stalk, choroid fissure is present, that closes by 7th week.
- Later, optic stalk forms optic nerve, whereas hyaloid vessels form central artery and vein of retina.

Congenital Retinal Detachment

- It involves separation of pigmented epithelium from neuronal layers of the retina.
- Congenital retinal detachment mostly occurs as an autosomal recessive disorder.
- It results in permanent blindness from birth.

Sclera and Choroid

- Sclera (white of eye) is opaque, fibrous protective outermost layer of eyeball.
- Choroid is a vascular coat of eyeball that lies between outer sclera and inner retina.
- During the 6th and 7th weeks, mesenchyme that surrounds external surface of optic cup condenses into two layers:
  a. Outer fibrous layer that forms sclera.
  b. Inner vascular layer that forms choroid.
- Choroid is anteriorly continuous with ciliary body and posteriorly with pia and arachnoid mater.
- Sclera is anteriorly continuous with substantia propria or stroma of the cornea and posteriorly with dura mater covering optic nerve.

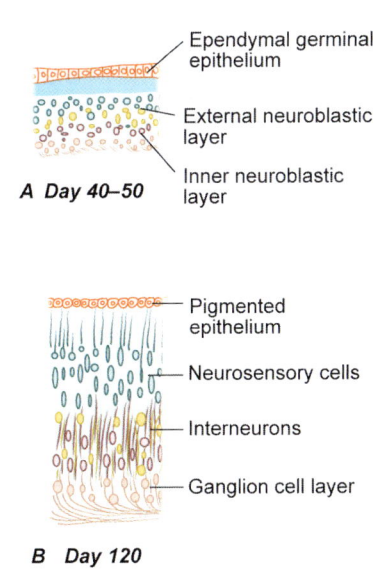

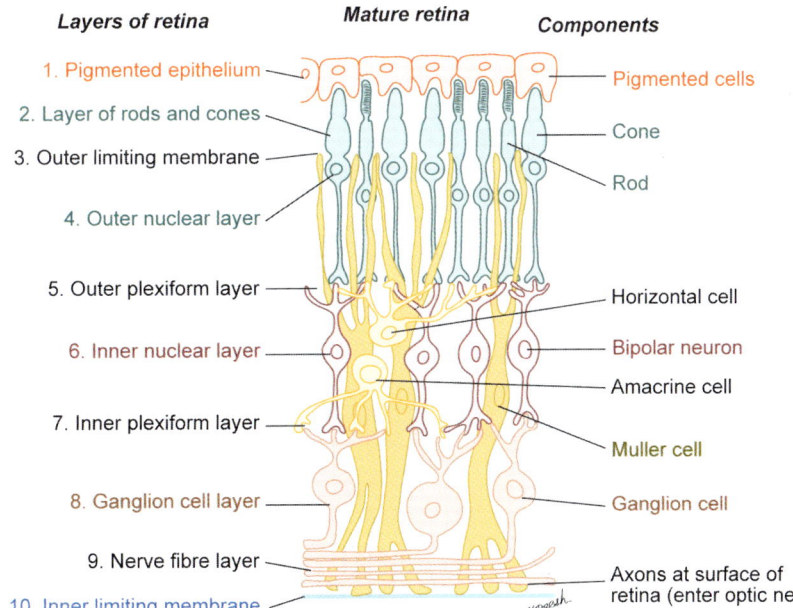

Fig. 23.6: Histogenesis of retina

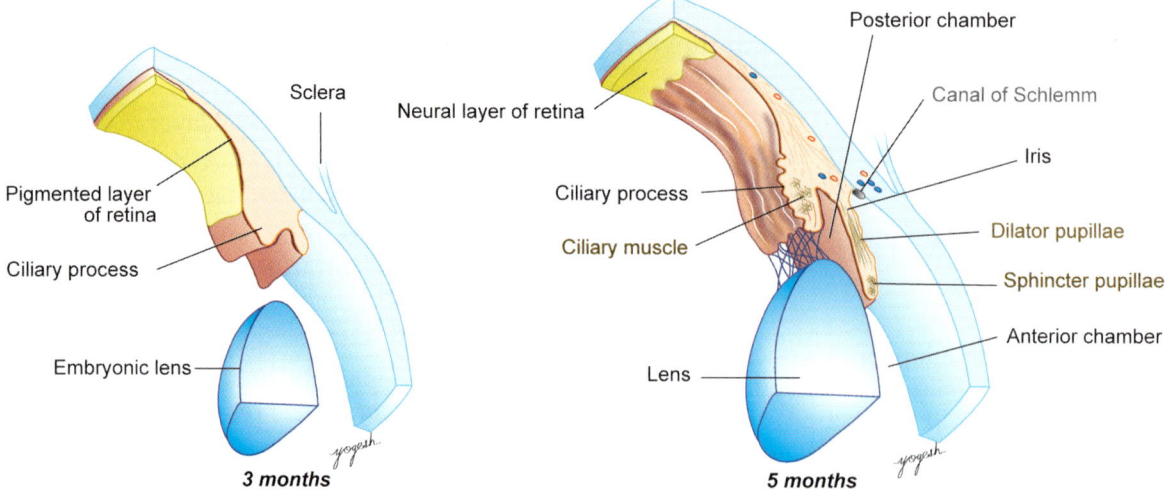

Fig. 23.7: Development of the iris and ciliary body

Ciliary Body

- Ciliary body is a ring-shaped mass that divides eyeball and separates aqueous humour from vitreous.
- It consists of *ciliary muscle* that controls shape of the lens.
- Ciliary body shows folding of epithelium called *ciliary processes* that secret the *aqueous humour*.
- Mesoderm surrounding the anterior part of optic cup forms *ciliary muscle* and connective tissues of ciliary body.
- Pigmented epithelial lining of inner aspect of ciliary body and ciliary processes is derived from outer layer of the optic cup; hence, continuous with pigmented layer of retina.
- The nonpigmented layer of epithelium covering deeper side of ciliary body is derived from inner layer of optic cup and continuous with neuronal layers of retina.

Iris

- Iris is a thin, circular structure in eyeball that controls size of the pupil.
- Iris shows anterior limiting layer, stroma, sphincter and dilator papillae muscles, and posterior pigmented epithelium.
- Iris develops from anterior extension of optic cup.
- Epithelium (anterior and posterior) of iris is derived from double layered optic cup.
- Neuroectodermal cells of optic cup also give rise to muscles of the iris.
- Stoma of the iris is derived from neural crest cells.
- Color of eye/pigmented layer of cornea depends on genetic constitution of an individual.

Anterior and Posterior Chambers of Eye

- Anterior and posterior chambers are similar to subarachnoid space of brain.^{MCQ}
- Mesoderm located between lens and cornea splits to form spaces. These spaces split into anterior and posterior chambers by developing *iris* and *pupillary membrane*.
- As pupillary membrane disappears, anterior chamber communicates with posterior chamber through pupil.
- Epithelium of ciliary process starts secreting *aqueous humour* that fills anterior and posterior chambers of eyeball.
- Sclera of sinus venosus forms a network of trabecular meshwork at sclerocorneal junction along the circumference of anterior chamber. These later form canal of Schlemm and drain aqueous humour. [Canal is named after Friedrich Schlemm (1795–1858), a German anatomist.]

Vitreous

- Vitreous occupies chamber of eyeball called *vitreous chamber*.
- Vitreous is a transparent, gelatinous mass that forms about 45% volume of the eyeball.
- Vitreous develops as follows:
  - *Primary vitreous humour* develops from neural crest cells of optic cup.
  - *Secondary vitreous humour* replaces the primary vitreous. Secondary vitreous humour is derived from inner layer of optic cup and lens vesicle.
- Vitreous humour is supplied by hyaloid artery that later gets obliterated.^{NEXT}

Accessory Structures of Eyeball

Extraocular Muscles

- Each eyeball has 6 extraocular muscles, namely superior rectus, inferior rectus, medial rectus, lateral rectus, superior oblique, and inferior oblique muscles (levator palpebrae superioris muscle for eyelid).
- All extraocular muscles are derived from *preoccipital myotomes* and hence, supplied by 3rd, 4th and 6th cranial nerves.^{NEXT}

Eyelids and conjunctival sac

- Eyelids are developed by folds of surface ectoderm that raise above and below the cornea.
- These ectodermal folds contain some mesoderm that gives raise to tarsal plate and other connective tissue of eyelids.
- Eyelashes and glands of eyelids develop from surface ectoderm.
- Surface ectoderm that lines inner surface of eyelids and covers eyeball form conjunctival sac.
- Eyelids remain fused till 28th week of IUL and later get separated.^{MCQ}

Lacrimal apparatus

- It consists of lacrimal gland, lacrimal sac and nasolacrimal ducts.
- Lacrimal gland is derived from 15 to 20 buds that grow at superolateral angle of conjunctival sac.
  - Nasolacrimal duct and lacrimal sac develop from naso-optic furrow (nasolacrimal furrow) (refer to Chapter 12, development of face).
  - Lacrimal canaliculi develop from canalization of ectodermal buds that raise from medial margins of eyelids. Later these canaliculi develop communication with lacrimal sac.

CONGENITAL ANOMALIES OF EYE

1. *Anophthalmia* is absence of eyeball due to failure of optic vesicle formation.
2. *Microphthalmia* is small eye due to under developed optic vesicle. It may be due to rubella virus, cytomegalovirus, toxoplasma or other intrauterine infections. PAX6 gene performs key-regulatory role in the development of eye. PAX6 gene mutation results in aniridia or microphthalmia.
3. *Cyclopia* is a presence of single median eye. It occurs due to fusion of two optic vesicles (synophthalmia). Single eye may be connected with face by a tubular stalk called *proboscis*. Inhibition of sonic hedgehog (SHH) gene may result in cyclops.
4. *Coloboma of iris*: Due to failure of fusion of choroid fissure, iris shows a cleft on inferior side (keyhole appearance). This condition is called coloboma of iris (coloboma = missing part, Greek) (Clinical image 23.10).
5. *Persistent papillary membrane:* Pupil may be covered partially or completely by persistent papillary membrane.
6. *Congenital aniridia* is complete absence of *iris* due to an arrest of development of optic cup.
7. *Congenital aphakia* is absence of *lens* of eyeball due to failure of formation of lens vesicle.
8. *Coloboma of eyelid* is absence of part of the eyelid.
9. Mutation of PAX2 gene results in optic nerve colobomas and renal aplasia.
10. Entropion is inward-turned eyelids, whereas ectropion is outward turned eyelids.
11. *Epicanthus* is a crescentic fold of skin that extends from upper eyelid to canthus. It is a feature of Mongolian races and Down syndrome (trisomy 21).
12. *Cryptophthalmos* is absence of eyelids and palpebral fissures. The eyeball is covered by skin.
13. *Congenital ptosis* (drooping of eyelid) occurs due to failure of development of levator palpebrae superioris muscle.

Table 23.1 Development of eye

Part	Embryological source
1. Cornea	Epithelium: Surface ectoderm^{NEXT} Other layers: Neural crest
2. Lens	Lens vesicle (surface ectoderm)
3. Retina	Optic cup (neuroectoderm)
4. Optic nerve	Optic stalk (neuroectoderm)
5. Sclera and choroid	Mesoderm surrounding optic cup
6. Ciliary body and muscle	Mesoderm
7. Iris	Mesoderm
8. Muscles of iris	Neuroectoderm optic cup
9. Extraocular muscles	Preoccipital myotomes
10. Eyelids, conjunctival sac	Surface ectoderm
11. Lacrimal glands	Surface ectoderm
12. Lacrimal sac and nasolacrimal duct	Ectoderm of naso-optic furrow

Some Interesting Facts

- The following parts of eye are also derived from neural crest cells: Trabecular meshwork, stroma of cornea, iris, ciliary body, choroid, melanocytes of conjunctiva, and muscle layer of orbital blood vessels, meningeal sheath of optic nerve, *sclera*, and part of vitreous.^{NEXT}
- Epithelium of cornea and conjunctiva, crystalline lens, lacrimal and tarsal glands are derived from *surface ectoderm*.^{NEXT}
- Iris and ciliary body epithelia, *epithelium and muscles of iris (constrictor and dilator pupillae)*, retina, vitreous, optic nerve, *optic cup*, vesicle are derived from *neuroectoderm*.^{NEXT}
- Optic cup forms retina.^{NEXT}
- Melanocytes of iris develop from neural crest cells.^{NEXT}
- Ocular structures (sclera, iris, corneal stroma) develop from somatic layer of lateral plate mesoderm.^{NEXT}

Clinical Embryology

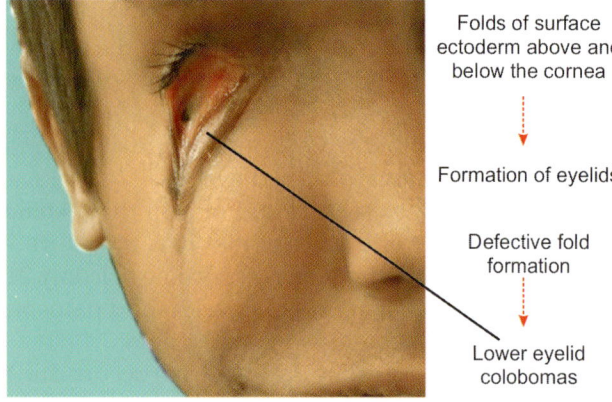

Clinical image 23.1: Lower eyelid colobomas is defect in the formation of eyelid. It is caused by failure of fusion of the mesodermal lid folds. As compared to upper lid colobomas, lower lid defects are encountered less frequently but when they occur, they are seen in the lateral half of the lid in association with Treacher Collins syndrome (mandibulofacial dysostosis) which is autosomal dominant with variable penetrance and expressivity (Image courtesy: *Dr Rohit Rao*)

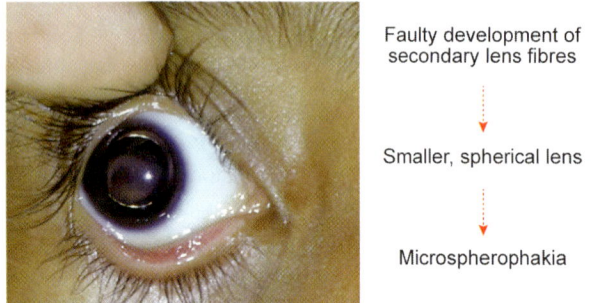

Clinical image 23.2: *Microspherophakia*. In microspherophakia, lens of the eye is smaller than normal and spherically shaped. With widely dilated pupil, entire lens equator can be visualised at the slit lamp examination. Faulty development of the secondary lens fibers during embryogenesis may produce microspherophakia. The spherical shape of the lens results in increased refractive power (highly myopic eye), causing secondary angle-closure glaucoma. Microspherophakia is most often seen as a part of Weill-Marchesani syndrome. This condition may also occur as an isolated hereditary abnormality or, occasionally, in association with Peters anomaly, Marfan syndrome, Alport syndrome, Lowe syndrome, or congenital rubella (Image courtesy: *Dr Rohit Rao*)

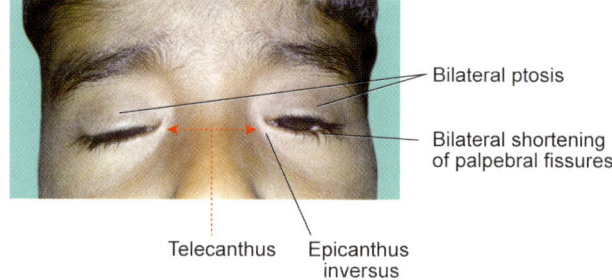

Clinical image 23.3: *Blepharophimosis*. It is an uncommon dysmorphic syndrome, which primarily affects the soft tissues of the mid-face. It is a condition that shows bilateral shortening of palpebral fissures (eyelid opening) with bilateral ptosis and epicanthus inversus syndrome. In blepharophimosis, the eyes are also spaced more widely apart than usual (telecanthus). Autosomal dominant inheritance with up to 50% happened sporadically (Image courtesy: *Dr Rohit Rao*)

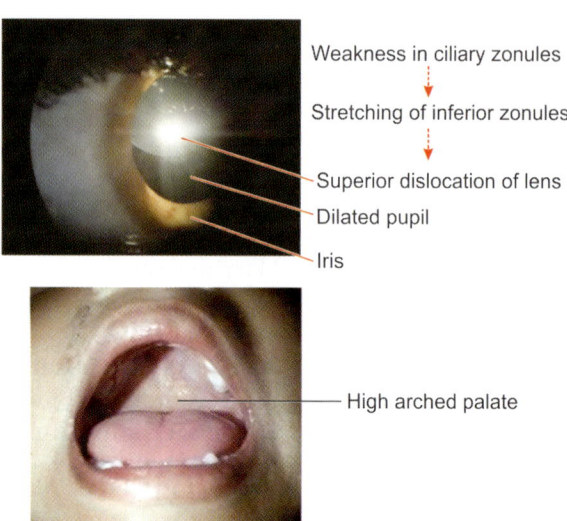

Clinical image 23.4: *Superior dislocation of lens* may be due to Marfan syndrome. In Marfan syndrome, the lens dislocates superiorly because of weakness in the ciliary zonules (the connective tissue strands that suspend the lens within the eye), and stretching of inferior zonules. In the same case, high arched palate (that another typical feature of Marfan syndrome) is observed (Image courtesy: *Dr Rohit Rao*)

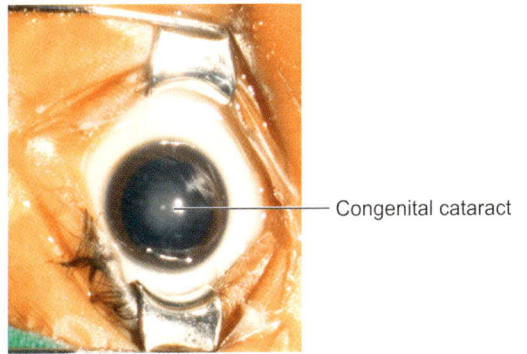

Clinical image 23.5: *Congenital cataract*. In the present case, congenital cataract is present in the form of lamellar or zonular form (the common morphological form in congenital cataract) (Image courtesy: *Dr Subashini K*)

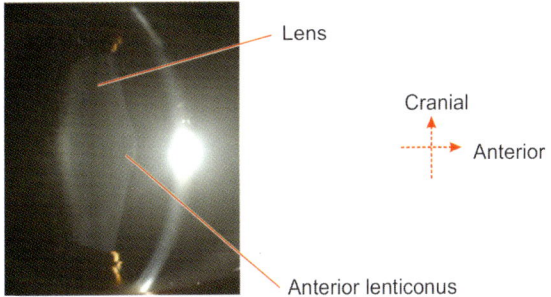

Clinical image 23.6: *Anterior lenticonus*. Lenticonus (a rare congenital anomaly) is characterised by a transparent, localised, conical protrusion on crystalline lens capsule, may be anterior or posterior. It causes a decrease in visual acuity and irregular refraction (Image courtesy: *Dr Subashini K*)

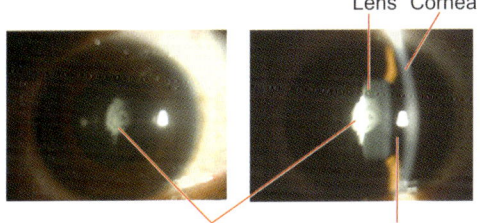

Clinical image 23.7: *Congenital cataract*. In the present case, congenital cataract is present in the form of posterior polar cataract. A dense plaque (disc-shaped opacity with onion-like ringed appearance like an onion) in the central posterior part of the lens is present (Image courtesy: *Dr Subashini K*)

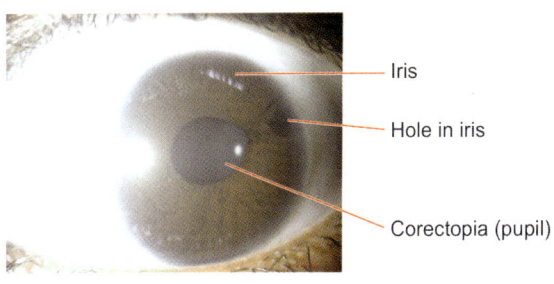

Clinical image 23.8: *Rieger's anomaly* (anterior segment dysgenesis). Rieger's anomaly is a congenital anomaly of the eye caused by anterior segment dysgenesis. It shows atrophy of the iris stroma, with hole or pseudo-hole formation and corectopia (displacement of pupil from its normal central position) or polycoria (one pupillary opening in the iris). It is associated glaucoma (Image courtesy: *Dr Subashini K*)

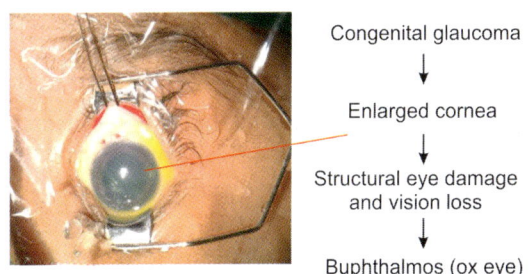

Clinical image 23.9: *Buphthalmos* (ox eye). Congenital glaucoma results in enlarged cornea and haze. Glaucoma is an elevated pressure within the eye that leads to structural eye damage and vision loss. Congenital glaucoma is also associated with horizontal breaks in the Descemet membrane called Haab's striae (Descemet's tears) (Image courtesy: *Dr Subashini K*)

• Development of Eye

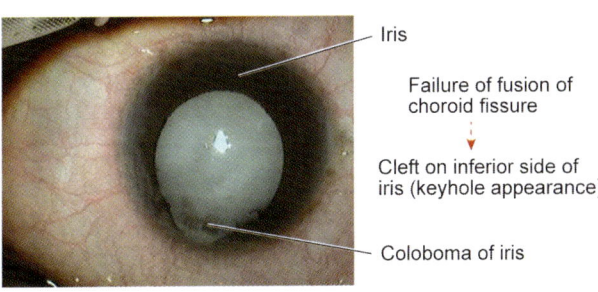

Clinical image 23.10: *Coloboma of iris* (Image courtesy: *Dr Rohit Rao*)

Chapter 24

Development of Ear

eSmartQuiz

Chapter Outline

- Development of internal ear
  - Membranous labyrinth
  - Bony labyrinth
  - Histogenesis of internal ear
- Middle ear
- External ear
  - External acoustic meatus
  - Auricle
- Molecular regulation
- Developmental anomalies

INTRODUCTION

- Ear is the organ of special sense that helps in hearing as well as maintenance of equilibrium.
- Anatomically, ear, has three parts: External ear, middle ear and internal ear.
- External ear includes auricle and external acoustic meatus. Tympanic membrane separates external ear from middle ear.
- Middle ear communicates anteriorly with nasopharynx through auditory tube and posteriorly with mastoid antrum through aditus.
- Internal ear consists of outer bony labyrinth and inner membranous labyrinth.
- Bony labyrinth lies in petrous part of temporal bone and it contains perilymph.
- Membranous labyrinth has cochlear duct, saccule, utricle and three semicircular ducts. Cochlear duct possesses organ of Corti that is responsible for hearing.
- Saccule and utricle possess maculae, whereas semicircular canals possess cristae ampullaris. Maculae and cristae ampullaris help to maintain equilibrium.
- Development of ear involves all three germ layers:
  - Surface ectoderm forms internal and external ear.
  - Endoderm forms middle ear.
  - Mesoderm forms connective tissue, cartilages bone (ossicles), and muscles of ear.

DEVELOPMENT OF INTERNAL EAR

- Inner ear develops from an ectodermal *otic vesicle* (Fig. 24.1, Scanning electron micrograph 24.1).
- Developmentally, internal ear consists of membranous labyrinth and bony labyrinth.

Membranous Labyrinth

Stages of Development (Flowchart 24.1)

- In the 4th week, surface ectoderm shows two thickenings called *otic placodes* (Fig. 24.1).
- Otic placode appears on each side of underlying rhombencephalon.
- Otic placode invaginates into underlying mesenchyme to form *otic pit*.
- Soon, otic pit forms *otic vesicle* or *otocyst* and lose the contact with surface ectoderm to move deep toward rhombencephalon.
- Oval-shaped otic vesicle gives rise to membranous labyrinth.
- Otocyst (otic vesicle) is divided into (Fig. 24.2):
  1. Dorsal vestibular part
  2. Ventral cochlear part
- Cochlear part gives rise to saccule and cochlear duct (organ of Corti).
- Vestibular part gives rise to utricle, semicircular ducts, endolymphatic duct, and endolymphatic sac.

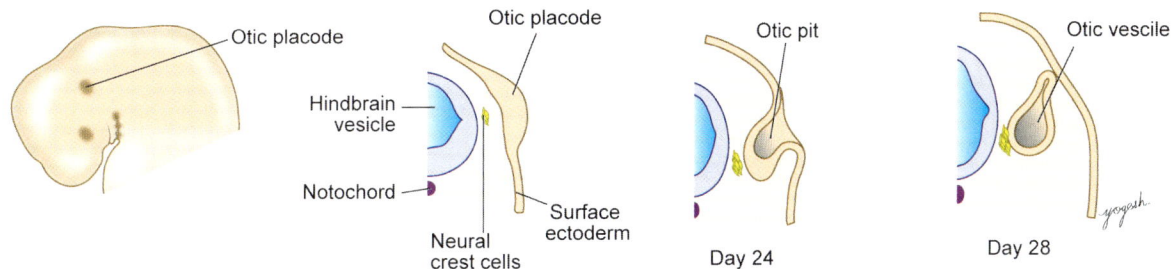

Fig. 24.1: Formation of otic vesicle

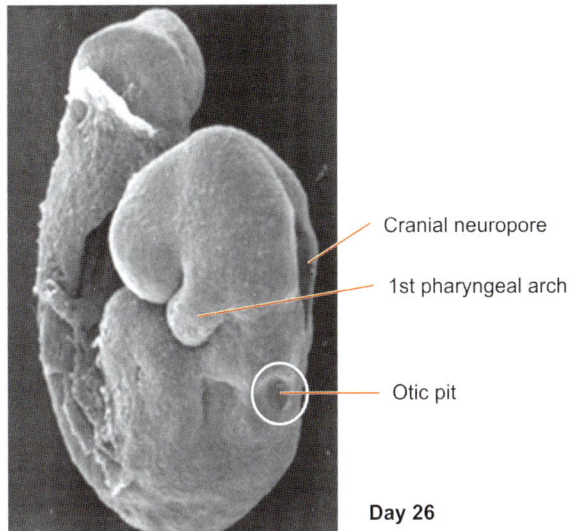

Scanning electron micrograph 24.1: The otic pit forms as this thickened (placodal) ectoderm invaginates. [Species: Mouse, approximate human age: 26 days, dorsolateral view]

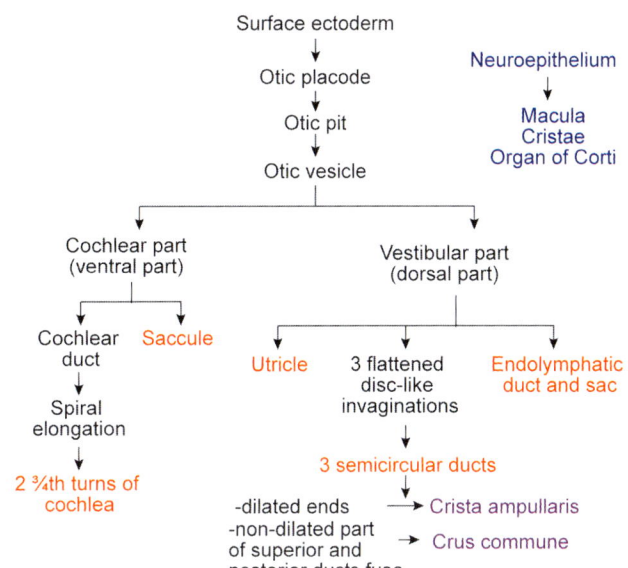

Flowchart 24.1: Development of membranous labyrinth. *Note:* Semicircular canals develop in the following sequence: First superior, then lateral (horizontal) followed by posterior

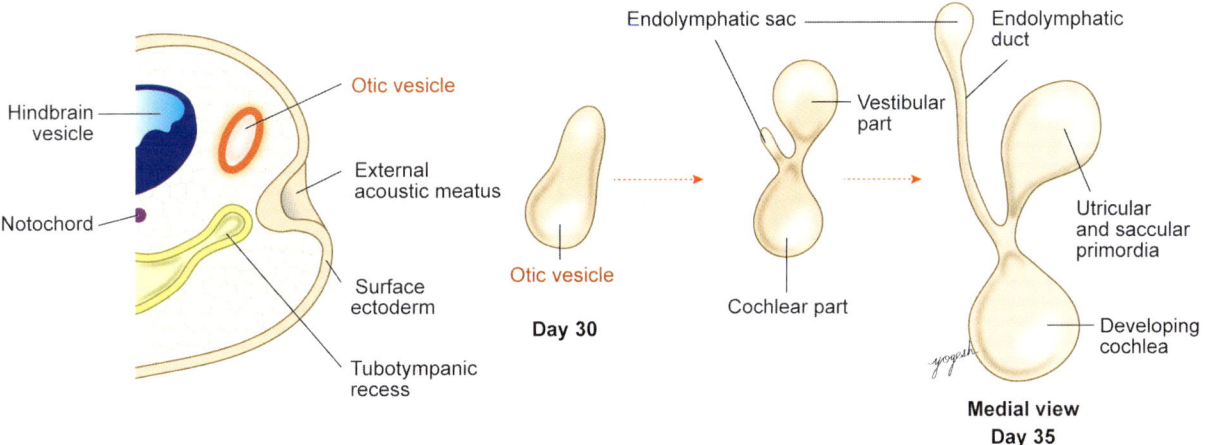

Fig. 24.2: Early development of otic vesicle

- Epithelium of membranous labyrinth modifies to form:
  1. Cristae of semicircular ducts for sense of equilibrium
  2. Macula of utricle for sense of equilibrium
  3. Organ of Corti of cochlea for hearing
  4. Macula of saccule for equilibrium

- Neural crest cells migrated toward otic vesicle give rise to bipolar neurons of vestibulo-cochlear ganglion.
- Peripheral process of bipolar neurons reaches the otic vesicle and gets communicated with saccule, utricle, semicircular ducts, and spiral organ of Corti (Fig. 24.3).

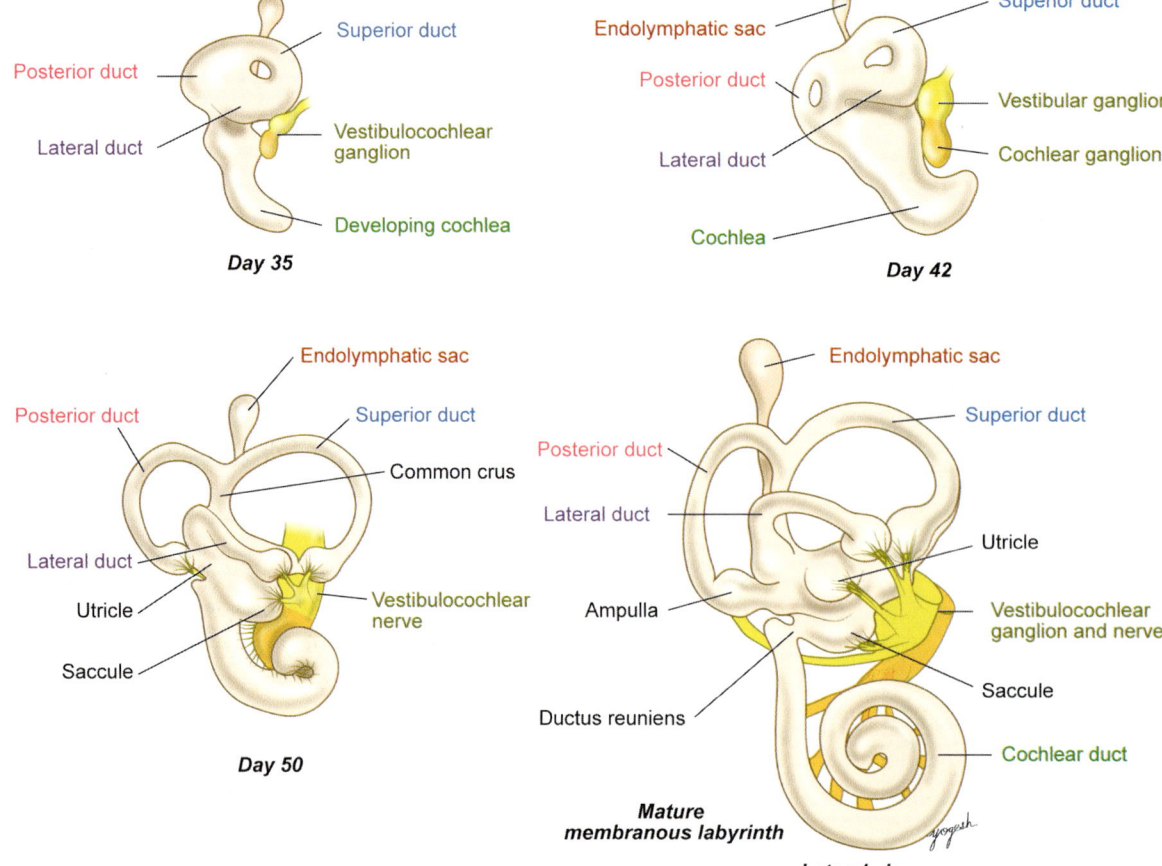

Fig. 24.3: Development of membranous labyrinth

- Central processes of bipolar neurons grow toward vestibular and cochlear nuclei of hindbrain to form vestibulocochlear nerve.

Bony Labyrinth

- Mesenchymal tissue surrounding the otic vesicle (membranous labyrinth) condenses to form *otic capsule* (Fig. 24.4).

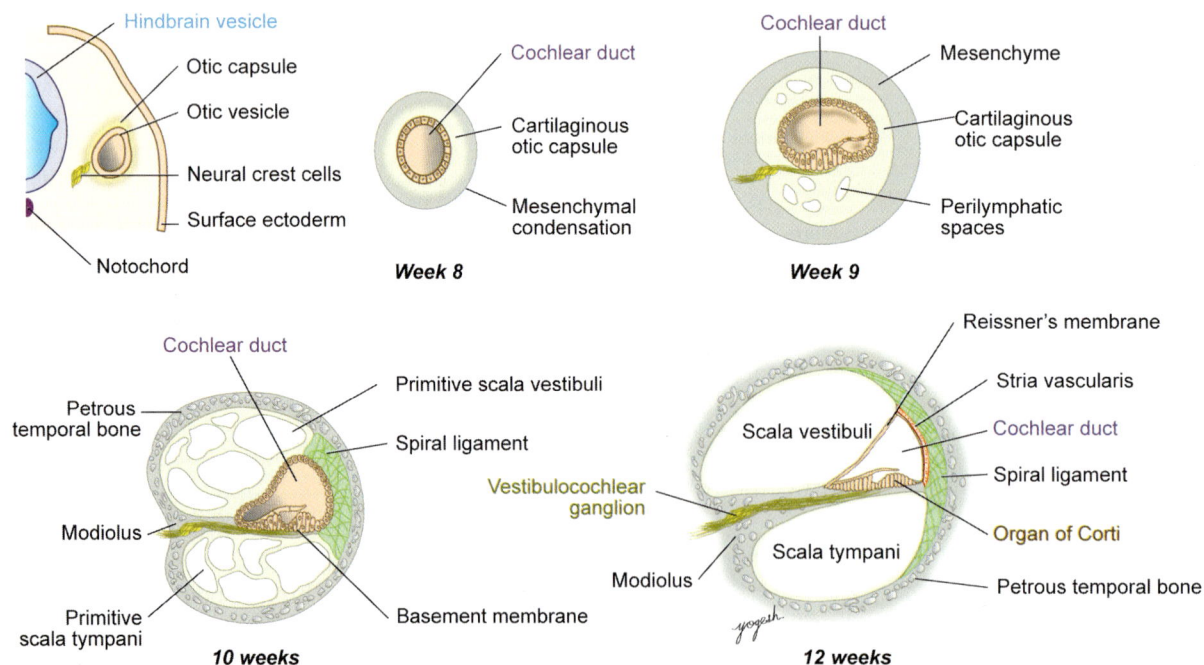

Fig. 24.4: Development of cochlea

- Otic capsule soon gets converted into cartilage.
- Space between membranous labyrinth (otic vesicle) and otic capsule is filled with loose *periotic tissue*.
- Periotic tissue disappears leaving behind a space surrounding membranous labyrinth that soon gets filled with *perilymph*.
- Membranous labyrinth becomes filled with *endolymph*.
- Periotic tissue, surrounding the otic vesicle and saccule degenerates to form a cavity called *vestibule*.
- Periotic tissue surrounding the semicircular ducts also disappears to form *semicircular canals*.
- Due to incomplete resorption of mesenchymal periotic tissue around cochlear duct, *scala tympani* and *scala vestibuli* (two spaces) are formed.
- Scala tympani is separated from cochlear duct by *basilar membrane*; whereas scala vestibuli is separated from cochlear duct by vestibular or *Reissner's membrane*.
- At the end of cochlea, scala vestibuli and scala tympani communicates with each other through an aperture called *helicotrema*.
- Cochlear duct is connected with the bony cochlear canal by spiral ligament.
- Vestibular membrane and basilar membrane meet at the *modiolous*.

Histogenesis of Internal Ear

Histogenesis of Semicircular Canals

- Auditory vesicle is lined by low columnar epithelium. Later, it becomes flattened except in ampullae.
- Cells in the ampulla produce *apical hair cells* and *cupula* (gelatinous mass). The hairs of hair cells and cupula form *crista* of the ampulla.
- In the utricle and saccule, hair cells with covering gelatinous mass form *maculae*.

Note: Cristae are more sensitive for rotational movements of head, whereas maculae are more sensitive for linear acceleration.

Histogenesis of Cochlea

- Cells of cochlear duct facing toward scala tympani get thickened in two areas and form outer and inner ridges separated by spiral sulcus.
  - A. Outer ridge forms inner hair cells, 3–4 rows of outer hair cells, *inner and outer rod cells*.
  - B. Inner ridge forms *membrana tectoria* (fibrillated gelatinous mass) that gives attachment to flagella of outer and inner hair cells.
- *Reissner's or vestibular membrane* is derived from dorsal surface of cochlear duct.
- External surface of cochlear duct forms a thick vascular zone, hence called *stria vascularis*.
- By 6th month of IUL, cochlear histogenesis completes.

MIDDLE EAR

- Middle ear cavity is endodermal in origin (Fig. 24.5).
- In 5th week, from the dorsal part of first pharyngeal pouch with a contribution from second pouch, a diverticulum called *tubotympanic recess* develops.
- Each tubotympanic recess grows laterally toward external ear.
- In 6th month of IUL, tubotympanic recess comes in contact with floor of first pharyngeal cleft (future external acoustic meatus). Still a thin rim of mesenchyme persists between endodermal pouch and ectodermal cleft. The combination of all 3 germ layers forms eardrum *(tympanic membrane)*.
- Mesenchyme of the second arch is displaced laterally by mesenchyme of the third arch. Thus, third arch comes in contact with first arch.
- A narrow part of tubotympanic recess lies between the second and third arches and it forms the *auditory tube*.
- The lateral part of the tubotympanic recess widens to form *primary tympanic cavity*.
- Formation of definitive tympanic cavity
  - *Primary tympanic cavity* extends laterally to enclose ear ossicles, muscles, nerves, and blood vessels to form *definitive ear cavity*.
  - Dorsal extension of tympanic cavity forms *tympanic antrum*.

Ear Ossicles

- By the end of 7th week, mesenchyme forms 3 condensations in the roof of tympanic cavity as follows:
  - Two from first arch (Meckel's cartilage) that later develop into malleus and incus.
  - One from second arch (Reichert's cartilage) that later develops into stapes.
- Ossicles remain embedded in the surrounding mesenchyme until 8 months.
- On degeneration of mesenchyme surrounding ossicles, mucous lining of primary tympanic cavity extends and envelopes the ossicles.

Muscles of Middle Ear

- Mesenchyme of the first arch forms **tensor tympani** muscle, and hence, supplied by *trigeminal nerve* (nerve of the 1st pharyngeal arch).[MCQ]
- Mesenchyme of the second arch forms *stapedius* muscle and hence, supplied by facial nerve (nerve of the 2nd pharyngeal arch).[MCQ]

Formation of Round and Oval Windows

- Parts of the bony labyrinth remain thin at two places:
  1. Opposite to stapes and this thin part of bony labyrinth forms *oval window* (fenestra vestibuli).
  2. Just below the stapes and this second thin part of bony labyrinth forms *round window* (fenestra cochleae).
- Fenestra vestibuli opens into the vestibule, whereas fenestra cochleae open into the scala tympani.
- Fenestra vestibuli gets closed by foot plate of stapes, whereas fenestra cochleae by a membrane called *secondary tympanic membrane*.

Formation of Tubal Tonsil

- Pharyngeal opening of tubotympanic recess is indicated by pharyngeal opening of the Eustachian (auditory) tube.
- The opening is surrounded by a considerable amount of lymphoid tissue, that forms a *tubal tonsil*.

EXTERNAL EAR

External Acoustic Meatus (Fig. 24.5)

- Dorsal part of the first pharyngeal cleft invaginates to form funnel-shaped portion called *primary meatus*.
- Primary meatus extends deep toward primary tympanic cavity.
- Medial cells of the primary meatus grow further to form as solid cord (medial plate).
- By 7th month, solid cord hollows out and touches primary tympanic cavity.
- On touching the primary tympanic cavity, the hollowed-out portion of solid cord forms *secondary meatus*.
- Cells of solid cord coming in touch with primary tympanic cavity form *outer (cuticular) layer of tympanic membrane*.
- The handle of malleus and chorda tympani nerve are trapped between ectoderm of meatal plug and endoderm of tympanic cavity and lies in the mesodermal components of tympanic membrane.
- Tympanic membrane lies horizontal at the birth and it faces downward, forward, and medially in later life.^{MCQ}

Auricle (Fig. 24.6, Scanning electron micrograph 24.2)

- At about 6th week of IUL, 6 small tubercles or hillocks appear around the dorsal part of first pharyngeal cleft; 3 on cranial side called *mandibular tubercles* and 3 on caudal side called *hyoid tubercles*.
- These hillocks fuse and expand to form the definitive ear auricle (ear pinna) as follows:
  1. 1st hillock forms tragus
  2. 2nd hillock forms crus of helix
  3. 3rd hillock forms helix
  4. 4th hillock forms antihelix
  5. 5th hillock forms antitragus
  6. 6th hillock forms lower part of helix and ear lobule.
- The development of external ear is completed by 4th month.

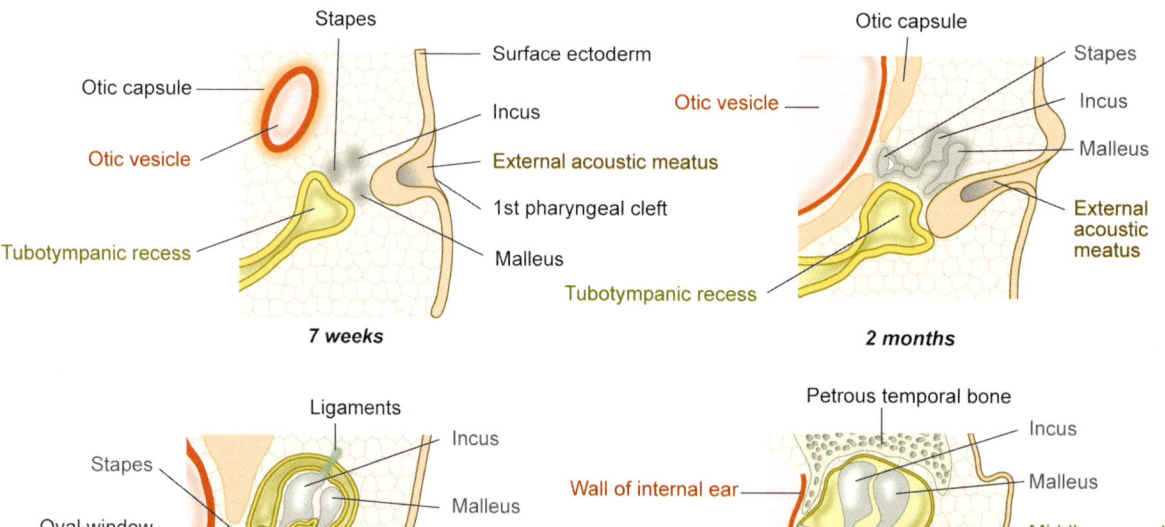
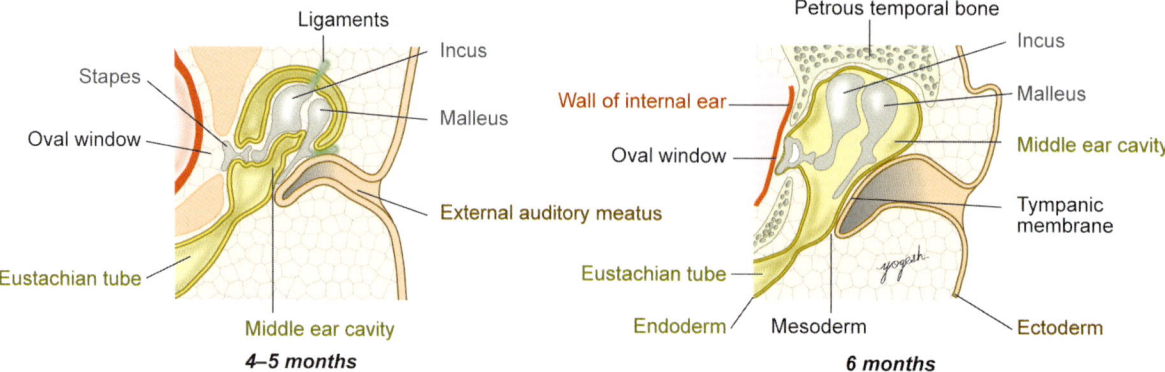

Fig. 24.5: Development of middle ear

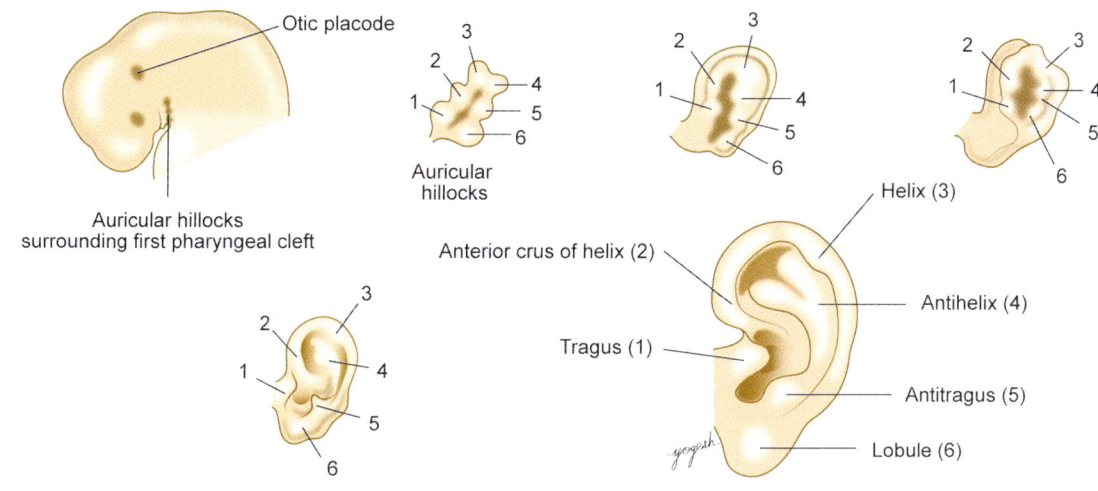

Fig. 24.6: Development of external ear

Some Interesting Facts

- Middle ear, ear ossicles, mastoid antrum and internal ear assume adult size at birth.^{MCQ}
- Internal ear appears earlier than middle and external ear (early in the 4th week).
- Failure of canalization of meatal plate is the most common cause of congenital deafness.
- Mastoid air cells develop by the age of 2 years.

MOLECULAR REGULATION

Following proteins/genes or factors are important in the molecular regulation of ear development.
1. Wnt proteins and bone morphogenic proteins for development of otic placode.
2. Retinoic acid for anteroposterior differentiation of otic vesicle.
3. Wnt and SHH genes for membranous labyrinth.
4. Noggin and PAX2 genes for cochlea.

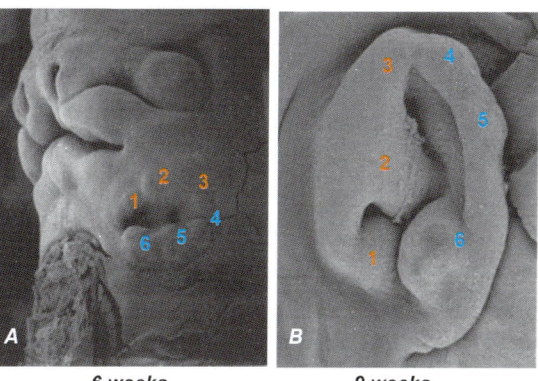

Scanning electron micrograph 24.2: Development of external ear at 6 weeks (A) and 9 weeks (B). The developing external ears are initially more caudal than the lower jaw. Growth of the lower jaw places the external ear in a relatively higher and more vertical orientation. Six hillocks fuse and expands to form the definitive ear auricle (ear pinna) as follows: 1st forms tragus, 2nd forms crus of helix, 3rd forms helix, 4th forms antihelix, 5th forms antitragus, 6th forms lower part of helix and ear lobule [Species: Human, lateral view]

DEVELOPMENTAL ANOMALIES

External Ear

- Developmental anomalies may result from nonunion or absence of primordial hillocks. It may cause partial or total absence of auricle and isolated nodule.
- Abnormal position of ear
- Auricle migrates and changes its position due to developing mandible. Hence, mandibular malformation (agnathia/micrognathia) results in abnormally low position of auricle. Hence, called *mandibulofacial dysostosis*.
- *Microtia* is suppressed development of auricle, whereas *anotia* is absence of auricle (Table 24.1).

External of Auditory Meatus

- Atresia of external auditory meatus may occur due to failure of meatal plate to canalize.
- Abnormal curvature of meatus: Tympanic membrane may not be fully visible due to congenitally accentuated curvature of meatus.

Middle Ear

- Malformation of ossicles: Defective malleus and incus may be observed in 1st arch syndrome.
- *Congenital fixation of stapes*: Stapes may be congenitally fixed with the margins of the fenestra vestibuli. It results into severe conductive deafness.
- Abnormal course of facial nerve: Bulging facial canal in the middle ear may be present.

Internal Ear

- *Rubella virus infection*: Rubella infection in the second month of pregnancy affects mostly cochlear and vestibular development and to some extent organ of Corti. Hence, children born to a mother with rubella infection may perceive only deep frequency sounds.

- *Thalidomide* may cause malformations of semicircular canals.

Table 24.1 Development of ear

Adult structures	Embryonic source
External ear	
Auricle	6 ectodermal hillocks: *1st arch*: (1) Tragus, (2) crus of helix, (3) helix
	2nd arch: (4) Antihelix, (5) antitragus, (6) lobule
External acoustic meatus	1st pharyngeal cleft
Middle ear	
Middle ear cavity	Tubotympanic recess
Muscles	Tensor tympani – 1st pharyngeal arch
	Stapedius – 2nd pharyngeal arch
Ear ossicles	Malleus, incus – 1st pharyngeal arch
	Stapes – 2nd pharyngeal arch
Auditory tube, mastoid antrum	Tubotympanic recess
Tympanic membrane	Outer cuticular layer – ectoderm of 1st pharyngeal cleft
	Middle fibrous layer – mesoderm
	Inner mucous layer – endoderm of 1st pharyngeal pouch
Internal ear	
Membranous labyrinth	Otic vesicle
• Utricle, semicircular ducts, endolymphatic duct	Vestibular (dorsal) part of membranous labyrinth
• Saccule, ductus reuniens, cochlear duct	Cochlear (ventral) part of membranous labyrinth
Bony labyrinth	
• Vestibule, semicircular canals, scala tympani, scala vestibuli	Mesenchyme around otic vesicle (otic capsule)

Chapter 25

Endocrine System

eSmartQuiz

Chapter Outline

- Pituitary Gland
  - Stages of development
  - Clinical aspects
- Pineal gland
- Adrenal gland
  - Stages of development
  - Congenital anomalies
- Chromaffin cells

Competency:
- **AN43.4:** Describe the development and developmental basis of congenital anomalies of pituitary gland and thyroid gland. Note: No specific competency is given for endocrine glands.

INTRODUCTION

- Endocrine glands are ductless glands. They secrete hormones directly into the blood.
- Hormones reach the target organ through circulation and get attached to specific receptors for exerting a specific effect.
- The major endocrine glands are:
  1. Pituitary gland
  2. Pineal gland
  3. Thyroid gland
  4. Parathyroid gland
  5. Adrenal gland
  6. Islets of Langerhans in pancreas
  7. Testis and ovary
  8. Hypothalamus (in addition to many other functions, hypothalamus controls secretions of anterior pituitary gland)
- In this chapter, development of pituitary gland, pineal gland, and adrenal gland is described. For development of thyroid gland and parathyroid gland, read Chapter 11, for pancreas read Chapter 15, for gonads read Chapter 21.

PITUITARY GLAND (HYPOPHYSIS CEREBRI)

- Pituitary gland is an unpaired endocrine gland located in a bony fossa called *sella turcica* of the sphenoid bone.
- It consists of two major parts: *Adenohypophysis* (anterior pituitary) and *neurohypophysis* (posterior pituitary).

Summary (Examination Guide) (Figs 25.1, 25.2, Flowchart 25.1, Practice Fig. 25.1)

- Anterior lobe of pituitary gland develops from Rathke's pouch that arises from ectoderm of stomodeum.
- Anterior lobe consists of pars distalis, pars intermedia, and pars tuberalis.
- Cavity of the Rathke's pouch forms intraglandular cleft.
- Neurohypophysis develops from evagination of the floor of 3rd ventricle (diencephalon).

Stages of Development

1. Adenohypophysis develops form *Rathke's pouch*.
   - *Ectoderm* of stomodeum becomes thicker on day 21 of IUL. This thickened ectoderm invaginates and grows toward diencephalon in the form of *Rathke's pouch*.
   - By 2nd month of IUL, the Rathke's pouch loses its contact with stomodeum.
   - Cells of thick anterior wall of Rathke's pouch proliferate to form *pars distalis*, posterior thin wall forms *pars intermedia*.

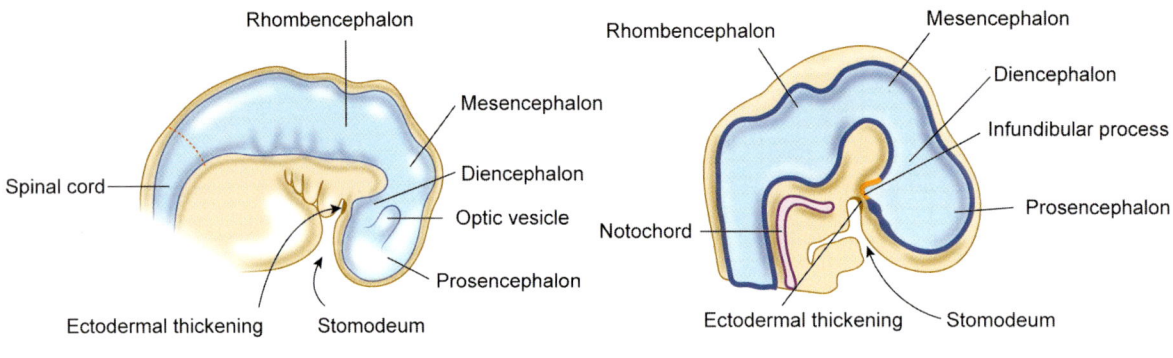

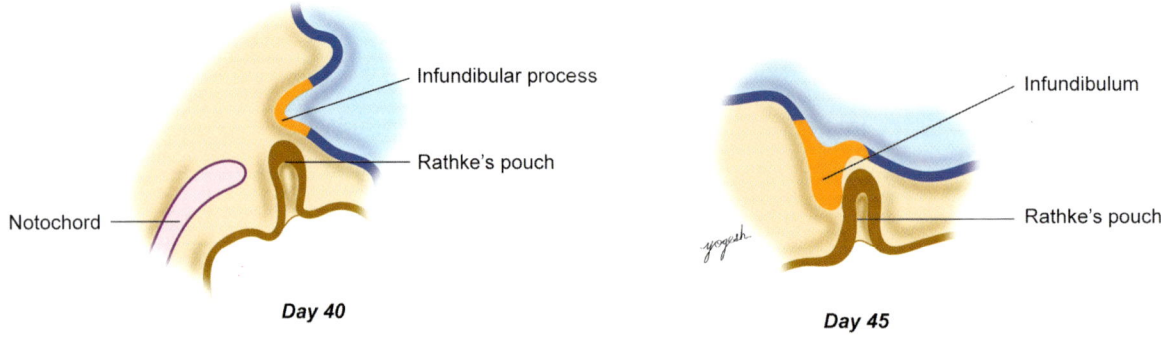

Fig. 25.1: Development of pituitary gland

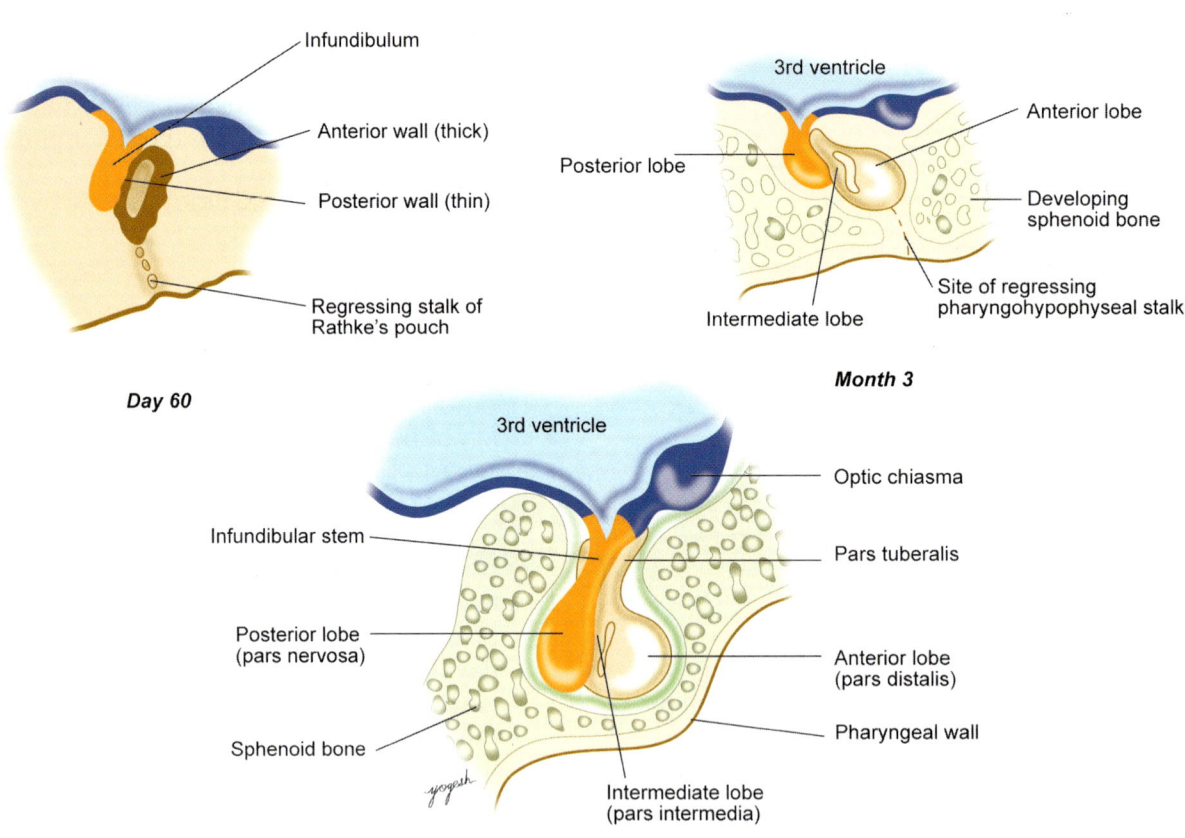

Fig. 25.2: Development of pituitary gland

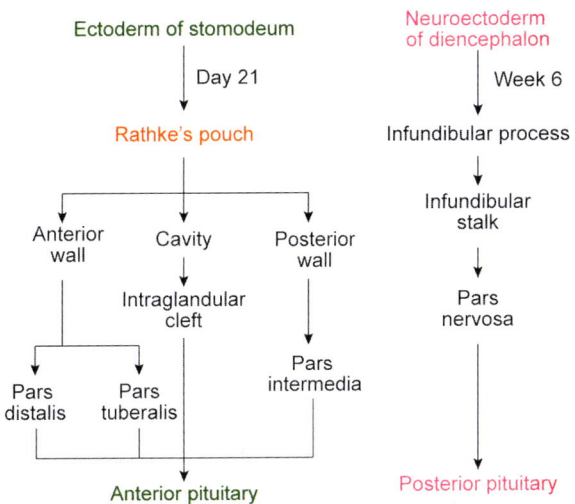

Flowchart 25.1: Development of pituitary gland

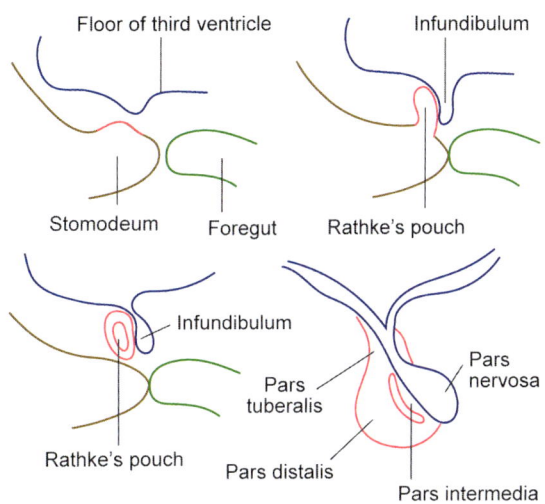

Practice Fig. 25.1: Development of pituitary gland

- The cavity of the pouch forms *intraglandular cleft* which is not recognisable in the adult human gland.
- Upward proliferation of anterior wall forms *pars tuberalis*.

2. Neurohypophysis develops from *infundibular process of diencephalon*.
   - During 6th week of IUL, an infundibular process arises from the diencephalon in the floor of 3rd ventricle.
   - Infundibular process grows toward stomodeum (Rathke's pouch) and fuses with Rathke's pouch.
   - Infundibular process forms *pars nervosa* (posterior pituitary) neurohypophysis.
   - The connecting stalk between pars nervosa and diencephalon (later hypothalamus) forms *infundibulum*.

3. Histogenesis of pituitary gland
   - Histogenesis of pituitary gland begins in the 4th month of IUL.
   - Acidophils appear earlier followed by basophils and chromophobes.
   - Neuroglial cells start appearing in neurohypophysis by the 4th month. This is followed by axonal colonization from supraoptic and paraventricular nuclei of hypothalamus.

Clinical Aspects

1. *Craniopharyngiomas*: Rathke's pouch passes through the craniopharyngeal canal from the stomodeum to the sella turcica and eventually loses contact with the stomodeum. *Remnants of Rathke's pouch* in craniopharyngeal canal may give rise to a tumor called *craniopharyngioma*. Craniopharyngioma is seen in relation to the sphenoid bone in the roof of nasopharynx. It may occur as childhood onset in 5–14 years of age or as adult onset between 50–70 years of age.
2. *Accessory pituitary gland*: It may be seen in relation to posterior wall of nasopharynx as pharyngeal hypophysis.
3. Pituitary agenesis or hypoplasia may be seen.

Box 25.1: Pineal gland (epiphysis cereberi)

Development of pineal gland

- Pineal gland is called the third eye of human body or principal seat of soul.
- Pineal gland develops as an evagination from diencephalon in the **roof** of 3rd ventricle (Fig. 25.3).[MCQ]
- Pineal gland is made up of pinealocytes (modified neuroglial cells).
- Pinealocytes secrete melatonin hormone.
- Melatonin inhibits the secretion of gonadotrophin-releasing hormone (GnRH).
- For functional and structural details of the pineal gland, refer Textbook of Human Histology, Yogesh Sontakke, CBS Publishers & Distributors Pvt. Ltd.

ADRENAL GLAND

- Adrenal glands (suprarenal glands) are the masses of glandular tissue located at upper pole of each kidney.
- Adrenal gland consists of superficial cortex and deep medulla.

Summary (Examination Guide) (Figs 25.4 to 25.6, Flowchart 25.2, Practice Fig. 25.2)

- *Adrenal cortex*: It develops from coelomic epithelium (mesoderm) that forms suprarenal ridge. Initially formed cortex gets replaced by definitive cortex which differentiates into zona glomerulosa, zona fasciculata, and zona reticularis.
- *Adrenal medulla*: It develops from sympathochromaffin cells derived from neural crest cells.

Stages of Development

Adrenal cortex is mesodermal in origin and medulla is neuroectodermal (neural crest) derivative.[MCQ]

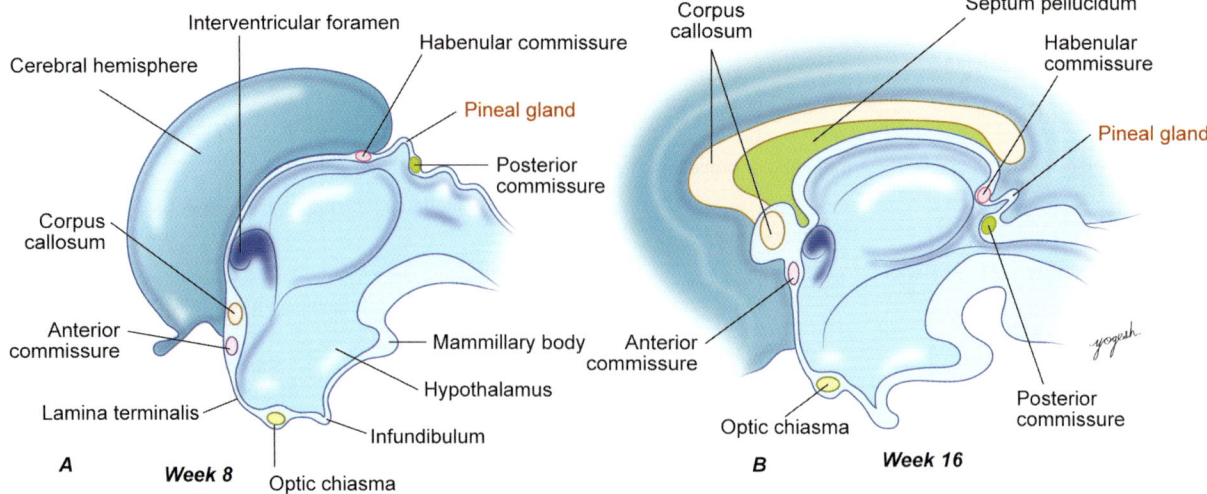

Fig. 25.3: Developing pineal gland and diencephalon

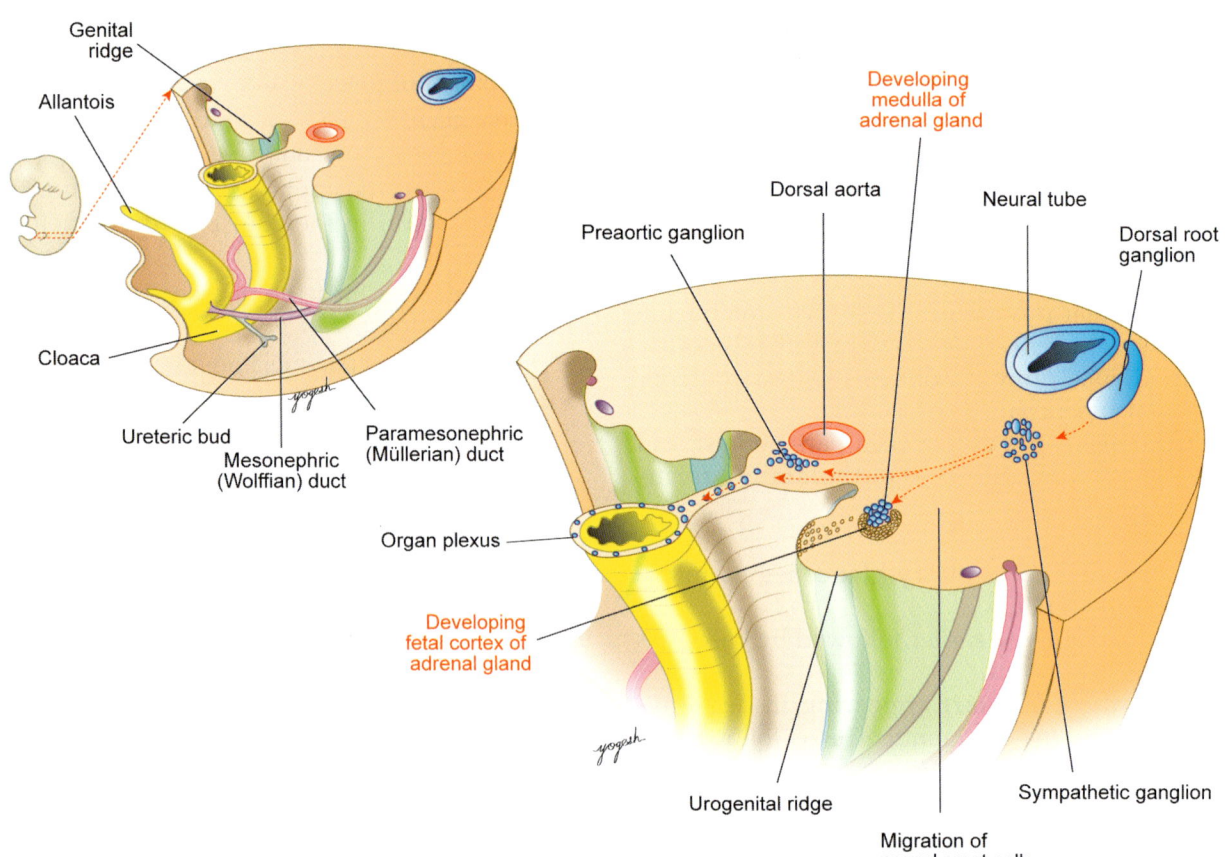

Fig. 25.4: Cross-section of embryo showing developing adrenal gland

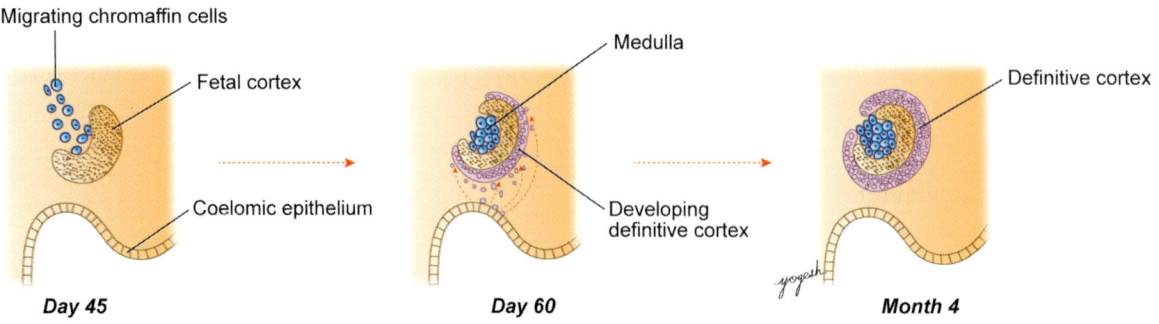

Fig. 25.5: Development of adrenal gland

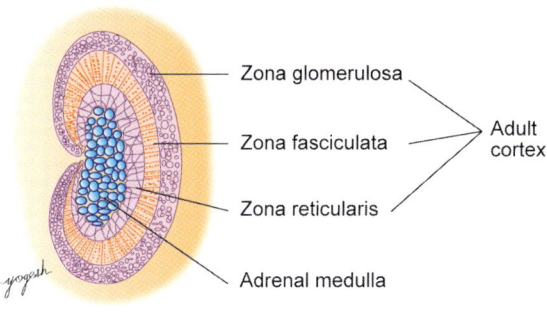

Age: 2 years

Fig. 25.6: Developed adrenal gland

Flowchart 25.2: Development of adrenal gland

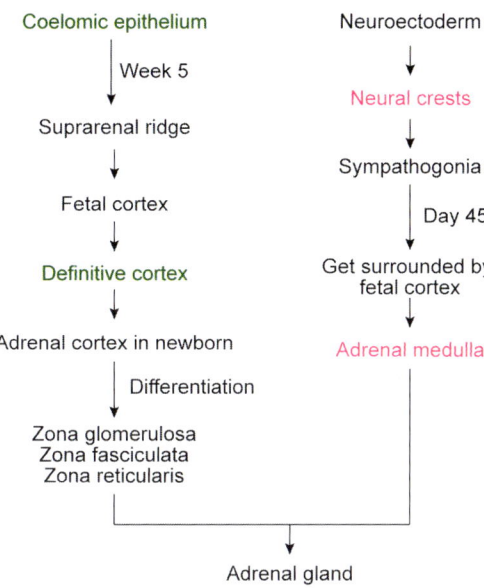

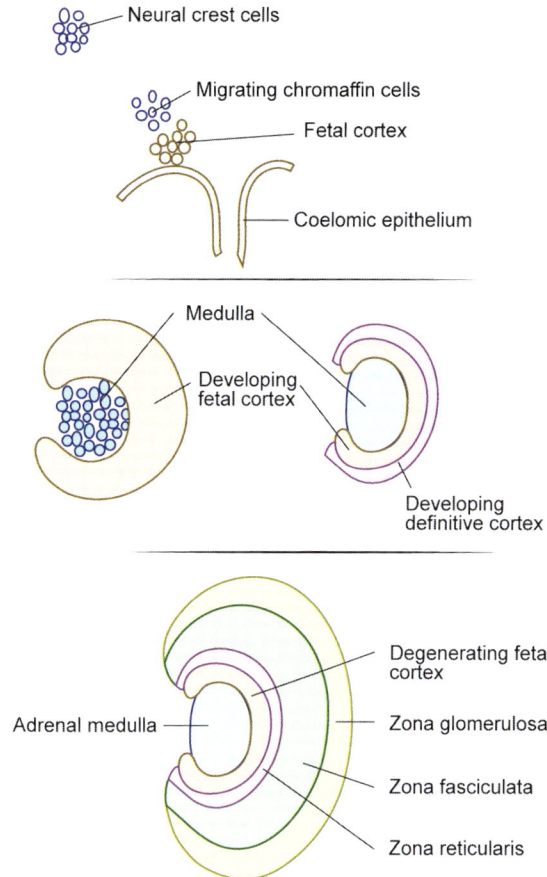

Practice Fig. 25.2: Development of adrenal gland

1. Development of adrenal cortex
   - In the 5th week of IUL, the *coelomic epithelium* in relation with developing gonad proliferates to form a *suprarenal ridge*.
   - In the 2nd month, the suprarenal ridge forms acidophilic cells that surround the primitive adrenal medulla. These acidophilic cells form *fetal cortex*.
   - In the 3rd month, a second wave of cells (small basophilic) arises from suprarenal ridge. These small basophilic cells surround fetal cortical cells and form *definitive cortex*.
2. Development of adrenal medulla
   - By the 45th day of gestation, sympathogonia accumulate near the fetal cortical cells. Sympathogonia arise from *neural crest cells* (neuroectoderm).
   - Sympathogonia invade fetal adrenal cortical cells and form clusters and cords of cells.
   - These sympathogonia differentiate to form *adrenal medulla*.
   - Differentiation of definitive cortex begins in fetal life.
   - At the birth, only zona glomerulosa and zona fasciculata are present.
3. Changes after birth
   - Proportional weight of fetal adrenal gland is 10–20 times larger than that of the adult adrenal gland.
   - At the birth, adrenal cortex forms only 15–20% of adrenal parenchyma.
   - The size of adrenal gland in fetus is almost of same size as that of the adult.
   - Fetal cortex regresses completely by the second year of life and thus, adrenal gland reduces in size.^MCQ
   - Zona reticularis appears at the end of the third year of life.^NEXT
   - Preganglionic sympathetic neurons terminate in relation to cells of medulla.
   - *Note:* Cells of medulla correspond the postganglionic sympathetic neurons.

Congenital Anomalies

1. *Ectopic adrenal gland*: Ectopic adrenal tissue may be present deep to the renal capsule, or fused with the kidney or liver.
2. *Congenital adrenal hyperplasia*: It involves deficiency of 21 hydroxylase enzyme (essential for steroid hormone synthesis). It results in elevation of androgens and causes pseudointersexuality as follows:

In male: It causes early development of secondary sexual characters and the condition is called adrenogenital syndrome.

In female: It causes enlargement of clitoris and the condition is called pseudohermaphroditism.

Box 25.2: Chromaffin cells

- Chromaffin cells or pheochromocytes are neuroendocrine cells derived from neural crests.
- Staining property: These cells show brown pigmentation on staining with chromium salts (affinity for chromium).
- *Note:* Enterochromaffin cells of Kulchitsky lie in gastrointestinal tract. Though these cells have similar chemical property similar to adrenal medulla, but enterochromaffin cells are derived from endoderm.
- Location of chromaffin cells
  1. Para-aortic bodies (organ of Zuckerkandl)
  2. Sympathetic ganglia
  3. Adrenal medulla
- *Pheochromocytoma* is a tumor of chromaffin cells. It produces a large quantity of adrenalin and noradrenalin. It causes hypertension.

Chapter 26

Skeletal System

eSmartQuiz

Chapter Outline

- Formation of cartilage
- Formation of bone
  - Intramembranous ossification
  - Endochondral ossification
  - Development of typical long bone
  - Anomalies of bone formation
- Achondroplasia
- Development of axial skeleton
  - Development of vertebral column
  - Development of ribs
  - Development of sternum
  - Development of skull
- Costal element and transverse element
- Fontanelles

Competencies:
- AN79.4: Describe the development of somites.
- AN79.5: Embryological basis of nucleus pulposus.

INTRODUCTION

- Skeletal system consists of bones and cartilages that can be grouped into two parts:
  1. *Axial skeleton*: It includes skull, vertebrae, ribs, and sternum.
  2. *Appendicular skeleton*: It includes pectoral and pelvic girdles, and bones of upper and lower limbs.
- Skeletal system develops from intraembryonic mesoderm.
- The intraembryonic mesoderm is divided into paraxial, intermediate, and lateral plate mesoderm.
- The *paraxial mesoderm* consists of
  - *Preotic part*: It lies cranial to otic capsules and forms unsegmented *somitomeres*.
  - *Postotic part*: It lies caudal to otic capsules and forms segmented *somites*.
- Each somite differentiates into dermatome for dermis of skin, myotome for skeletal muscles, and sclerotome for vertebrae.
- For the details about somites, read Chapter 8.
- Dermatome forms dermis at the back of the head and trunk, whereas in other parts dermis is derived from the lateral plate mesoderm.^{NEXT}

FORMATION OF CARTILAGE

- Cartilages are derived from mesenchymal tissue (Fig. 26.1).

Stages of Formation

1. *Mesenchymal cells* become closely packed (to form mesenchymal condensation) in the region of cartilage formation (Fig. 26.1A).
2. Mesenchymal cells differentiate to *chondroblasts* (Fig. 26.1B).
3. Chondroblasts deposit intercellular matrix and differentiate to form *chondrocytes* (Fig. 26.1C).
4. Depending on the type and amount of the fibres in the matrix, the following cartilages are formed:
   a. *Hyaline cartilage*: Fine collagen fibres in the matrix.
   b. *Elastic cartilage*: Elastic fibres in the matrix.
   c. *Fibrocartilage*: Dense collagen fibres in the matrix.
5. Mesenchymal cells surrounding the cartilage form *perichondrium*.

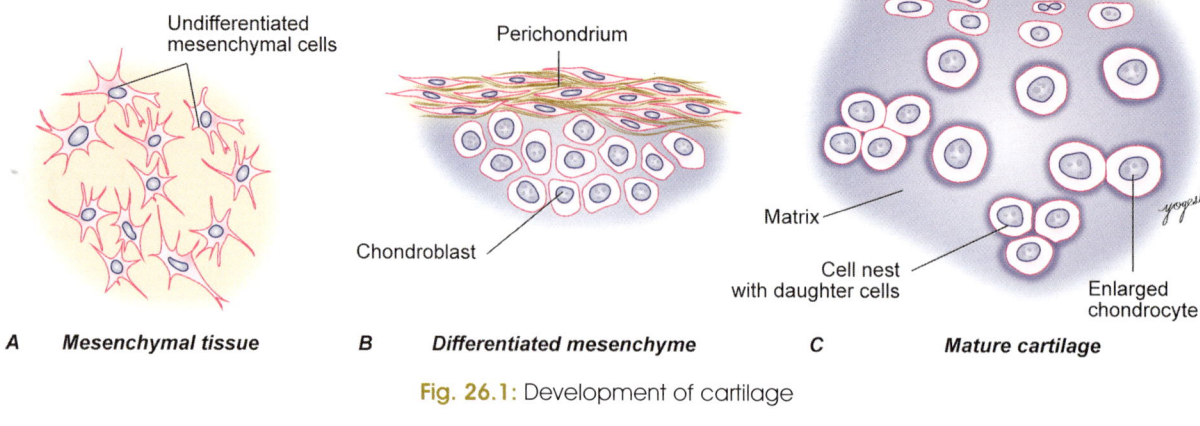

Fig. 26.1: Development of cartilage

FORMATION OF BONE

- Bones are mesodermal derivatives (except in the facial skeleton – formed by neural crest contribution).
- The process of formation of bone is called *ossification*.
- Ossification may be
  a. *Intramembranous ossification* that involves the direct conversion of mesenchymal tissue to bone.
  b. *Endochondral (cartilaginous) ossification* that involves the conversion of mesenchyme to a cartilage which is later replaced by bone.

Intramembranous Ossification

- In intramembranous ossification, the mesenchymal tissue forms bone (Fig. 26.2, Flowchart 26.1).

Steps of formation

1. Mesenchymal condensation: Star-shaped mesenchymal cells condense and differentiate to spindle-shaped fibroblasts that form a fibrous membrane (Fig. 26.2A).
2. Osteoid formation: Fibroblasts differentiate to osteoblasts that laydown the early bone matrix and forms uncalcified bone (osteoid) (Fig. 26.2B).
3. Calcification of osteoid: Osteoblasts deposit calcium salts in intercellular matrix and thus convert osteoid into calcified bony spicules (Fig. 26.2B).
4. Formation of woven bone: Trapped osteoblasts in the matrix get differentiated to osteocytes. Spicules fuse with each other to form plates of compact bones. Arrangement of collagen bundles running in different directions produces woven bone appearance (Fig. 26.2C, D).
5. Formation of Haversian system: Waves of calcification and trapping of osteocyte processes in bony canaliculi form Haversian system.
6. Stage of bone modelling and remodelling: Fusion of progressively growing bone gives a primitive shape to a bone model. Continuous deposition and reabsorption of bone give the definitive shape to bone.

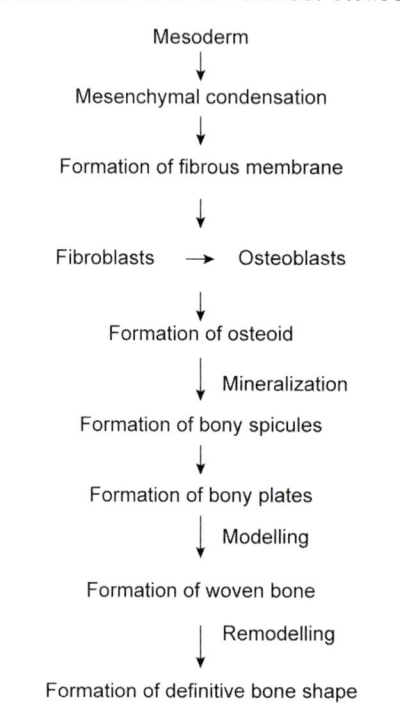

Flowchart 26.1: Intramembranous ossification

- Bones formed by membranous ossification are called *membranous bones*.
- Examples: Bones of skull vault, mandible, clavicle (partly).

Endochondral Ossification

- It involves conversion of mesenchymal tissue into cartilage that later replaced by bone (Fig. 26.3, Flowchart 26.2).
- The bones developed by cartilaginous ossification are called *cartilaginous bones*.
- Examples: All long bones (except clavicle), base of the skull, vertebrae, ribs.

Stages of endochondral ossification

1. Mesenchymal condensation: Mesenchymal cells form condensed mesenchymal tissue at the site of bone formation (Fig. 26.3A).

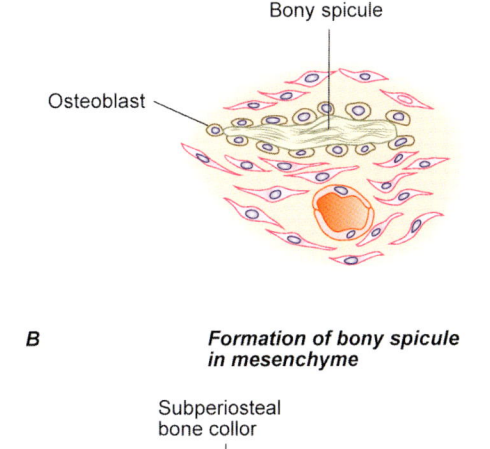
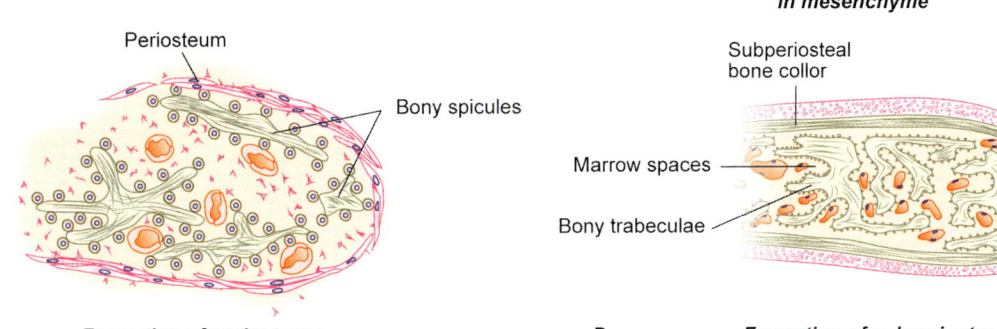

Fig. 26.2: Intramembranous ossification

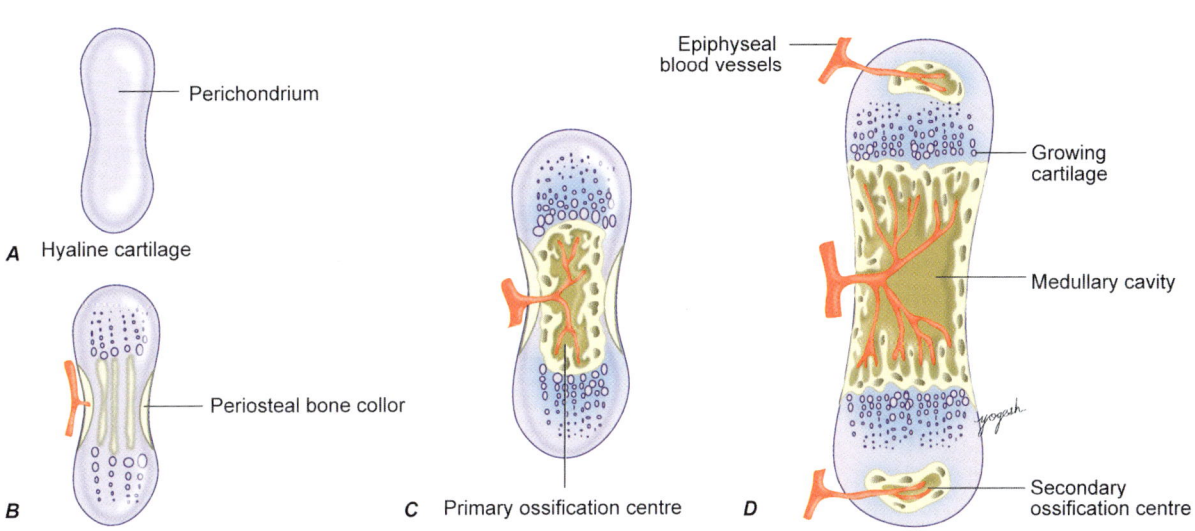

Fig. 26.3: Endochondral ossification (development of long bone)

2. Formation of cartilaginous model: At the site of mesenchymal condensation, chondroblasts appear and deposit hyaline cartilage. This cartilage is surrounded by a vascular mesenchyme that forms perichondrium (Fig. 26.3A).
3. Stage of cartilage hypertrophy: At the site of bone formation, the cells of cartilage increase in size (hypertrophy) and chondroblasts get converted to chondrocytes on the deposition of cartilage matrix (Fig. 26.4).
4. Stage of calcification: Hypertrophied cartilaginous cells start secretion of alkaline phosphatase and deposit calcium in intercellular matrix. Soon, chondrocytes lose nutritional source and die due to calcified matrix to leave behind *primary areolae* (Fig. 26.4).
5. Formation of periosteal buds: Perichondral vessels and osteogenic cells invade calcified matrix to form periosteal bud.
6. Formation of secondary areolae: Periosteal bud removes calcified matrix from the wall of primary areolae and forms large cavities called secondary areolae.
7. Formation of osteoid: Osteogenic cells (osteoblasts) form a gelatinous matrix along the wall of secondary areolae. This newly formed mass is called *osteoid*.
8. Formation of bone lamella: Intercellular gelatinous matrix of osteoid gets calcified to develop a lamella of bone.
9. Formation of trabecular bone: Osteoblasts lay another layer of lamella over the first one and so on.

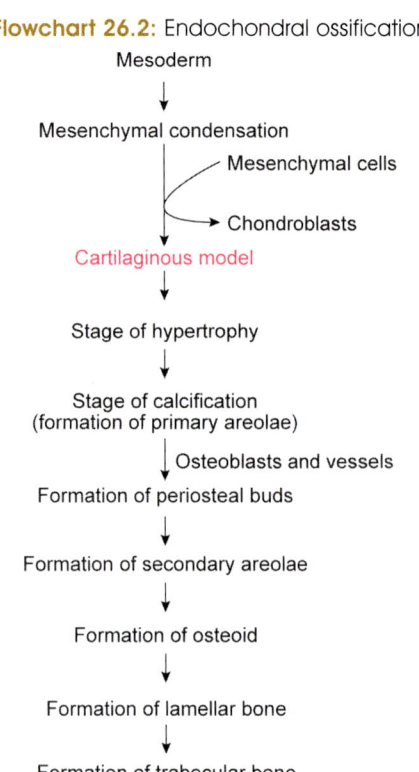

Flowchart 26.2: Endochondral ossification

Osteoblasts trapped in the lamellae form osteocytes. The multilamellar portion is called trabecular bone.

Development of Typical Long Bone

Formation of long bone shows various stages as follows:
1. Stages of mesenchymal condensation
2. Formation of cartilaginous model
3. Stage of endochondral ossification
4. Stage of bone growth
5. Stage of remodelling

- The calcification in the cartilaginous model of long bones starts in shaft at the *primary centre of ossification* (diaphysis).
- On the appearance of the primary centre of ossification, the periosteum produces a calcified bone on the surface of cartilage by intramembranous ossification. This periosteal bone is called *periosteal collar*.
- After the birth, cartilages at ends of the long bone starts ossification (secondary centres) to form *epiphysis*.
- Diaphysis and epiphysis are separated by a plate of *epiphysis cartilage*.

Growth of long bone

1. Increase in thickness and formation of bone marrow: Periosteal collar increases in the thickness by deposition of more layers on outer surface of bone. Simultaneously, osteoblasts remove lamellae from the inner surface of bone, leaving behind a *bone marrow cavity*.

2. Increase in length: The length of bone increases by lengthening of epiphyseal cartilage and its simultaneous conversion into new bone.
   - In the developing bone, epiphysial cartilage shows the zone of resting cartilage, zone of proliferation, zone of calcification, and zone of ossification (Fig. 26.4).
   - The terminal portion of diaphysis (active site of bone formation) is called *metaphysis*.
   - On completion of bone growth, epiphyseal cartilage stops proliferation and epiphysis fuses with diaphysis.
   - Cartilages show interstitial growth (deposition of intercellular substance), whereas bones show oppositional growth (growth on the surface and ends).

Some Interesting Facts

- Mandible, clavicle, occipital bone, temporal bone, and sphenoid bone show membranocartilaginous ossification.
- Bones of cranial vault and facial bones are membranous bones.
- The clavicle is the first bone in the body to ossify.

Anomalies of Bone Formation

1. *Osteogenesis imperfecta* (brittle-bone disease): It involves lack of collagen type I fibres and defective calcification; hence, bones break easily. Other symphonies include short height, hearing loss, blue sclera, and loose joints. *NEXT*
2. Achondroplasia (Box 26.1).
3. *Cleidocranial dysostosis*: It is a congenital anomaly that involves partial or complete absence of clavicles. It also involves skull vault, causing large fontanelles and delayed closure of sutures. Due to the absence of clavicles, affected individual can bring both the shoulders close together.
4. *Dyschondroplasias* (enchondromatosis): It involves excessive proliferation of cartilages at growth plates in the long bones. These cartilages form abnormal cartilage masses with the metaphysis.

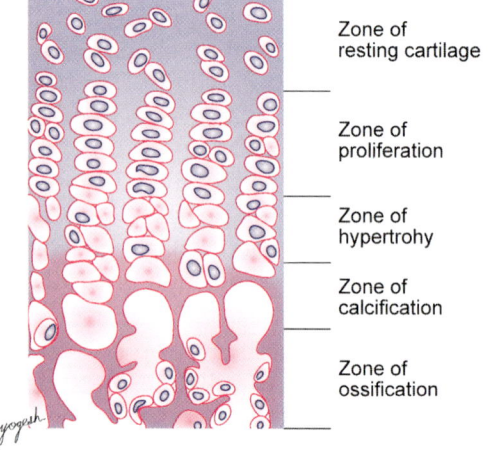

Fig. 26.4: Epiphyseal cartilage of developing bone

> **Box 26.1:** Achondroplasia (dwarfism)
>
> ***Q. Write a short note on achondroplasia.***
> - It is a genetic disorder that causes dwarfism.
>
> **Cause**
> - It is inherited as autosomal dominant disease due to mutation of fibroblast growth factor receptor 3 (FGFR 3) gene.
>
> **Signs and symptoms**
>
> The affected individual shows the following features:
> – Disproportionate shortening (dwarf)
> – Proportional large head
> – Short-curved arms and legs
> – Dorsal lordosis (convex curvature of vertebral column)
> – Short fingers and toes

DEVELOPMENT OF AXIAL SKELETON

- Axial skeleton consists of skull, vertebrae, ribs, and sternum.

Development of Vertebral Column

- Vertebral column develops from *sclerotomes* of somites (Figs 26.5 to 26.9).^{MCQ}
- Development of vertebral column takes place in 3 essential stages: Precartilage stage, chondrification stage, ossification stage.

Precartilage stage
- Cells of sclerotome migrate in three directions as follows (Fig. 26.6):
  1. Ventromedial group
     It is divided into two portions:
     a. Densely arranged cells
     b. Loosely arranged cells
  2. Dorsal group covers the neural tube and forms vertebral arch and spine of vertebrae.
  3. Venterolateral group forms costal elements.
- Resegmentation of sclerotomes: Each sclerotome is divided into cranial and caudal portions by a transverse line called intrasegmental boundary or von Ebner's fissure. Later, the caudal segment of each sclerotome fuses with the cranial segment of the sclerotome caudal to it, with each of the two segments of the sclerotome contributing to a vertebra. This process is called resegmentation of the sclerotomes. Hence, the vertebrae are intersegmental in development.^{MCQ}

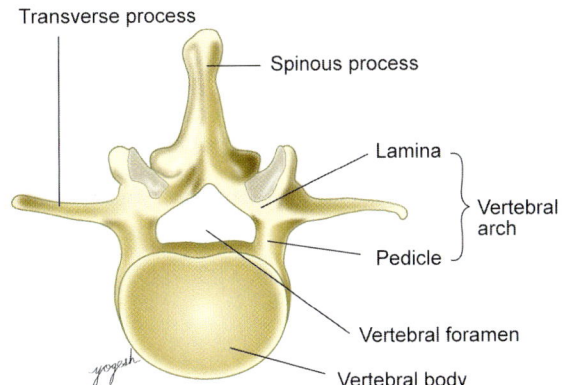

Fig. 26.5: Parts of typical vertebra

- At the intrasegmental boundary, the fibrous intervertebral discs develop. Notochordal cells form a gelatinous core called nucleus pulposus, whereas the surrounding annulus fibrosus develops from sclerotomal cells that are left in the region of the resegmentating sclerotome.
- The sclerotomes of the first four somites (occipital somites) fuse to form the occipital bone of skull. Eight cervical somites form only seven cervical sclerotomes. The sclerotome of the 1st cervical sclerotome fuses with the caudal half of the 4th occipital sclerotome and contributes to the base of the skull. The caudal half of the 1st cervical sclerotome fuses with the cranial half of the 2nd cervical sclerotome to form the 1st cervical vertebra (atlas).
- Notochord regresses slowly except at intervertebral disc, it forms nucleus pulposus.^{NEXT}

Chondrification stage
- During the 6th week of IUL, chondrification of mesenchymal vertebrae begins.

Ossification stage
- Ossification of vertebrae begins in intrauterine life and continues up to 25 years of age.

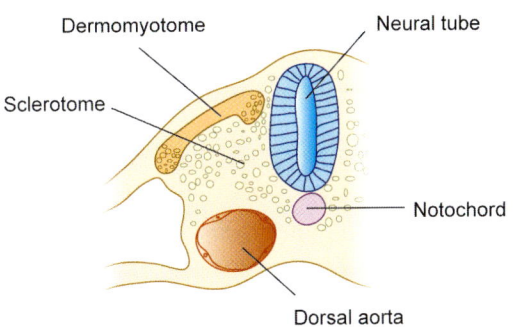
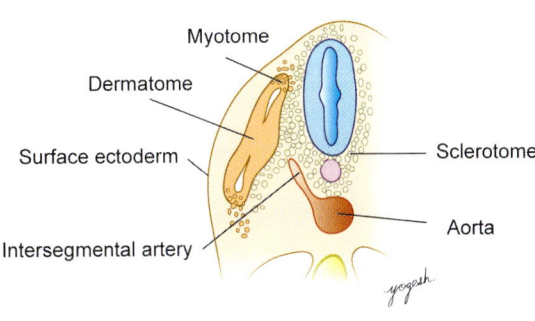

Fig. 26.6: Sclerotome

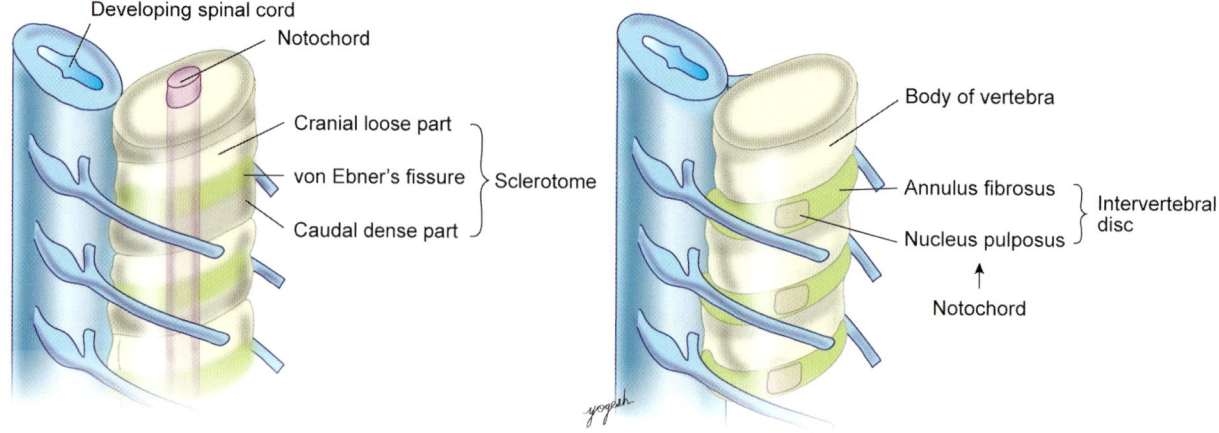

Fig. 26.7: Role of sclerotome in the formation of body of vertebrae

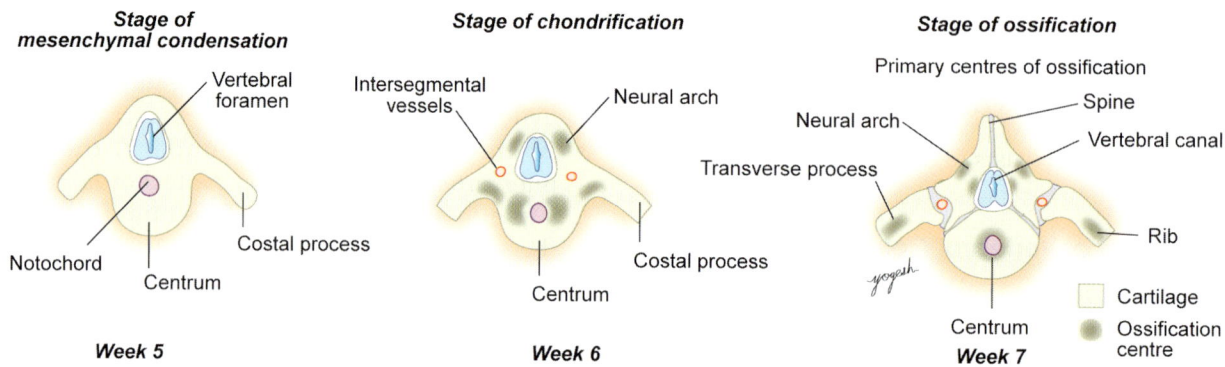

Fig. 26.8: Development of vertebra

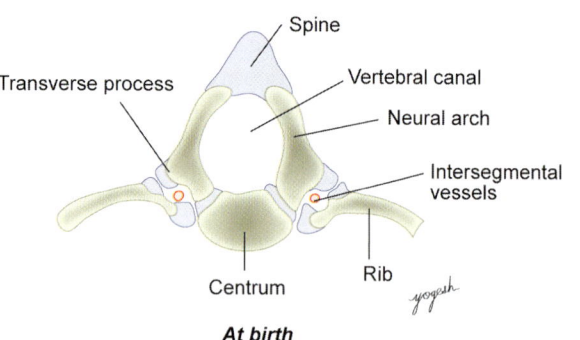

Fig. 26.9: Vertebra at birth

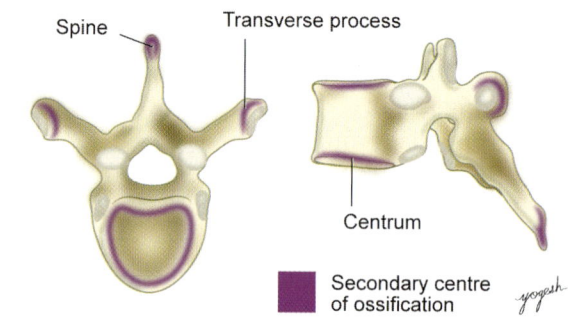

Fig. 26.10: Secondary centres of ossification for vertebra

- 3 primary centres: 1 for centrum, 1 for each half of the vertebral arch. At birth, each vertebra has 3 parts (body and two halves of vertebral arch) connected by cartilages (Fig. 26.8).
- 3–6 years: 2 halves vertebral arches fuse with each other as well as with centrum. Thus, vertebral arch (neural arch) of developing vertebra forms pedicle, laminae, spine, and articular processes.
- Secondary centres: Total 5 centres: 1 for tip of each transverse process, 1 for tip of spinous process and 1 for upper and 1 for lower surface of body of vertebra (Fig. 26.10).
- 25 years: All secondary centres fuses with rest of the vertebra.

Box 26.2: Costal element and transverse element (Fig. 26.11)

- Each vertebra shows transverse and costal elements that have different derivatives in different regions.

Derivatives of costal element
- In cervical region: Anterior root, anterior tubercle, costotransverse bar, and posterior tubercle[MCQ]
- In thoracic region: Rib[MCQ]
- In lumbar region: Transverse process
- In sacral region: Anterior two-thirds of lateral mass

Transverse element
- In cervical region: Posterior root
- In thoracic region: Transverse process[MCQ]
- In lumbar region: Mammillary process, accessory mammillary process[MCQ]
- In sacral region: Posterior one-third of lateral mass

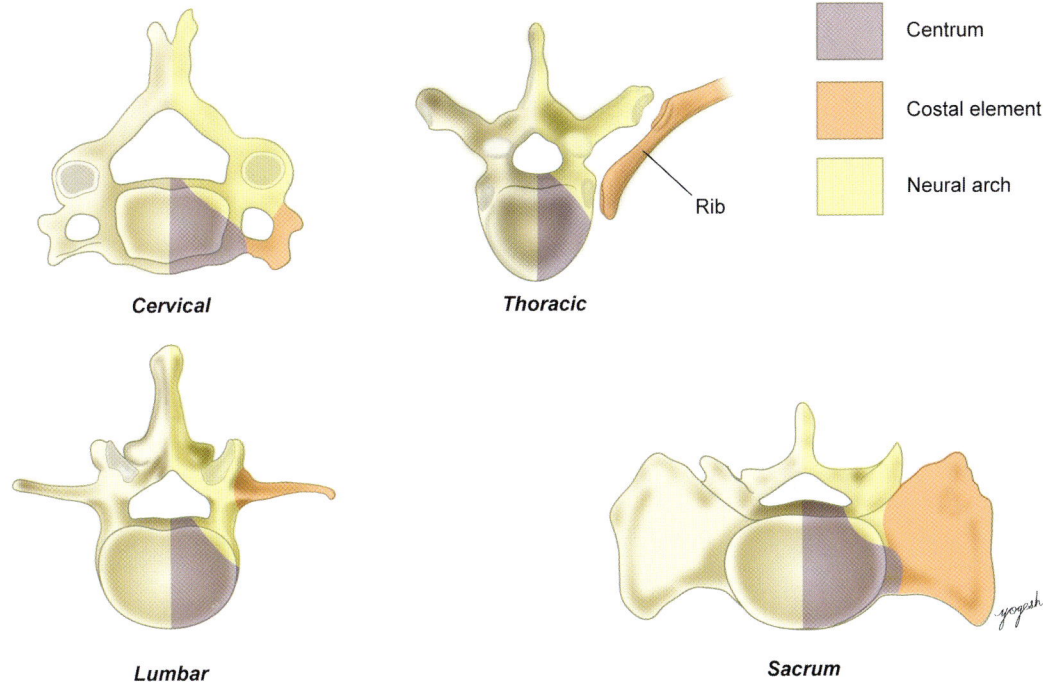

Fig. 26.11: Contribution of centrum, costal element, and neural arch in the formation of vertebrae

Congenital Anomalies of Vertebral Column

1. *Spina bifida:* Two halves of vertebral arch (neural arch) fail to fuse. For details, read Chapter 22. Spina bifida is the most serious vertebral defect. Rachischisis is the most serious form of spina bifida.^{MCQ}
2. *Hemivertebra:* Usually, vertebral body ossifies from two primary centres. Failure of one of these primary centres (abnormal sclerotome) may result in absence of half of the vertebral body (hemivertebra) and absence of corresponding rib. Hemivertebra is invariably associated with congenital scoliosis (lateral bending of vertebral column).
3. *Klippel-Feil syndrome:* It is congenital fusion of one or more cervical vertebra.^{NEXT}
4. *Occipitalization of atlas vertebra:* In this condition, atlas vertebra fuses with the occipital bone.
5. Sacralization of 5th lumbar vertebra: It involves fusion of 5th lumbar vertebra with sacrum.
6. Lumbarization of 1st sacral vertebra: It involves fusion of 1st sacral vertebra with 5th lumbar vertebra. Here, 1st sacral vertebra remains separated from rest of the sacrum.
7. *Spondylolisthesis:* It is a slippage (displacement) of vertebral body. Failure of formation of articular facet may cause spondylolisthesis. It commonly involves anterior displacement of 5th lumbar vertebra over the sacrum.

Development of Ribs

- Ribs are derived from ventral extensions of costal elements of the thoracic vertebrae.^{MCQ}
- Costal elements (arches) that later ossify to form the ribs.
- The mesenchyme near the junction of transverse process and costal arch undergo differentiation to form costotransverse joint.

Accessory ribs

- *Cervical rib:* It develops from costal element of the 7th cervical vertebra. It produces superior thoracic outlet syndrome due to compression of lower trunk of brachial plexus and subclavian artery.^{MCQ}
- *Lumbar rib:* It is occasionaly present but remains asymptomatic in most of the cases.

Development of Sternum

- Sternum develops from mesodermal condensation (lateral plate mesoderm) in the anterior body wall (Fig. 26.12).

Stages of development

1. *Formation of sternal bars:* In midline, the lateral plate mesoderm of anterior body wall forms two mesenchymal sternal bars that undergo chondrification and develop cartilaginous sternal bars.
2. *Formation of cartilaginous sternum model:* Two cartilaginous sternal bars fuse in the midline to form cartilaginous sternum model that has manubrium, body and xiphoid process. Body consists of four fused segments called sternebrae.
3. Ossification of sternum
    - Ossification centres for sternum appear before birth except for the xiphoid (occurs in childhood).
    - For manubrium: A pair of ossification centres appears in 5th month of IUL.

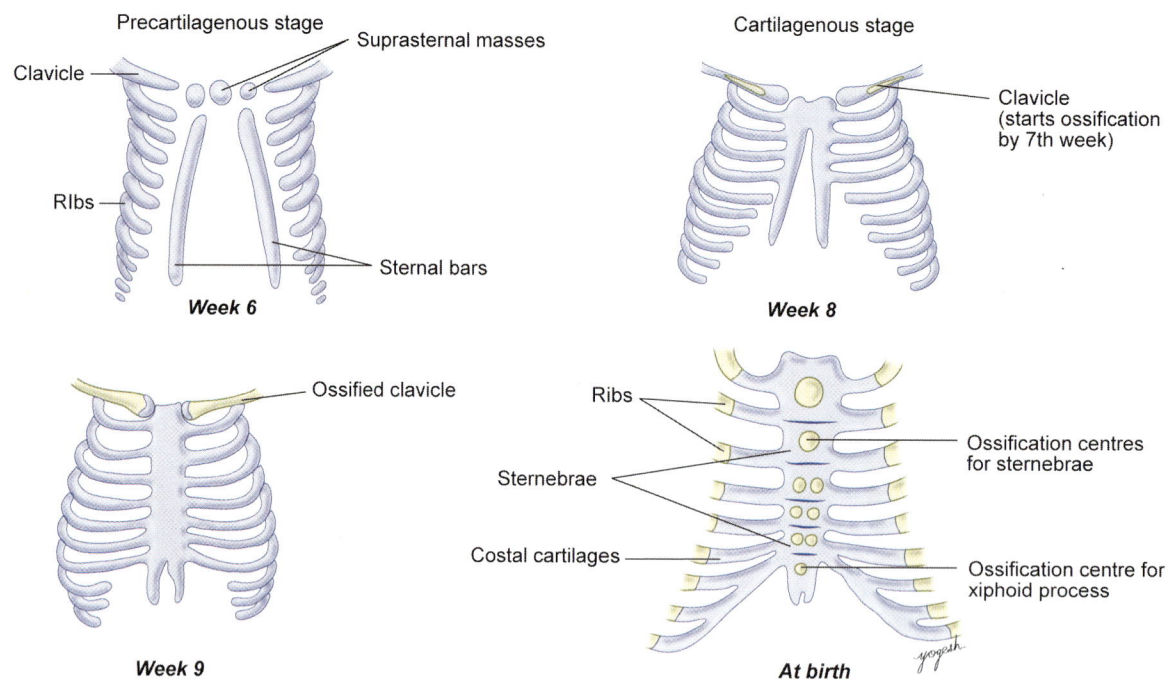

Fig. 26.12: Development of sternum

- For body: 4 pairs of ossification centres appear in 6th, 7th, 8th, 9th month of IUL (from above downwards). Each pair of centres fuses to form sternebrae. Fusion of four sternebrae takes place from below upward and completes by 25 years of age.
- For xiphoid process – centre appears in 3rd year of life and fuses with body by 40 years.

Abnormalities of sternum
1. *Bifid sternum:* Failure of fusion of two sternal bars may result in sternal foramen, sternal cleft, bifid sternum or bifid xiphoid process.
2. *Funnel chest:* Due to abnormally short central tendon of diaphragm, lower part of sternum and ribs are drawn inwards into the thorax. This condition is called *funnel chest.*^MCQ Funnel chest is the most common congenital anomaly of the chest.
3. *Pigeon chest* (pectus carinatum): It involves forward projection of upper part of sternum and ribs.

Development of Skull (Cranium)

- Mesenchyme surrounding the developing brain condenses to form cranium (skull). Skull consists of
  1. *Neurocranium:* These bones enclose and protect the brain.
  2. *Viscerocranium:* These bones form facial skeleton.
- Neurocranium is divided into:
  – *Chondrocranium:* It forms bones of skull base.
  – *Membranous neurocranium:* It forms bones of skull vault.
- Viscerocranium is also divided into cartilaginous and membranous viscerocranium.

Chondrocranium (Fig. 26.13)
- At the 6th week of IUL, the cartilaginous neurocranium (chondrocranium) forms by fusion of several cartilages.
- Endochondral ossification starts forming the bones of skullbase.
- The cartilages are as follows:
  – Parachordal cartilage (basal plate) appears around the cranial end of notochord. It forms base of occipital bone and boundaries of foramen magnum.
  – Hypophyseal cartilage appears around the pituitary gland and forms body of sphenoid bone.
  – Trabeculae cranae form body of ethmoid bone.
  – Ala orbitalis forms lesser wing of sphenoid bone.
  – Otic capsule forms bony labyrinth, petrous and mastoid part of temporal bone.
  – Nasal capsule contributes to ethmoid bone.
  – Ala temporalis forms greater wing of sphenoid bone.

Membranous neurocranium
- Membranous ossification develops calvaria (cranial vault) on sides and top of the brain.
- The bones of skull vault are separated by sutures (fibrous joints).
- At 6 places, the sutures are wide and they form a gap called *fontanelles*. Modelling of fetal cranium during birth passage is possible due to the fontanelles.

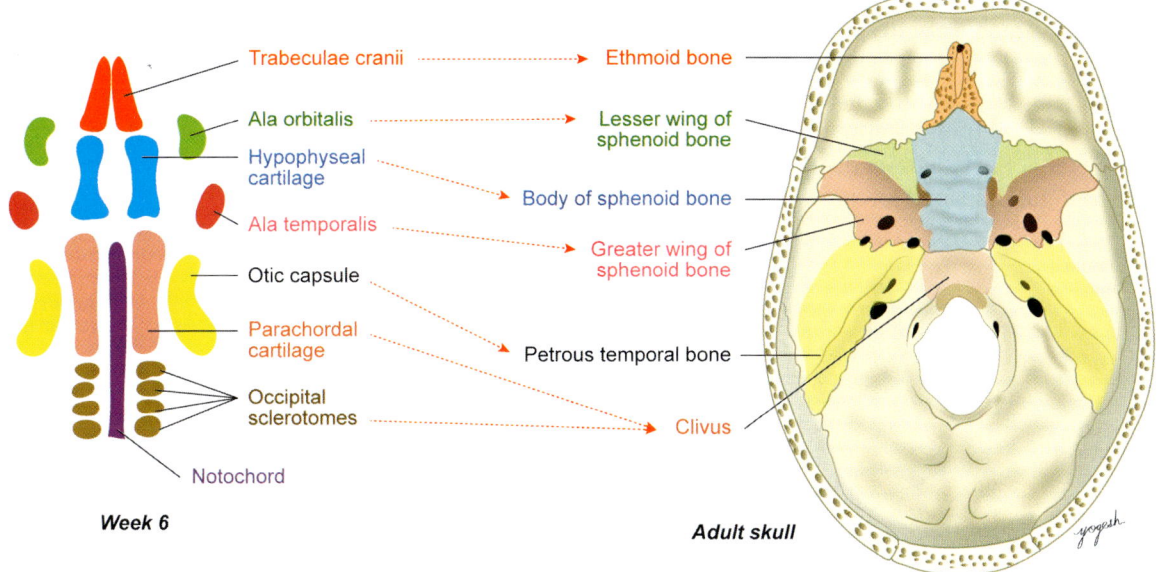

Fig. 26.13: Developmental components of chondrocranium and their derivatives

Cartilaginous viscerocranium
- Cartilaginous viscerocranium is constituted by contribution from first and second pharyngeal arch cartilages as follows:
  a. First arch cartilage forms malleus and incus.^{MCQ}
  b. Second arch cartilage forms stapes and styloid process of temporal bone.^{MCQ}

Membranous viscerocranium
- Intramembranous ossification forms the following bones.
  Squamous part of temporal bone
  Maxillary and zygomatic bones
  Mandible (mandibular condyle and chin of mandible shows endochondral ossification)

Cranium in newborn
- In newborn, the cranium is large in proportion to that of the rest of body skeleton.
- In newborn, neurocranium is larger than viscerocranium because of:
  1. Underdeveloped jaw bone.
  2. Absence of paranasal air sinuses.
  3. Underdeveloped facial bones.

Anomalies of Skull
1. *Anencephaly:* Major portion of brain, skull and scalp are absent in anencephaly. Anencephaly is most severe birth defect in stillborn babies.
2. *Cleidocranial dysostosis:* It involves absence of clavicle, nonclosure of metopic suture (between frontal bones), prominent forehead and abnormal teeth.
3. *Scaphocephaly:* Early closure of sagittal suture results in scaphocephaly. It shows boat-shaped skull (long narrow head).^{MCQ}

Box 26.3: Fontanelles (Fig. 26.14)

- Fontanelles are soft membranous gaps present in the skull vault of newborn.
- There are 6 fontanelles at birth as follows:
  – *Anterior fontanelle* between frontal and parietal bones. Anterior fontanelle is the largest fontanelle.^{MCQ}
  – *Posterior fontanelle* between occipital and parietal bones.
  – *Anterolateral (sphenoid) fontanelle* between greater wing of sphenoid, squamous temporal, frontal, and parietal bones.
  – *Posterolateral (mastoid) fontanelle* between parietal, occipital, squamous temporal, and occipital bones.
- Closure of fontanelle
  – All fontanelles close within 3–4 months after birth.
  – Anterior fontanelle closes by 2–3 years of age.^{MCQ}
- Function of fontanelles
  – Allow moulding of skull during the birth passage of body.
  – Permit growth of skull bones to increase the cranial capacity.
  – Accommodate developing brain.
- Clinical aspects
  1. Closure of fontanelles gives an idea about the age of the newborn.
  2. Appearance of fontanelle gives an idea of intracranial pressure.
     – Bulging fontanelles indicate increased intracranial pressure.
     – Depressed fontanelles indicate dehydration cases.

4. *Brachycephaly:* Early closure of coronal suture results in short skull (brachycephaly).
5. *Plagiocephaly:* Early closure of coronal and lambdoid sutures on one side results into grossly unequal curvatures of skull (plagiocephaly).
6. *Trigonocephaly:* Early closure of metopic suture results in triangular-shaped forehead (trigonocephaly).
7. *Hydrocephalus:* In this condition, the skull bones may be widely separated due to increased intracranial pressure.
8. *Hand-Schüller-Christian disease:* It is a defect of reticuloendothelial system (Langerhans cell histiocytosis) associated with lytic bone lesions of the skull.^{NEXT}

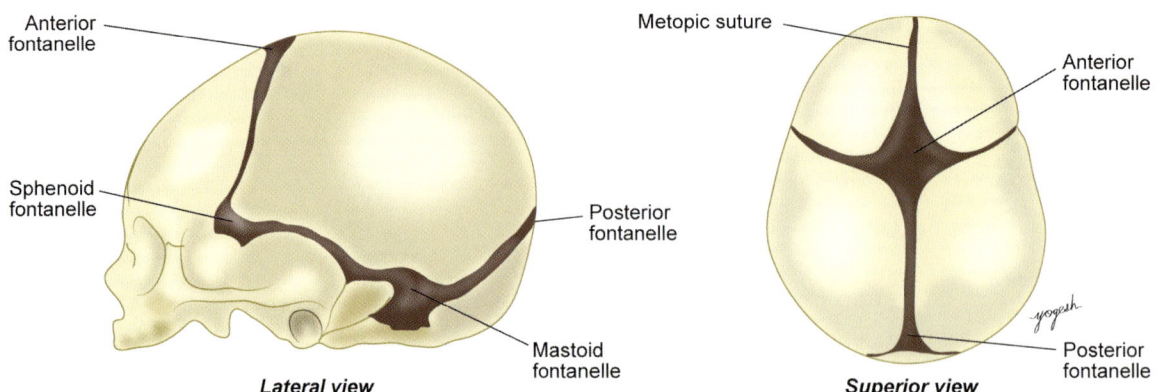

Fig. 26.14: Skull of the newborn showing fontanelles

Clinical Embryology

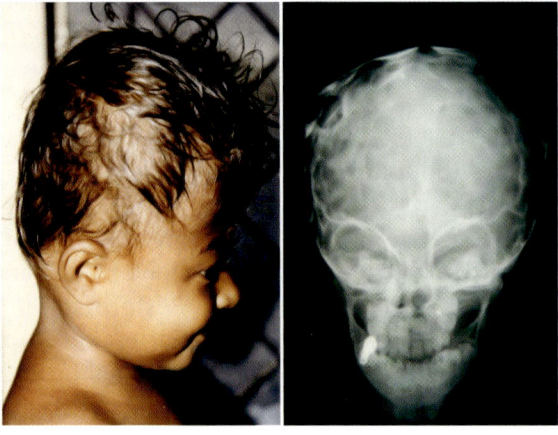

Clinical image 26.1: *Scaphocephaly*. Craniosynostosis involves premature ossification (fusion) of sutures. It causes alternation of the growth pattern of the skull and abnormal head shape. Scaphocephaly (premature fusion of sagittal sutures) is the most common craniosynostosis and is characterized by a long, narrow head that resembles an inverted boat (skaphe meaning 'light boat or skiff' and kephale meaning 'head' in Greek) (Image courtesy: *Dr Kumaravel S*)

Chapter 27

Muscular System

eSmartQuiz

Chapter Outline

- Development of skeletal muscles
  - Histogenesis of skeletal muscle
- Development of individual group muscle
  - Muscles of body wall
  - Extraocular muscles
  - Muscles of tongue
  - Muscles of pharyngeal arches
  - Muscles of limbs
  - Congenital anomalies of skeletal muscles
- Duchenne muscular dystrophy
- Development of smooth muscles
- Development of cardiac muscle

INTRODUCTION

- All the muscles of the body are derived from mesoderm except muscles of iris, arrector pili of skin, and myoepithelial cells of glands.^{NEXT} These are derived from ectoderm (neural crest).
- Muscles are classified as follows:
  A. Striated muscles: These show cytoplasmic striations of actin and myosin filaments. These are of two types:
    1. Skeletal muscles: These are responsible for the movement of bones and are derived from paraxial mesoderm (somites).
    2. Cardiac muscles: These are in myocardium and develop from splanchnopleuric mesoderm.
  B. Smooth muscles: These do not show cytoplasmic striations (hence, smooth) and develop from splanchnopleuric mesoderm.
- Skeletal muscles are voluntary, whereas cardiac and smooth muscles are involuntary.

DEVELOPMENT OF SKELETAL MUSCLES

- Skeletal muscles develop from somites.

Histogenesis of Skeletal Muscle

- Each *somite* has dorsolateral dermomyotome and venteromedial sclerotome
- Dermomyotome differentiates into superficial dermatome and deep myotome.
- Mesenchyme of myotome differentiates into *myoblasts* (primordial muscle cells).
- Myoblasts elongate and fuse at ends with each other to form multinucleated *myotube* (syncytium)
- Myotubes synthesize muscle proteins (actin, myosin, troponin, and so on) and become muscle fibers. Muscle proteins push the nuclei to periphery (Fig. 27.1).
- Adjacent muscle fibers form bundles, fascicle and complete muscle.

Some Interesting Facts

1. Extraocular muscles develop from *preotic myotomes*.^{MCQ}
2. Muscles of tongue (except palatoglossus) develop from *occipital myotomes*.^{MCQ}
3. Skeletal muscle looses mitotic activity after birth, but they can undergo hypertrophy.

DEVELOPMENT OF INDIVIDUAL GROUP MUSCLE

The skeletal muscles can be grouped on the basis of development into the following groups:
1. Muscles of trunk (body wall)
2. Muscles of branchial arches
3. Extraocular muscles
4. Muscles of tongue
5. Muscles of limbs

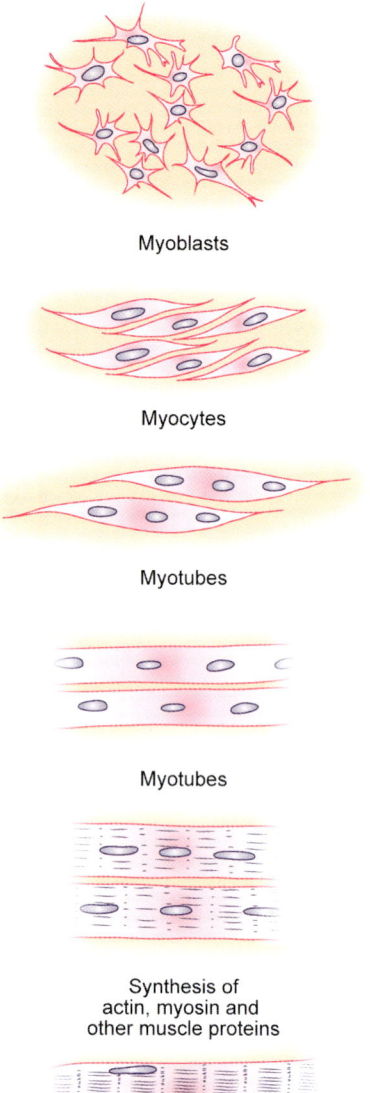

Fig. 27.1: Histogenesis of muscle fiber

- Muscles of ventral midline longitudinal column (rectus abdominis, rectus sternalis, infrahyoid muscles). These are also called strap muscles.
- Developmentally, scalene group of muscles corresponds to the intercostal muscles of thoracic cage.^{MCQ}
- Muscles of diaphragm correspond to transverse thoracic muscle (innermost muscle column).^{MCQ}
- Similarly, muscles of pelvic diaphragm develop from innermost muscle column.^{MCQ} Morphologically, medial fibers of levator ani represent the downward continuation of rectus abdominis muscle (longitudinal column).^{NEXT}
- Nerve supply: Muscle of epimere are supplied by dorsal ramus of spinal nerve, whereas muscles of hypomere are supplied by ventral ramus of spinal nerve (Fig. 27.2).

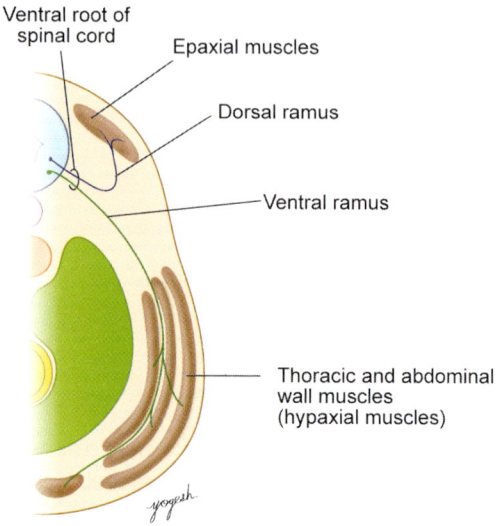

Fig. 27.2: Nerve supply of trunk muscles

Extraocular Muscles

- Extraocular muscles develop from 3 preotic myotomes (Fig. 27.3).^{MCQ}
- Nerve supply:$^{MCQ, Viva}$
  3rd cranial nerve: Inferior oblique, levator palpabrae superioris, medial rectus, and inferior rectus.
  4th cranial nerve: Superior oblique.
  6th cranial nerve: Lateral rectus.

Muscles of Tongue

- All the muscles of tongue (extrinsic and intrinsic) except palatoglossus are derived from 4 occipital myotomes.
- Hypoglossal nerve (precervical nerve) supplies the derivatives of occipital (precervical) myotomes.^{MCQ}
- Occipital myotomes migrate from cervical region to developing tongue along the epipericardial ridge. During migration, hypoglossal nerve traverses superficial to external and internal carotid arteries.$^{Clinical fact}$

Muscles of Body Wall

- Muscles of body wall develop from myotomes of somites.
- Each myotome has two parts:
  A. Epaxial part (epimere): It is a smaller dorsal part. It forms extensor muscles of vertebral column; for example, erector spinae.
  B. *Hypomere* (hypaxial part): It is a larger ventral part. It forms the following muscles of the body wall:
    – Intercostal muscles
    – Muscles of anterior abdominal wall
    – Muscles of neck (longus coli, longus capitis and scalene muscles)

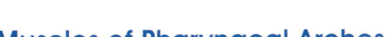

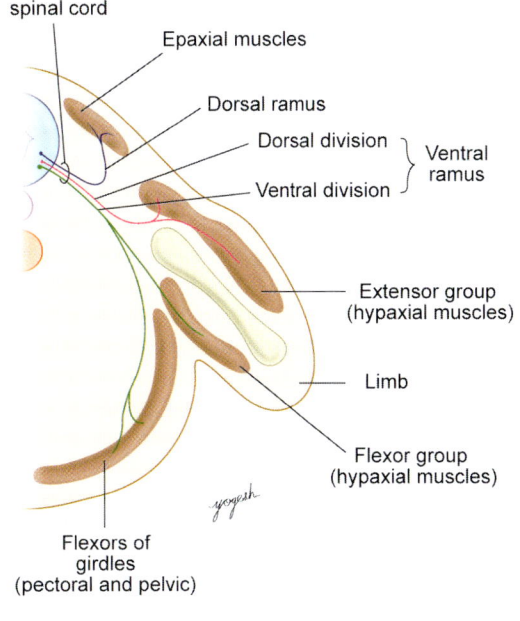

Fig. 27.3: Myotomes

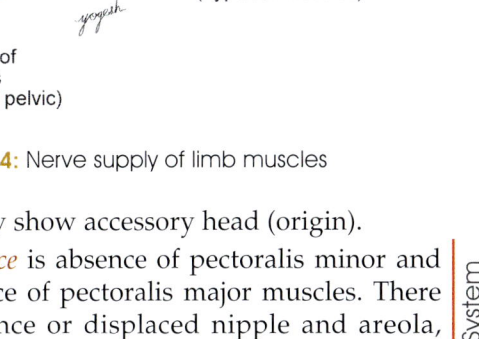

Fig. 27.4: Nerve supply of limb muscles

Muscles of Pharyngeal Arches

- Muscles of pharyngeal arches develop from mesoderm of pharyngeal arches.
- The muscular derivatives of pharyngeal arches are as follows:*High yielding facts, NEXT*
  - 1st arch: Muscle of mastication (temporalis, masseter, lateral, and medial pterygoid), tensor tympani, tensor veli palatini, anterior belly of digastric, and mylohyoid
  - 2nd arch: Muscles of facial expression, posterior belly of digastric, stapedius, and stylohyoid
  - 3rd arch: Stylopharyngeus
  - 4th arch: Cricothyroid, constrictors of pharynx, muscles of palate except tensor veli palatini
  - 6th arch: Intrinsic muscles of larynx except cricothyroid

Muscles of Limbs

- In the 5th week, myotomes of limb bud form anterior and posterior condensations.
- Anterior mesenchymal condensation forms flexor and pronator muscles in upper limb, whereas extensor and adductor muscles in lower limb.
- Posterior mesenchymal condensation forms extensor and supinator muscles in upper limb, whereas flexor and abductor muscles in lower limb (Fig. 27.4).

Congenital Anomalies of Skeletal Muscles

1. Duchenne muscular dystrophy: Box 27.1.
2. A skeletal muscle may be partially or completely absent.
3. A muscle may show accessory head (origin).
4. *Poland sequence* is absence of pectoralis minor and partial absence of pectoralis major muscles. There may be absence or displaced nipple and areola, syndactyly (fused fingers) or brachydactyly (less number of fingers).
5. *Congenital torticollis:* Excessive stretching of sternocleidomastoid muscle during delivery causes shortening of this muscle (torticollis).*MCQ*

DEVELOPMENT OF SMOOTH MUSCLES

- Mesenchymal tissue differentiates into myoblast that later forms spindle-shaped smooth muscle cells.
- Smooth muscles are derived from the following sources:
  1. Splanchnopleuric mesoderm forms smooth muscles of gastrointestinal tract and respiratory tract.*MCQ*
  2. Intermediate mesoderm forms smooth muscles in urogenital system.*MCQ*
  3. Surrounding mesenchyme forms smooth muscles in developing vessels and lymph vessels.
  4. Neuroectoderm of optic cup forms muscles of iris (sphincter and dilator pupilae) and ciliaris muscle.*MCQ*
  5. Arrector pili muscles of skin and myoepithelial cells of mammary gland are derived from ectoderm.*MCQ*
  6. Serum response factor (SRF) (transcription protein) is responsible for smooth muscle cell differentiation. Myocardin and myocardin-related transcription factors are cofactors that enhance the activity of SRF.

DEVELOPMENT OF CARDIAC MUSCLE

- The cardiac muscle develops from mesenchyme of myoepicardial mantle (part of splanchnic mesoderm).

Histogenesis of cardiac muscle

- In cardiac muscle development, each myoblast elongates and gives rise to numerous side branches.
- These side branches of adjacent cells come in contact with each other.
- At the point of contact, cell membrane modifies to form *intercalated disc*.
- Thus, cardiac muscle does not form true syncytium.

Some Interesting Facts

- First occipital myotome disappears soon after its formation.
- Rectus sternalis in thorax represents its abdominal counterpart rectus abdominis. ^{NEXT}
- Myoepithelial cells of secretory acini of glands, myoid cells of seminiferous tubules and myofibroblasts of healing wound are also contractile (nonmuscular) cells. ^{MCQ}

Box 27.1: Duchenne muscular dystrophy (DMD)

Q. Write a short note on Duchenne muscular dystrophy.

- DMD is a hereditary muscular dystrophy (progressive weakening of muscle)

Cause

- It is X-linked recessive disorder.
- Mutation of gene responsible for production of protein dystropin (essential for maintenance of cell membrane of muscle fiber).

Incidence

- 1 in 4000 males at birth.
- Most common type of muscular dystrophy.

Signs and symptoms

- Severe progressive muscle degeneration.
- Loss of ability to walk by 9–12 years of age.
- Death by the age of 20 years due to respiratory failure.

Treatment

- No cure treatment is available.
- Steroids can be given to slow down muscle dystrophy.
- Other supportive measure (breathing assistance, braces and so on) may be required.

Clinical Embryology

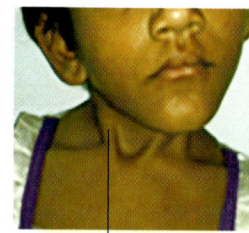
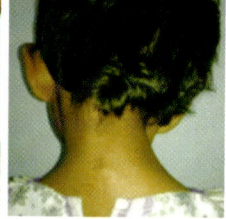

Contracted sternocleidomastoid muscle

Clinical image 27.1: Congenital muscular torticolis or wry neck. Tortus meaning twisted in Latin. Affecting right sternocleidomastoid muscle causes tilt of chin to opposite side [Image courtesy: *Dr Uday Kumbhar*]

Chapter 28

Fetal Period: Nine Weeks to Birth

eSmartQuiz

Chapter Outline

- Growth of fetus
  - Changes in 3rd month
  - Changes in 4th month
  - Changes in 5th month
  - Changes in 6th month
  - Changes in 7th month
  - Changes in 8th month
  - Changes in 9th month
- Factor influencing growth

INTRODUCTION

- Embryologically prenatal period is divided into:
  1. Germinal/ovular period: It consists of first two weeks of development after fertilization.
  2. Embryonic period: It extends from 3rd week to 8th week of development.^{NEXT}
  3. Fetal period (organ growth): It extends from 9th week (3rd month) up to the termination of the pregnancy.

Gestation

- The period of development in the uterus, between conception and birth is called *gestation*.
- Length of gestational period in humans: 280 days = (40 weeks or 9 months ± 7 days).
- Gestation means menstrual age in Latin.
- Gestational period (menstrual age) begins from the date of onset of last menstrual period (LMP).

Use of gestational period

- It can be used to calculate the expected date of delivery as follows:

  (LMP or Date of onset of last menstrual period) + 9 months 7 days = Expected date of delivery (EDD)^{Viva}
- Thus, embryologically the age of fetus (fertilization age) is 14 days less than the gestational age.
- *Note*: 14 days are considered as duration of the last menstrual cycle up to fertilization.

GROWTH OF FETUS

- In the fetal period, fetus grows rapidly to give shape of the newborn.
- All body parts undergo considerable growth and cellular and functional differentiation.
- Major events during fetal period are listed below.

Changes in 3rd Month (9–12 Weeks) (Fig. 28.1)

1. At beginning of the 3rd month, head is about half of the fetal size. Body grows in crown-to-rump (CR) length and doubles by the 12th week.
2. Face: Broad face, widely spaced eyes, low sets of ears, fused eyelids.
3. Limbs: By the 12th week, the upper limb develops to take their normal shape, but lower limbs lag.
4. External genitalia: It remains undifferentiated till 9th week.
5. Umbilical hernia: Intestinal loop returns to the abdominal cavity by 10th week.^{MCQ}

Changes in 4th Month (13–16 Weeks) (Fig. 28.1)

1. Head: It becomes comparatively smaller due to growth of other body parts.
2. CR length: Length of fetus increases rapidly.
3. Limbs: Limbs increase in length. Lower limb obtains its normal shape. Movements of limbs can be seen on ultrasound examination.

Changes in 5th Month (17–20 Weeks) (Fig. 28.1)

1. CR length: Increases slowly up to 190 mm.
2. Quickening: Mother can feel fetal movements (quickening).
3. Vernix caseosa: Fetal skin is covered by greasy, cheese-like material (*vernix caseosa*) secreted by sebaceous glands.^MCQ
4. Lanugo: By the end of 5th month, the fetus is fully covered by fine brown hairs *(lanugo)*.^MCQ
5. Eyebrows and hairs on head become visible.

Changes in 6th Month (21–24 Weeks) (Fig. 28.1)

1. Skin: Due to the absence of subcutaneous tissue, skin is wrinkled, translucent, and pink.
2. Lungs: Alveoli starts secreting surfactant.
3. Weight: Fetus starts gaining weight.

Changes in 7th Month (25–29 Weeks) (Fig. 28.2)

1. Lungs: Fetus is *viable with supporting measures* as lung maturation is going on.
2. Blood formation: Bone marrow takes over the function of hematopoiesis from spleen.
3. CNS: Nervous system is matured to control respiration.

Changes in 8th Month (30–34 Weeks) (Fig. 28.2)

1. Skin: On the deposition of subcutaneous fat, skin becomes smooth.
2. Weight: Body weight increases rapidly.

Changes in 9th Month (35–38 Weeks) (Fig. 28.2)

1. Termination: Delivery takes place on 266 days (38 weeks) of fertilization age or 280 days (40 weeks) of gestational age (after onset of last menstruation).^NEXT
2. Testis: In male fetus, testes reach scrotum by the end of 9th month.^NEXT
3. Fingernails: By 28th week, fingernails grow beyond fingertip.^NEXT

FACTORS INFLUENCING GROWTH

Following factors play a major role in growth of the fetus:

1. *Nutrition*: Maternal nutrition has the highest impact on growth of the fetus. Maternal malnutrition causes fetal growth retardation.
2. *Genetic factors:* Growth depends on genetic constitution. Chromosomal/genetic abnormalities may lead to fetal growth retardation.
3. *Placenta:* Placental disorder affects the fetal growth due to insufficient uteroplacental blood flow.
4. *Multiple pregnancies:* Each fetus tends to be smaller than the normal single pregnancy due to distribution of available resources (nutrition and space).
5. Smoking, alcohol and drugs (teratogens) may produce adverse fetal outcome.

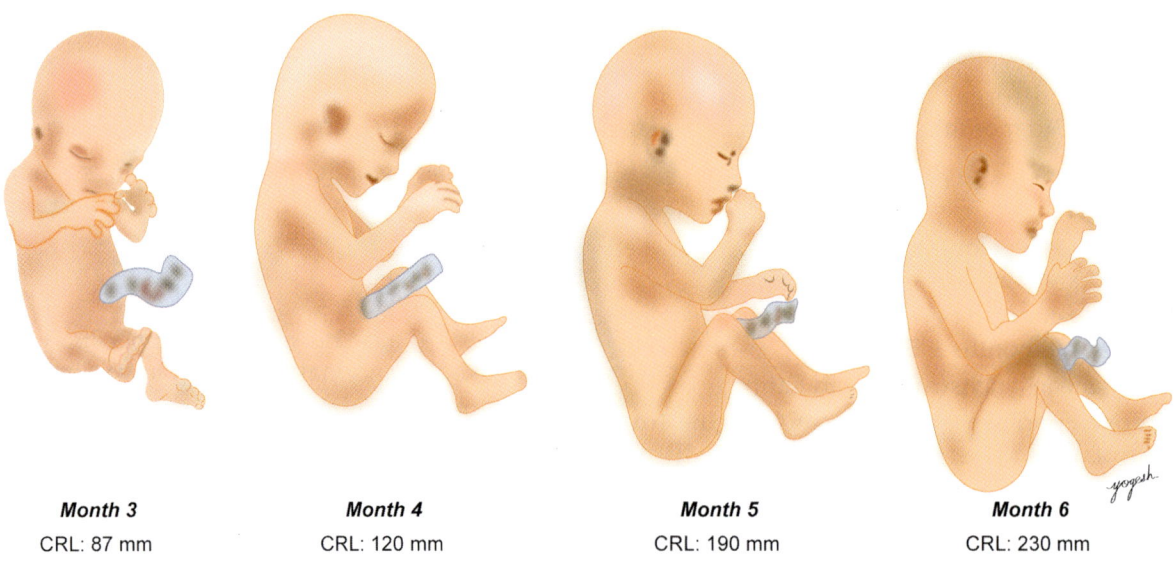

| Month 3 | Month 4 | Month 5 | Month 6 |
| CRL: 87 mm | CRL: 120 mm | CRL: 190 mm | CRL: 230 mm |

Fig. 28.1: Fetus of 3rd to 6th month of intrauterine life

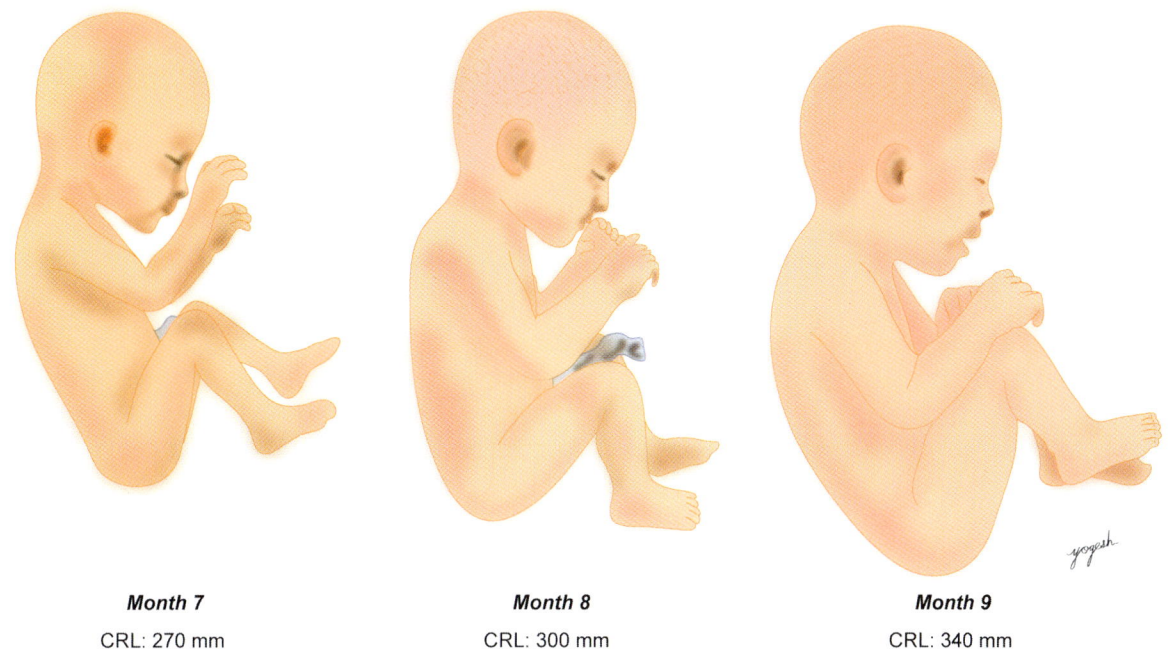

Month 7	Month 8	Month 9
CRL: 270 mm	CRL: 300 mm	CRL: 340 mm

Fig. 28.2: Fetus of 7th to 9th month of intrauterine life

Clinical Embryology

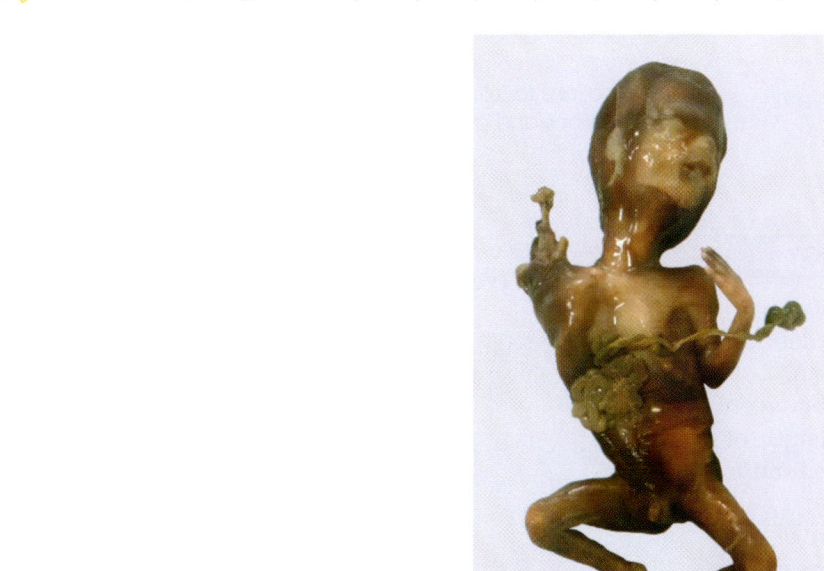

Clinical image 28.1: Fetus of second trimester (Image courtesy: *Dr Haritha Sagili*)

Chapter 29

Clinical Applications and Ultrasonography in Embryology

eSmartQuiz

Chapter Outline

Clinical applications in embryology
- Criteria for estimation of age in embryo
- Prenatal diagnosis
  - Amniocentesis
  - Chorionic villus sampling
  - Maternal blood screening
  - Percutaneous umbilical blood sampling
  - Fetoscopy

Ultrasonography in embryology
- Principle of ultrasonography
- Grey scale of ultrasound in obstetrics
- Ultrasound frequency
- Types
- Purpose of antenatal ultrasonography
- Classification of fetal sonographic examinations
- Indications for ultrasound examination
- Guidelines and parameters for ultrasonography

CLINICAL APPLICATIONS IN EMBRYOLOGY

- Obstetrics is the branch of the medicine that deals with the care of pregnant woman, unborn baby, labour, and immediate period following the childbirth.
- The period of development in the uterus, between conception and birth is called *gestation*. Length of gestational period: 280 days = (40 weeks or 9 months ± 7 days).
- During obstetrics practice, determination of the gestational age is important for the following reasons:
  1. For antenatal assessment of fetal wellbeing.
  2. For planning of termination of pregnancy.
  3. For taking decision about mode of delivery (normal vaginal or cesarean section).
  4. For taking decision about chorionic villus sampling or amniocentesis.
- Criteria for determination of age varies according to the age of the conceptus.

CRITERIA FOR ESTIMATION OF AGE IN EMBRYO

- The age of embryo (up to 8 weeks) can be determined by number of somites and crown to rump length.
- *Crown to rump length (CR length)*: It is also called sitting length. It is measured from top of the skull (vertex) to the bottom of buttock (Table 29.1).
- *Crown to heel length (CHL)*: It is measured from top of the skull (vertex) to the heel.

Table 29.1 Estimation of age in embryo

Age (days)	Number of somites	CR length (mm)
20–21	1–7	1.5–3
22–23	7–13	2–3.5
24–25	13–19	2.5–4.5
26–27	19–24	3–5
28–30	24–35	4–6

Estimation of Age in Fetus (9–38 weeks)

- Fetal age can be determined by using the following parameters (Table 29.2):
  1. Crown to rump length (CR length)
  2. Foot length
  3. Weight of fetus

PRENATAL DIAGNOSIS

- Pregnancy outcome depends on multiple factors such as genetic constitution, maternal factors and so on.

Table 29.2	Fetal parameters for age estimation (approximate values)	
Age (in weeks)	Crown to rump length (mm)	Weight (g)
9	50	8
10	61	14
12	87	45
16	120	200
20	190	460
24	230	820
28	270	1300
32	300	2100
36	340	2900
38	360	3400

- Prenatal diagnosis is the application of available techniques to assess the status of fetus *in utero* and to detect the congenital malformations.
- The methods of prenatal diagnosis are classified as noninvasive methods, minimal invasive methods and invasive methods.
- Noninvasive methods include prenatal checkup and ultrasound examination. Minimal invasive techniques include maternal blood screening. Invasive methods include amniocentesis, chorionic villus sampling, fetoscopy, and fetal blood sampling.

Amniocentesis

- Amniotic fluid (20 ml) is collected under ultrasound guidance during 14–20 weeks of IUL.
- Cells are assessed from amniotic fluid for chromosomal or genetic abnormalities.
- Amniotic fluid is also assessed for α-fetoprotein and other biochemical parameters.

Chorionic Villus Sampling (CVS)

- Chorionic villus tissue is collected under ultrasound guidance during 9–12 weeks of IUL.
- Cells are assessed for genetic and metabolic abnormalities.

Maternal Blood Screening

- Maternal blood screening (16 weeks onward) includes assessment for circulating fetal cells, β-hCG (human chorionic gonadotropin), α-fetoprotein, estriol and inhibin A.

Percutaneous Umbilical Blood Sampling

- It is performed under ultrasound guidance to collect fetal blood, usually in Rh incompatibility cases and for assessment of chromosomal aberrations.

Fetoscopy

- It is the visualization of the fetus using endoscope usually in second trimester to detect severe structural damage.
- For details about prenatal diagnosis, read *Principles of Clinical Genetics* by Dr Yogesh Sontakke.

ULTRASONOGRAPHY IN EMBRYOLOGY

- Ultrasonography is a noninvasive technique useful for prenatal assessment.
- *Ultrasound examination during pregnancy* was introduced in Sweden in 1973.

PRINCIPLE OF ULTRASONOGRAPHY

- In ultrasound examination, transducer generates ultrasound waves and record echoes generated by medium (here, tissue).
- Transducer has piezoelectric material that can generate ultrasound of typical wavelength (2–18 MHz) on electric stimulus.
- The material on the surface of transducer enables the sound to be transmitted efficiently into the body.
- To enhance the transmission, water-based gel is placed between the skin and the transducer probe.
- Returning sound waves (echoes) vibrate the transducer that in turn generates electric pulses.
- These electric pulses are carried to the scanner that generates the image depending on the time required for the sound wave to come back from the object (for example, uterus), strength of the echo and focal length of phased array.
- Depending on the strength of the echoes, scanner generates different shades of grey to produce an image.
- 2D image (slice of body) can be generated by sweeping or rotating transducer mechanically. 3D images can be generated by acquiring a series of adjacent 2D images.
- *Doppler ultrasonography* is useful to study blood flow and muscle motion of fetus.^{NEXT} In Doppler ultrasonography, different detected speeds are represented in color for easy interpretation.
- Doppler shifts cells fall in audible sounds. It is represented by audibly distinctive pulsing sound (*pulsed Doppler*) to measure the velocity.
- In Doppler ultrasonography, use of specific color has not set with any standard. Some use red for artery, whereas some use red to indicate flow towards transducer.
- World Health Organization (1988) declared that diagnostic ultrasound is safe (harmless) and capable of providing clinically relevant information about most parts of the body and even ultrasound is safe for fetus.

GREY SCALE OF ULTRASOUND IN OBSTETRICS

- On ultrasonography, substance may be
  - Hyperechoic: It gives white color on screen. For example, fat containing tissue.
  - Hypoechoic: It gives grey scale. For example, soft tissue.

- Anechoic: It gives black color. For example, clear fluid (amniotic fluid), blood vessels.
- Acoustic shadow: Gas does not echo sound waves; hence, it produces black color.
- Bones appear as black (anechoic) with bright hyperechoic rim as ultrasound does not penetrate the bone.^MCQ
- Cartilage appears white (hyperechoic) as ultrasound penetrates cartilage.^MCQ
- Usually, Doppler shows red for flow towards probe and blue for flow away from probe. (BART: Blue away, red toward).^MCQ
- Muscles are hypoechoic, whereas other connective tissues are hyperechoic.

ULTRASOUND FREQUENCY

- High frequency probes (10–15 MHz) are suitable for superficial structures (2–4 cm depth).
- Mid-frequency probes (5–10 MHz) are suitable for deeper structures (5–6 cm).
- Low frequency probes (2–5 MHz) are suitable for more deeper structures (~10 cm depth).
- With decreasing frequency of probe; quality of image also decreases.

TYPES

According to the method of ultrasonography technique, it is classified as:

A. *Transabdominal sonography*: It is performed across the abdominal wall.

B. *Transvaginal sonography*: It is performed through vagina. It is also called endovaginal sonography.

PURPOSE OF ANTENATAL ULTRASONOGRAPHY

- The ultrasonography during pregnancy is targeted for the following purposes:
  1. Confirmation of pregnancy (presence of gestational sac).
  2. Estimation of gestational age of fetus.
  3. Detection of multiple pregnancies.
  4. Detection of fetal anomalies.
  5. Monitoring of fetal growth and development.
  6. Detection of ectopic pregnancy.
  7. To guide surgical procedures (amniocentesis, chorionic villus sampling).

CLASSIFICATION OF FETAL SONOGRAPHIC EXAMINATIONS

A. First Trimester Examination

- It includes evaluation of presence, size, location, and number of gestational sac(s).
- The gestation sac is examined for presence of a yolk sac and embryo/fetus.

B. Second and Third Trimester Examination

- It includes an evaluation of fetal wellbeing, fetal presentation/position, volume of amniotic fluid, cardiac activity, placental position and fetal morphometric parameters (biometry).

C. Limited Examination

- It includes a specific targeted examination. For example, fetal heart activity in bleeding patient.

D. Specialized Examinations

- It includes detailed anatomic examination for suspected anomaly on the basis of history.

INDICATIONS FOR ULTRASOUND EXAMINATION

First Trimester Ultrasound Examination

Indications for the first trimester ultrasound examination include:

1. Confirmation of the pregnancy.
2. Detection of the ectopic pregnancy.
3. Detection for cause of vaginal bleeding.
4. Determination of gestational age.
5. Detection of multiple gestation.
6. Confirmation of cardiac activity.
   - Gestational sac is seen in 3rd–5th week after menstruation.^MCQ
   - Embryonic cardiac activity is identifiable by 6–6.5 weeks (embryonic length 2 mm or more).^NEXT
   - In addition to above indications, adnexal masses, uterus, and cervix are also screened for the presence of any abnormalities.

Second and Third Trimester Examination

Indications for second and third trimester ultrasound examination include:

1. Evaluation of fetal anatomy, growth, and anomalies.
2. Determination of gestational age.
3. Evaluation of abdominal pain, vaginal bleeding, and ectopic pregnancy.
4. Evaluation of fetal presentation, position of placenta, amniotic fluid abnormalities, and premature rupture of membranes.
5. Evaluation of hydatidiform mole, uterine abnormalities
6. To guide amniocentesis and chorionic villus sampling.

GUIDELINES AND PARAMETERS FOR ULTRASONOGRAPHY

Some important parameters and guidelines for the ultrasound examination in obstetrics are as follows (Table 29.3):

1. To visualize cervix and internal os, transvaginal ultrasound may be helpful.

Table 29.3	Fetal parameters in second and third trimesters (Handlock)			
Gestational age (weeks)	BPD (mm)	Head circumference (mm)	Abdominal circumference (mm)	Femur length (mm)
13	21	82	60	11
16	32	124	99	20
20	46	177	150	33
24	59	224	197	44
28	71	266	240	54
32	81	301	281	62
36	89	328	318	70
38	92	338	336	74

BPD: Biparietal diameter.

2. *Gestational sac*
   - It can be detected during 3–5th week after menstruation.
   - Mean diameter of gestational sac is useful for the determination of gestational age.
   - Growth rate of gestational sac is 1 mm per day.
   - It is suitable only up to gestational sac diameter 14 mm for gestational age determination, after that embryo can be identified.^{MCQ}

3. *Yolk sac*
   - It becomes visible by 5th–6th week and useful only for confirmation of pregnancy.^{MCQ}
   - It becomes 6 mm by 10th week (maximum size), then gradually decreases in size and becomes nondetectable by the end of third week.

4. *Crown to rump length (CRL)* (Clinical image 29.1)
   - It is the distance between highest point of skull and lowest point of buttocks.
   - It is most accurate for gestational age determination in **first** trimester.
   - It is suitable up to 84 mm size, after that biparietal diameter is useful.^{MCQ}

5. In second and third trimesters, gestational age determination depends on biparietal diameter, head circumference, abdominal circumference, and femur length. Use of multiple parameters is recommended.

6. *Biparietal diameter:* It is the diameter of axial plane through skull of the fetus (embryo) (Clinical image 29.2).

7. *Head circumference*: It is obtained in the same plane of biparietal diameter. The tracings for head circumference should follow the outer perimeter of skull (Clinical image 29.2).

8. *Abdominal circumference*: It should be measured at the level of bifurcation of portal vein or at the level of stomach (Clinical image 29.3).

9. *Femur length:* For measurement of the femur length, both femoral condyles should be visualized simultaneously. The ultrasound transducer should be perpendicular to the long axis of the femur. It is measured from tip of the greater trochanter to the lateral epicondyle (Clinical image 29.4).

Further Reading

- Babuta S, Chauhan S, Garg R, Bagarhatta M. Assessment of fetal gestational age in different trimester from ultrasonographic measurements of various fetal biometric parameters. *J ASI* 2013;60: 40–6.
- Butt K, Lin K. Determination of gestational age by ultrasound. *J Obstet Gynaecol Can* 2014;36(2):171–81.
- Handlock FP, Deter RL, Harrist RB, et al. Estimating fetal age: Computer-assisted analysis of multiple fetal growth parameters. *Radiology* 1984;152:497–501.
- Handlock FP, Deter RL, Harrist RB, et al. Fetal head circumference: Accuracy of real time ultrasound measurement of term. *Perinatol Nenatal* 1982;6: 97–100.
- Handlock FP, Deter RL, Harrist RB, et al. Fetal head circumference: Relation to menstrual age. *AJR* 1982; 139: 367–70.
- Ihnatsenka B, Boezaarrt AP. Ultrasound: Basic understanding and learning the language. *Int J Shoulder Surg* 2010; 4(3):55–62.
- Obstetrics ultrasound examinations by the America Institute of Ultrasound in Medicine. 2013.

Clinical Embryology

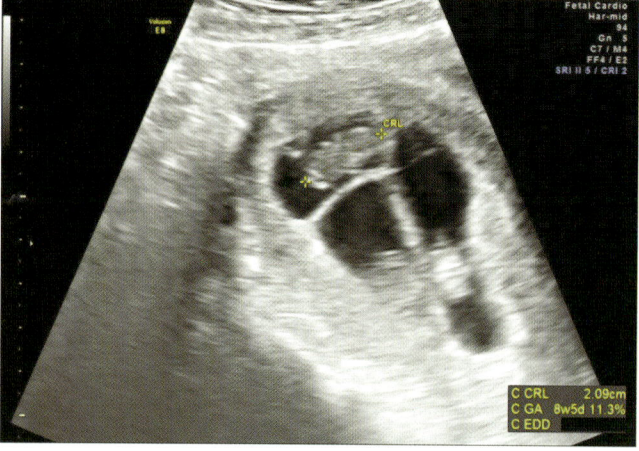

Clinical image 29.1: Ultrasonographical measurement of crown to rump length (CRL). It is the distance between highest point of skull and lowest point of buttocks. It is most accurate for gestational age determination in first trimester (Image courtesy: *Dr Mamatha Gowda*)

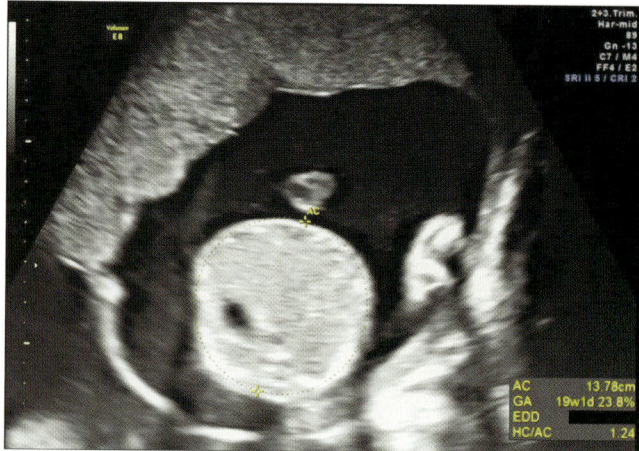

Clinical image 29.3: Ultrasonographical measurement of abdominal circumference (AC) (Image courtesy: *Dr Mamatha Gowda*)

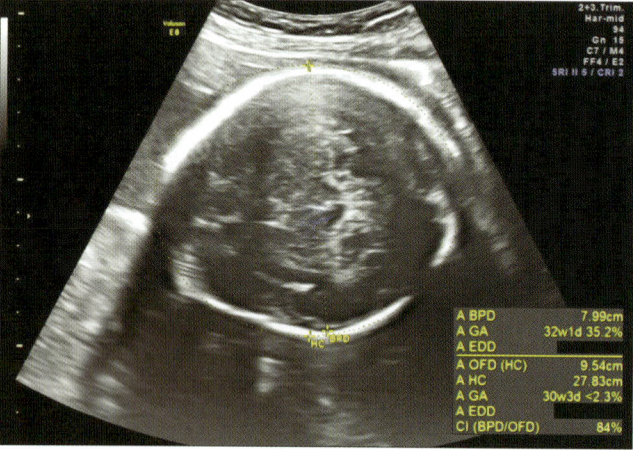

Clinical image 29.2: Ultrasonographical measurement of biparietal diameter (BPD) and head circumference (HC). BPD is the diameter of axial plane through skull of the fetus (embryo). Head circumference is obtained in the same plane of biparietal diameter. The tracings for head circumference should follow the outer perimeter of skull (Image courtesy: *Dr Mamatha Gowda*)

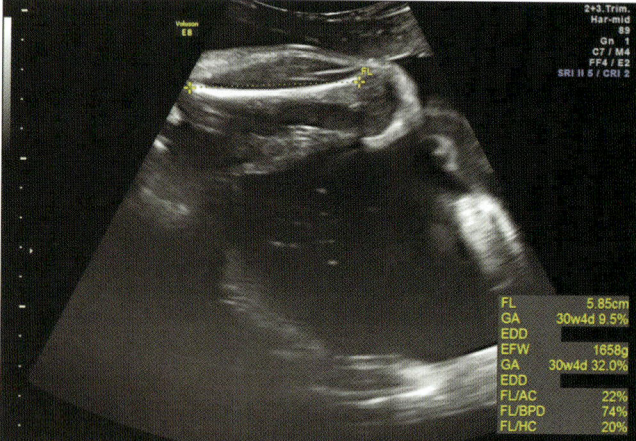

Clinical image 29.4: Ultrasonographical measurement of femur length: For measurement of the femur length, both femoral condyles should be visualized simultaneously. The ultrasound transducer should be perpendicular to the long axis of the femur. It is measured from tip of the greater trochanter to the lateral epicondyle (Image courtesy: *Dr Mamatha Gowda*)

Chapter 30

Twinning (Multiple Pregnancy)

eSmartQuiz

Chapter Outline

- Classification of twins
  - Dizygotic twins
  - Monozygotic twins
- Classification of twins according to degree of separation
  - Diamniotic dichorionic twins
  - Diamniotic monochorionic
  - Monoamniotic monochorionic twins
  - Conjoined twins

Competency:
- **AN80.4:** Describe embryological basis of twinning in monozygotic and dizygotic twins.

INTRODUCTION

- As in human, only one ovum is released in one menstrual cycle, usually, *singleton pregnancy* is seen.
- When the mother gives birth to **two or more** offspring in a single pregnancy, it is called *multiple pregnancy*. Multiple pregnancy, in dogs, cats, and so many other mammals is common.
- When the mother gives birth to two offspring in a single pregnancy, it is called *twinning*.
- *In vitro* fertilization enhances the chances of multiple pregnancy (incidence of twins in IVF: 21 twins/1000 births). *Clinical fact*

CLASSIFICATION OF TWINS

- Multiple pregnancy is classified as per the number of offspring born as follows:
  1. Twins: 2 offspring
  2. Triplets: 3 offspring
  3. Quadruplets: 4 offspring
  4. Quintuplets: 5 offspring
- Multiple pregnancy can be classified according to the genetic relationship of the offspring as follows:
  1. *Monozygotic twins*: These twins are produced by fertilization of a *single oocyte* by one sperm (one zygote).
  2. *Dizygotic twins*: These twins are produced by fertilization of *two different oocytes* by *two different sperms* (two zygotes).
  3. *Trizygotic twins*: These are produced by fertilization of multiple oocytes by different sperms (3 zygotes).
- Differences between monozygotic and dizygotic twins are listed in Table 30.1.

Some Interesting Facts

- *Superfecundation:* In polyovulatory animal, multiple ova are discharged and may get fertilized by sperms from *different male partners*. In such case, resultant fetuses are of *same* gestational age.
- *Superfetation*: In some animals, ova released during pregnancy, may get fertilized and produce another offspring of *different* gestational age.

Dizygotic (Fraternal) Twins

Q. Write a short note on dizygotic twins.

- *Definition*: Dizygotic twins are produced by the fertilization of two different oocytes by two different sperms (two zygotes) (Fig. 30.1).
- Fraternal means unlike.
- Incidence: 7–10 per 1000 births, incidence increases with increasing maternal age.

Features

1. The dizygotic twins (diovular/divitelline) are phenotypically dissimilar, even may have different gender (one male and other female offspring).

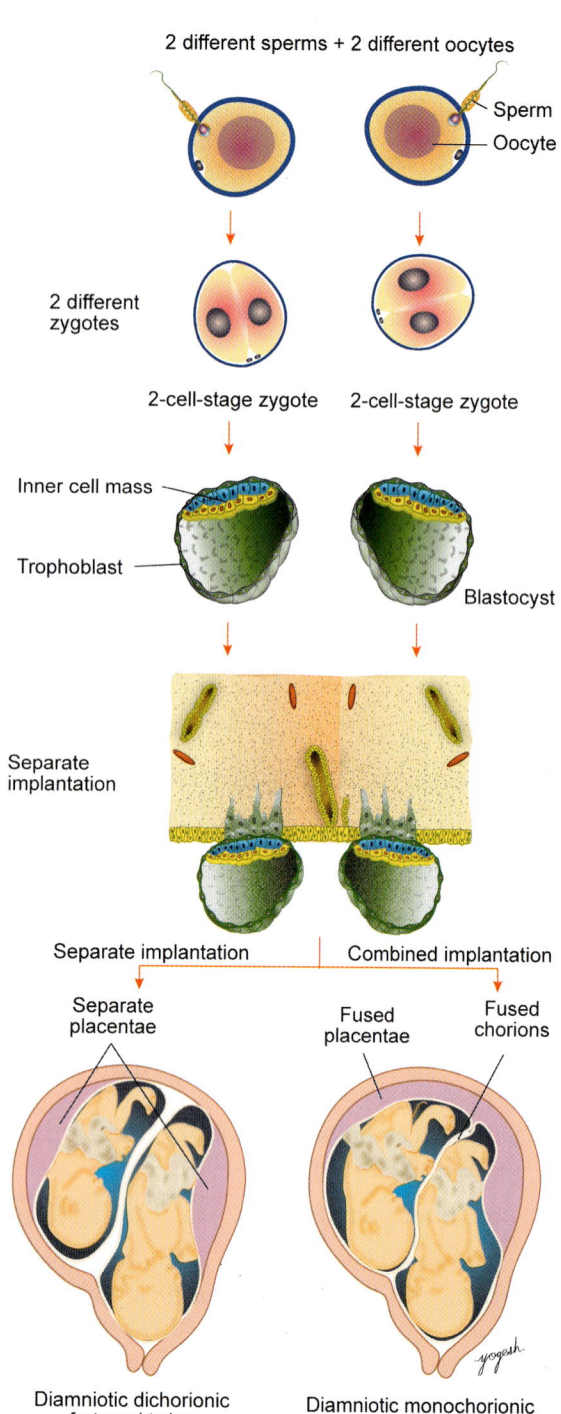

Fig. 30.1: Fraternal twins

2. The dizygotic twins are genetically and phenotypically dissimilar.
3. Dizygotic twins do not share placenta (except occasionally), chorion and amnion.
4. They have two different gestational sacs.
5. As placentae may be close to each other, occasionally fused placentae may be observed.
6. About 2/3rds of human twins are dizygotic.

Monozygotic (Identical) Twins

Q. Write a short note on monozygotic twins.

- *Definition*: Monozygotic twins (monoovular/monovitelline) are produced by fertilization of one oocyte by one sperm (single zygote). The resultant zygote forms blastocyst with inner cell mass. This inner cell mass (embryoblast) divides into two parts and produce monozygotic twins (Fig. 30.2).
- Incidence: 3 in 1000 births.

Features

1. Monozygotic twins are phenotypically similar (they have same gender).
2. They are genetically similar.
3. They may share placenta, amniotic cavity and chorionic sac.
4. About 1/3rd of human twins are monozygotic twins.

CLASSIFICATION OF MONOZYGOTIC TWINS ACCORDING TO DEGREE OF SEPARATION

- Monozygotic twins can be classified based on degree of separation as follows:

1. Diamniotic Dichorionic Twins

- These are also called bichorial, diamniotic twins.
- In monozygotic twins, after first few divisions, cells of zygote get separated and form two embryos with separate chorionic and amniotic sac.
- *Note*: Dizygotic twins are also diamniotic.
- *Up to 3rd day* of fertilization, separation of cells results in diamniotic dichorionic twins.^{NEXT}
- These twins have separate placenta.
- Incidence is 25% of twin pregnancies.

2. Diamniotic Monochorionic Monozygotic Twins

- They are also called diamniotic monochorial twins.
- Mechanism: If separation of inner cell mass of blastocyst takes place on *4th–7th day*, diamniotic monochorionic twins are produced.^{NEXT}
- These twins have a common chorionic sac and single placenta but two amniotic sacs.
- Incidence is 70–75% of monozygotic twin pregnancies.

3. Monoamniotic Monochorionic Twins

- They are also called monoamniotic, monochorial twins.
- Mechanism: If the separation of inner cell mass takes place on *9th day* of fertilization, monoamniotic monochorionic twins are produced.^{NEXT}

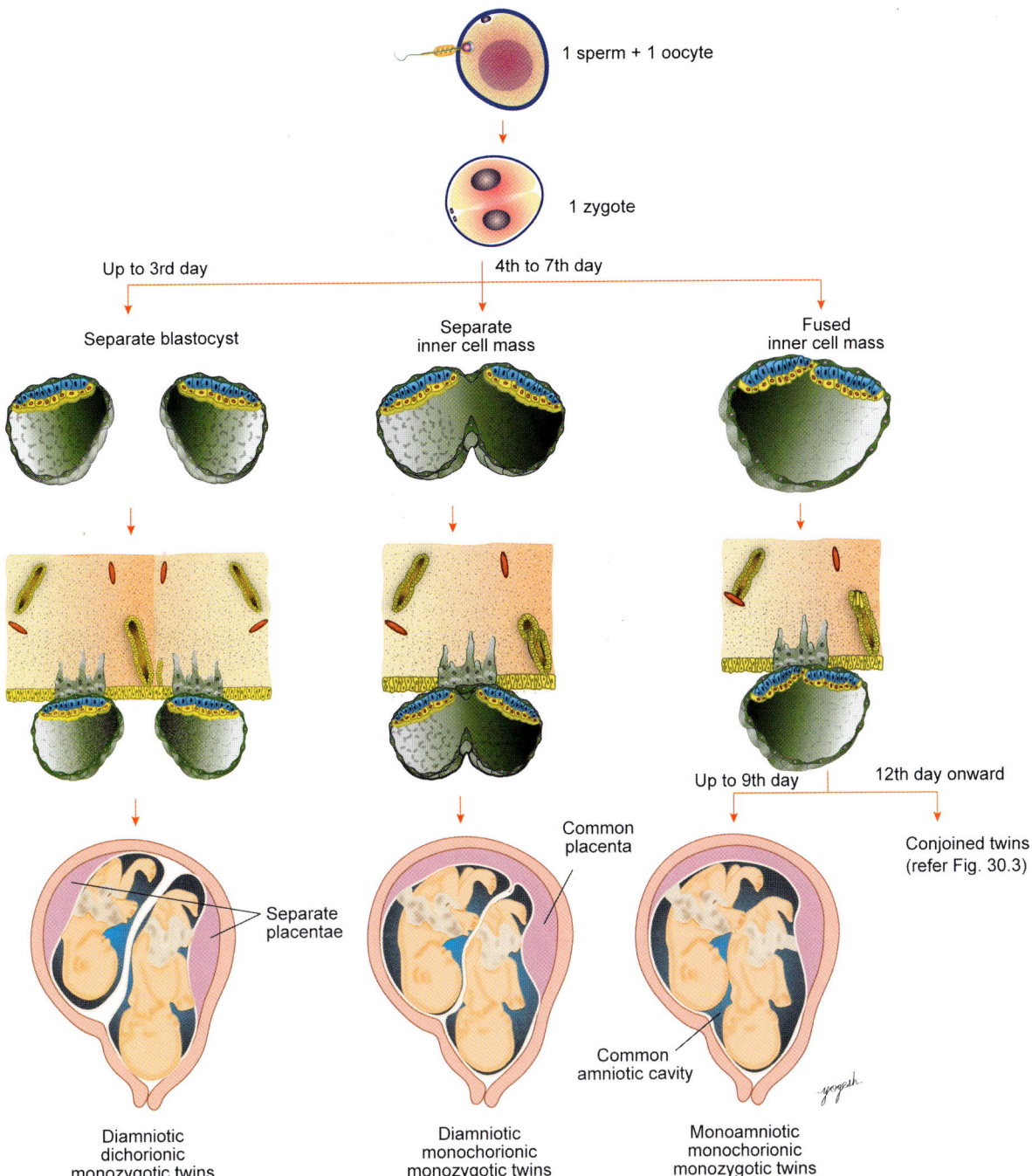

Fig. 30.2: Monozygotic twins

- They have common placenta, chorionic cavity, and amniotic cavity.
- Incidence is 1–2% of monozygotic twin pregnancies.

4. Conjoined (Siamese) Twins (Fig. 30.3)
- If the separation occurs *after 12th day* of fertilization, monozygotic twins form conjoined twins.
- Conjoined twins have joined bodies.
- Incidence: 1 in 400 monozygotic twins.

Classification of conjoined monozygotic twins
Based on the site and extent of fusion, conjoined twins are classified as follows:

1. Craniopagus: Fusion of heads (skulls).
2. Thoracopagus: Fusion of anterior thoracic walls and abdominal walls up to umbilicus.
3. Omphalopagus: Fusion of lower abdominal walls.
4. Cephalothoracopagus: Fusion of head and thoracic walls.
5. Pyopagus: Fusion of sacral regions.
6. Ischiopagus: Fusion at the pelvis. These twins are classically joined with the vertebral axis at 180° (Clinical image 30.1).
7. Parasitic twin: Conjoined twin that have one large and another smaller (parasitic) twin.

Q. List the differences between monozygotic and dizygotic twins.

Table 30.1 Differences between monozygotic and dizygotic twins

Origin	Monozygotic twins	Dizygotic twins
Cause	1 sperm + 1 oocyte = 1 zygote	2 different sperm + 2 different oocyte = 2 different zygotes
Incidence	Less common (3 in 1000 births)	More common (7–10 in 1000 births)
Phenotype	Similar	Dissimilar
Genotype	Similar	Dissimilar
Sex	Similar	May or may not be similar
Placenta	Usually single, shared by twins	Usually different placentae
Chorionic sac	May be single	Always different
Amniotic sac	May be single	Always different

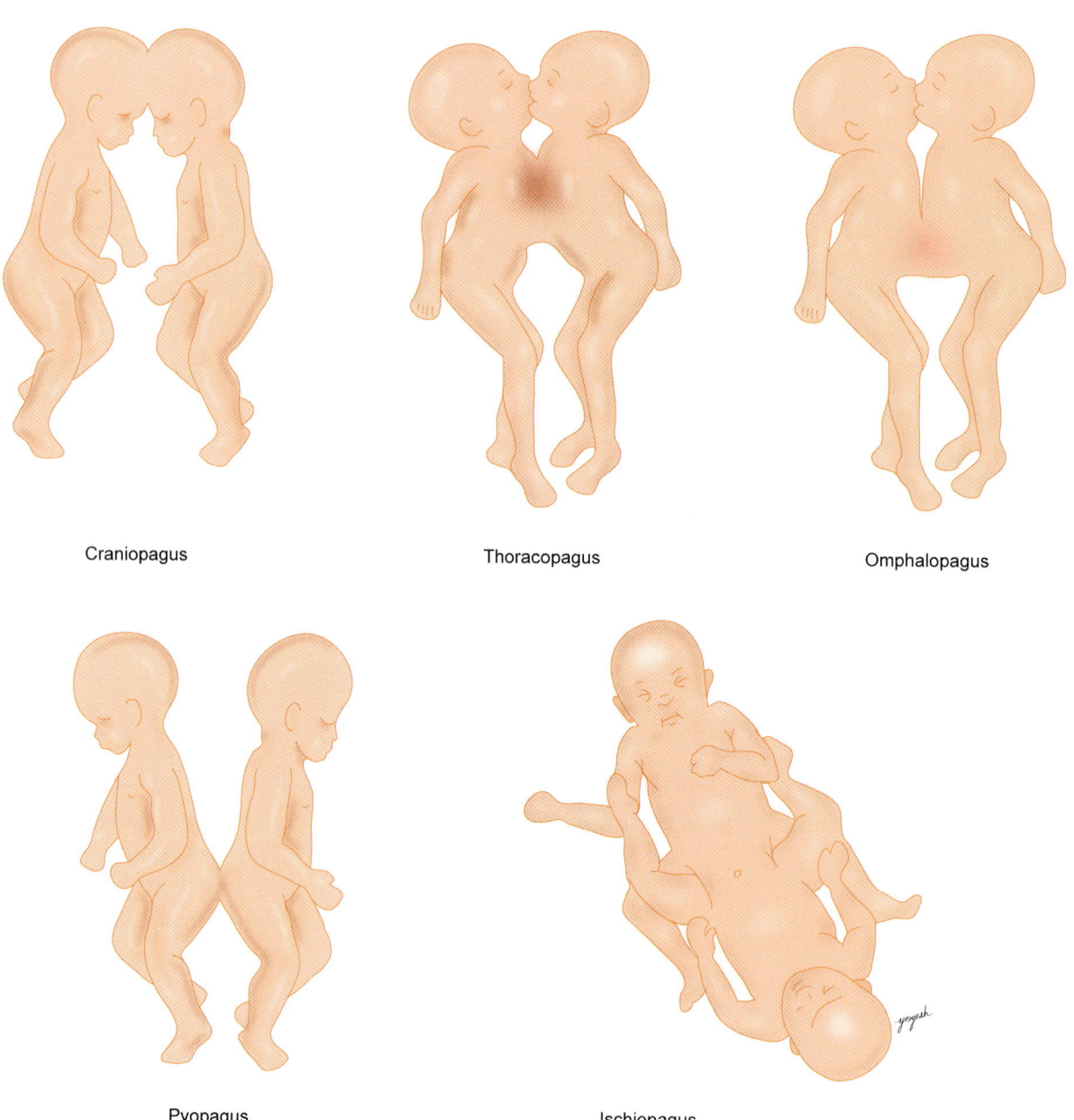

Craniopagus Thoracopagus Omphalopagus

Pyopagus Ischiopagus

Fig. 30.3: Conjoined twins

Clinical Embryology

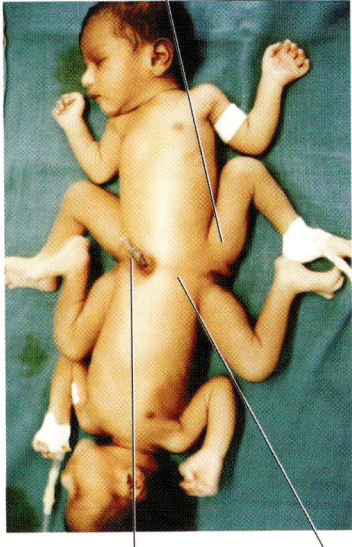
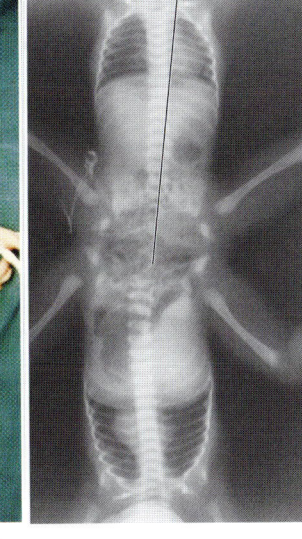
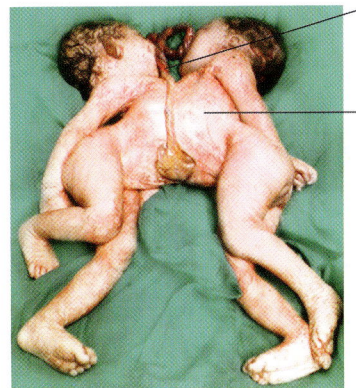

Clinical image 30.1: Ischiopagus tetrapus twins (phenotype on the left and radiological features on the right). Ischiopagus twins are united dorsally at the sacrum and coccyx. The twins are classically joined with the vertebral axis at 180°. Ischiopagus tetrapus (quadripus) shows four lower limbs and they are continuous anteriorly with each other. Limbs are oriented at right angles to the axes of the thorax. *Ischiopagus dipus* shows two shared lower limbs, *ischiopagus tripus* twins have three shared lower limbs. *Note*: In pygopagus, twins are joined ventrally at the buttocks and facing away from each other. Parapagus twins are joined side-by-side. (Image courtesy: *Dr Kumaravel S*)

Clinical image 30.2: Conjoined twins: *Thoracopagus*. Thoracopagus is the most common form of conjoined twins. It involves fusion of anterior thoracic wall up to the umbilicus. A common pericardial sac is present in 90% of thoracopagus twins and conjoined hearts in 75% cases (Image courtesy: *Dr Haritha Sagili*)

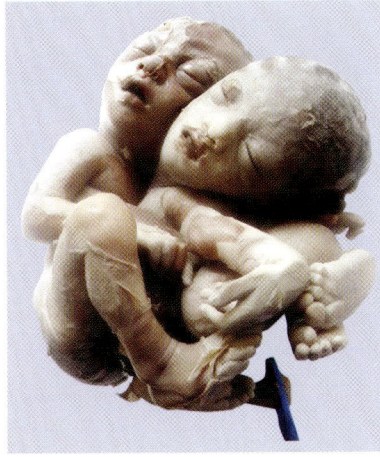

Clinical image 30.3: Conjoined twins: *Thoracopagus*. It involves fusion of anterior thoracic wall up to the umbilicus. (Image courtesy: *Dr Mamatha Gowda*)

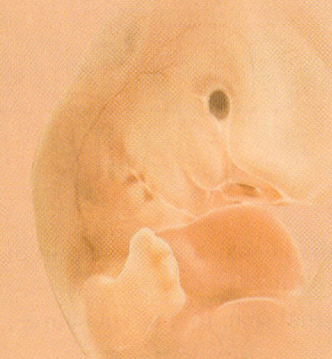

Annexures

Annexure I

EMBRYONIC REMNANTS *NEXT, High yielding facts*

Remnant after birth	Embryonic source
Ligamentum arteriosum	Ductus arteriosus
Ligamentum teres hepatis	Left umbilical vein
Fossa ovalis	Septum primum
Annulus fossa ovalis	Septum secundum
Ligamentum venosum	Ductus venosus
Meckel's diverticulum	Vitellointestinal duct
Median umbilical ligament	Urachus
Medial umbilical ligament	Distal part of umbilical arteries
Superior vesicle artery	Proximal part of umbilical arteries
Superior aberrant ductules Inferior aberrant ductules Tubules of paradidymis Efferent ductules of testis	Mesonephric tubules in male
Tubules of epoöphoron Tubules of paroöphoron	Mesonephric tubules in female
Duct of epoöphoron (Gartner's duct)	Mesonephric duct in female
Organ of Rosenmuller (epoöphoron)	Mesonephric tubules
Appendix of testis, prostatic utricle	Paramesonephric ducts in male

Annexure II

PLACENTA PREVIA

Q. Write a short note on placenta previa.

Definition: If the placenta is implanted partially or completely over the lower uterine segment, it is called placenta previa. *Previa* means in front of (Latin). Here, it indicates the position of placenta in relation to the internal os cervix uteri.

Incidence

0.5–1% hospital deliveries.
Incidence increases with increasing maternal age beyond 35.

Types

There are four types of the placenta previa depending on encroachment over lower uterine segment as follows:

- Type I (low-lying): Only a lower margin of placenta encroaches on to the lower uterine segment.
- Type II (marginal): Placenta encroaches the margin of internal os but does not cover it.
- Type III (incomplete or partial central): Placenta covers the internal os partially.
- Type IV (central or total): Placenta completely covers the internal os.
- Type I and II are considered as minor degree, whereas type III and IV are considered as major degree of placenta previa.

Diagnosis: Ultrasonographical examination in third trimester is useful for detection of placenta previa.

Complications: Placenta previa is one of the commonest causes of antepartum hemorrhage (bleeding from the genital tract after 28 weeks of the pregnancy but before birth of the baby).

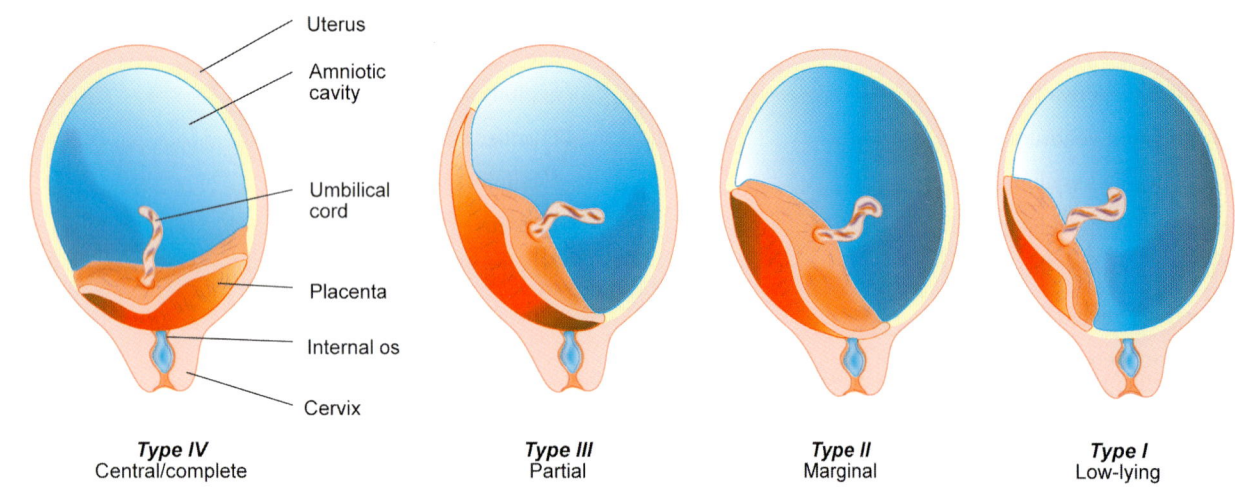

Fig. AII.1: Placenta previa

Annexure III

HERMAPHRODITE

Q. Write a short note on hermaphroditism.

Hermaphrodite

- *A hermaphrodite* is a person who phenotypically (physical characteristics) does not entirely resemble male or female and shows the characteristics of both the sexes. Hence, also called *intersex*.
- Hermaphrodites include ambiguous external genitalia and mosaic karyotypes (46,XX/46,XY, 46,XX/47,XXY or 45,X/XY mosaic).

True Hermaphrodites

- The *true hermaphroditism* is a rare condition. This individual has both testes and ovaries (usually combined as ovotestes) and external ambiguous genitalia (neither completely male nor completely female).
- Both testes and ovaries are usually nonfunctional.
- Genotype: Mostly 46,XX in 80% cases or 46,XX/46,XY mosaics or may have SRY translocations.
- The uterus is present and breasts are frequently developed. Most of these individuals are brought up as females. Most of these individuals menstruate except in XY mosaic cases.

Pseudohermaphrodite

- It is defective sexual development due to mutations or chromosomal anomalies affecting autosomes or sex chromosomes.
- Pseudohermaphrodites have gonads of one sex and external genitalia and genital tract of another sex.
- For example:
  1. Male pseudohermaphrodites: These are genetically male (46,XY) individuals with testes and external genitalia that resembles female.
  2. Female pseudohermaphrodite: These are genetically female (46,XX) individuals with ovaries and external genitalia that resembles male.
- Pseudohermaphrodites usually have abnormal levels of sex hormones or anomalies in the sex hormone receptors.
- The differences between male and female pseudohermaphrodites are listed in Table AIII.1.

Table AIII.1 Differences between male and female pseudohermaphrodites

Feature	Male pseudohermaphrodite	Female pseudohermaphrodite
Gonads	Testes	Ovaries
Genotype	46,XY	46,XX
Phenotype	Male	Female
External genitalia	Resembles that of female	Resembles that of male
Phallus	Phallus remains rudimentary and looks similar to clitoris	Excessive enlargement of clitoris resembling penis
Labioscrotal swellings	Scrotal swellings fail to fuse, giving an appearance of labia majora	Partial fusion of labia majora, giving an appearance of a scrotum
Cause	Lack of androgen receptors (hence androgens produced by fetal testes are ineffective in inducing differentiation of male genitalia)	Congenital adrenal hyperplasia with excessive production of androgens. Excessive production of androgens masculinises external genitals

Annexure IV

DERIVATIVES OF NEURAL CREST CELLS
NEXT, High yielding facts

Dorsal mass
A. Neuroblast cells
- Dorsal root ganglia
- Sensory ganglia of V, VII, IX and X cranial nerves
- Skeletal elements of pharyngeal arches
- Odontoblast of teeth
- Parafollicular cells of thyroid gland

B. Spongioblast cells
- Satellite cells in ganglion
- Schwann cells

C. Pluripotent cells
- Melanocytes

Ventral mass
A. Sympatho-chromaffin organ
B. Sympathoblasts
- Sympathetic ganglionic neurons
- Parasympathetic ganglionic neurons (ciliary, pterygopalatine, submandibular and otic)

C. Chromaffin cells
- Chromaffin cells of medulla of adrenal gland
- Para-aortic body
- Argentaffin cells in respiratory system
- Enterochromaffin cells in gut

Other derivatives
- Facial bones and vault of skull
- Dermis of face and neck
- Muscles of ciliary body
- Sclera and choroids of eyeball
- Substantia propria and posterior epithelium of cornea
- Pharyngeal arch cartilages
- Semilunar valves in heart
- Spiral and bulbar septum in heart

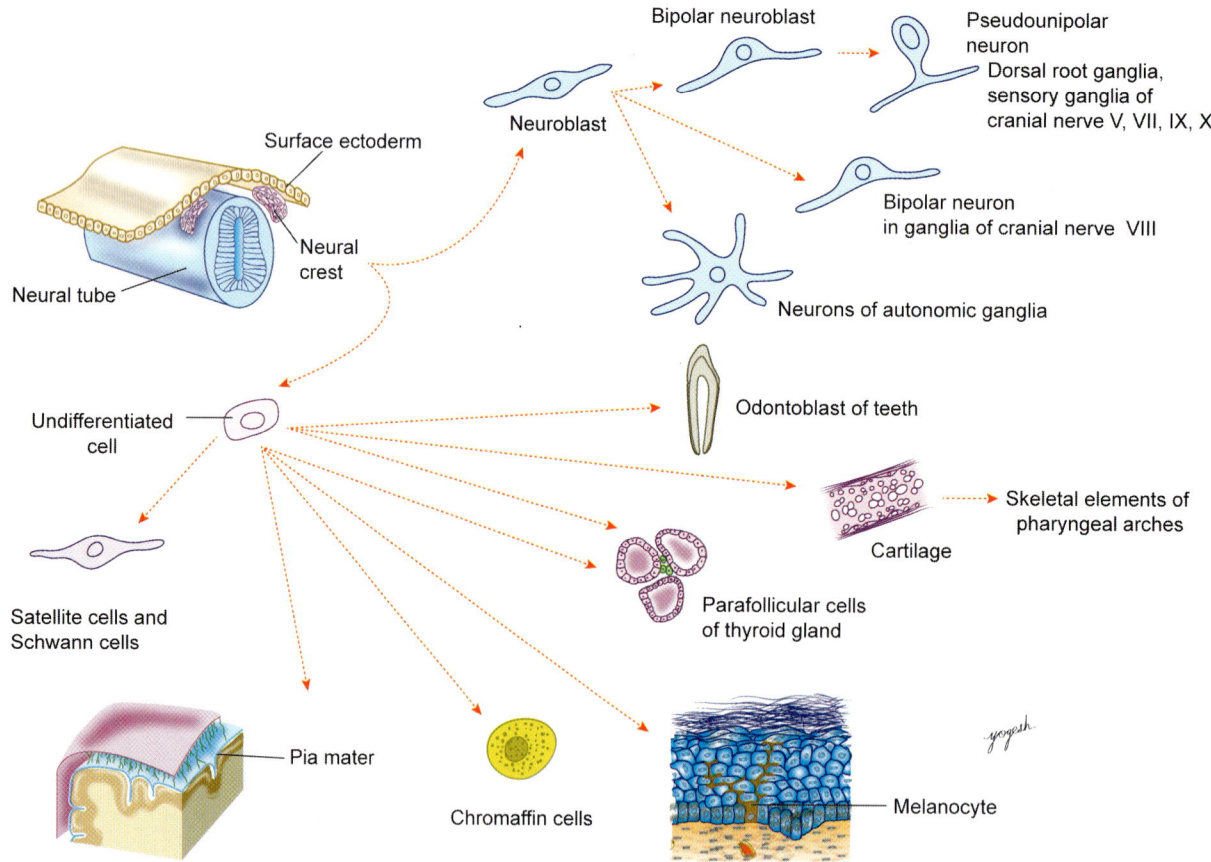

Fig. AIV.1: Derivatives of neural crest cells

Annexure V

MISCELLANEOUS

- Fetal viability
- Contraception
- Teratogenesis
- Fertility, infertility, sterility
- Surrogate motherhood
- Sex ratio
- Abortion
- Pregnancy test
- Development of limbs

Competencies:

- **AN13.8:** Describe development of upper limb.
- **AN20.10:** Describe basic concept of development of lower limb.
- **AN76.2:** Explain the terms – phylogeny, ontogeny, trimester, viability (for phylogeny, ontogeny, and trimesters, refer Chapter 1).
- **AN77.5:** Enumerate and describe the anatomical principles underlying contraception
- **AN77.6:** Describe teratogenic influences; fertility and sterility, surrogate motherhood, social significance of sex-ratio.
- **AN78.5:** Describe in brief abortion; decidual reaction, pregnancy test (for decidual reaction, refer Chapter 9)

FETAL VIABILITY

- *Definition*: Fetal viability is defined as the potential of the fetus to survive outside the uterus after birth (natural or induced) with or without the support.
- It is a stage of fetus at which it becomes capable of living in the external environment.
- Nonviable fetus is delivered live but not able to survive.
- The viability of a fetus increases with increase in gestational age (Table AV.2).
- Babies with gestational age <21 weeks or body weight <500 g are not viable.^NEXT
- Usually, it is considered that the fetus crossed 28 weeks of gestation and becomes viable (recently taken as 24 weeks).^NEXT

Intrauterine growth retardation (IUGR) and prematurity are the important causes of perinatal deaths due to less viability.

- Fetuses with gestational age 20 weeks or fetal weight less than 500 g are considered as previable fetuses. They can survive only with extreme medical care.
- Fetuses with gestational age 21 weeks or more, crown to rump length 210 mm or more, foot length 45 mm or more and weight 500 g or more are considered as viable fetuses.
- Even fetuses born between 26 to 28 weeks have difficult survival because of less maturity of lungs and central nervous system.

Factors influencing chance of survival

1. Gestational age
2. Weight of newborn
3. Environmental factors
4. Medical support system
5. Oxygen supply

Investigation

- **Viability scan:** It is an ultrasound examination for assessing the cardiac activity of the fetus.
- Viability is mainly based on lung maturity of the fetus. To promote lung maturity and surfactant production, *steroids* are given to the mother during the last trimester (after 7 months of pregnancy).

Table AV.2 Percentage of survival

Completed weeks of gestation at birth	≤21	22	24	26	27	30	34
Percentage of survival	0%	0–3%	40–70%	80–90%	>90%	>95%	>98%

CONTRACEPTION

- Contraception is the method that prevents pregnancy by the following means:
  1. By separating sperms and ovum
  2. By stopping ovum production
  3. By preventing implantation.

Methods of Contraception

- Methods of contraception are of two types:
  1. Permanent methods
  2. Temporary methods.

Permanent methods

- These are vasectomy (male sterilization) and tubectomy (female sterilization)

Temporary methods

- These include barrier methods [condoms (for male or female)], intrauterine device, hormonal contraceptives, behavioural methods (withdrawal, avoiding fertile dates).
- *Barrier methods* include use of male or female condom, diaphragm, or contraceptive sponge.
- *Intrauterine devices* (copper T) act by damaging sperms (copper is spermicidal) and prevents implantation.
- *Hormonal contraceptives* include oral pills, implants under skin, injection, patches, and intrauterine hormonal devices.

  Hormones (progesterone and estrogen) interfere in normal menstrual cycle, inhibits ovulation, thickens cervical mucous, and induces menstruation.
- *Behavioral methods* include withdrawal method or coitus interruptus (withdrawal before ejaculation) and avoiding unprotected intercourse during fertile dates of a month.
- *Emergency contraception* or *morning after pills* are taken to prevent unwanted pregnancy after unprotected intercourse. For example, progestin (Brand name – I pill) should be taken within 72 hours after intercourse. It inhibits ovulation, prevents fertilization, and prevents implantation.

TERATOGENESIS

- Teratogenesis is the formation of developmental congenital anomalies in the fetus or embryo due to the exposure to the teratogens (*Teratos* = monster in Greek).
- It is the induction or production of malformation in a developing embryo or fetus (Table AV.2).
- *Teratogens* are substances that may cause birth defects in the embryo or fetus.

Table AV.2 Teratogens and associated congenital malformation

Alcohol	*Fetal alcohol syndrome*: Intra-uterine growth retardation, mental retardation, microcephaly, ocular anomalies
Phenytoin	*Fetal hydantoin syndrome*: IUGR, microcephaly, mental retardation, cleft lip/palate, inner epicanthal folds, eyelid ptosis
Lithium carbonate	Heart and major vessel anomalies
Vitamin A (large doses)	Facial anomalies, neural tube defects
Tetracycline	Stained teeth, hypoplasia of enamel
Cytomegalovirus	Microcephaly, hydrocephaly, microphthalmia
Herpes simplex virus	Microcephaly, retinal detachment
Ionizing radiation	Microcephaly, mental retardation, skeletal malformations
Warfarin	Nose, eye, hand defects
Thalidomide	Phocomelia, meromelia, multiple defects

Rubell virus: IUGR, postnatal growth retardation, mental retardation, eye defects, cardiac anomalies, deafness

- Susceptibility for teratogens depends on genotype, environmental factors, developmental stage, and quantity and duration of teratogen exposure.
- *Teratology* is the study of abnormal development of fetus or embryo and its causes.
- *Major teratogens*
  1. Alcohol
  2. Cigarettes
  3. Medications (isotretinoin, lithium, chemotherapy)
  4. Ionizing radiations
  5. Drugs and chemicals (amphetamines, cocaine, heroin, marijuana)
  6. Infections (TORCH infection)
  7. Maternal health and nutrition (diabetes, phenylketonuria)
  8. Folic acid deficiency
- Causes of congenital anomalies are
  - Genetic factors (chromosomal aberrations)
  - Environmental factors such as drugs, viruses and nutritional deficiency.
  - Multifunctional inheritance that includes both genetic and environmental factors together.
- Principles in teratogenesis
  1. Tetragenesity of an agent depends on the period of development dose of the agent and genetic constitution of the embryo.
  2. Critical period of development: Organogenesis takes place during 3rd to 8th week of development. This period is more critical and may induce anomalies on exposure of teratogenic agents.
  3. There is dose – development relationship of teratogens and anomalies.
  4. Genetic constitution of the embryo plays an important role in teratogenesis. For example, only one-third of the embryo exposed to the phenytoin shows fetal hydantoin syndrome.

FERTILITY, INFERTILITY, STERILITY

Fertility

- *Fertility* is the natural capability of an individual to produce offspring.
- *Fertility rate* is the number of offspring born per couple.
- Fertility depends on nutrition, sexual behavior, consanguinity, culture, hormonal levels, and emotions.
- *General fertility rate* is the number of births in a year divided by the number of women aged 15–44 years, times 1000.

$$\text{General fertility rate} = \frac{\text{Number of births in a year}}{\text{Women aged 15 – 44 years}} \times 1000$$

- Females are fertile in a period from menarche (beginning of menses) to menopause (cessation of menses).
- Males are fertile from puberty till death but fertility in both males and females decreases with advancing age.

Infertility

- *Definition:* Infertility is a failure to conceive after 1 year of physical contact without contraception.

- Infertility is the inability of a person to produce live offspring by natural means.
- There may be male infertility or female infertility.

Causes
- There are various causes of infertility.
- Some of them are as follows:
  1. Presence of antisperm antibodies
  2. Sexually transmitted infections
  3. Genetic causes such as gene mutations
  4. Other associated disorders: Diabetes mellitus, hypothyroidism, hypopituitarism, and so on
  5. Azoospermia, asthenozoospermia
  6. Pelvic inflammatory disease, tuberculosis, and tubal ligation.

Sterility
- *Sterility* is the physiological inability to conceive.
- Sterility may be due to the following reasons:
  1. Menopause
  2. Before puberty
  3. Tubectomy
  4. Vasectomy
  5. Absence of uterus (surgical removal or congenital absence).

SURROGATE MOTHERHOOD

- *Surrogacy* is a legal arrangement where a female agrees to become pregnant and give birth to a child for another couple.
- Surrogacy is a method of assisted reproductive technology.
- *Surrogacy (regulation) Bill, 2016* is the lawful control of surrogacy in India.
  It includes:
  – Prohibition of commercial surrogacy
  – Allows altruistic surrogacy to Indian married couple who cannot bear children
  – Prohibition of commercial surrogacy
  – Surrogate mother should be a close relative of the couple who wants to have her child
  – There are National Surrogacy and State Surrogacy Board to control surrogacy related issues.

Procedure
- There are the following two methods:
  1. *Traditional surrogacy*: In this, sperms are artificially inseminated to the surrogate mother.
  2. *Gestational surrogacy*: In this, *in vitro* fertilized ovum is transferred to the surrogate mother. If sperms or ovum are not available from the desired couple, donors may be used.

SEX RATIO

- The *sex ratio* is the ratio of males-to-females in a population.
- The sex ratio of India is 107.48 in 2019, that is, 107.48 males per 100 females or 930 females per 1000 males.^{MCQ}
- This ratio is more in rural area (929 females per 1000 males in rural and 949 females per 1000 males in urban area).

Social Significance of Sex Ratio
- **Gender discrimination:** In many Indian societies, orthodox people feel males are better than females, and hence, there is a tendency of sex determination by sonography and forced abortions of female fetuses (sex-selective abortion) and female infanticide.
  It will worsen the condition due to increasing sex ratio.
- **Laws:** India has laws against sex determination and sex-selective abortion to make safe environment for female fetuses and infants (Pre-Conception and Pre-Natal Diagnostic Techniques/PCPNDT Act, 1994).
  Laws against dowry also helps for changing social vision against females.
- **Physical abuse:** In India, females are less in number than males. It results in female physical abuse by surplus men.
- **Antisocial behavior:** Surplus men may not have women to marry. They will not have families and may get deviated to antisocial activities and violence.
- **Homosexual behavior:** Surplus men may deviate toward homosexuality.

Solutions for maintaining normal sex ratio
1. Education and social awareness
2. Laws against prenatal sex determination, dowry, and abuse
3. Preference and facilities to girls such as free education, job opportunities, and so on
4. Prevent human trafficking
5. Protection of families and old-age people with single girl child.

ABORTION

- *Abortion* is the termination of the pregnancy before the period of viability, which is considered to occur at 28th week of gestation.^{MCQ}

Types of abortion
Abortions are classified as spontaneous or induced.

A. Spontaneous Abortion/Miscarriage
- It occurs naturally as accident.
- It may be isolated (only once) or recurrent.
- Spontaneous abortions occur due to fetal chromosomal abnormalities, maternal diabetes mellitus, hormonal problems, infections, uterine abnormalities, and so on.
- It may be
  1. *Threatened abortion*: It is a state where abortion has started but has not progressed to a state from which recovery is possible.
  2. *Inevitable abortion*: It is a state where abortion has reached to the state from which recovery is impossible.
  3. *Complete abortion*: It is an abortion in which all products of conception are expelled from the uterus.
  4. *Incomplete abortion*: It is an abortion in which a part of conceptus is left inside the uterus.

5. *Missed abortion*: It is an abortion in which dead fetus is retained inside the uterus for few days.

B. Induced Abortions

- It is the purposeful termination of a pregnancy before the fetus becomes viable.
- It may be legal or illegal (criminal).
- *Legal abortion* follows medical termination of pregnancy Act, 1971 in India.
- *Reasons of induced abortion*
  1. To save the life of pregnant woman.
  2. Because of unsuitable age or health of the pregnant woman.
  3. To avoid legal issues, socioeconomic stress.
  4. To avoid birth of child as a result of rape.
  5. To avoid birth of abnormal child.
  6. To fulfil wish of a couple within the limits of law.
- In induced abortion, under guidance of a medical professional, a combination of two drugs, mifepristone and misoprostol, is used.
- Mifepristone prevents attachment of fertilized egg to the lining of uterus or detaches the attached ovum. Mifepristone is a synthetic steroid and progesterone receptor antagonist. Misoprostol causes uterine contractions.
  - This method is useful between 5th and 9th week of pregnancy. The side effects include pain, heavy bleeding, severe cramping, vomiting, and so on.
  - Other methods include vacuum aspiration, dilation and suction curettage, dilatation and evacuation.

PREGNANCY TEST (URINE PREGNANCY TEST)

Introduction

- Human chorionic gonadotropin (hCG) is a hormone produced by trophoblasts that later forms placenta.
- The hCG starts circulating in the maternal blood from the implantation, that is, from 7th day after fertilization.
- The hCG is similar to the luteinizing hormone of pituitary gland and helps in the maintenance of corpus luteum.
- Corpus luteum secretes progesterone and estrogen that maintain pregnancy.
- The hCG is a polypeptide hormone (237 amino acids).
- The hCG starts secreting in the urine of pregnant female after implantation, that is, from one week prior to next due menstruation.

Principle

- The beta subunit of hCG (β-hCG) is detected from the urine by *enzyme linked immune sorbent assay* (ELISA).
- β-hCG ELISA tests are positive when the maternal serum levels of β-hCG are 25 mU/mL or more. It can be positive after 7–10 days after conception.

Procedure

- Collect at least 1 mL of urine in a dry, clean container. First morning urine sample is preferred.
- Apply few drops of urine at a given site of test strip.

Interpretation and Reaction

- If the urine sample contains hCG, a complex is formed with monoclonal anti-hCG antibody and continues to migrate along the membrane to the test (T) line of the strip.
- At this line, this complex becomes bound to a fixed polyclonal anti-hCG antibody and the result will be indicated by a colored marker line.
- Unbound monoclonal anti-hCG antibodies migrate further and become bound with polyclonal anti-hCG at control (C) line.
- Thus, *two bands*, one at Test (T) line and another at control (C) line indicates *positive result*.
- Only one band at control (C) line indicates negative results.
- Weak colored band indicates invalid result.
- **Positive result**
  It may occur in the following conditions:
  1. Pregnancy
  2. Patient with gestational and nongestational trophoblastic disease
  3. Trophoblastic neoplasm such as choriocarcinoma, hydatidiform moles
  4. Germ cell tumors in males (seminoma)
  5. Teratomas
  6. For few days after spontaneous abortions
  7. Retained placental fragments

Note: This test cannot distinguish between normal and ectopic pregnancy. *Viva*

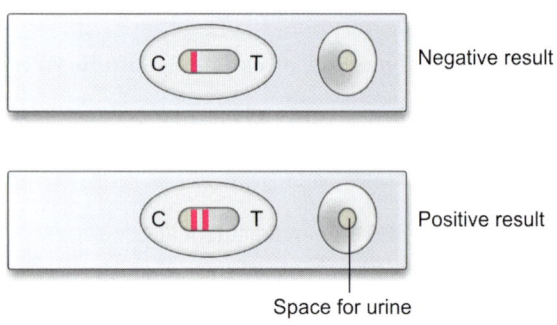

Fig. AV.1: Pregnancy test: C: Control line, T: Test line

DEVELOPMENT OF LIMBS

Limbs develop from mesenchyme of limb buds as follows (Figs AV.1, AV.2, SEM AV.1, AV.2):

Formation of limb bud primordia

- At the end of 4th week, small elevations of limb bud primordia appear on the ventrolateral body wall.

Formation of limb bud

- In second month, limb primordia enlarge as paddle-shaped outgrowths on surface ectoderm to form *limb buds*.
- Forelimb bud grows faster than lower limb buds.

Formation of limbs

- In the 6th week, limb bud shows thickening at the tip called *apical ectodermal ridge*. Limb bud starts diff-

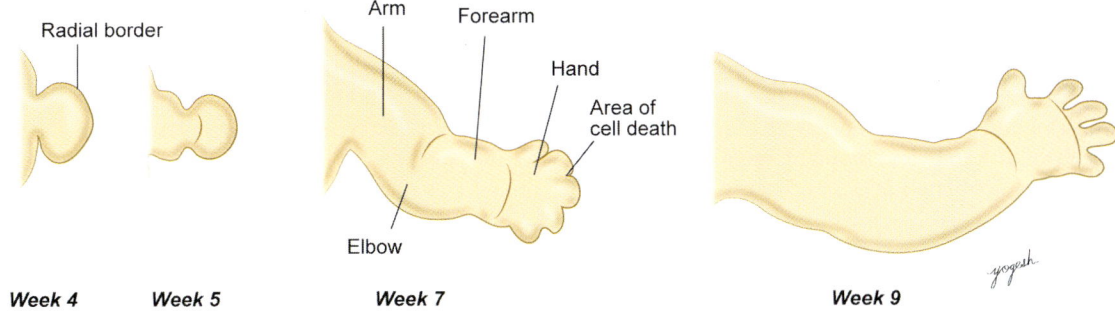

Fig. AV.1: Development of upper limb

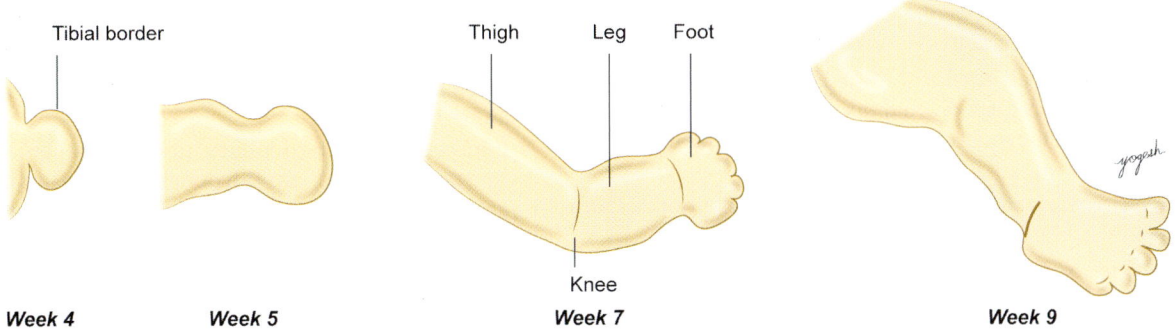

Fig. AV.2: Development of lower limb

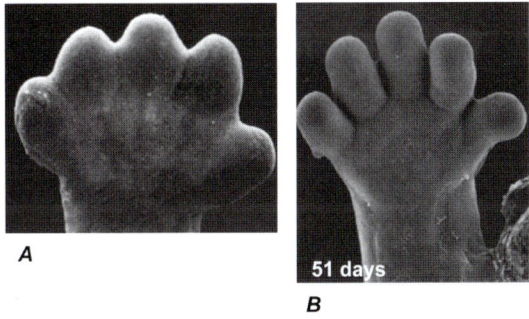

Scanning electron micrograph AV.1: Development of hand. During the seventh and eighth weeks of development the digits of hand become apparent: (A) 48 days; (B) 51 days. [Species: Human]

erentiation to form arm-forearm-hand and thigh-leg-foot in respective limb buds.
- Chondroblasts forms cartilaginous models for development of limb bones.
- Myoblasts form muscle masses.
- Hand differentiates to form palm and digits and foot differentiates to form sole and toes.

Rotation of limbs
- In the 7th week, upper limbs rotate laterally through 90° along their long axes and extensor surface comes to lie on dorsal aspects of the arm.
- Lower limbs rotate medially through 90° along their long axes and extensor surface comes to lie on ventral aspect of leg.
- Rotation makes preaxial border laterally in upper limb (thumb) and medially in lower limbs (greater toe).

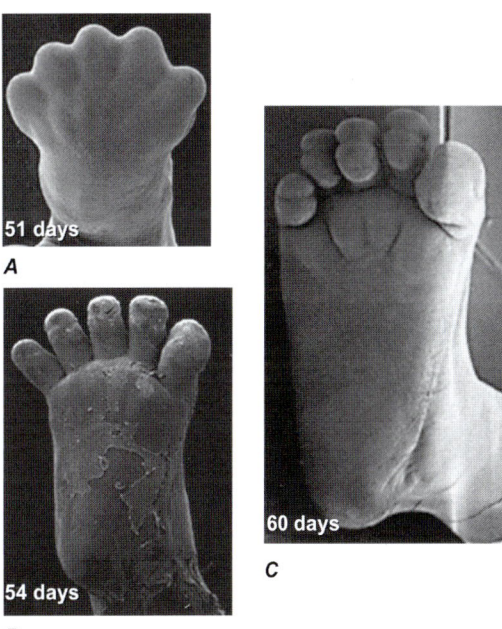

Scanning electron micrograph AV.2: Development of foot. Development of the foot is like that of the hand. It starts approximately 3–4 days later: (A) 51 days; (B) 54 days; (C) 60 days [Species: Human]

Blood supply and nerve supply
- Limb buds are supplied by axis artery. For detailed development of axis artery of limbs, refer to Chapter 19.
- Dermatome is the area of skin supplied by a single spinal nerve.

- Upper limb receives supply from C4–8 and T1–2 spinal nerves.
- Lower limb receives supply from L2–5 and S1–2 spinal nerves.
- As the limb elongates, sensory nerves also migrate out.
- For further details of limb development, refer Textbook of Human Anatomy, Volume 1 and 3 by Yogesh Sontakke.

Anomalies of Limbs

1. *Amelia:* It is complete absence of all four limbs.
2. *Phocomelia:* It involves rudimentary hands and feet that are directly attached to the trunk.^{MCQ}
3. *Meromelia:* It is shortening of all the segments of the limb.
4. *Syndactyly* (fused or webbed digits): It results due to failure of differentiation between two or more digits.^{MCQ}
5. *Polydactyly* (supernumerary digits): In this condition, there is an extra digit or phalanx on the hand or foot. Polydactyly is the most common anomaly of fingers and toes.
6. *Brachydactyly:* In this condition, there is an abnormal shortness of the fingers due to absence of phalynx.
7. *Cleft hand or foot* (Lobster-claw deformity): In this condition, one or more central digits are absent resulting in a wide cleft in hand or foot. Remaining digit may be separate or fused.
8. *Club hand* (congenital absence of radius): In this condition, radius is absent, ulna is bowed and hand deviates to lateral side.^{MCQ}
9. *Club foot* (talipes equinovarus): In this condition, the foot is turned inward and it remains inverted (adducted and plantar flexed).^{MCQ}
10. *Congenital dislocation of hip:* Due to lax joint capsule of hip joint and underdeveloped acetabulum at birth, dislocation of hip may occur. Its incidence is 1 in 1500 newborn and more common in females.
11. *Sirenomelia* (sympodia): In this condition, the lower limbs are fused. Foot may be separated or fused.^{MCQ}

DEVELOPMENT OF JOINTS

- The mesenchymal tissue between two bones differentiates to form joint.
- Type of joint depends on the differentiation of mesenchyme:
  - If mesenchyme differentiates into fibrous tissue – fibrous joint (syndesmosis).
  - If mesenchyme differentiates into cartilage – cartilaginous (primary or secondary cartilaginous joint).
  - If mesenchyme differentiates into three layers as outer two layers continuous with perichondrium of cartilages at ends of bones and middle layer degenerates to form joint cavity and synovial membrane – synovial joint.

Muscles of Limbs

- In the 5th week, myotomes of limb bud form anterior and posterior condensations.
- Anterior mesenchymal condensation forms flexor and pronator muscles in upper limb, whereas extensor and adductor muscles in lower limb.
- Posterior mesenchymal condensation forms extensor and supinator muscles in upper limb, whereas flexor and abductor muscles in lower limb.

Clinical Embryology

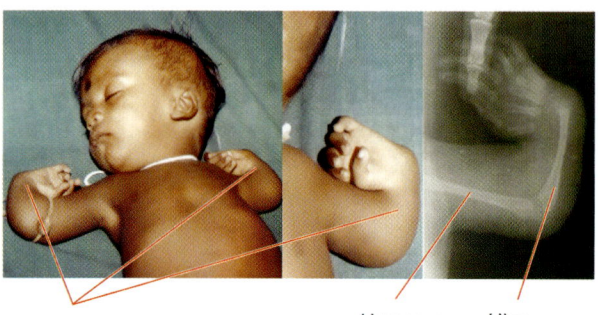

Growing limb bud
↓
In 6–12 weeks of gestation damage at the apical ectoderm of the limb bud
↓
Arrest of radial longitudinal development
↓
Radial aplasia

Clinical image AV.1: A case of bilateral radial aplasia (absence of radius). Incidence is 1 in 30,000 births and it occurs bilaterally in 50% of cases (Image courtesy: *Dr Kumaravel S*)

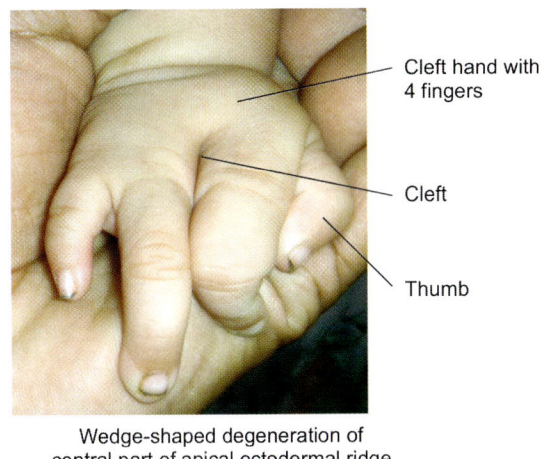

Wedge-shaped degeneration of central part of apical ectodermal ridge
↓
Cleft hand

Clinical Image AV.2: Cleft hand of the right side with four fingers. Cleft hand (lobster-claw deformity) is characterized by the absence of 1 or more central digits of the hand and V-shaped cleft in the centre of the hand. Incidence is 1:10,000 to 1:90,000 and more common in males than in females (5:1). It is inherited as an autosomal dominant disorder in 70% cases (Image courtesy: *Dr Kumaravel S*)

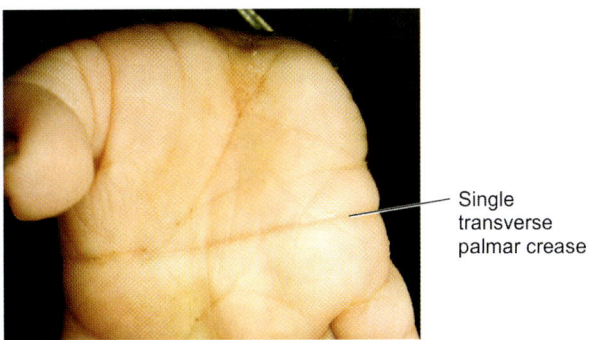

Clinical image AV.3: Single transverse palmar crease. Usually, in humans, two transverse palmar creases are present (proximal and distal). In the present case, a single transverse palmar crease (Simian crease) formed by the fusion of the two palmar creases is present. Here, it is associated with Down syndrome (facial features are not shown). It is present in 1.5% of the general population in at least one hand. The individual may be asymptomatic or may be associated with genetic chromosomal abnormalities such as Down syndrome, cri du chat syndrome, Klinefelter syndrome, Wolf-Hirschhorn syndrome, Noonan syndrome, Patau syndrome and Edward syndrome (Image courtesy: *Dr Kumaravel S*)

Index

A

Abdominal circumference 301
Abembryonic pole 31
Abortion 314
    complete 314
    incomplete 314
    inevitable 314
    spontaneous 314
    threatened 314
    induced 315
Accessory pancreatic tissue 146
Accretionary growth 2
Achalasia cardia 128
Achondroplasia 284, 285
Acrosine 28
Acrosome reaction 28
Adenohypophysis 275
Adrenal gland 277, 279
Afferent columns 245
Age
    conceptional 3
    fertilization 3
    gestational 2
    menstrual 2
    somite 3
Agenesis 70, 156
Aglossia 123
Agnathia 115
Alar lamina 241, 247, 249
Alar plates 252
Albinism 89
Allantoenteric diverticulum 54
Allantoic diverticulum 83
Allantois 54
Allocortex 254
Alpha zones 78
Amastia 94
Amelia 317
Amelogenesis imperfecta 120
Amenorrhea 13
Amnio-ectodermal junction 41, 68
Amniocentesis 84, 299
Amnion nodosum 84
Amniotic fluid index 84
Ampulla 209
Anal canal 136
Anaphase 4
Anastomosis
    postcostal 192
    post-transverse 192
    precostal 192
Anchoring villi 55, 77
Anencephaly 84, 245, 289
Angiogenesis 64, 186
Angora 90
Animal pole 31
Ankyloglossia 123
Ankyloglossia superior 124
Annulus ovalis 176
Anodontia 120
Anonychia 93
Anophthalmia 265
Anorchism 223
Anotia 273
Anovulation 13, 23
Anterior commissure 255
Anterior intestinal portal 126
Anterior lenticonus 267
Anterior neuropore 60
Anterior spina bifida 245

Anti-Müllerian substance 220
Anus
    ectopic 137
    imperforate 137
Aorta
    coarctation of 190
Aortae
    dorsal 187
    ventral 187
Apical ectodermal ridge 315
Aplasia 70
Appendicular skeleton 281
Appendix 135
Apple-peel atresia 135
Apposition stage 119
Appositional growth 2
Arch
    branchial 96
    cartilage third 100
    first 99
    fourth 100
    pharyngeal 96
    sixth 100
Arches
    arteries of 102
    pharyngeal 97
    derivatives of 98
    nerves of 101
Archipallium 254
Arrector pili 89
Arteries
    aortic arch 188
    pharyngeal arch 187
    umbilical 192, 202
    vitelline 190
    accessory renal 210, 212
    first aortic arch 187
    median sacral 210
    pharyngeal arch 187
    vertebral 192
Artificial insemination 38
Ascending tract 242
Aspermia 19
Asthenozoospermia 19
Astrocytes 242
Athelia 94
Atresia 70
    congenital laryngeal 152
    duodenal 131
    esophageal 128
    intrahepatic biliary 143
Atrial septal defects 178
Atrium
    left 173
    right 172
Atrophy 70
Auricle 272
Autosomes 4
Auxetic growth 1
AV node 180
Axial skeleton 281
Axis artery of lower limb 193
Axis artery of upper limb 193
Axon 242
Azoospermia 19

B

Barr body 220
Basal cell layer 88
Basal lamina 246, 248, 249

Basal part 253
Basal plate 74, 241
Bell stage 118
Beta zone 78
Bifid sternum 288
Bilaminar germ disc 41
Billings method 22
Biparietal diameter 301
Bladder
    extrophy 217
    hourglass 215
    urinary 213
Blastocoel 31
Blastomeres 29
Blastopore 49, 51
Blepharophimosis 266
Blood island 64
Body ciliary 264
Bone 282
    lamella 283
    labyrinth 270
Brachycephaly 290, 317
Brainstem functional columns of 245
Brittle-bone disease 284
Bronchial tree 149
Bronchus
    left principal 153
    right principal 153
    secondary 154
    tracheal 152
Buccopharyngeal membrane 50
Bud
    cystic 144
    division of hepatic 141, 142
    formation of hepatic 141
    growth of hepatic 142
    hepatic 144
    lung 149
    stage 118
    ureteric 226
Bulbopontine extension 247, 248
Bulboventricular chamber 179
Bulboventricular loop 172
Bulbs sinovaginal 227
Bulbus cordis 179
Buphthalmos 267
Bursa
    inguinal 222
    omental 166

C

Camerous fluid 83
Canal/s
    atrioventricular 175
    inguinal 222
    pulp 118, 120
    uterovaginal 227
    vaginal 227
    pericardio-peritoneal 150
    pericardioperitoneal 159
    semicircular 271
Cap stage 118
Capacitation 18, 28
Cardiac muscle 293
Cardiospasm 128
Cartilage 281
    arch second 100
    hypophyseal 288
    parachordal 288
    Reichert's 100

Cartilaginous bones 282
Cartilaginous viscerocranium 289
Caudal dysgenesis 55
Caudal intestinal portal 131
Caudal neuropore 236
Caudal pharyngeal complex 105
Cavity/ies
    pleural 150
    chorionic 43
    definitive mouth 117
    primary tympanic 271
    primitive mouth 117
Caecum 135
Cell/s
    cardiac progenitor 168
    chromaffin 239, 280, 311
    dendritic 88
    ependymal 243
    follicular 225
    Langerhans 87, 89
    microglial 243
    multipotent 2
    neural crest 239, 279, 311
    neuroblast 239, 242, 311
    pluripotent 2, 239, 311
    primordial germ 218
    primordial muscle 291
    progenitor heart 168
    rod 271
    Sertoli 221
    spongioblast 239, 311
    totipotent 2
Cementoblasts 120
Cementum 118, 120
Central artery of retina 260
Central vein of retina 260
Cephalic flexure 239
Cephalothoracopagus 305
Cerebellar
    cortex 251
    lobes 250
    peduncles 251
    plate 250
Cerebellum 250, 251
    evolutionary aspect of 250
    histogenesis of 250
Cerebral
    aqueduct 250
    aqueduct of Sylvius 250
    cortex 253
    hemispheres 254
    hemispheres lobes of 254
Cerebrum 253
Cervical flexure 239
Cervical mucus 12
Cervical rib 288
Cetrorelix 36
Chamber, vitreous 264
Chambers of eye 264
Cheeks 112
Chemotaxis 26
Chiasmata 5
Chimera 29
CHL 298
Chondrification stage 285
Chondroblasts 281
Chondrocranium 288
Chondrocytes 281
Chordomas 54
Chorion 43, 76

Chorion frondosum 77
Chorion laevae 77
Chorionic plate 74
Chorionic villi
   definitive 55
      development of 55
      primary 55
Chorionic villus sampling 299
Choroid 263
Choroid plexus 248
Choroidal fissure 259
Chromatin 4
Chromosomes 4
Ciliary beats 31
Circumvallate papillae 122
Cleavage 29
Cleft hand or foot 317
Cleft lip 115
Cleft oblique facial 115
Cleft palate 115
   complete 115
   incomplete 115
   unilateral complete 115
Clefts pharyngeal 97
Cleidocranial dysostosis 284, 289
Cloaca 126, 135, 206
Cloacal exstrophy 139
Cloacal membrane 50
Clomiphene citrate 23
Club foot 317
Club hand 317
Cochlea 271
Coelom intraembryonic 158
Collodion babies 88
Coloboma of eyelid 265
Coloboma of iris 265, 267
Complete mole 32
Congenital
   adrenal hyperplasia 279
   alopecia 90
   aniridia 265
   aphakia 265
   cataract 262, 267
   dislocation of hip 317
   hepatic fibrosis 143
   hydrocoele 224
   megacolon 137
   ptosis 265
   torticollis 292
Conjunctival sac 265
Connecting stalk 43, 68
Contraception 312
Contraceptives 312, 313
Conus cordis 179
Convergence 53
Copula of His 122
Cornea 260
Corona radiata 24
Corpus albicans 24
Corpus callosum 255
Corpus hemorrhagicus 24
Corpus luteum 24
Cortex hippocampal 254
Costal element 287
Costotransverse joint 288
Cotyledons 74
CR length 298
Cranial neuropore 236
Craniopagus 305
Craniopharyngiomas 277
Cranium in newborn 289
Crater nipple 94
Crista 271
Crista terminalis 176
CRL 301
Crossover 5

Crown to heel length 298, 301
Cryptophthalmos 265
Cryptorchidism 223, 233
Cumulus 20
Cupula 271
Cuticle 92
Cyanotic lips 182
Cyclopia 265
Cyst
   branchial 103
   cervical 103
   dentigerous 120
   urachal 215
Cytokinesis 4
Cytotrophoblast 40
Cytotrophoblast shell 55, 77

D

Decidua 45, 74
Decidua
   basalis 45, 74
   capsularis 74
   parietalis 74
   reaction 12, 33, 47, 75
Definitive
   ear 271
   gonad 219
   oral cavity 117
   yolk sac 85
Dental cuticle of Nasmyth 119
Dental lamina 118
Dentine 118
Dentinogenesis imperfecta 120
Dermal papillae 89
Dermatoglyphics 89
Dermis 89
Dermomyotome 64
Deutoplasm 24
Development 1
Dexter 177
Dextrocardia invertus 177
Diaphragm 160
   eventration of 163
Diaphysis 284
Diencephalon 252, 277
Differentiation 2
Diplotene 5
Disease
   Caroli's 143
   Hand-Schüller-Christian 290
   Hirschsprung's 137
   hyaline membrane 156
   polycystic liver 143
Diverticulum
   laryngotracheal 150
   Meckel's 134
   respiratory 149
Doppler ultrasonography 300
Dorsal mesentery 68, 131
Dorsal mesogastrium 129
Down syndrome 6
Duchenne muscular
   dystrophy 293, 294
Duct/s
   atresia of 144
   coelomic 158
   ejaculatory 221
   genital 226
   inversion of pancreatic 146
   mesonephric 207, 226
   Müllerian 207, 227
   nasolacrimal 110
   of Cuvier 194
   omphaloenteric 66
   paramesonephric 207, 227
   patent vitellointestinal 139
   thyroglossal 106
   vitellointestinal 66, 68, 83, 85, 131,
   Wolffian 207
Ductus arteriosus 202

Ductus venosus 202
Duodenal diverticula 131
Duodenum 131
Dwarfism 285
Dyschondroplasias 284
Dyskeratosis congenita 93
Dysmenorrhoea 13

E

E-cadherin 54
Ear ossicles 271
Ectoderm 56
Ectodermal anal pit 137
Ectopia cordis 177, 184
Ectopia vesicae 216, 217
Ectopic pregnancy 33
EDD 3
Efferent columns 245
Egg freezing 39
Egg pickup 36
Eisenmenger's complex 183
Elastic cartilage 281
Emboly 53
Embryoblast 31, 40
Embryonic organizer 54
Embryotroph 43
Eminence hypobranchial 122
Enamel 118
Encephalocele 245, 256, 258
Enchondromatosis 284
Endochondral ossification 282
Endoderm 50, 69
Endodermal cloaca 136
Endolymph 271
Endometrium 9, 74
Endovaginal sonography 45
Enterochromaffin cells of
   Kulchitsky 280
Enterocystoma 134
Entropion 265
Epiblast 40, 48
Epiboly 53
Epicanthus 265
Epidermal ridges 88
Epidermolysis bullosa 95
Epididymis 221
Epiglottis 122
Epimere 291
Epiphysis 284
Epiphysis cereberi 277
Epispadias 232
Epithalamus 252
Epithelium
   coelomic 279
   germinal 225
   inner dental 118
   of lens 262
   olfactory 113
   outer dental 118
Epitrichium 88
Eponychium 92
Estrogen 12, 13
Estrogenic phase 10
Exocelomic cavity 41
Exomphalos 135
Expected date of delivery 3
External acoustic meatus 272
External ear 272, 273
Extraembryonic coelom 43
Extraocular muscles 265, 292
Eyelids 265

F

Face, development of 109
Facial colliculus 248
Factor testis determining 219
Female pseudohermaphrodite 310
Femur length 301
Fertile period 7

Fertility 313
Fertilization 25, 37
   effects of 29
   stages of 28
Fetal circulation 202
   peculiarities of 202
   cotyledons 79
   heartbeat 202
   viability 312
Fetomaternal organ 73
Fetoplacental circulation 55
Fetoscopy 299
Fetus as graft 46
FGF8 54
Fibrocartilage 281
Filum terminale 243
Fimbriae 227
First polar body 21
Fissure ventral median 241
Fistula
   congenital rectovesical 215
   congenital vesicovaginal 215
   rectal 138
   rectovaginal 229
   rectovestibular 139
   thyroglossal 107
   tracheoesophageal 128, 152
   umbilical fecal 134
   urachal 215
   vitelline 134
Floating villi 78
Flocculonodular lobe 250
Floor plates 241
Foldings of embryo 65
Folds
   anal 229
   cloacal 229
   definitive urethral 230
   of Rathke 136
   urethral 229
Follicle-stimulating hormone 36
Follicular fluid 22
Follicular phase 9
Fontanelles 288
Foramen
   ovale 176, 202
   primum 176
   secundum 176
   of Luschka 248
Foregut 70, 126
Formation
   of auricles 172
   of bile canaliculi 142
   of limb bud 315
   of limb bud primordia 315
   of limbs 315
   of S-loop 172
   of zygote 28
Frontal lobe 254
FSH 12
Funnel chest 288

G

G0 phase 6
G1 phase 6
G2 phase 6
Gallbladder
   agenesis of 144
   double 144
   floating 144
   intrahepatic 144
   septate 144
   sessile 144
Gamete 4
Gamete intrafallopian transfer 38
Gametogenesis 15
Ganirelix 36
Gastroschisis 72, 135, 139
Gastrulation 48
Gender discrimination 314

General somatic afferent 246
General somatic efferent 245
General visceral afferent 246
General visceral efferent 245
Genitalia
    female external 230
    male external 229
Genomic imprinting 47
Genotype 4
Germination 120
Gestation 295, 298
Gestational period 296
Gestational sac 301
Gland
    accessory pituitary 277
    apocrine sweat 91
    eccrine sweat 91
    ectopic adrenal 279
    parotid 124
    pineal 277
    salivary 124
    sebaceous 91
    sublingual 124
    submandibular 124
    sweat 90
    thyroid 106, 107
Gonadotropin 36
Gonadotropin-releasing hormone 36
Gonads 218
Graafian follicle 20
Grey matter 242
Groove
    definitive urethral 230
    laryngotracheal 127, 149
    nasolacrimal 110
    neural 236
    primitive urethral 229
Growth 1
Gubernaculum testis 222
Gynecomastia 94

H

Habenular commissure 255
Hair peg 89
Harelip 115
Harlequin fetuses 89
Harlequin ichthyosis 95
Hatching of blastocyst 32
Haversian system 282
Head circumference 301
Head fold 66
Heart tube 169
Helicotrema 271
Hematopoiesis 148
Hemiglossia 123
Hemivertebra 288
Hensen's node 48
Hermaphrodite 310
Hernia
    congenital diaphragmatic 163
    congenital hiatal 163
    congenital inguinal 224
    congenital umbilical 135
    physiological umbilical 132
    proboscoid umbilical 167
    retrosternal 163
Heuser's membrane 41
Hindgut 70, 126
Hippocampal commissure 255
Hofbauer cells 82
Holoprosencephaly 55, 58, 257
HPO axis 12
Human chorionic gonadotropin 82
Humour aqueous 264
Hyaline cartilage 281
Hyaloid vessels 259
Hydatidiform mole 32
Hydrocele en bisac 234
Hydrocephalus 245, 290
Hydrops fetalis 86
Hydroureter 213
Hyoid tubercles 272
Hyperspermia 19
Hypertelorism 115
Hypertrichosis 90
Hypoblast 40
Hypomenorrhea 13
Hypomere 292
Hyponychium 92
Hypophysis cerebri 275
Hypoplasia 156
Hypospadias 231, 232, 233
Hypospermia 19
Hypothalamo-pituitary-ovarian axis 12
Hypothalamus 252
Hyrtl's anastomosis 83

I

Ichthyosis 89
Imperforate hymen 229
Implantation 32
    abdominal 33
    abnormal 33
    interstitial 33
    process of 32
    site of 32
    tubal 33
In vitro fertilization 35
Increta placenta 80
Induced ovulation 23
Induction 6
Infantile hemangioma 95
Inferior vena cava 199
Infertility 313
Infundibular process 252
Inhibin 12
Iniencephaly 245
Intercalated disc 293
Intermaxillary segment 113
Internal ear 273
    histogenesis of 271
Interstitial cells of Leydig 221
Intervillous space 76, 77
Intracervical insemination 38
Intracytoplasmic sperm injection 38
Intraembryonic coelom 63
Intraembryonic mesoderm 50
Intraretinal space 263
Intrauterine insemination 38
Iris 264
Ischiopagus 305
Isolated dextrocardia 177
Isomerism 148

K

Kidney/s 208
    anomalies of ascent of 211
    congenital polycystic 211
    horseshoe 211
    lobulated 211
    pancake 211
Klinefelter syndrome 6
Koller's sickle 51

L

Lacunar stage 41
Langhans layer 79
Lanugo 90, 296
Larygoptosis 152
Laryngeal web 152
Laryngocele 152
Larynx 149
Lateral folds 68
Lateral horn 242
Layer
    ependymal cell 240
    mantle 240
    marginal 240
    splanchnopleuric 159
Lens 260
    pit 259
    placode 259
    vesicle 259
Leptotene 5
Lesser omentum 142
Leuprorelin 36
LH 12
LH surge 13, 22
Ligament/s
    falciform 142
    periodontal 118
    peritoneal 142
Ligamentum arteriosum 189
Ligamentum teres hepatis 83
Limbic lobe 254
Liquefaction of semen 26
Liquor amnii 83
Liquor folliculi 11, 20
Lobe
    azygos 156
    of Wrisberg 156
    Riedel's 143
    tracheal 152
Long bone 284
Louise Brown 3
Lower eyelid colobomas 266
Lower lip 111
Lumbar rib 288
Lumbarization 288
Lung/s 149
    congenital polycystic 157
    ectopic 157
Lunula 92
Luschka 121
Luteal phase 9
Luteinizing hormone 13, 36
Luteinization 24
Lymphatic system 203

M

M phase 6
Macroglossia 124
Macrostomia 115
Maculae 271
Male pseudohermaphrodite 233, 310
Malformation
    Arnold-Chiari 255
    Dandy-Walker 255
Mammillary body 252
Mammary buds 93
Mammary pit 94
Mammary ridges 93
Mandibular tubercles 272
Mandibulofacial dysostosis 104, 273
Maternal blood screening 299
Maternal inheritance 29
Mature neurons 242
Meconium 138
Medial nasal prominence 110
Median umbilical ligament 54
Medulla oblongata 246
Medullary plate 56
Medullary velum 251
Meiosis 5, 6
Meiotic spindle 23
Melanoblasts 88
Membrana tectoria 271
Membrane
    amniochorionic 85
    anal 215, 229
    basilar 271
    buccopharyngeal 61, 109, 117, 126
    cloacal 61, 126
    fetal 85
    hymenal 227
    Nitabuch's 79
    oropharyngeal 61
    persistent papillary 265
    pupillary 264
    Reissner's 271
    secondary tympanic 272
    tympanic 98, 271
    urogenital 215, 229
    pharyngeal 98
Membranous bones 282
Membranous labyrinth 268
Membranous neurocranium 288
Membranous viscerocranium 289
Meningocele 244
Meningomyelocele 244
Menkes syndrome 90
Menometrorrhagia 13
Menopause 7
Menorrhagia 13
Menstrual bleeding 9, 12
Menstrual cycle 7
    disorders of 13
    duration of 9
    hormonal synchronization in 12
    ovarian changes in 10
    phases of 9
Menstrual phase 9
Menstruation 7
Meromelia 317
Mesencephalon 236
Mesenchyme 4
Mesenteries 129, 163
Mesentery
    dorsal 163
    ventral 163
Mesocardium 172, 181
Mesoderm
    intermediate 62, 205
    lateral plate 62, 205
    paraxial 62, 205, 281
    splanchnic 149
    splanchnopleuric 43, 153
Mesodermal differentiation 62
Mesogastrium ventral 163
Mesonephric tubules 226
Mesonephros 208
Mesovarium 225
Metameres 62
Metanephric blastema 208
Metanephric cap 209
Metanephros 208, 209
Metaphase 4
Metaphysis 284
Metencephalon 246
Metrorrhagia 13
Microcephaly 255
Microglossia 124
Microphthalmia 265
Microspherophakia 266
Microstomia 115
Midbrain 249, 250
Middle cerebellar peduncle 248
Middle ear 271, 273
Midgut 70, 126
Milk lines 93
Miscarriage 314
Mitosis 4
Mittelschmerz 22
Modiolous 271
Molar pregnancy 32
Monorchism 223
Morula 30, 31
Mosaics 29
Multiple pregnancies 296
Multiplicative growth 1
Muscle/s
    cardiac 291
    ciliary 264
    of body wall 291
    of limbs 292
    of pharyngeal arches 292
    of tongue 292
    skeletal 291
    smooth 291
    striated 291
Myelencephalon 246

Myelination 243
Myelinogenesis 243
Myelomeningocele 244, 256
Myoblasts 291
Myocele 64
Myoepicardial mantle 168, 169
Myometrium 9
Myotome 64, 291

N

Naegele's formula 3
Nail field 93
Nail plate 92
Nails 92
Nasal pit 110
Nasal placodes 109
Natal teeth 120
Nerve
 optic 263
Neural crest 57, 60, 236
 cells 56
Neural folds 56, 60, 236
Neural groove 56, 60
Neural plate 56
Neural tube 56, 235, 239
 defects 243
 differentiation of 236
 flexures of 239
 formation of 56
 histogenesis of cells in 241
Neurenteric canal 51, 54
Neuroblast 241
 apolar 242
 bipolar 242
 multipolar 242
 unipolar 242
Neurocranium 288
Neuroectoderm 60, 235, 236, 265, 279
Neurohypophysis 277
Neurons 242
Neuropores 56
Neurulation 56, 236
Non-disjunction 6
Notochord 51
 definitive 54
significance of 54
Notochordal
 canal 51
 plate 54
 process 51
Nucleus pulposus 54
Nutrition 296

O

Obstruction ureteric 213
Occipital lobe 254
Occipitalization 288
Odontoblasts 118
Olfactory bulb 254
Olfactory pit 110
Olfactory placode 109
Oligo-ovulation 13, 23
Oligodendrocytes 242
Oligohydramnios 84
Oligomenorrhea 13
Oligozoospermia 19
Olivary group of nuclei 248
Omphalocele 135, 139
Omphalopagus 305
Ontogeny 1
Oocyte 21
 retrieval 36
Oogenesis 20, 23
Oogonia 15, 225
Ooplasm 23
Optic chiasma 255
Optic cup 259, 265
Optic stalk 259
Optic sulcus 252, 259
Optic vesicle 259
Organ of Zuckerkandl 280

Organizer 6
Ossification 282
 endochondral 282
 intramembranous 282
Ossification stage 285
Osteogenesis imperfecta 284
Osteoid 282, 283
Otic capsule 270
Otic pit 268
Otic placodes 268
Otic vesicle 268
Otocyst 268
Oval window 272
Ovarian cycle 7
Ovarian stimulation 36
Ovary 224
 anomalies of 226
 descent of 225
Ovulation 22
 tests for 22
Ovum 24
 lifespan of 27
 structure of 23
Ox eye 267

P

Pachytene 5
Palate
 definitive 115
 primary 114
 secondary 114
Palatogenesis 114
Paleopallium 254
Pancreas
 annular 145
 divided 145
Para-aortic bodies 280
Paramesonephric ducts 227
Pars distalis 275
Pars intermedia 275
Pars nervosa 277
Pars tuberalis 277
Parthenogenesis 29
Partial mole 32
Patent ductus arteriosus 189
Pelvic ostium 227
Penis primitive 229
Percutaneous umbilical blood sampling 299
Pericardial bar 51, 63
Pericardium 181
Periderm 88
Perilymph 271
Perimetrium 9
Perineal body 215
Period
 alveolar 156
 canalicular 155
 embryonic 2, 60
 fetal 2
 germinal 2
 organogenic 60
 prenatal 2
 pseudoglandular 155
 terminal sac 155
Perionychium 92
Periosteal buds 283
Periosteal collar 284
Periotic tissue 271
Perivitelline space 24
Persistent truncus arteriosus 180
Phallus 229
Pharyngeal apparatus 97
Pharyngeal bursa 121
Pharynx 121
Phenotype 4
Pheochromocytoma 280
Phocomelia 317
Phrygian cap 144
Phylogeny 1, 77
Piebaldism 89
Pigeon chest 288

Placenta 73, 202, 296
Placenta
 accreta 80
 battledore 80
 bidiscoid 79
 circumvallate 80
 discoid 79
 functions of 80
 lobed 79
 membranacea 79
 previa 33, 309
 succenturiate 79
 velamentous 80, 86
Placental barrier 79, 81
Placental septae 73
Plagiocephaly 290
Plate medullary 236
Plate vaginal 227
Pleura
 parietal 153
 visceral 153
Pleural cavity 159
Pleuropericardial opening 160
Poland sequence 292
Polydactyly 317
Polyhydramnios 84
Polymastia 94
Polymenorrhea 13
Polyspermy 28
Polysplenia 148
Polythelia 94
Pons 248
Pontine flexure 239
Pontine nuclei 248
Posterior commissure 255
Posterior grey horn 242
Posterior intestinal portal 126
Posterior neuropore 60
Pouch/es
 fifth 105
 first 104
 fourth 105
 Hartmann's 144
 of Lushka 121
 pharyngeal 96, 97, 103
 Rathke's 275, 277
 second 105
 third 105
Prechordal plate 43
Pregnancy test 315
Premaxillary part 114
Prenatal diagnosis 298
Preoccipital myotomes 265
Prepuce 230
Prevention 244
Primary
 amenorrhea 14
 follicle 20
 heart field 168
 lens fibers 261
 meatus 272
 oocytes 20
 spermatocyte 17
 stem villi 43
 villi 76
 yolk sac 41, 84
Primitive
 anterior nares 110
 follicle 225
 germ cells 15
 gonads 219
 groove 50
 gut 126
 heart field 168
 oral cavity 117
 pit 49
 sex cords 219
 streak 48
Proboscis 115
Process/es
 ciliary 264
 frontonasal 109
 lateral palatine 114
 mandibular 109

 maxillary 109, 110
 median palatine 114
Processus vaginalis 222
Progestational phase 9, 11
Progesterone 12, 13
Proliferative phase 9, 10
Prometaphase 4
Pronephros 208
Prophase 4
Prosencephalon 236
Prostate 229
Pseudohermaphrodite 310
Puberty 7
Pulsed Doppler 299
Purkinje fibres 181
Pyopagus 305

Q

Quadruplets 303
Quickening 296
Quintuplets 303

R

Rachischisis 245, 256
Rami chorii 78
Ramuli chorii 78
Rauber's sickle 51
Red nucleus 249
Reissner's membrane 271
Renal agenesis 211
Renal collar 199
Renaud's residual body 17
Reproduction 1
Reproductive biology 1
Rete testis 221
Retina 263
Retinal detachment 263
Retrognathia 115
Rhombencephalic isthmus 246
Rhombencephalon 236
Ribs 288
Ridge genital 219
Ridge gonadal 219
Ridge suprarenal 279
Riegerís anomaly 267
Rohr's fibrinoid stria 79
Roof 241
Rubella virus 273

S

S phase 6
SA node 180
Sac
 lesser 165
 pericardial 158
Sacralization 287
Sacrococcygeal teratoma 54, 58
Scala tympani 271
Scala vestibuli 271
Scaphocephaly 289, 290
Sclera 263
Sclerotome 64, 285
Screening 244
Scrotum 222
Second polar body 21, 28
Secondary
 amenorrhea 14
 areolae 283
 heart field 168
 lens fibers 262
 meatus 272
 oocyte 15
 spermatocyte 17
 villi 55, 76
 yolk sac 43, 84
Segment
 bronchopulmonary 154
 intermaxillary 110
Sella turcica 275
Semicircular canals 271
Sensory roots 242

separation   159
septum
    aorticopulmonary   180
    dorsal median   241
    interatrial   175
    intermedium   175
    primum   175
    secundum   176
    sinus   173
    spiralling of   180
    spurium   173
    tracheoesophageal   149
    transversum   162, 163
    urorectal   135
    urorectal   126
sequestration   157
Serotina   74
Sex chromosomes   4
Sex ratio   314
Sinus/es
    definitive urogenital   215
    inferior petrosal   197
    paranasal air   114
    sigmoid   197
    superior petrosal   197
    transverse   172, 197
    urachal   215
    urogenital   215
    venarum   176
    venosus   173
Sinusoids   142
Sirenomelia   55, 317
Situs inversus   53
Skeletal muscle   291
Skin, aplasia of   89
Skull   288
Smooth muscles   292
Snail gene   53
Somatopleuric layer   63
Somite   62, 63, 283, 291
    preoccipital   63
Somitomeres   62, 63, 281
Spemann organizer   54
Sperm   18, 24
    lifespan of   27
Spermatid   17, 18
Spermatogenesis   16, 23
Spermatogonia   15, 16, 18, 221
Spermatozoa   18
Spermatozoon   17
Spermiation   17
Spermiogenesis   17
Spina bifida   244, 288
    cystica   244
    occulta   244, 256
Spinal cord   240
    central canal of   241
    functional columns of   243
    positional changes in   243
    recession   243
Spinnbarkeit cervical mucus
        method   22
Splanchnopleuric layer   63
Spleen
    accessory   148
    lobulated   148
Spondylolisthesis   288
Spongioblast   241
Stapedius   271
Stenosis   152
    duodenal   131
    esophageal   128
    tracheal   152
Sterility   314
Sternal bars   288
Sternum   288
Stomodeum   96, 117
Stratum
    basale   9
    compactum   9
    functionale   9
    germinativum   88
    spongiosum   9

Striated nuclei   253
Substantia nigra   249
Sulcus
    bulboventricular   172
    labio-gingival   118
    limitans   241, 246
    linguo-gingival   117
    terminalis   122
Superior dislocation of lens   266
Superior pallium   253
Suppressed ovulation   23
Surface ectoderm   60, 61
Surgical sperm extraction   38
Surrogacy   314
Surrogate motherhood   314
Swellings genital   229
Sympatho-chromaffin organ   239, 311
Sympathoblasts   239, 311
Synapsis   5
Syncytiotrophoblast   40
Syncytium   291
Syndactyly   317
Syndrome
    amniotic band   86
    DiGeorge   104, 183
    Goldenhar   107
    Gorlin   89
    Holt-Oram   183
    Klippel-Feil   288
    nevoid basal cell carcinoma   89
    oculo-auriculo-vertebral   107
    persistent mullerian duct   234
    Pierre Robin   104
    Potter   84
    premenstrual   13
    Prune-belly   217
    Taussig-Bing   183
    Treacher Collins   104
    first arch   104
Syringomyelia   245

T

Tail fold   66
Teeth
    development of   118
    successional   118
    superadded   118
Tela choroidea   248
Telencephalic flexure   239
Telencephalon
    commissures of   255
Telophase   4
Temporal lobe   254
Teratogen   4
Teratogenesis   313
Teratology   313
Teratoma   15
Teratozoospermia   19
Tertiary follicle   20
Test-tube baby   35
Testis   220
    anomalies of   222
    descent of   221
    ectopic   224
Tetralogy of Fallot   182
Thalamus   252
Thalidomide   274
Theca externa   21
Theca interna   21
Thoracopagus   305
Thymic involution   106
Thymus development of   106
Thyroid lingual   124
Tongue
    bifid   123
    development of   121
    tie   123
Tonsil
    palatine   105
Tonsillar buds   105
Tonsillar crypts   105
Tooth
    impaction of   120
    structure of   118

Tourneux fold   136
Trabeculae   76
Trabecular bone   283
Trachea   149
    agenesis of   152
Tracts descending   242
Transabdominal sonography   300
Transposition of great vessels   180
Transvaginal sonography   45, 300
Transverse element   287
Trichorrhexis nodosa   90
Trigeminal nerve   271
Trigone   226
Trigonocephaly   290
Trilaminar germ disc   64
Trimester   3
Triplets   303
Trophectoderm   31
Trophoblasts   40
True hermaphrodites   310
Truncal ridges   180
Truncus arteriosus   179
Truncus chorii   78
Tubal tonsil   272
Tube
    auditory   271
    fallopian   227
    laryngotracheal   149
    uterine   227
Tubercle
    genital   229
    Müllerian   227
Tuberculum impar   106
Tubotympanic recess   104, 271
Tubule primitive renal   209
Tubules seminiferous   221
Tunica albuginea   221
Twin/s   303
    acardiac   184
    conjoined   305, 306
    conjoined monozygotic   305
    diamniotic dichorionic   304
    diamniotic monochorionic
            monozygotic   304
    dizygotic   303
    fraternal   303
    ischiopagus tetrapus   306
    monoamniotic monochorionic   304
    monozygotic   303, 304
    parasitic   305
    Siamese   305
    trizygotic   303
Tympanic antrum   271

U

Ultrasonography, principle of   300
Ultrasound frequency   300
Umbilical
    cord   43, 81
    contents of   82
    hernia   296
    vesicle   66, 85
    vessels   82
Upper lip   111
Urachal
    cyst   55
    fistula   55
    sinus   55
Urachus   54
Ureter   212
Ureter blind   213
Ureter ectopic   212
Ureteric buds   208
Urethra   215
    female   215
    male   216
    penile   230
Urethral plate   230
Uterine cycle   7
Uteroplacental circulation   42, 76
Uterus   227
    absence of   228
    anomalies of   227

bicornuate   228
double   228
septate   228
unicornuate   228

V

Vacteral association   157
Vagina
    agenesis of   229
    anomalies of   228
    atresia of   229
    development of   228
    double   228
    septate   229
Valve
    aortic   180
    atrioventricular   180
    left venous   173
    of coronary sinus   176
    of heart   180
    of inferior vena cava   176
    pulmonary   180
    right venous   173
Vas deferens   221
Vasculogenesis   64, 185
Vein/s
    accessory hemizygos   201
    anterior cardinal   197
    azygos   200
    hemizygos   201
    posterior cardinal   197, 198
    primary head   197
    primary maxillary   197
    somatic   194
    subcardinal   198
    supracardinal   198
    umbilical   196, 202
    visceral   194
    vitelline   195
Ventral mesogastrium   129
Ventral motor roots   242
Ventricles   177
Ventricular septal defects   183
Vermiform appendix   135
Vermis   250
Vernix caseosa   88, 296
Vertebral column   285
Vesicle metanephric   209
Vesicles seminal   221
Vestibule   167, 271
Viability scan   312
Villi   43
Viscerocranium   288
Vitelline block   28
Vitelline cyst   134
Vitelline membrane   24
Vitiligo   89
Vitreous   264

W

Wharton's jelly   83
White matter   242
Woven bone   282

X

X chromosome inactivation   47

Y

Y chromosome   3
Yolk sac   46, 84, 301
    definitive   126
    functions of   85

Z

Zinc finger transcription factor   53
Zona pellucida   21, 24, 32
Zygote intrafallopian transfer   38
Zygotene   5

Free access to learn step-by-step drawing of embryology figures through videos on CBSiCentral App.

Companion Workbook for Textbook of Human Embryology

Second Edition

Yogesh Sontakke MBBS, MD

Additional Professor
Department of Anatomy
Jawaharlal Institute of Postgraduate Medical Education and Research (JIPMER)
(An Institution of National importance under the Ministry of Health and Family Welfare, Government of India)
Puducherry, India

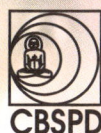

CBSPD

CBS Publishers & Distributors Pvt Ltd

New Delhi • Bengaluru • Chennai • Kochi • Kolkata • Lucknow • Mumbai
Hyderabad • Jharkhand • Nagpur • Patna • Pune • Uttarakhand

Preface

The second edition of **Textbook of Human Embryology** has been written to fulfil the requirements of students and teachers as per the latest Competency Based Undergraduate Curriculum for Indian Medical Graduate. It helps to train the students to achieve the required levels of the given competencies: Knows (K), knows how (KH), and shows how (SH), with the help of included domains of learning, knowledge (K) and skills (S).

To fulfil the need for curriculum, requirements of the students and the field of medicine, it is essential for every learner to convert embryology knowledge into presentable format in the examinations. Students face the problem in revision and focusing on the practice of figures. Each book on the embryology contains thousands of images. It is very difficult to select the figures to be practiced. To solve these student's concerns, this Workbook has been prepared to help out the students for making them aware about practicing selected figures and flowcharts for preparation of theory examinations.

The students should keep in mind that while writing a short or brief answer questions in the examination about embryology, if they support answer by a selected figure and flowchart, the explanations will be easy and presentable.

In a given time frame of examination, students should be very selective for the figure drawings and writeups. This Workbook will help for preferential selection of the figures and flowcharts for the rapid revisions. This book will help to consolidate the knowledge of the subject they have received from the textbook and will help to get prepared for the examinations. ***Always read a complete textbook for getting better knowledge and generating perfect concepts of the subject.***

For any suggestions, please write at dryogeshas@rediffmail.com

Yogesh Sontakke

Chapter 1
Introduction

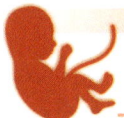

Flowchart 1.1: Stages of human life

```
                    Stages of human life
                            |
            ┌───────────────┴───────────────┐
      Prenatal period                 Postnatal period
      Sperm + Ovum                    Newborn
            ↓ Fertilization                 ↓
      Zygote                          Neonate    Up to first 4 weeks
            ↓ Germinal period               ↓
            ↓ First 2 weeks           Infant     1 month to 1 year
      Germ disc                             ↓
            ↓ Embryonic period        Child      > 1 to 12 years
            ↓ 3rd to 8th week               ↓
      Embryo                          Puberty    > 12 to 16 years
            ↓ Fetal period            (pubescent)
            ↓ 9th week to birth             ↓
      Fetus                           Adolescent > 16 to 20 years
            ↓                               ↓
      Newborn                         Adult      > 20 to 40 years
                                            ↓
                                      Middle age > 40 to 60 years
                                            ↓
                                      Old age    60 years onward
```

- *Ontogeny* is a branch of science that deals with complete life cycle (prenatal and postnatal growth and development) of an organism. Phylogeny deals with an evolutionary history and relationship among organisms.
- *Expected Date of Delivery* (EDD): A normal, full-term pregnancy lasts from 37 to 42 weeks. Expected date of delivery can be determined by counting 280 days after the first day of last menstrual period (LMP) or 266 days after conception.

Chapter 2
Menstrual Cycle

Flowchart 2.3: Uterine/Menstrual cycle

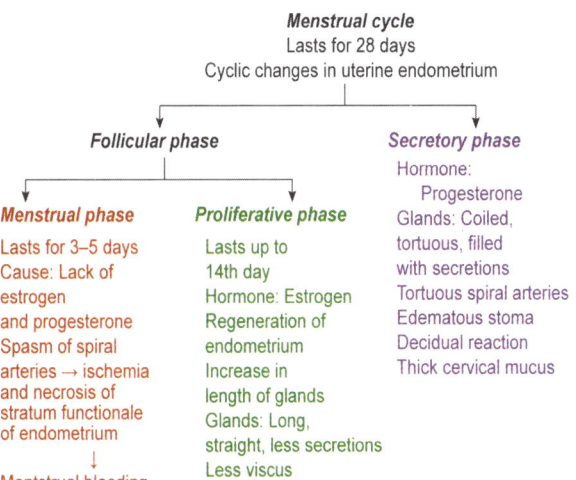

Flowchart 2.5: Ovarian cycle

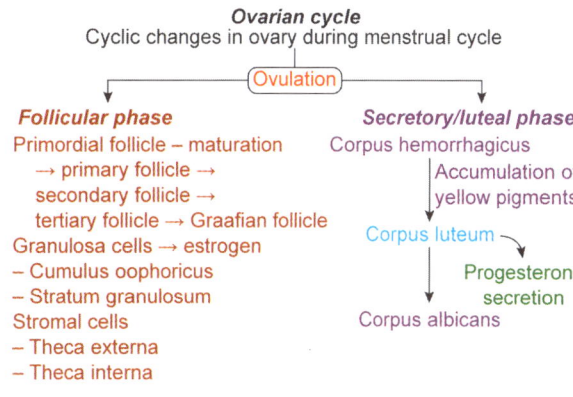

Menstrual cycle is a rhythmic change in uterus starting from puberty until menopause.
Stratum functionale = Stratum compactum + Stratum spongiosum.
Menstruation in female is under the influence of hypothalamo-pituitary-ovarian axis (HPO axis).
Amenorrhea is the absence of menstruation in a menstrual cycle in a woman of reproductive age.
Primary amenorrhea is an absence of menstruation since birth of a woman.
Secondary amenorrhea occurs when menstrual cycle stops in a woman who had menstruation before.

Chapter 3
Gametogenesis

Flowchart 3.1: Stages in spermatogenesis

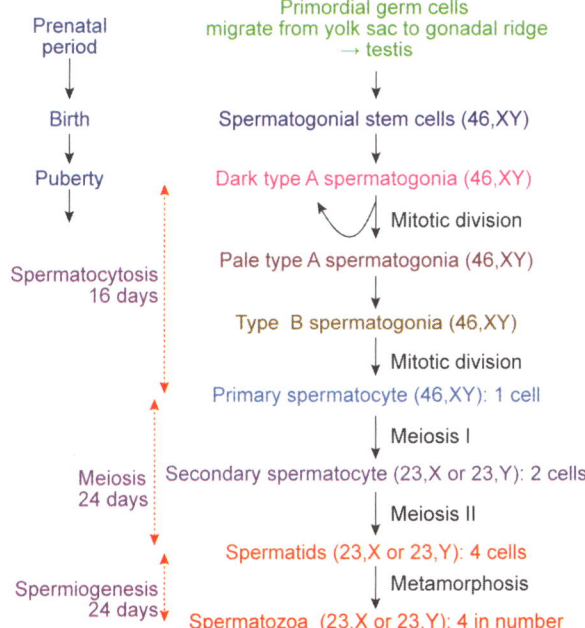

Flowchart 3.3: Stages in oogenesis

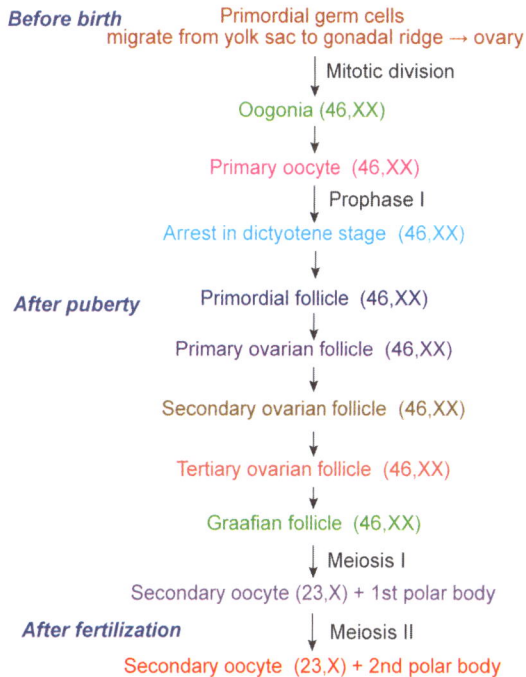

Gametogenesis is a process of formation of gametes (sperms in male and ovum in female) from germ cells by cell division.

Teratoma is a tumor that consists of tissues derived from all germ layers.

Spermatogenesis is a process of formation of sperms (male gametes) from spermatogonia in seminiferous tubules of testis.

Spermatocytosis is a conversion of spermatogonia → primary spermatocyte.

Spermiogenesis is the process of metamorphosis of spermatids by which they get converted into a spermatozoon.
Capacitation is a process of conversion of immature spermatozoa to mature spermatozoa.

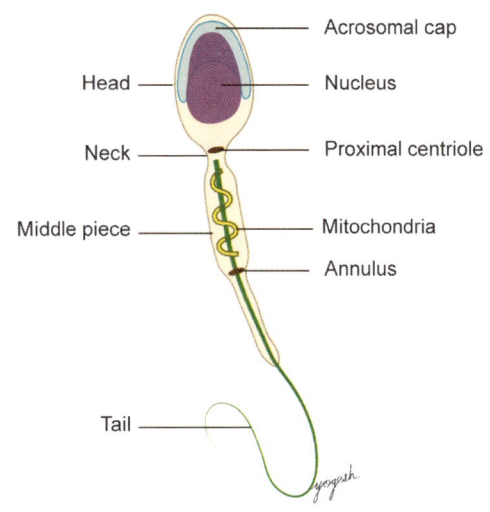

Practice Fig. 3.2: Structure of sperm

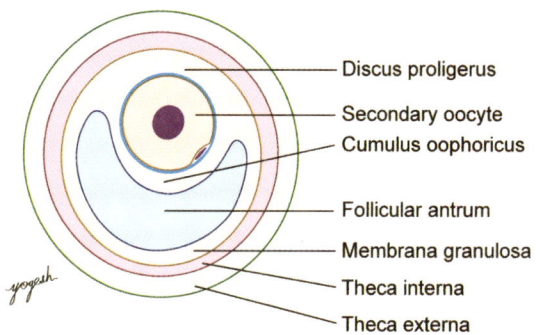

Practice Fig. 3.4: Graafian follicle

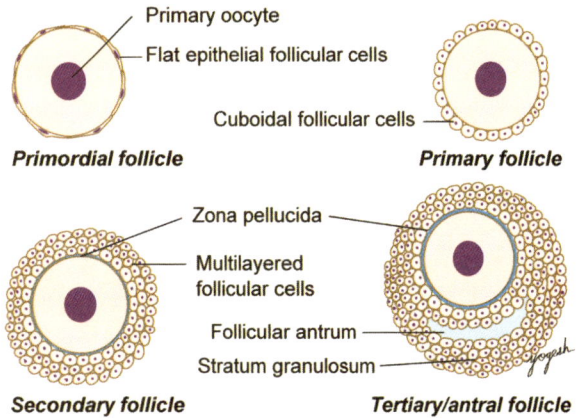

Practice Fig. 3.3: Developing ovarian follicles

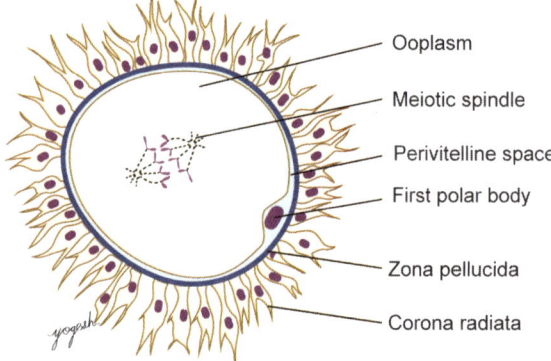

Practice Fig. 3.5: Structure of ovum

Oogenesis is a process of formation of a mature ovum from primordial germ cells.

Ovulation is a process of release of ovum from Graafian follicle. It takes place 14 days prior to onset of next menstrual bleeding.

Zona pellucida: It is a glycoprotein coat that surrounds vitelline membrane. It prevents implantation.

Chapter 4
First Week of Development

Fertilization is the process of fusion of two mature germ cells, an ovum and a spermatozoon (haploid cells) to form a single cell, zygote (diploid cell).

- *Stages of fertilization*:
  1. Approximation of gametes
  2. Contact and fusion of gametes
  3. Consequences or effects of fertilization.

Lifespan: After ejaculation, sperms are viable for 24–48 hours in female reproductive tract (maximum up to 4 days). Ovum is viable for 24–48 hours after ovulation.

Cleavage is a process of repeated mitotic segmentation of zygote within zona pellucida to give rise to small cells called blastomeres.

Implantation is a process of penetration of product of conceptus (blastocyst) into the uterine endometrium. Usually, implantation occurs in the upper part of body of the uterus in mid-sagittal plane, mostly, it happens on the posterior uterine wall (55%) or anterior uterine wall (45%).

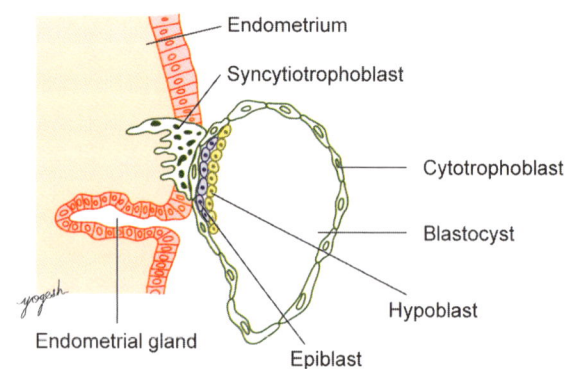

Practice Fig. 4.4: Implantation

Draw well-labelled diagrams of: 1. Structure of sperm, 2. Graafian follicle, 3. Developing ovarian follicles, 4. Structure of ovum

Flowchart 4.3: Process of fertilization

Sexual intercourse → Oxytocin release
↓
Uterine contractions
↓ 2–7 hours   Ovum
Aspiration of gametes ← Uterine tube contractions
↓ Chemotaxis
Sperms attracted towards ovum
↓
Contact and fusion of gametes
↓
Release of acrosomal enzymes
↓
Disintegration of zona pellucida and corona radiata
↓
Fusion of sperm with vitelline membrane
↓
Induction of calcium wave
↓
Vitelline block → Prevention of polyspermy
↓
Nuclear fusion
↓
Formation of zygote

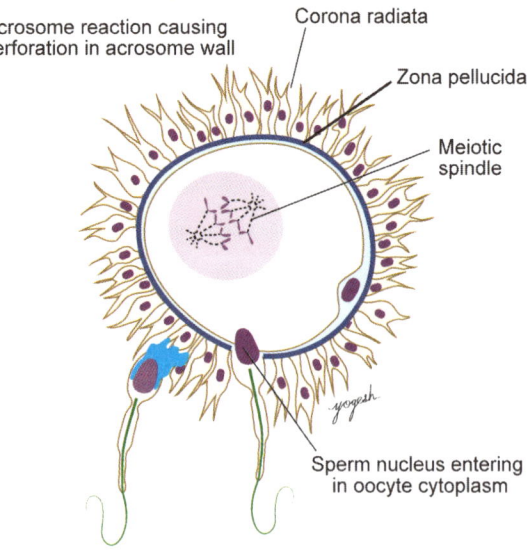

Practice Fig. 4.1: Fertilization

Flowchart 4.5: Cleavage and formation of morula

Cleavage
– Repeated mitotic segmentation of zygote → blastomeres
– Lasts for 6–7 days after fertilization

Diploid zygote
1st cleavage ↓ 30 hours after fertilization
2-cell stage
2nd cleavage ↓ 40–50 hours after fertilization
4-cell stage
3rd cleavage
Compaction ↓ 72 hours after fertilization
8-cell stage
4th cleavage ↓ 96 hours after fertilization
16-cell stage (morula)
↓   ↓
Inner embryoblast   Outer trophoblast
↓   ↓
Embryo   Placenta

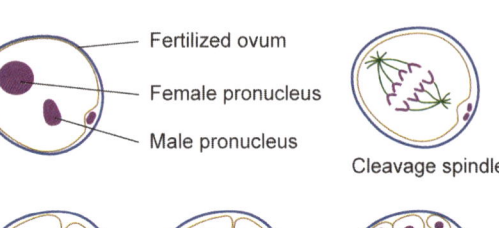

Practice Fig. 4.2: Cleavage and formation of morula

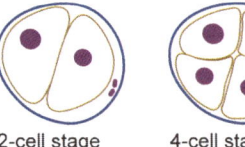

Flowchart 4.7: Process of implantation

Fertilization
↓ by 6th day
Zona pellucida disappears
↓ Diffusion of uterine fluid
Hatching of blastocyst
↓
Trophoblast attaches with endometrium
↓
Release of proteolytic enzymes
↓
Erosion of endometrium
↓
Blastocyst burrows within endometrium
↓ by 9th day
Formation of fibrin plug
↓
Closure of penetration defect

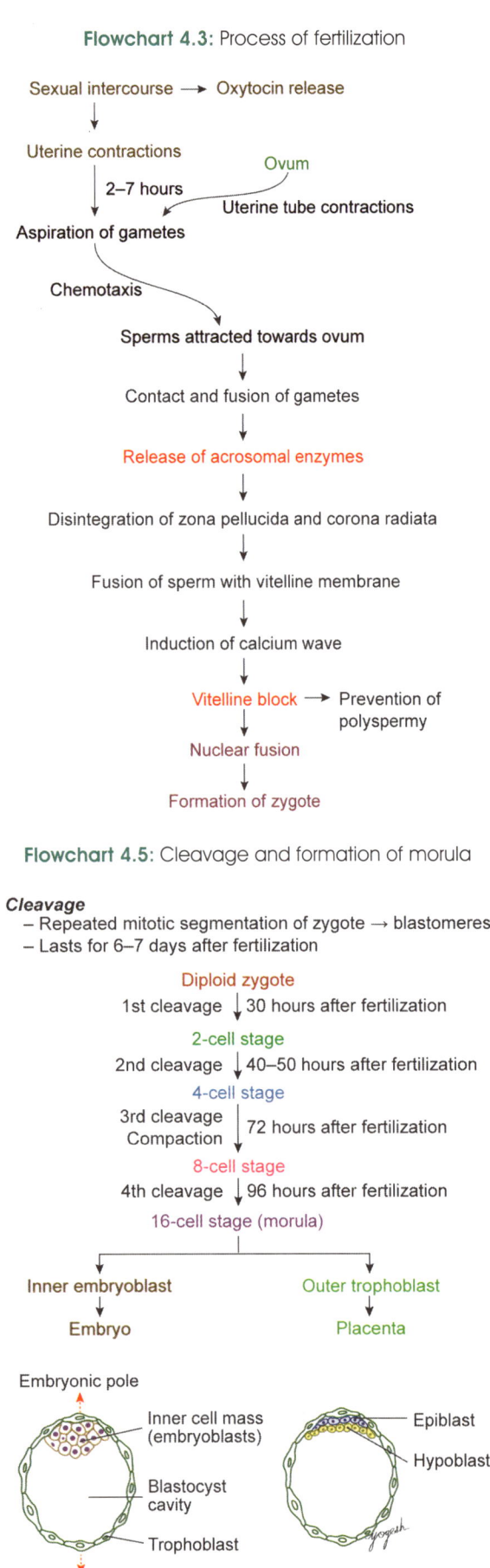

Practice Fig. 4.3: Blastocyst

Draw well-labelled diagrams of: 1. Fertilization, 2. Cleavage and formation of morula, 3. Blastocyst

Chapter 5
Assisted Reproduction Technology

In vitro fertilization is a process of fertilizing ovum outside the body.

Intracytoplasmic sperm injection (ICSI) is a procedure that involves a direct transfer of a single sperm into cytoplasm of oocyte.

Artificial insemination is the deliberate introduction of sperm into uterus or cervix by means other than sexual intercourse. It is of two types: Intrauterine insemination (IUI), and intracervical insemination (ICI).

Flowchart 5.1: Stages of *in vitro* fertilization

Stage 1: Ovarian stimulation
Injectable GnRH, FSH, LH
↓
Stage 2: Oocyte retrieval
hCG → induction of ovulation
USG guided aspiration
↓
Stage 3: In vitro fertilization
↓
Stage 4: Development of embryo
Fertilized ovum is incubated at 37°C till the stage of blastocyst
↓
Stage 5: Transfer of embryo
Embryo transfer through vaginal route using a catheter
↓
Stage 6: Luteal phase support
Injectable progesterone to maintain pregnancy

Chapter 6
Second Week of Development: Bilaminar Germ Disc

Flowchart 6.1: Trophoblastic changes in the second week

Day 8
Differentiation of trophoblast
– outer syncytiotrophoblast
– inner cytotrophoblast
↓
Day 9–10
Closure of penetration defect
↓
Formation of multinucleated trophoblastic mass
↓
Appearance of lacunar spaces in trophoblast
↓
Day 11–12
Enlargement and fusion of lacunar spaces
↓
Formation of syncytiotrophoblastic trabeculae
↓
Erosion of maternal vessels
↓
Filling of lacunar spaces with maternal blood
↓
Establishment of uteroplacental circulation
↓
Day 13–14
Formation of syncytiotrophoblastic villi
↓
Cytotrophoblastic invasion in villi
↓
Formation of primary stem villi

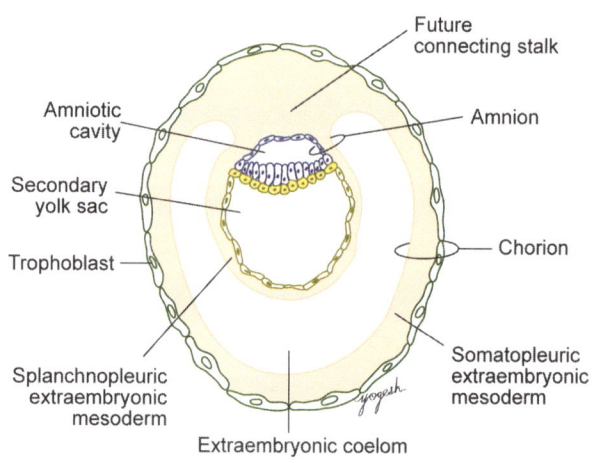

Practice Fig. 6.2: Formation of extraembryonic mesoderm, extraembryonic coelom, amnion and chorion

Draw well-labelled diagrams of formation of extraembryonic mesoderm, extraembryonic coelom, amnion and chorion.

Chorion: Trophoblast and somatopleuric layer of extraembryonic mesoderm together form the chorion and blastocystic cavity called the chorionic cavity.

Prechordal plate: Hypoblast cells become columnar in a small area near cranial end of germ disc (head end). This small circular area is called prechordal plate (also called prochordal plate).

Decidua: Stratum compactum sheds off during childbirth; hence, it is called decidua. Part of decidua that lies deep to blastocyst is decidua basalis, thus trophoblast invades only decidua basalis.

Genomic imprinting is a phenomenon that involves expression of a gene depending on its maternal or paternal origin.

Flowchart 6.2: Changes in embryoblasts in the second week

Day 8 — Differentiation of embryoblasts
– hypoblast
– epiblast
↓
Formation of amniotic cavity
↓
Formation of bilaminar germ disc

Day 9–10 — Formation of Heuser's membrane
↓
Blastocoel cavity → Primary yolk sac

Day 11–12 — Formation of extraembryonic mesoderm
↓
Formation of extraembryonic coelom
↓
Formation of connecting stalk
↓
Differentiation of embryoblasts
– Somatopleuric layer
– Splanchnopleuric layer
↓
Formation of chorion

Day 13–14 — Formation of secondary yolk sac
↓
Formation of prechordal plate

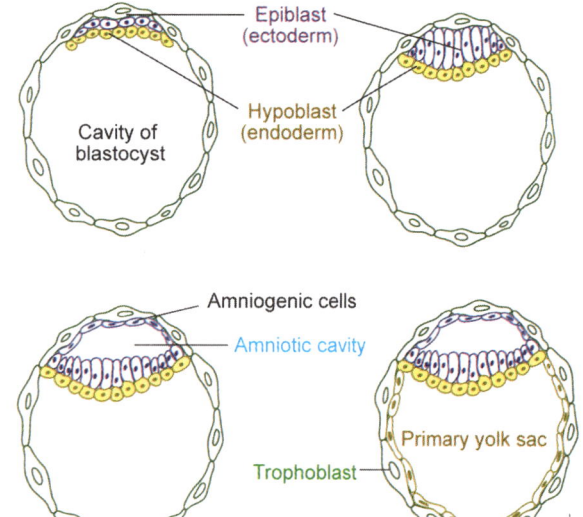

Practice Fig. 6.1: Formation of ectoderm, endoderm, amniotic cavity and primary yolk sac

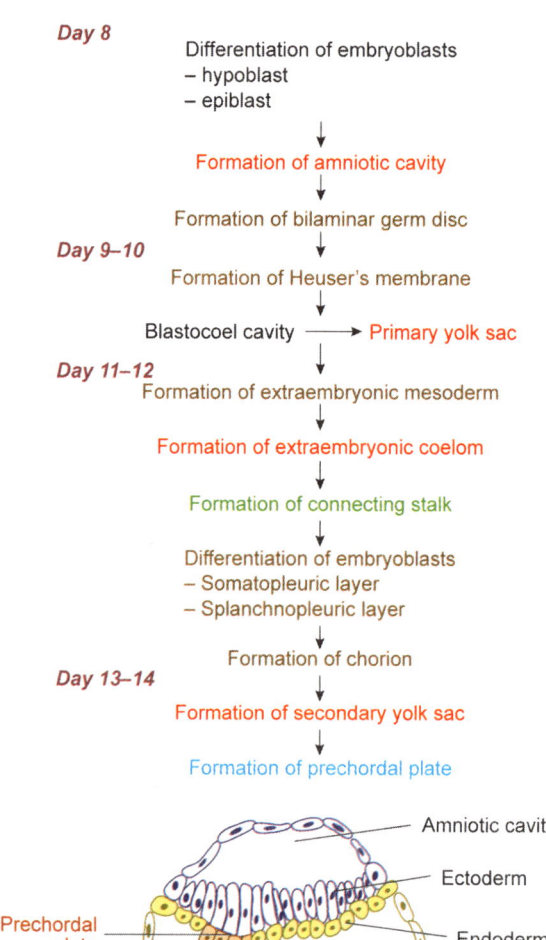

Practice Fig. 6.3: Formation of prechordal plate

Chapter 7
Third Week of Development: Trilaminar Germ Disc

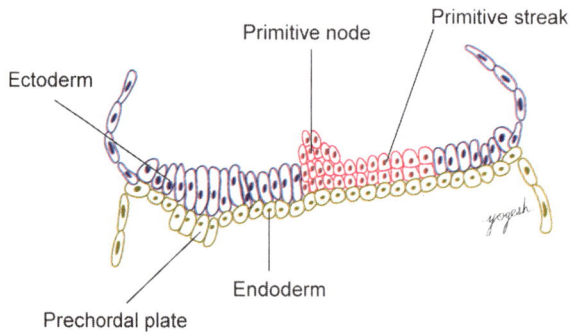

Practice Fig. 7.2: Bilaminar germ disc showing primitive node and primitive streak (longitudinal section)

Draw well-labelled diagrams of: 1. Formation of ectoderm, endoderm, amniotic cavity and primary yolk sac, 2. Formation of prechordal plate, 3. Bilaminar germ disc showing primitive node and primitive streak (longitudinal section).

Flowchart 7.1: Process of gastrulation.

Gastrulation = Bilaminar germ disc → trilaminar germ disc

Day 15: Primitive streak
↓
Formation of Hensen's node with blastopore and primitive groove
↓
Migration and invagination of epiblast cells
↓
Formation of
1. Embryonic definitive endoderm
2. Intraembryonic mesoderm
3. Definitive ectoderm

Bilaminar regions of trilaminar germ disc
↓
Germ disc area devoid of mesodermal cells
├── At cranial end → Buccopharyngeal membrane (break down in 4th week)
└── At caudal end → Cloacal membrane (break down in 7th week)

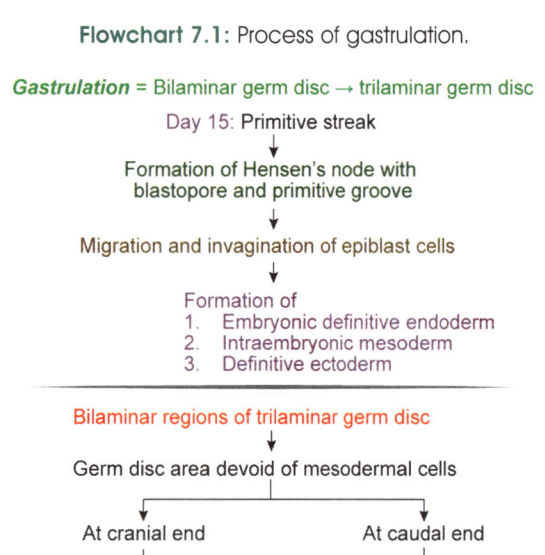

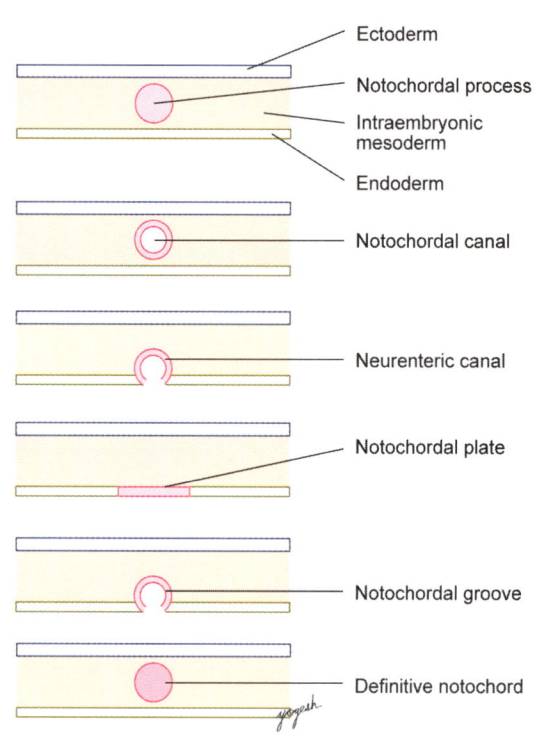

Practice Fig. 7.4: Formation of notochord

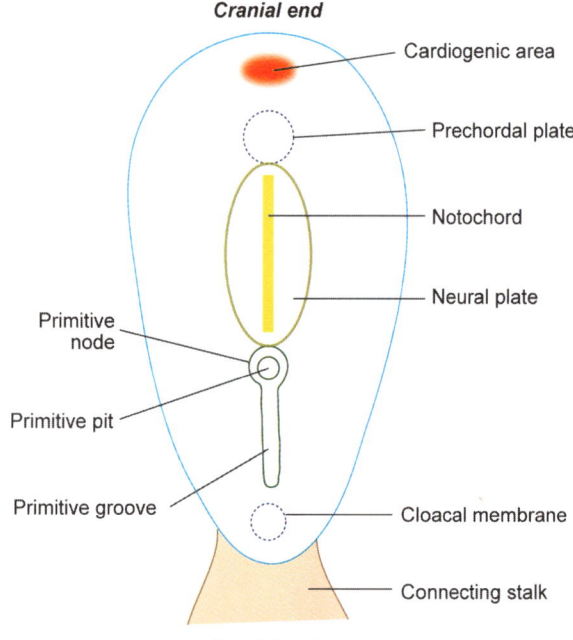

Practice Fig. 7.1: Germ disc showing notochord, primitive pit, primitive knot, primitive groove and cloacal membrane

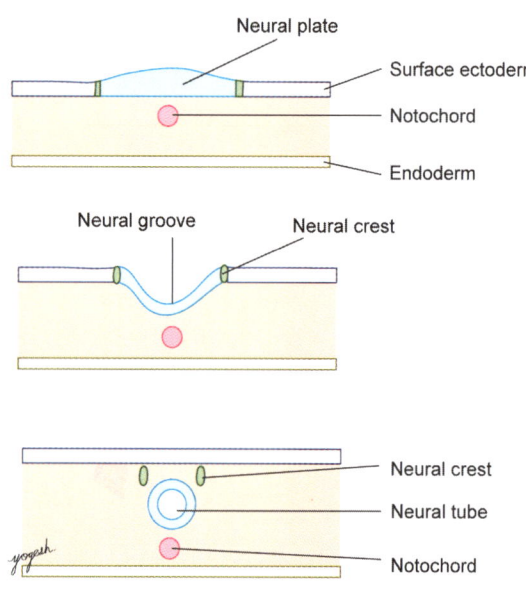

Practice Fig. 7.6: Formation of neural plate and neural crest

Chapter 8
Further Development of Embryo

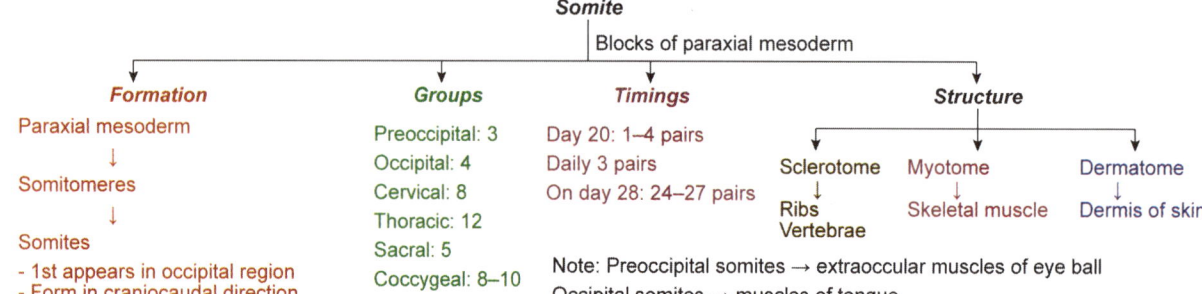

Flowchart 8.1: Somite

Somite — Blocks of paraxial mesoderm

Formation
Paraxial mesoderm
↓
Somitomeres
↓
Somites
- 1st appears in occipital region
- Form in craniocaudal direction

Groups
Preoccipital: 3
Occipital: 4
Cervical: 8
Thoracic: 12
Sacral: 5
Coccygeal: 8–10

Timings
Day 20: 1–4 pairs
Daily 3 pairs
On day 28: 24–27 pairs

Structure
Sclerotome → Ribs, Vertebrae
Myotome → Skeletal muscle
Dermatome → Dermis of skin

Note: Preoccipital somites → extraocular muscles of eye ball
Occipital somites → muscles of tongue

Draw well-labelled diagrams of: 1. Germ disc showing notochord, primitive pit, primitive knot, primitive groove and cloacal membrane, 2. Formation of notochord, 3. Formation of neural plate and neural crest.

Somite: From prechordal plate to primitive streak, the paraxial mesoderm undergoes condensation to form somitomeres. Later, somitomeres undergo segmentation to form somites. A somite is differentiated into three parts: Sclerotome, myotome, and dermatome.

Neuropores: Cranial open end of neural tube called anterior neuropore, closes by the 25th day of IUL (18–20 somite age). Caudal open end of neural tube called posterior neuropore, closes by the 27th day (25 somite age).

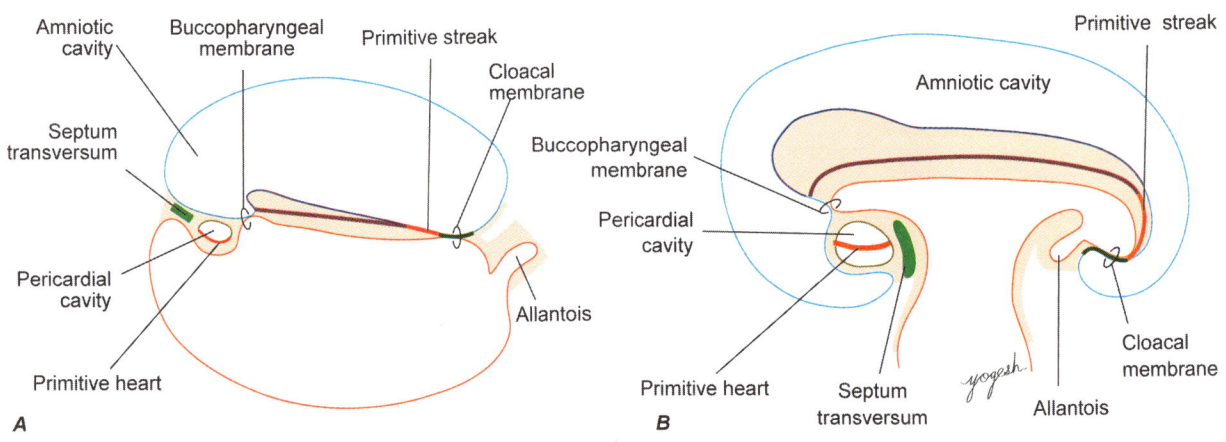

Practice Fig. 8.1: Head and tail folds of embryo

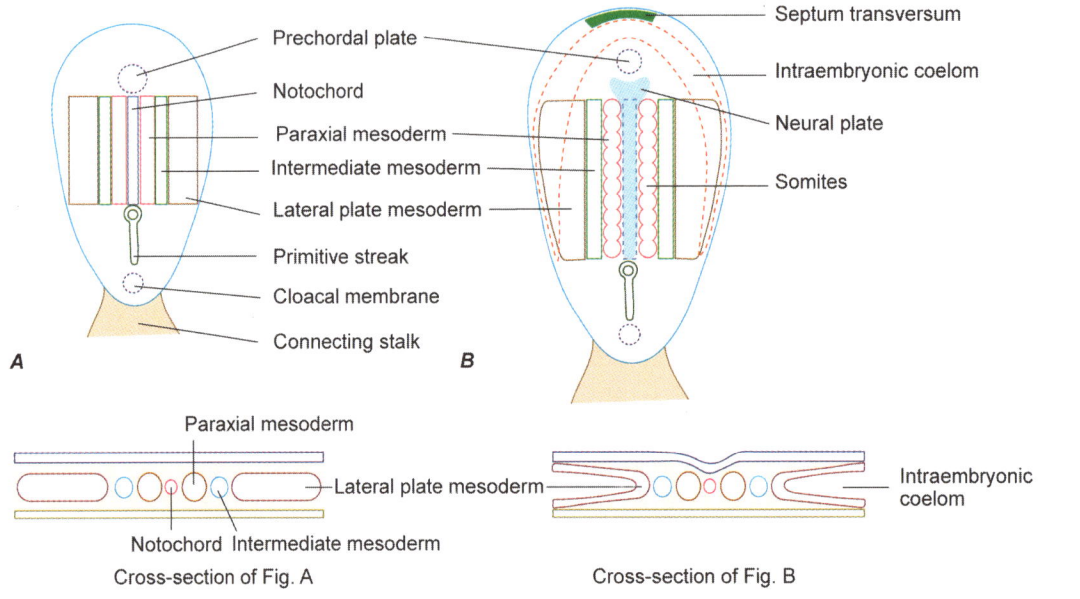

Practice Fig. 8.3: Subdivisions of intraembryonic mesoderm, intraembryonic coelom and somites

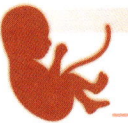

Chapter

9

Placenta and Umbilical Cord

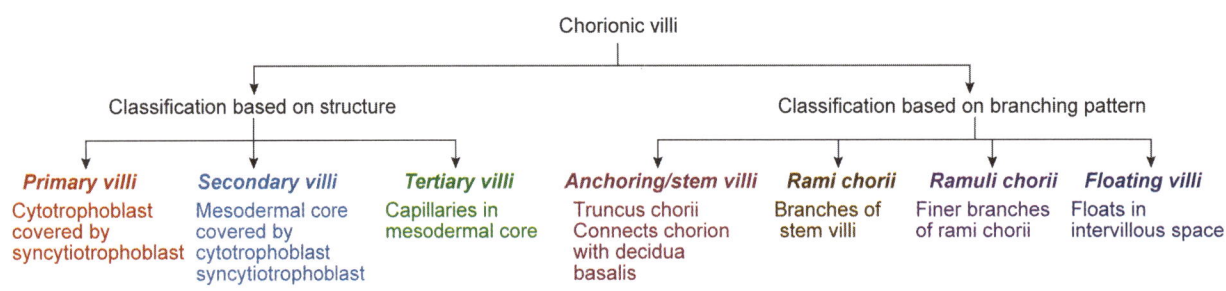

Draw well-labelled diagrams of: 1. Head and tail folds of embryo, 2. Subdivisions of intraembryonic mesoderm, intraembryonic coelom and somites.

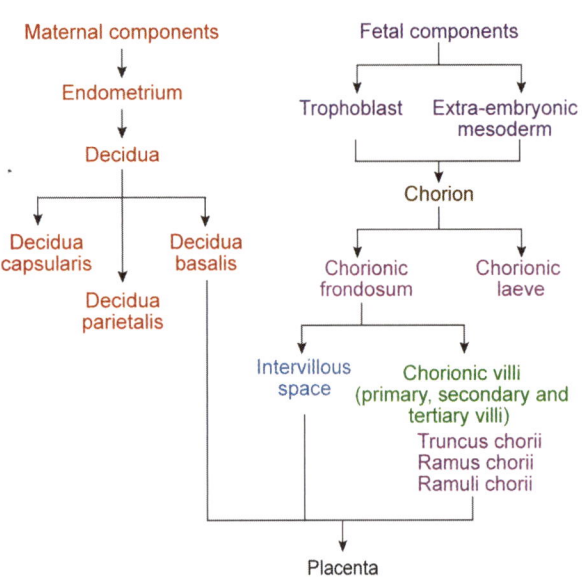

Flowchart 9.1: Structure of the placenta

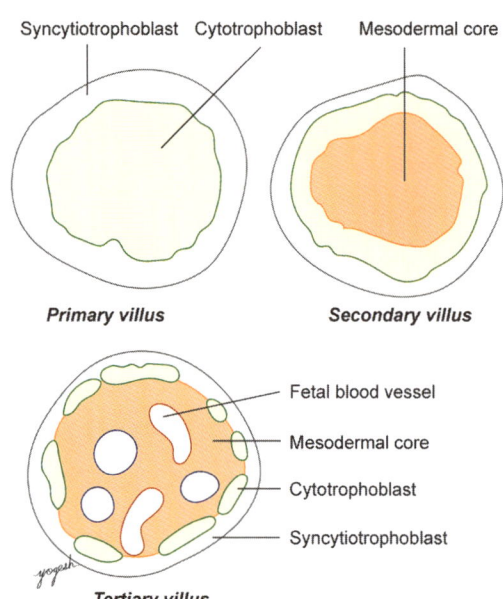

Practice Fig. 9.3: Placental villi

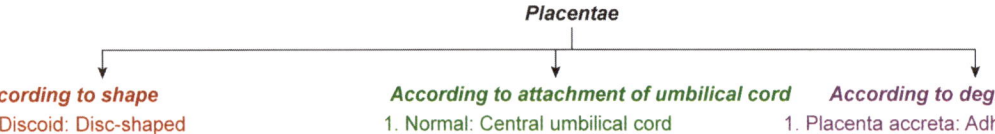

Flowchart 9.4: Classification of placentae

Placentae

According to shape
1. Discoid: Disc-shaped
2. Bidiscoid: Two discs
3. Lobed: Two or more lobes
4. Placenta succenturiata: Accessory lobe
5. Placenta membranacea: Diffuse
6. Circumvallate: Circular fold covering peripheral edge

According to attachment of umbilical cord
1. Normal: Central umbilical cord
2. Battledore placenta: Umbilical cord attached to margin
3. Velamentous: Umbilical cord attached to fetal membranes

According to degree of adhesion
1. Placenta accreta: Adhered with decidua basalis
2. Placenta increta: Penetrates myometrium
3. Placenta percreta: Penetrates uterine wall

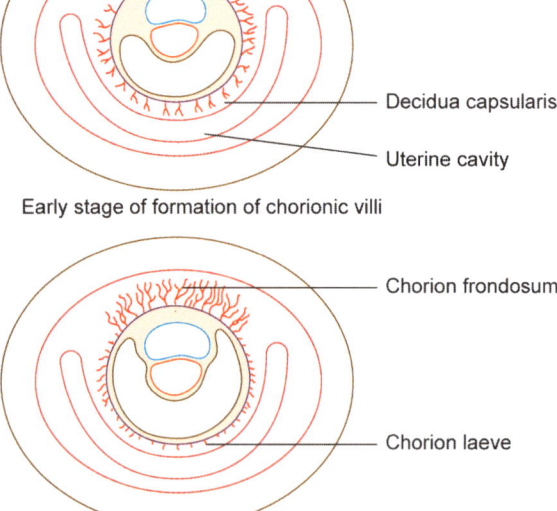

Decidua = Endometrium during pregnancy

Practice Fig. 9.1: Zones of decidua

Practice Fig. 9.4: Subdivisions of decidua, interstitial implantation

Placenta is an organ that performs exchange of nutrients and gases between mother and fetus. Thus, the placenta is a fetomaternal organ.

Uterine endometrium during pregnancy is called decidua. The cellular and vascular changes in the decidua during pregnancy are called decidual reaction.

Chorion: The syncytiotrophoblast, cytotrophoblast and extraembryonic mesoderm together form chorion.

Draw well-labelled diagrams of: 1. Placental villi, 2. Zones of decidua, 3. Subdivisions of decidua, interstitial implantation.

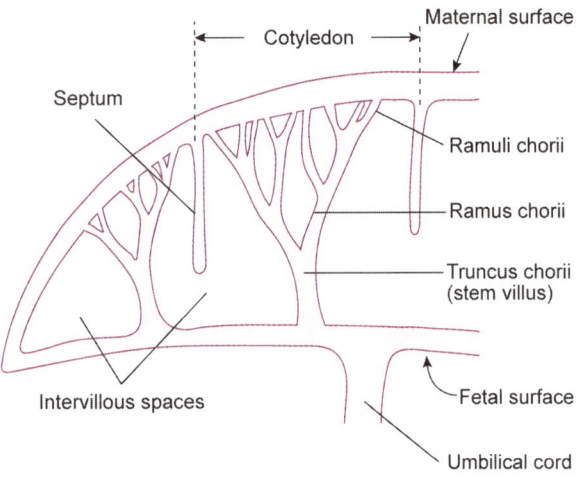

Practice Fig. 9.5: Arrangement of villi

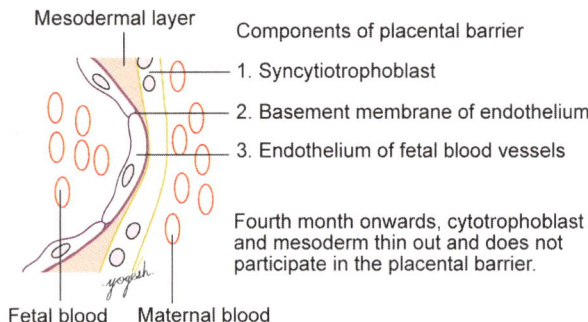

Practice Fig. 9.6: Placental barrier

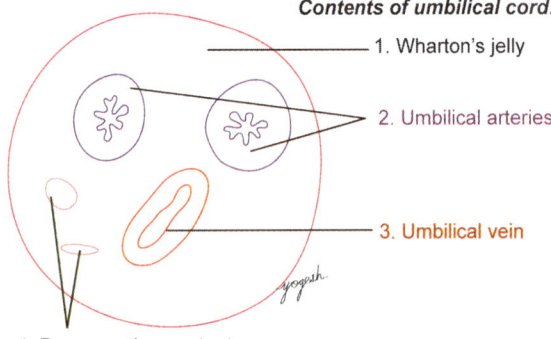

Practice Fig. 9.7: Structure of the umbilical cord

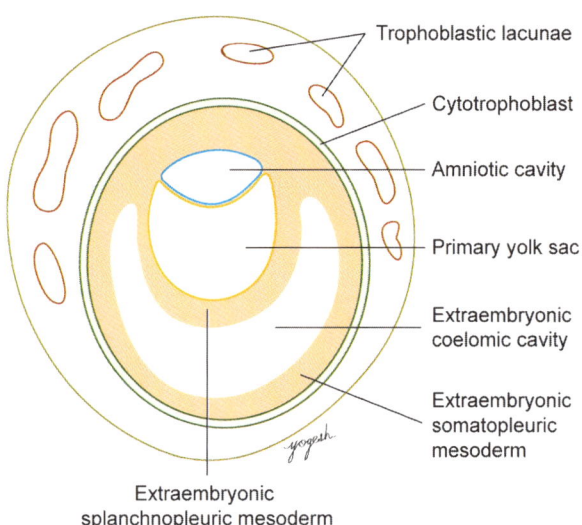

Practice Fig. 9.8: Yolk sac, amniotic cavity and extraembryonic coelomic cavity

Chapter 10
Integumentary System: Skin, its Appendages, and Mammary Gland

Flowchart 10.1: Development of skin

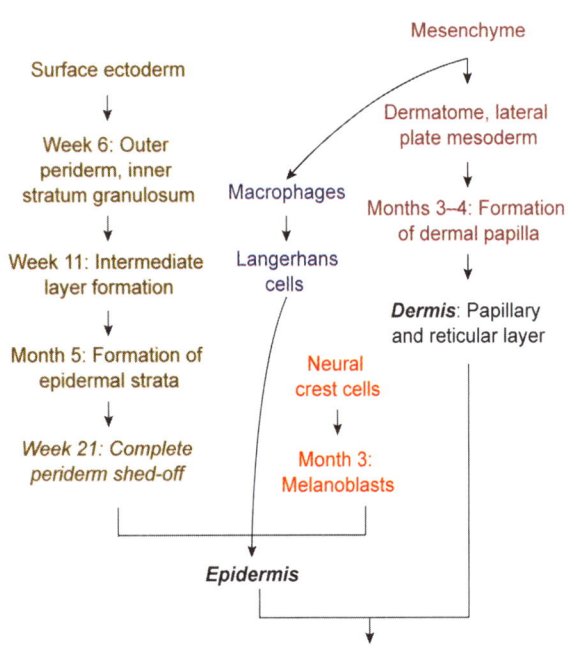

Flowchart 10.2: Development of hair

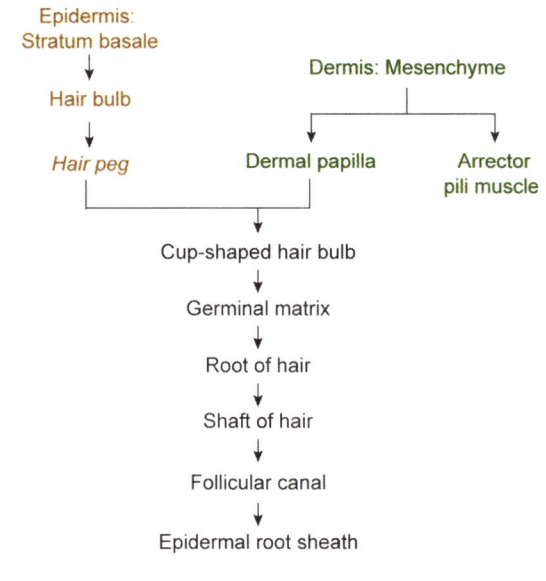

Draw well-labelled diagrams of: 1. Arrangement of villi, 2. Placental barrier, 3. Yolk sac, amniotic cavity and extraembryonic coelomic cavity.

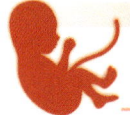

Chapter 11
Pharyngeal Apparatus

Pharyngeal arches: Thickened mesodermal bars present in the floor and lateral wall of the primitive pharynx are called pharyngeal arches.

Pharyngeal clefts: Depressions (grooves) on the surface ectoderm in between adjacent arches are called pharyngeal clefts.

Pharyngeal pouches: Endodermal depressions between adjacent pharyngeal arches in the floor and lateral wall of the primitive pharynx are called pharyngeal pouches.

Branchial cyst is a congenital cyst in the skin of the lateral part of the neck.

Caudal pharyngeal complex: It is formed by fusion of ventral part of the fourth pouch with a rudimentary fifth pouch. It shows three components: Thymic element (incorporated in developing thymus), lateral thyroid element (forms thyroid gland) and ultimobranchial body (forms parafollicular or C-cells of the thyroid gland).

In the floor of the primitive pharynx, over the first arch in the midline, there is a swelling called tuberculum impar. By the 24th day, just behind tuberculum impar, pharyngeal epithelium forms a depression (diverticulum) called thyroglossal duct.

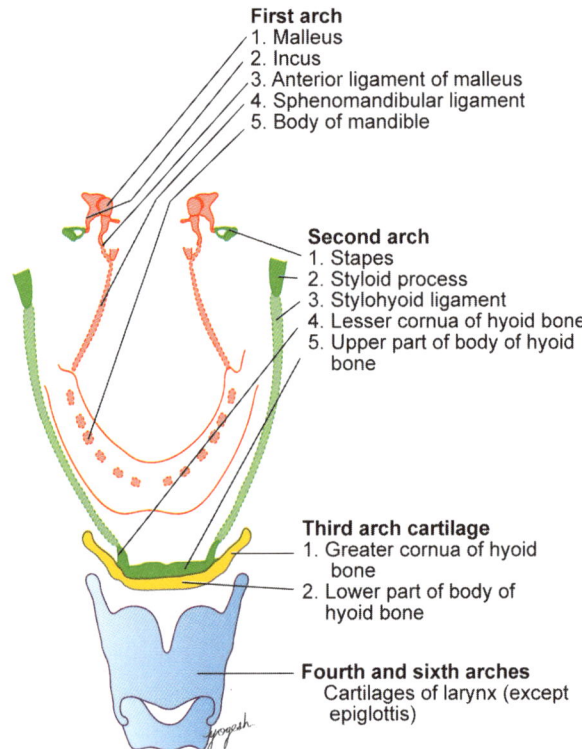

Practice Fig. 11.1: Structures derived from cartilages of the pharyngeal arches

Flowchart 11.4: Derivatives of 1st arch

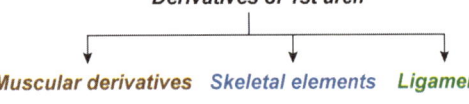

Muscular derivatives
Muscles of mastication
 Temporal
 Masseter
 Medial pterygoid
 Lateral pterygoid
Tensor veli palatini
Tensor tympani
Anterior belly of digastric
Mylohyoid

Skeletal elements
Incus
Malleus
Premaxilla
Zygomatic bone
Temporal bone

Nerves of first arch
Pretrematic: Chorda tympani
Posttrematic: Mandibular

Ligaments
Anterior ligaments of malleus
Sphenomandibular ligament

Flowchart 11.6: Third pharyngeal arch

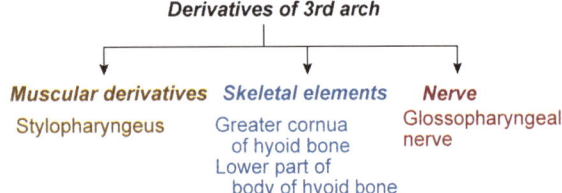

Muscular derivatives
Stylopharyngeus

Skeletal elements
Greater cornua of hyoid bone
Lower part of body of hyoid bone

Nerve
Glossopharyngeal nerve

Flowchart 11.7: Fourth and sixth arches

	Fourth arch	Sixth arch
Muscles	Cricothyroid Constrictors of pharynx Muscles of palate except tensor veli palatini	Intrinsic muscles of larynx except cricothyroid
Nerve	Superior laryngeal nerve	Recurrent laryngeal nerve
Skeletal elements	——— Laryngeal cartilages except epiglottis ———	

Note: Epiglottis is derived from hypobranchial eminence.

Flowchart 11.5: Second pharyngeal arch

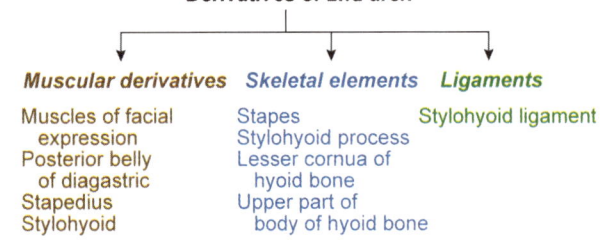

Muscular derivatives
Muscles of facial expression
Posterior belly of digastric
Stapedius
Stylohyoid

Skeletal elements
Stapes
Stylohyoid process
Lesser cornua of hyoid bone
Upper part of body of hyoid bone

Ligaments
Stylohyoid ligament

Nerves of second arch: Facial nerve

Flowchart 11.10: Development of the palatine tonsil

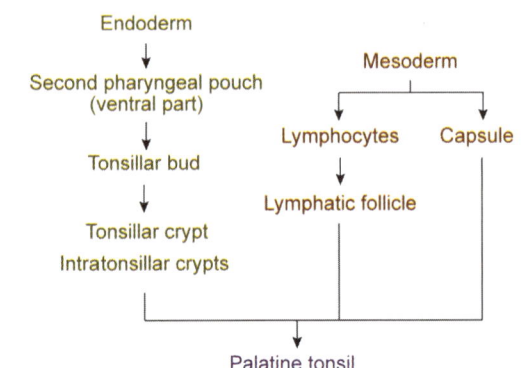

Draw a well-labelled diagram of structures derived from cartilages of the pharyngeal arches.

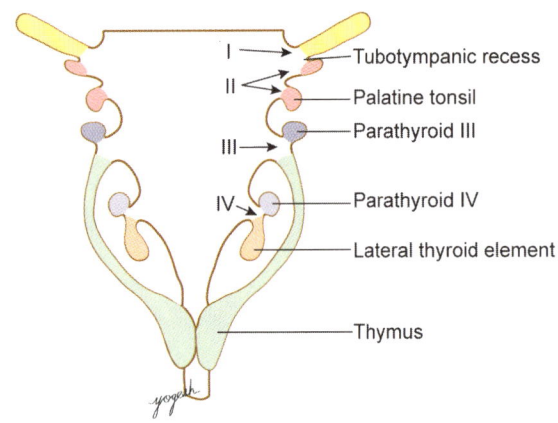

Practice Fig. 11.2: Derivatives of the pharyngeal pouches

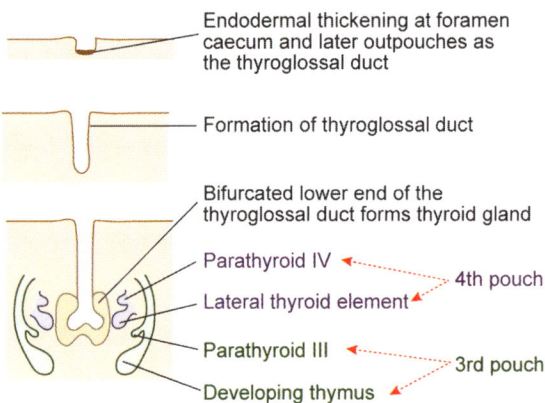

Practice Fig. 11.3: Development of thyroid gland

Chapter 12
Alimentary Tract I: Development of Face, Nose, Palate

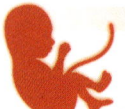

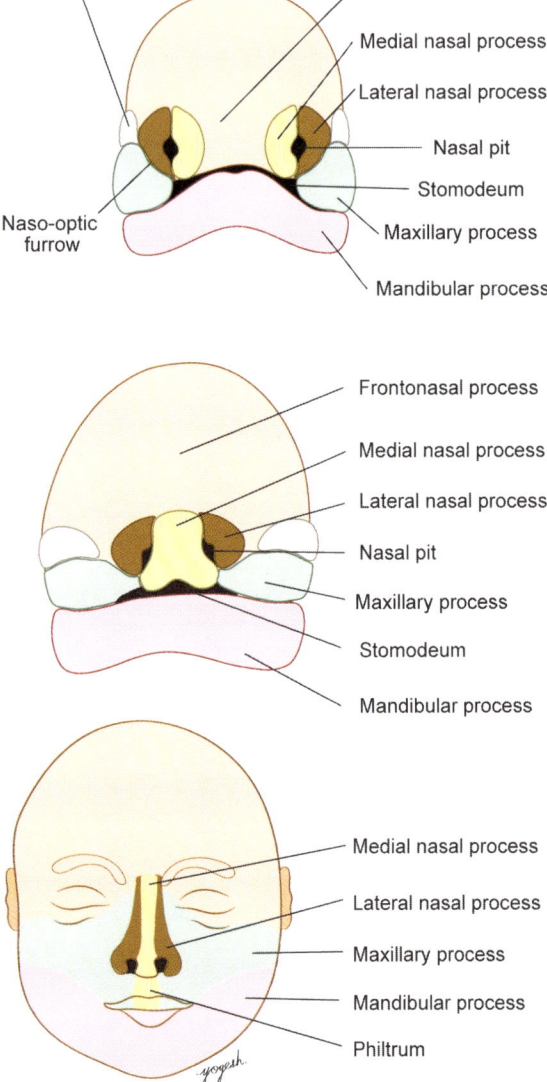

Practice Fig. 12.1: Development of the face

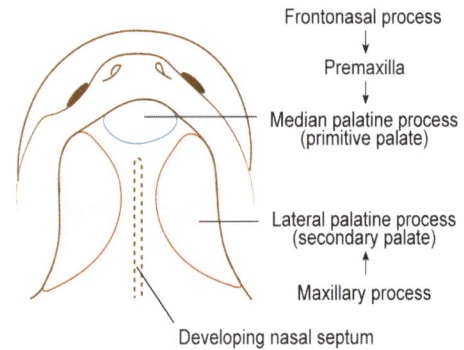

Practice Fig. 12.2: Development of palate

Flowchart 12.3: Cleft palate

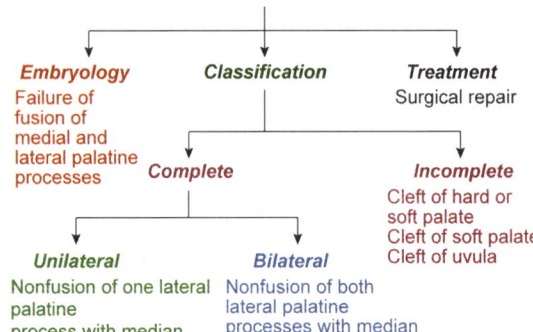

Draw well-labelled diagrams of: 1. Derivatives of the pharyngeal pouches, 2. Development of thyroid gland, 3. Development of the face, 4. Development of palate.

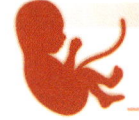

Chapter 13
Alimentary Tract II: Development of Teeth, Pharynx, Tongue and Salivary Glands

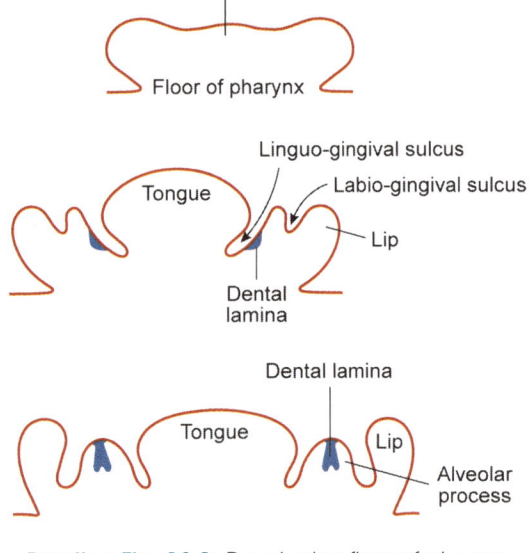

Practice Fig. 13.1: Developing floor of pharynx

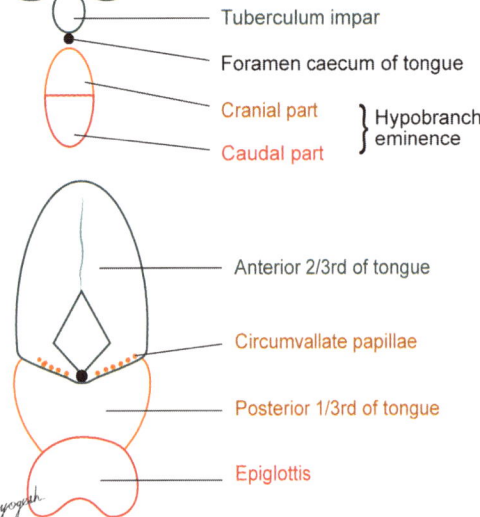

Practice Fig. 13.4: Development of tongue

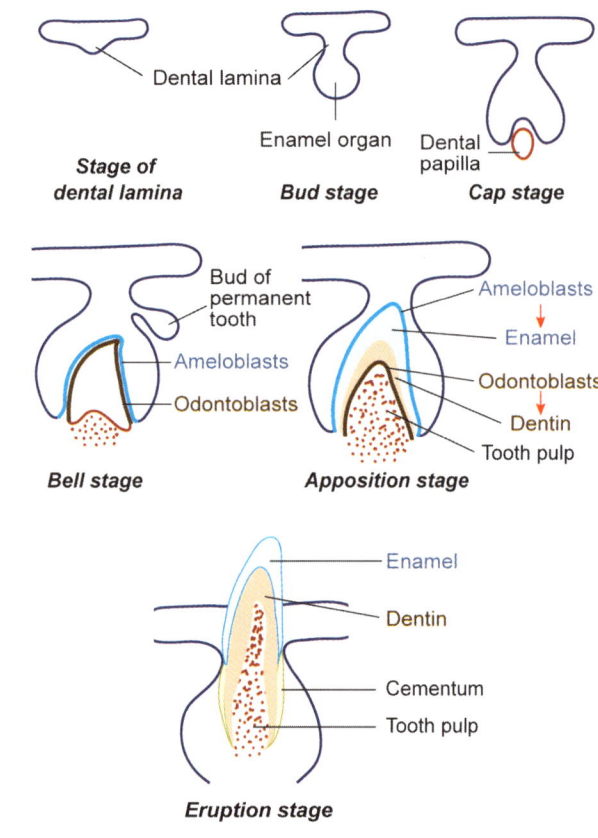

Practice Fig. 13.3: Development of tooth

Anodontia: Anodontia is a complete absence of teeth.

Amelogenesis imperfecta is a condition due to hypocalcification of enamel in vitamin D deficiency (rickets). The enamel becomes soft, friable and yellowish–brown in color.

Humans are diphyodont (having only two successive sets of teeth).

Tongue tie or ankyloglossia occurs due to incomplete formation of alveolo-lingual sulcus. The tongue is connected with a floor of mouth by short frenulum.

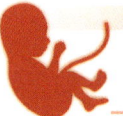

Chapter 14
Alimentary Tract III: Development of Intestine

Cranial part of the gut that lies in the head fold is foregut. Caudal part of gut that lies in the tail fold is hindgut. The part of gut that communicates with vitellointestinal duct is midgut.

Achalasia cardia or cardiospasm: Loss of the anglionic cells in Auerbach's plexus of the esophageal wall results in a failure of muscle relaxation in lower part of the esophagus.

Midgut undergoes 270° counterclockwise rotation.

Physiological umbilical hernia is the protrusion of midgut loop (herniation) outside the abdominal cavity through umbilical opening from 6th week to 12th week of intrauterine life.

Meckel's diverticulum is the persistent proximal part of vitellointestinal duct.

Meconium is the earliest stool of newborn.

Imperforate anus is the noncommunication of the distal part of gut with exterior. It may be due to failure of rupture of anal membrane.

Draw well-labelled diagrams of: 1. Developing floor of pharynx, 2. Development of tooth, 3. Development of tongue.

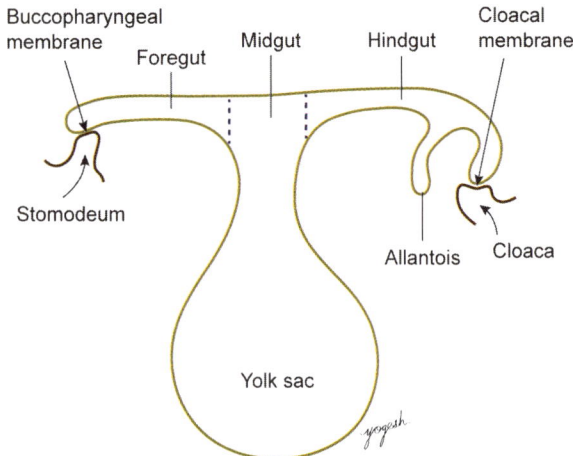

Practice Fig. 14.1: Parts of primitive gut

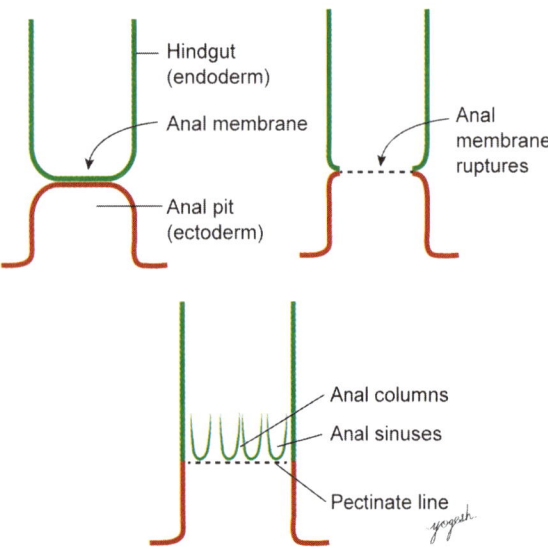

Practice Fig. 14.7: Development of anal canal

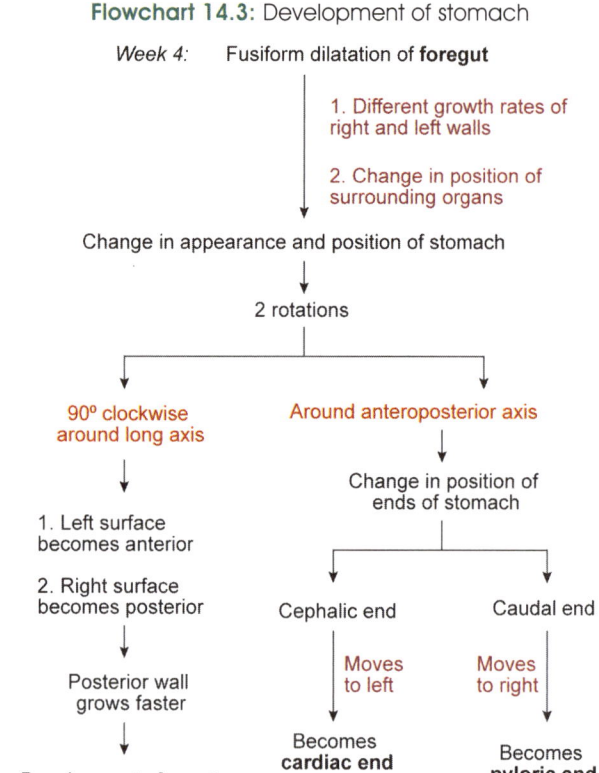

Flowchart 14.3: Development of stomach

Flowchart 14.5: Development of duodenum

Stages of development
- Rotation of stomach
- Shift duodenum to the right
- Mesoduodenum
- Zygosis
- Retroperitoneal duodenum

Blood supply
- Foregut: Proximal to opening of CBD: Celiac trunk
- Midgut: Distal to opening of CBD: Superior mesenteric art

Anomalies
- Duodenal stenosis – partial occlusion
- Duodenal atresia – complete occlusion
- Duodenal diverticula

CBD = Common bile duct

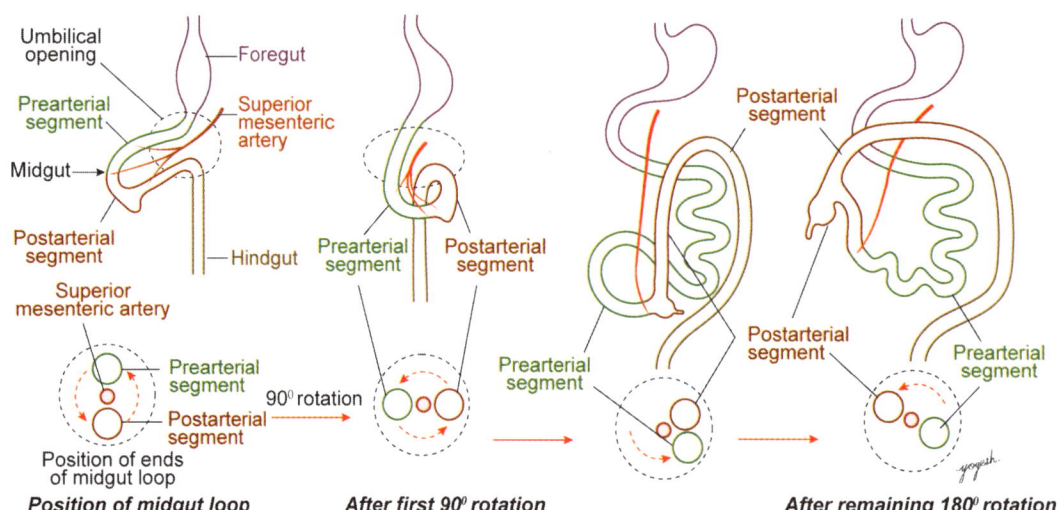

Practice Fig. 14.4: Rotation of gut

Draw well-labelled diagrams of: 1. Parts of primitive gut, 2. Development of anal canal, 3. Rotation of gut.

Chapter 15
Alimentary Tract IV: Development of Liver, Gallbladder, Pancreas and Spleen

Septum transversum (mesoderm) forms connective tissue of liver including fibrous capsule, Kupffer's cells, and blood vessels.

Riedel's lobe: It is a downward tongue-like extension of the right lobe of the liver.

Caroli's disease: It involves congenital cystic dilatation (ectasia) of intrahepatic biliary tree.

Annular pancreas is a congenital anomaly where second part of duodenum is surrounded by a ring of pancreatic tissue.

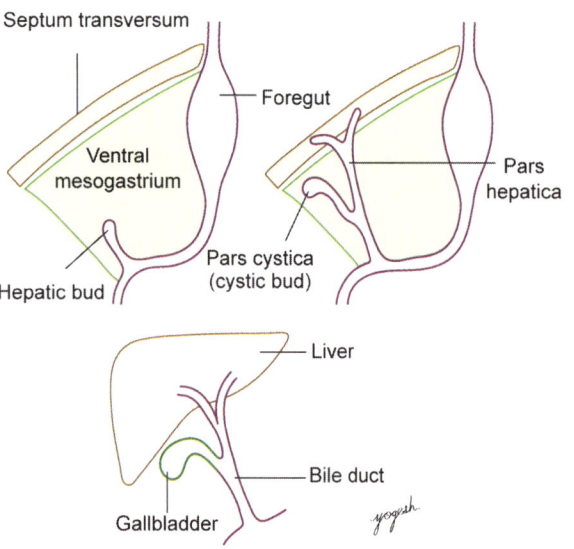

Practice Fig. 15.1: Development of liver and gallbladder

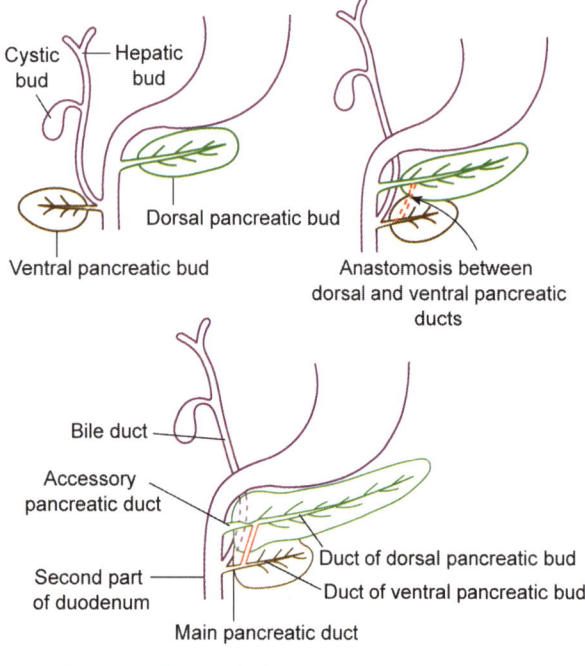

Practice Fig. 15.2: Development of pancreas

Flowchart 15.1: Development of liver

Distal end of foregut → outpouching → Liver bud

Hepatic bud:
- Rapid proliferation of cells
- Penetration of cells into septum transversum
- Epithelial cords of liver + Vitelline and umbilical veins
- Liver sinusoids
- Bulging of developing liver
- Division of ventral mesogastrium
  1. Lesser omentum
  2. Falciform ligament

1. Common bile duct
2. Right and left hepatic ducts

Cystic bud:
1. Cystic duct
2. Gallbladder

Flowchart 15.2: Development of pancreas

A. Parenchyma

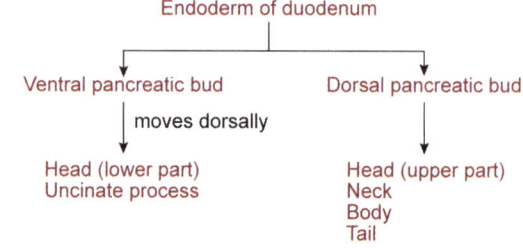

B. Islets of Langerhans

3rd week: Formation of Islets

Seventh week: Alpha-cells start secreting glucagon
Tenth week: Beta-cells start secreting insulin

C. Pancreatic ducts

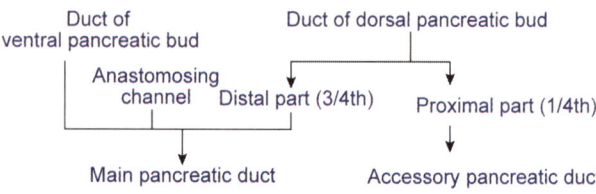

Draw well-labelled diagrams of: 1. Development of liver and gallbladder, 2. Development of pancreas.

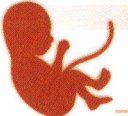

Chapter 16
Respiratory System

Maturation of lungs is divided into four phases or periods: Pseudoglandular period (6–16 weeks), canalicular period (16–26 weeks), terminal saccular period (26 weeks to birth), and alveolar period (32 weeks to 8 years).
Lung buds invaginate into pericardio-peritoneal canals that later form pleural cavities.
Tracheoesophageal fistula is an abnormal congenital communication between the trachea and esophagus.

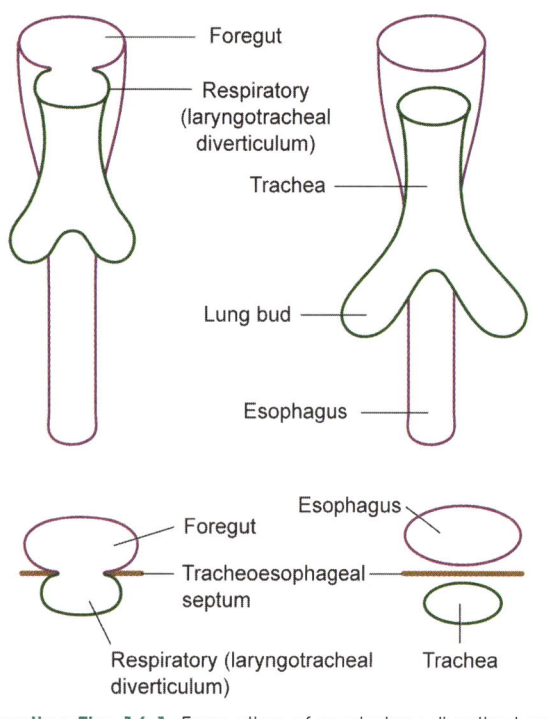

Practice Fig. 16.1: Formation of respiratory diverticulum

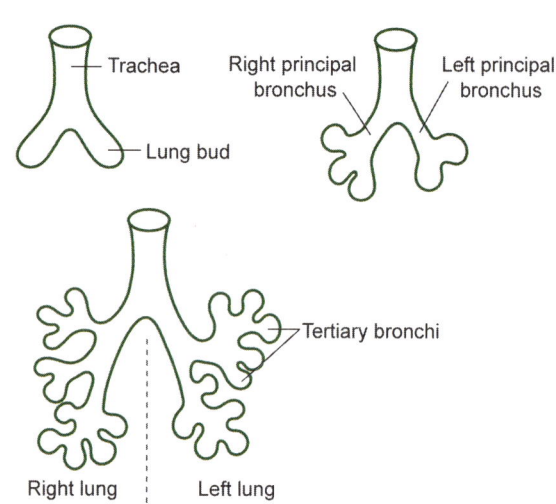

Practice Fig. 16.2: Development of lungs

Flowchart 16.3: Maturation of lung

6–16 weeks	Pseudoglandular stage	Lungs resemble exocrine glands
16–26 weeks	Canalicular period	Formation of respiratory bronchioles, alveolar ducts, primary alveoli
26–32 weeks	Terminal sac period	Thinning of blood–air barrier Increase in quantity of surfactant
32 weeks onwards	Alveolar period	Formation of definitive alveoli Increasing quantity of surfactant

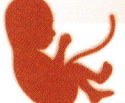

Chapter 17
Development of Body Cavities and Diaphragm

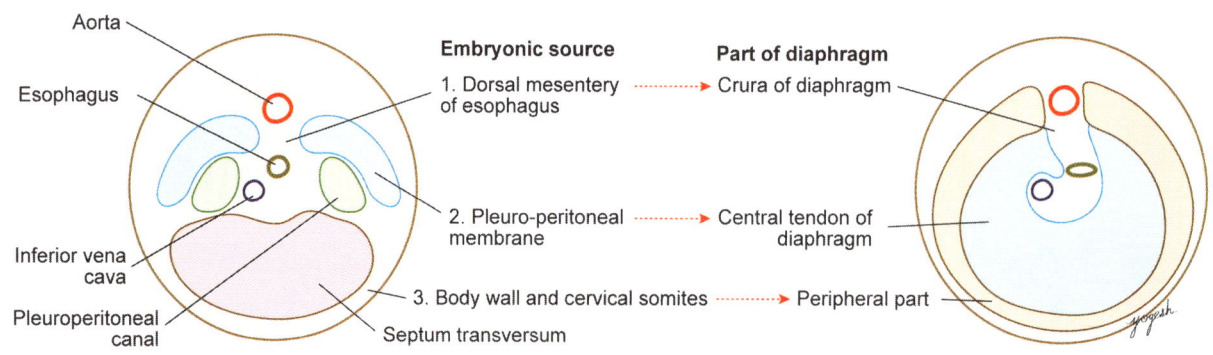

Practice Fig. 17.6: Development of diaphragm

Draw well-labelled diagrams of: 1. Formation of respiratory diverticulum, 2. Development of lungs, 3. Development of diaphragm.

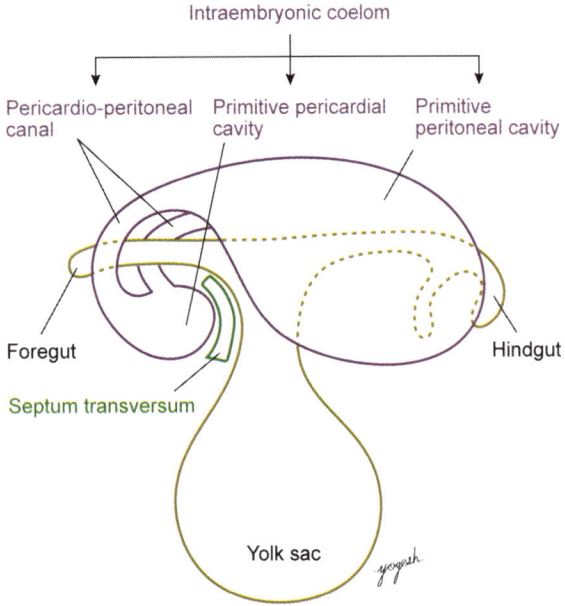

Practice Fig. 17.2: Relationship of intraembryonic coelom and gut tube

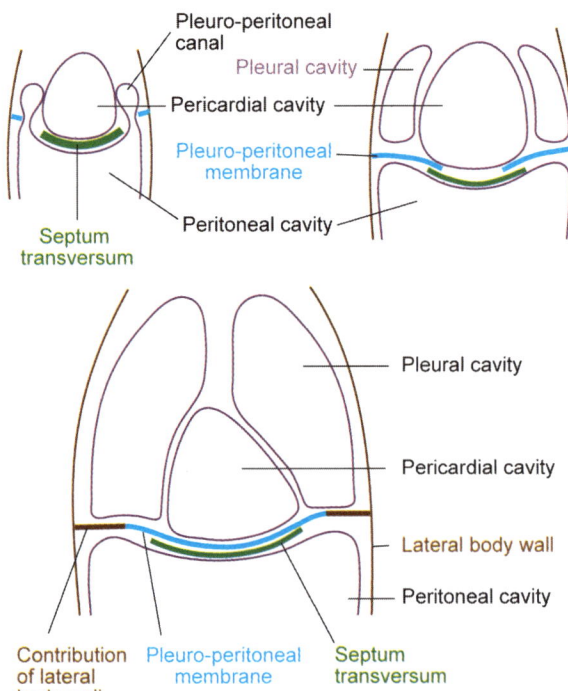

Note: Dorsal mesentery of esophagus also contributes to diaphragm.

Practice Fig. 17.4: Development of diaphragm and pleural cavity

Chapter 18
Cardiovascular System I: Development of Heart

Right atrium develops as follows: Rough trabeculated part of right atrium and right auricle from right half of primitive atrium, smooth part of right atrium (sinus venarum) from sinus venosus, crista terminalis, valve of inferior vena cava, and valve of coronary sinus develops from right venous valve, small area of most ventral smooth part develops from right half of atrioventricular canal.

Interatrial septum develops in 5th week of intrauterine life from septum primum and septum secundum.

Dextrocardia is a congenital condition in that heart points to right side rather than the usual left side.

Ventricular septal defect (VSD) is the most common congenital anomaly of the heart. VSDs are more common in males than in females. VSDs commonly involve the membranous part of interventricular septum.

Flowchart 18.6: Atrial septal defects (ASD)

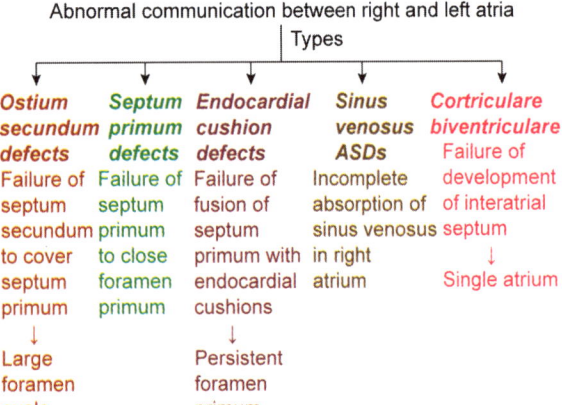

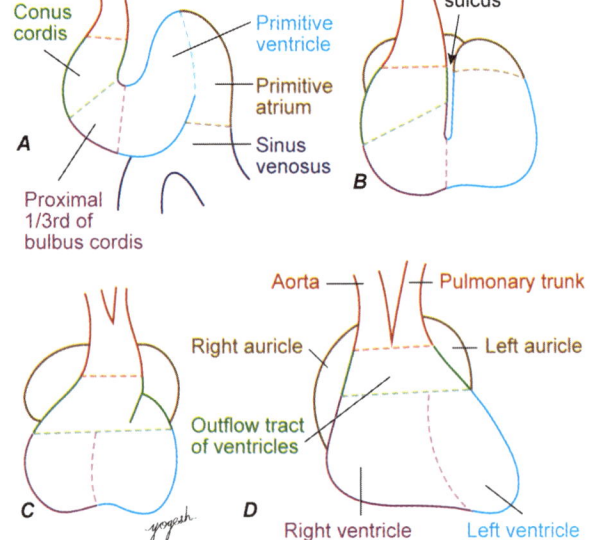

Practice Fig. 18.3: Establishment of external features of heart

Draw well-labelled diagrams of: 1. Relationship of intraembryonic coelom and gut tube, 2. Development of diaphragm and pleural cavity, 3. Establishment of external features of heart.

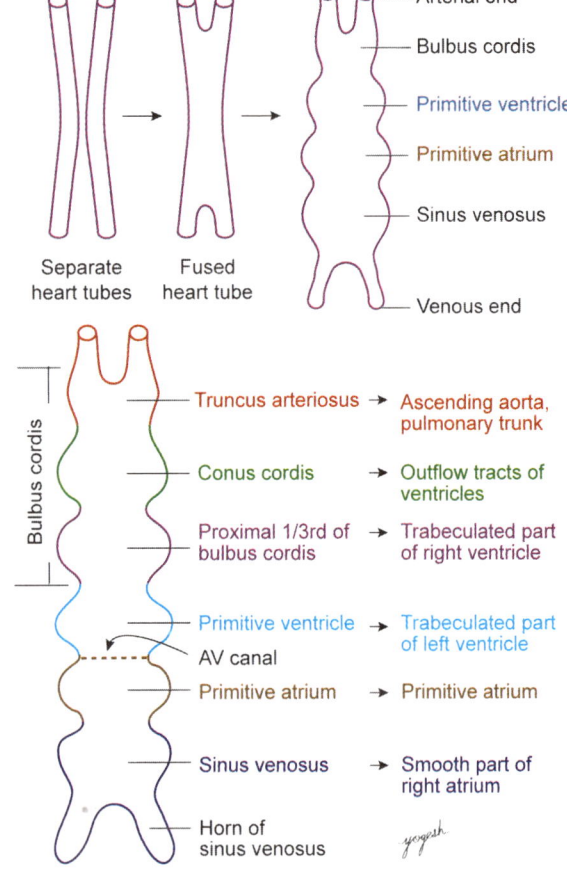

Practice Fig. 18.1: Parts of heart tube

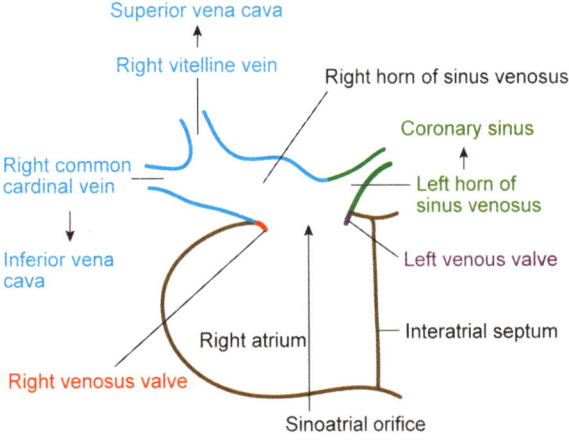

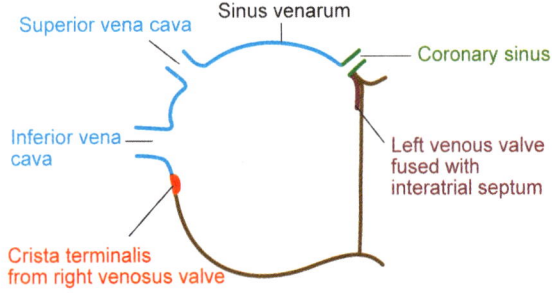

Practice Fig. 18.6: Absorption of sinus venosus into the right atrium

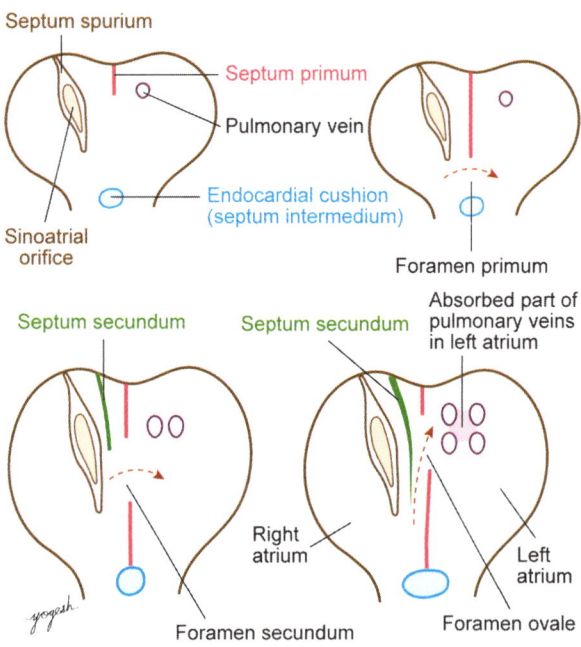

Practice Fig. 18.4: Development of interatrial septum

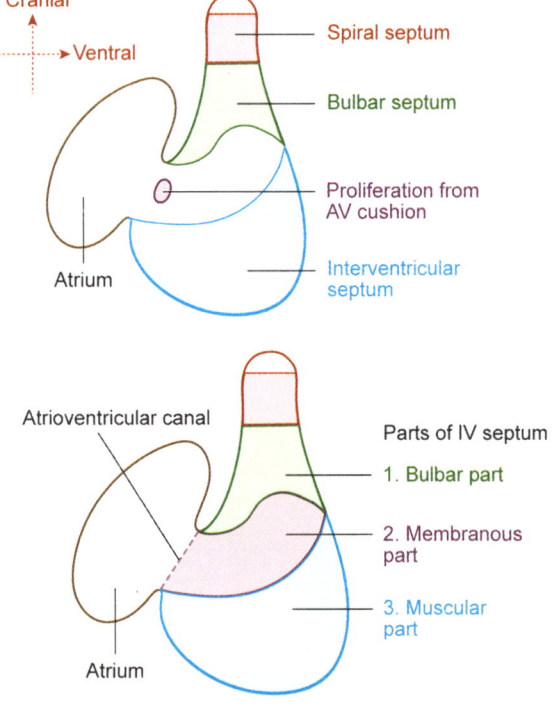

Practice Fig. 18.8: Development of interventricular septum

Flowchart 18.8: Fallot's tetralogy

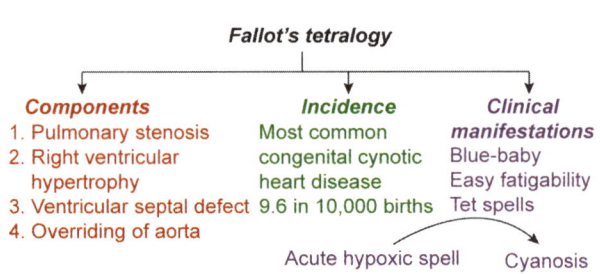

Draw well-labelled diagrams of: 1. Parts of heart tube, 2. Development of interatrial septum, 3. Absorption of sinus venosus into the right atrium, 4. Development of interventricular septum.

Chapter 19
Cardiovascular System II: Blood Vessels and Fetal Circulation

Initially, there are six pairs of aortic arch arteries. Later, fifth pair disappears along with fifth pharyngeal arch. First and second arch arteries mostly disappear leaving behind maxillary artery from first pharyngeal arch artery, and hyoid and stapedial arteries from second arch artery.

Flowchart 19.3: Patent ductus arteriosus

Patent ductus arteriosus
↓
Shunting of blood from aorta to pulmonary trunk
↓
Pulmonary hypertension

Normal closure	Incidence	Mechanism of closure
Physiological: Immediately after birth	8 in 10,000 births	First breathing ↓ Release of bradykinin from lungs ↓ Contraction of smooth muscles ↓ Closure of ductus arteriosus ↓ Ligamentum arteriosum
Anatomical: Within 3 months after birth		

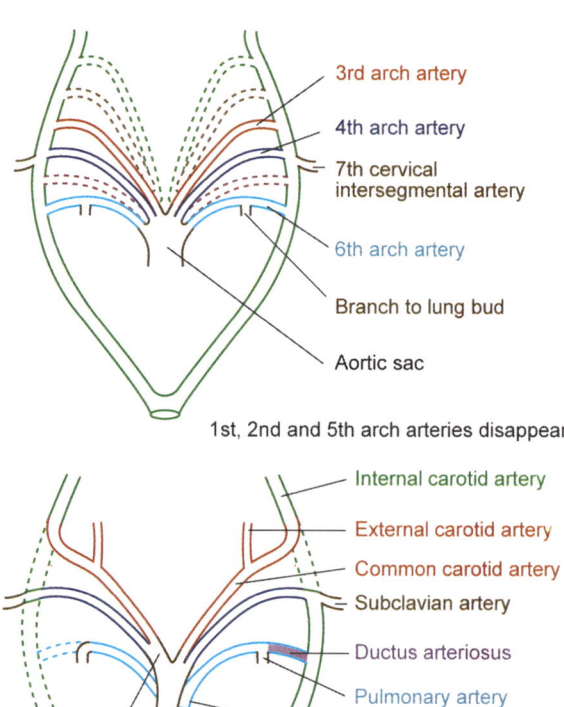

1st, 2nd and 5th arch arteries disappear

1st arch artery → Maxillary artery
2nd arch artery → Hyoid and stapedial arteries in fetal life

Practice Fig. 19.2: Fate of aortic arch arteries

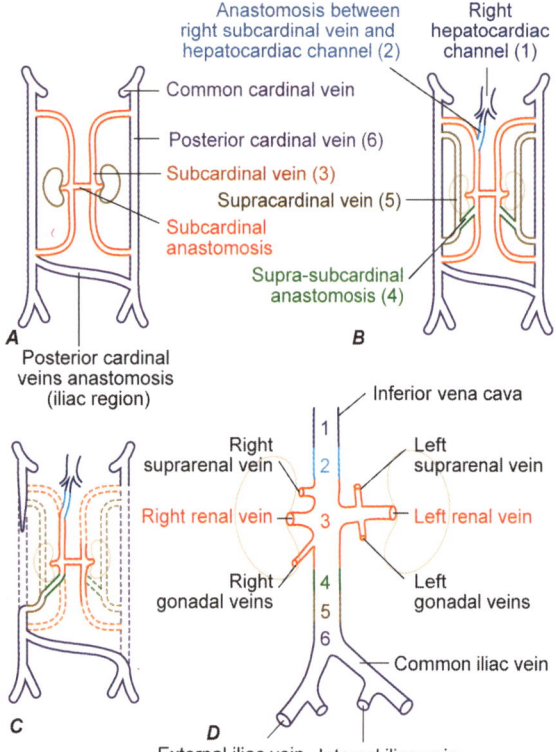

Practice Fig. 19.9: Development of inferior vena cava

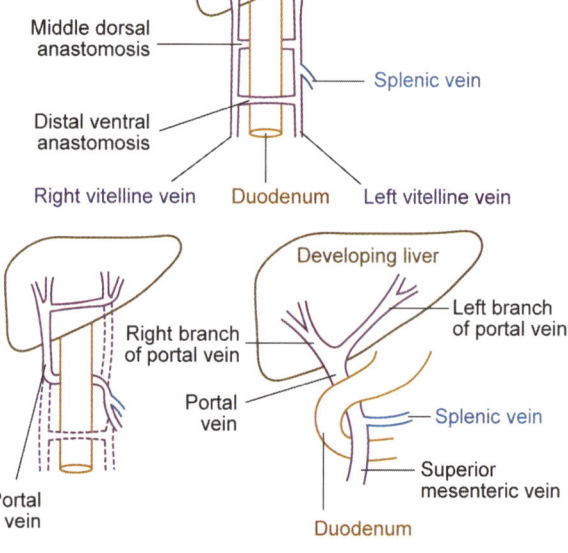

Practice Fig. 19.8: Development of portal vein

Table 19.8 Remnants of embryonic vessels [High yielding, NEXT]

Embryonic vessel	Remnant
Umbilical arteries	Superior vesical artery / Median umbilical ligament
Left umbilical vein	Ligamentum teres hepatis
Ductus venosus	Ligamentum venosum
Ductus arteriosus	Ligamentum arteriosum

Draw well-labelled diagrams of: 1. Fate of aortic arch arteries, 2. Development of portal vein, 3. Development of inferior vena cava.

Chapter 20
Urinary System: Kidney, Ureter, Urinary Bladder, Urethra

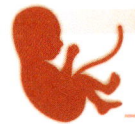

Urogenital ridge has two parts: Medial genital ridge and lateral nephrogenic cord. Nephrogenic cord extends from cervical to sacral segments of embryo.

Ureteric bud forms collecting part of kidney, whereas metanephric blastema forms secretory part.

Congenital polycystic kidney is failure to establish communication between secretory/excretory and collecting part of kidney. These cysts are filled with urine. Autosomal recessive polycystic kidney disease (ARPKD) (childhood) shows symptoms shortly after birth, whereas autosomal dominant polycystic kidney disease (ADPKD) (adult) is more common and develops in adulthood (30–40 years).

Ectopia vesicae is also called extrophy of urinary bladder that occurs due to failure of complete formation of lateral folds of embryo.

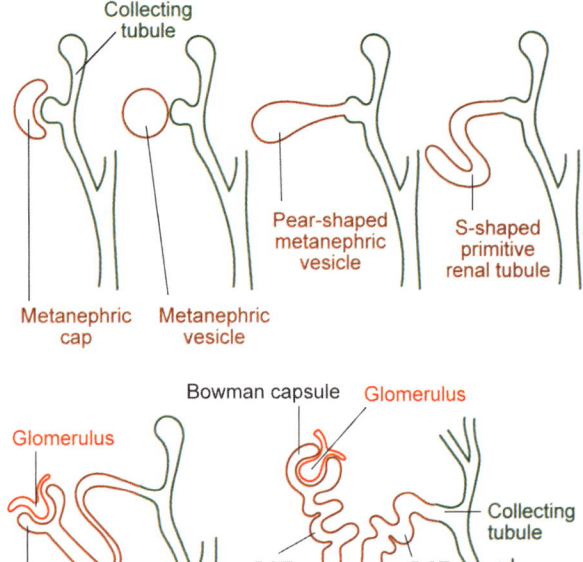

Practice Fig. 20.3: Development of nephron

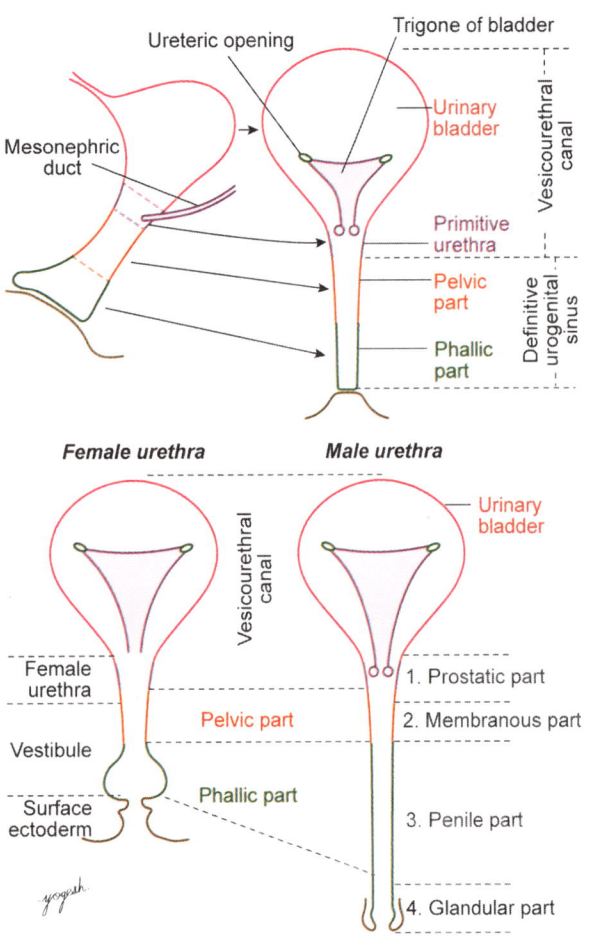

Practice Fig. 20.5: Development of urethra

- Y-chromosome determines testis formation as testis determining factor (TDF) is located on short arm of chromosome Y. TDF is controlled by SRY gene (sex determining region of Y chromosome). In the absence of TDF, cells of sex cords differentiate into follicular cells of ovary.

Flowchart 20.5: Development of kidney

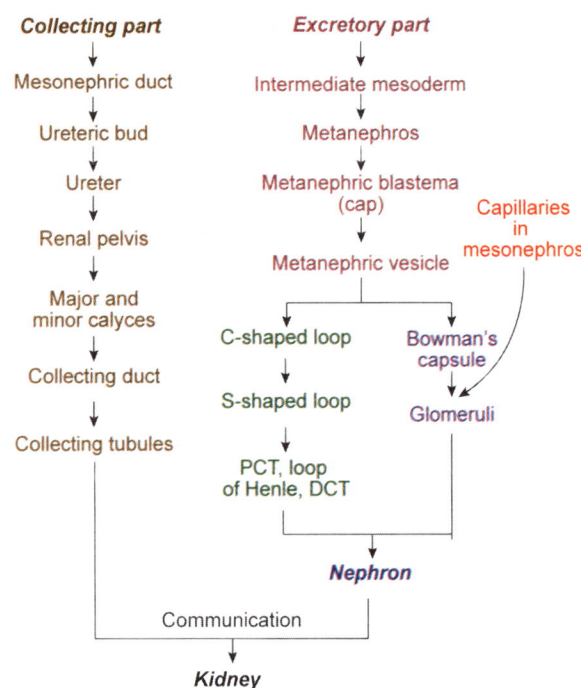

Draw well-labelled diagrams of: 1. Development of urethra, 2. Development of nephron.

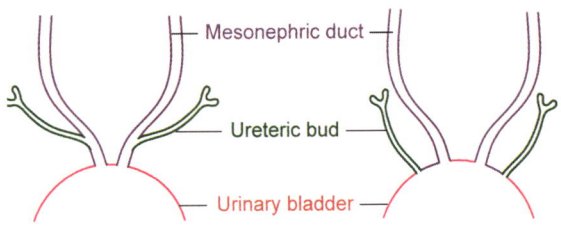

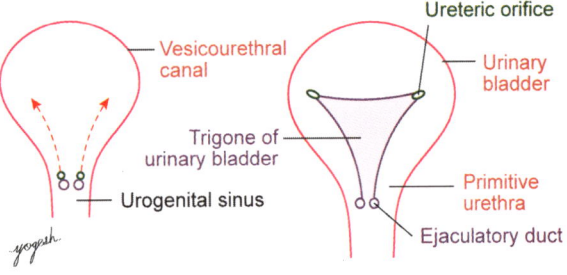

Practice Fig. 20.4: Development of urinary bladder

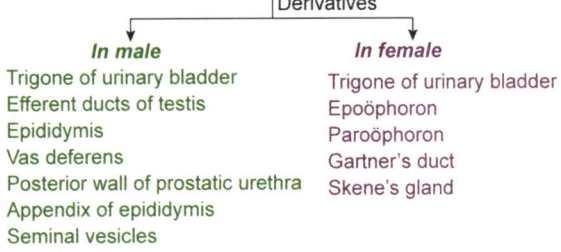

Flowchart 20.3: Mesonephric (Wolffian) duct

Mesonephric (Wolffian) duct
Paired ducts, develops in intermediate mesoderm
Derivatives

In male
Trigone of urinary bladder
Efferent ducts of testis
Epididymis
Vas deferens
Posterior wall of prostatic urethra
Appendix of epididymis
Seminal vesicles
Ejaculatory ducts

In female
Trigone of urinary bladder
Epoöphoron
Paroöphoron
Gartner's duct
Skene's gland

Flowchart 20.4: Paramesonephric duct

Paramesonephric duct
Paired duct develops in urogenital ridge
Fused part forms uterovaginal canal
Derivatives

In males
Appendix of testis
Prostatic utricle

In females
Uterine tubes
Uterus
Upper part of vagina

Chapter 21

Reproductive System: Male and Female Reproductive Organs

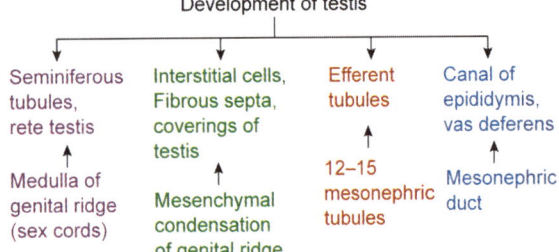

Flowchart 21.3: Development of testis

Development of testis
- Seminiferous tubules, rete testis ← Medulla of genital ridge (sex cords)
- Interstitial cells, Fibrous septa, coverings of testis ← Mesenchymal condensation of genital ridge
- Efferent tubules ← 12–15 mesonephric tubules
- Canal of epididymis, vas deferens ← Mesonephric duct

Remnant of paramesonephric duct → Appendix of testis
Remnant of mesonephros → Appendix of epididymis

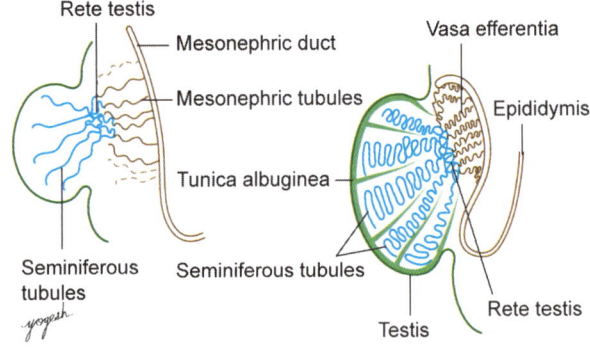

Practice Fig. 21.4: Development of testis

Cryptorchidism (undescended testis) is a failure of descent of testis that results in absence of one or both the testes from scrotum. In about 80% cases, testis descent during the first year of life.

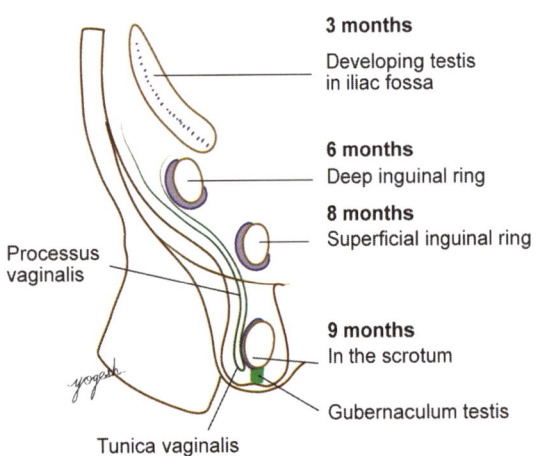

3 months — Developing testis in iliac fossa
6 months — Deep inguinal ring
8 months — Superficial inguinal ring
9 months — In the scrotum
Processus vaginalis
Gubernaculum testis
Tunica vaginalis

Practice Fig. 21.5: Descent of testis

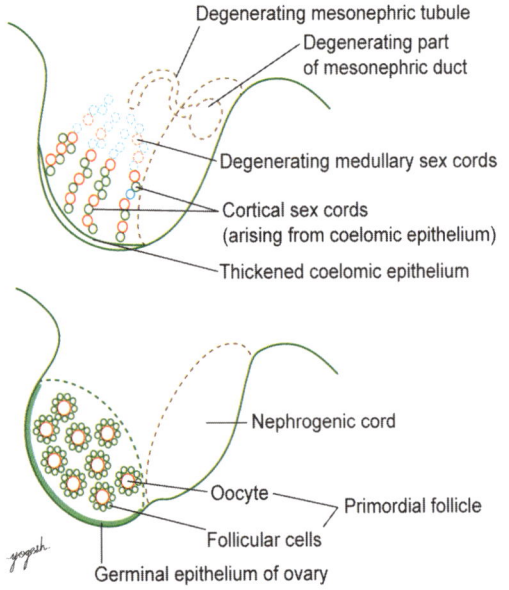

Degenerating mesonephric tubule
Degenerating part of mesonephric duct
Degenerating medullary sex cords
Cortical sex cords (arising from coelomic epithelium)
Thickened coelomic epithelium

Nephrogenic cord
Oocyte
Primordial follicle
Follicular cells
Germinal epithelium of ovary

Practice Fig. 21.6: Development of ovary

Draw well-labelled diagrams of: 1. Development of urinary bladder, 2. Development of testis, 3. Descent of testis, 4. Development of ovary.

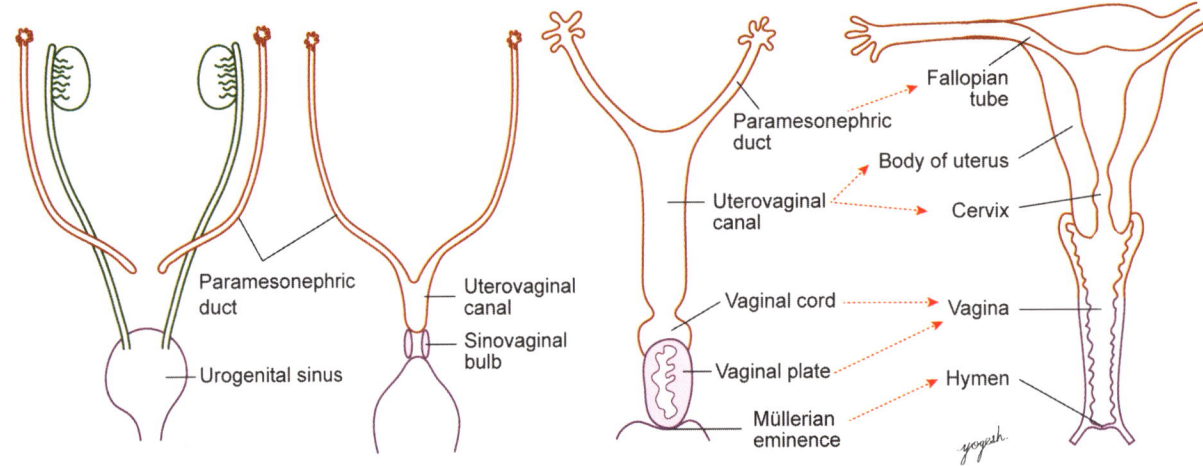

Practice Fig. 21.8: Development of uterus and vagina

Chapter 22
Nervous System

Myelination (myelinogenesis) is the process of formation of myelin around the axons.

Neural tube defects (NTDs) are a group of conditions formed owing to non-closure of neural tube.

Hydrocephalus is the excess of CSF in the ventricular system.

Practice Fig. 22.3: Developing brain vesicles

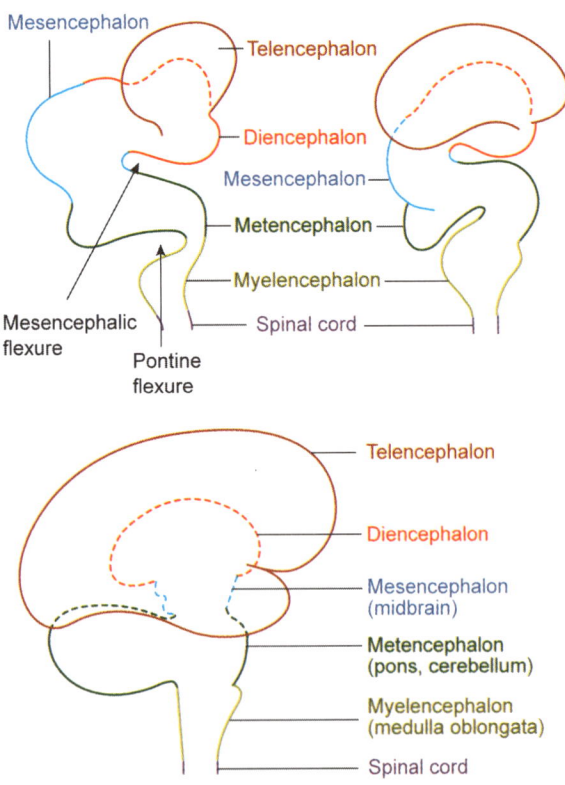

Practice Fig. 22.4: Further developing brain vesicles

Flowchart 22.5: Spina bifida

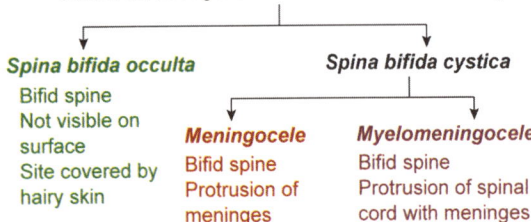

Spina bifida
Incomplete closure of neural tube in first 4 weeks
Cause: MTHFR gene defect or folic acid deficiency

Spina bifida occulta
- Bifid spine
- Not visible on surface
- Site covered by hairy skin

Spina bifida cystica

Meningocele
- Bifid spine
- Protrusion of meninges

Myelomeningocele
- Bifid spine
- Protrusion of spinal cord with meninges

Prevention
- Folic acid supplementation
- Increased maternal serum fetoprotein

Draw well-labelled diagrams of: 1. Development of uterus and vagina, 2. Developing brain vesicles, 3. Developing brain.

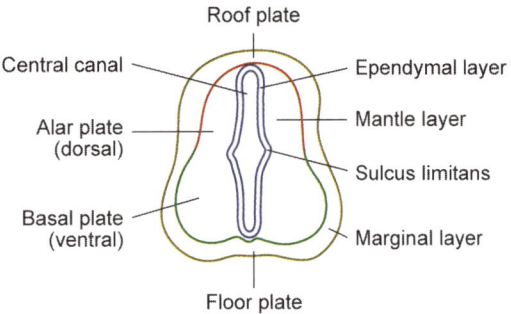

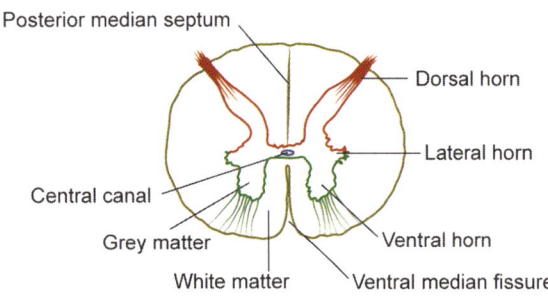

Practice Fig. 22.5: Development of spinal cord

Flowchart 22.6: Development of cerebellum

External differentiation of cerebellum

Metencephalon
↓
Proliferation of cells of *rhombic lip*
↓
Fusion of rhombic lips in midline
↓
Formation of cerebellar plate
↓ *Proliferation*
Primitive cerebellum
↓ *Differentiation*
Central vermis and bilateral cerebellar hemispheres
↓ *Development of fissures*
Separation of lobes and lobules

Cellular differentiation of cerebellum

3 layers of rhombic lips
(ependymal, mantle, marginal)
↓   ↓ Outward migration
Cerebellar nuclei   Formation of external
(dentate, emboliformis,   granular layer
globosus and fastigius)   ↓ *Differentiation*
                      Astrocytes, oligodendrocytes

Flowchart 22.4: Neural tube defects

Neural tube defects
Nonclosure of neural tube | Commonest birth defects
Cause: Folic acids deficiency, MTHFR enzyme deficiency

Spina bifida	***Anencephaly***	***Encephalocele***	***Iniencephaly***	***Rachischisis***
Spina bifida occulta	Failure of closure of anterior neuropore	Failure of formation of skull cap	Defective occipital bone	Failure of closure of posterior neuropore
Meningocele	Absence of major portion of brain	↓ Protrusion of brain and meninges	Spina bifida of cervical vertebrae	Exposure of neural tissue on the surface
Myelomeningocele			Retroflexion of neck	

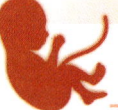

Chapter 23
Development of Eye

Table 23.1 Development of eye

Part	Embryological source
1. Cornea	Epithelium: Surface ectoderm[NEXT]
	Other layers: Neural crest
2. Lens	Lens vesicle (surface ectoderm)
3. Retina	Optic cup (neuroectoderm)
4. Optic nerve	Optic stalk (neuroectoderm)
5. Sclera and choroid	Mesoderm surrounding optic cup
6. Ciliary body and muscle	Mesoderm
7. Iris	Mesoderm
8. Muscles of iris	Neuroectoderm optic cup
9. Extraocular muscles	Preoccipital myotomes
10. Eyelids, conjunctival sac	Surface ectoderm
11. Lacrimal glands	Surface ectoderm
12. Lacrimal sac and nasolacrimal duct	Ectoderm of naso-optic furrow

Draw a well-labelled diagram of development of spinal cord. List the various components of eye and their embryological sources.

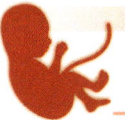

Chapter 24
Development of Ear

Table 24.1 Development of ear

Adult structures	Embryonic source
External ear	
Auricle	6 Ectodermal hillocks: *1st arch*: (1) Tragus, (2) crus of helix, (3) helix
	2nd arch: (4) Antihelix, (5) antitragus, (6) lobule
External acoustic meatus	1st pharyngeal cleft
Middle ear	
Middle ear cavity	Tubotympanic recess
Muscles	Tensor tympani – 1st pharyngeal arch
	Stapedius – 2nd pharyngeal arch
Ear ossicles	Malleus, incus – 1st pharyngeal arch
	Stapes – 2nd pharyngeal arch
Auditory tube, mastoid antrum	Tubotympanic recess
Tympanic membrane	Outer cuticular layer – ectoderm of 1st pharyngeal cleft
	Middle fibrous layer – mesoderm
	Inner mucous layer – endoderm of 1st pharyngeal pouch

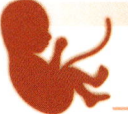

Chapter 25
Endocrine System

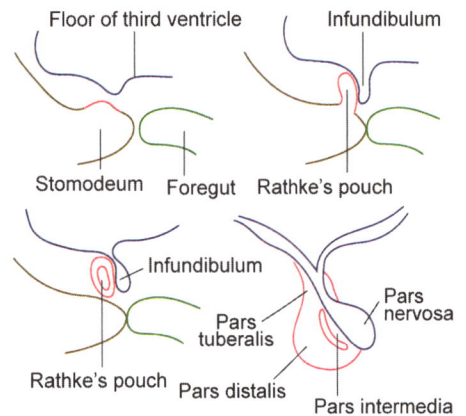

Practice Fig. 25.1: Development of pituitary gland

Flowchart 25.1: Development of pituitary gland

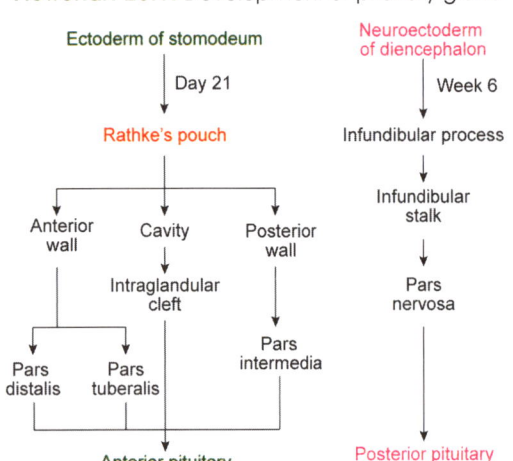

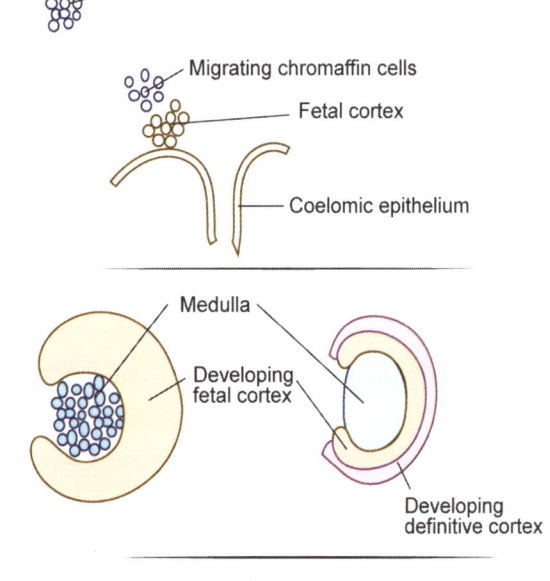

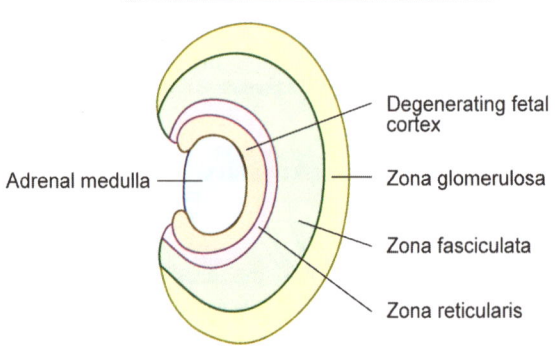

Practice Fig. 25.2: Development of adrenal gland

Draw well-labelled diagrams of: 1. Development of adrenal gland, 2. Development of pituitary gland.

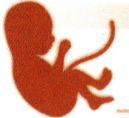

Chapter 30
Twinning

Multiple pregnancy can be classified as follows:
1. *Monozygotic twins*: These twins are produced by fertilization of a single oocyte by one sperm (one zygote).
2. *Dizygotic twins*: These twins are produced by fertilization of two different oocytes by two different sperms (two zygotes).
3. *Trizygotic twins*: These are produced by fertilization of multiple oocytes by different sperms (3 zygotes).

Diamniotic dichorionic twins: These are also called bichorial, diamniotic twins. Up to 3rd day of fertilization, separation of cells results in diamniotic twins dichorionic.

Diamniotic monochorionic monozygotic twins: They are also called diamniotic monochorial twins. Mechanism: If separation of inner cells mass of blastocyst takes place on 4th–7th day, diamniotic monochorionic twins are produced.

Monoamniotic monochorionic twins: They are also called monoamniotic, monochorial twins. Mechanism: If the separation of inner cell mass takes place by 9th day of fertilization, in monochorionic monoamniotic monozygotic twins are produced.

Conjoined (siamese) twins: If the separation occurs after 12th day of fertilization, monozygotic twins form conjoined twins. Conjoined twins have joined bodies. Conjoined monozygotic twins may be craniopagus (fusion of heads), thoracopagus (fusion of anterior thoracic walls and abdominal walls up to umbilicus), omphalopagus (fusion of lower abdominal walls), cephalo-thoracopagus (fusion of head and thoracic walls), pyopagus (fusion of sacral regions), and ischiopagus (fusion at the pelvis).

EMBRYONIC REMNANTS *NEXT, High yielding fact*

Remnant after birth	Embryonic source
Ligamentum arteriosum	Ductus arteriosus
Ligamentum teres hepatis	Left umbilical vein
Fossa ovalis	Septum primum
Annulus fossa ovalis	Septum secundum
Ligamentum venosum	Ductus venosus
Meckel's diverticulum	Vitellointestinal duct
Median umbilical ligament	Urachus
Medial umbilical ligament	Distal part of umbilical arteries
Superior vesicle artery	Proximal part of umbilical arteries
Superior aberrant ductules Inferior aberrant ductules Tubules of paradidymis Efferent ductules of testis	Mesonephric tubules in male
Tubules of epoöphoron Tubules of paroöphoron	Mesonephric tubules in female
Duct of epoöphoron (Gartner's duct)	Mesonephric duct in female
Organ of Rosenmuller (epoöphoron)	Mesonephric tubules
Appendix of testis, prostatic utricle	Paramesonephric ducts in male